Essential Oils
pocket reference

SIXTH EDITION

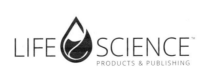

LIFE SCIENCE
PRODUCTS & PUBLISHING

Sixth Edition

Copyright © May 2014   Life Science Publishing
1-800-336-6308 • www.LifeSciencePublishers.com

ISBN 978-0-9894997-7-4

Printed in the United States of America

Contents

Acknowledgments

When D. Gary Young brought back 13 essential oils from Europe in 1985, virtually no written information was available about their usage and application. The essential oils that were sold in a few heath food and novelty stores were perfume grade with no suggested therapeutic usage.

This opened the door and led the way to a new and exciting frontier that propelled Gary into the research of an ancient knowledge that had been lost to the synthetic production of perfumes and food flavorings. His work began a resurgence of healing modalities from out of the dust of history. He was ridiculed and laughed at for his ideas about therapeutic usage, even though the medical world was beginning to awaken in Europe.

He has spent decades conducting clinical research on the ability of essential oils to combat disease and improve health. He has also developed new methods of application from which thousands of people have benefited, especially his integration of therapeutic-grade essential oils with dietary supplements and personal care products. In our research, we have found no evidence of anyone formulating these types of quality products with essential oils in North America prior to those formulated by Gary Young.

Gary grew up learning to love and work the land as a farmer and rancher in Idaho, which made it easy for him to see the vision of developing his own farms. That vision soon became reality as he purchased his first farm in 1992. His passion for extracting God's healing oils from Mother Nature's bounty made him one of the world's leading growers of aromatic herbs and plants for the distillation of essential oils.

With six privately owned farms and distillation operations in Utah, Idaho, France, Oman, and Ecuador, over 5,000 acres of purchased land under cultivation, and numerous partnerships and contract growers stretching to the far corners of the world, Gary has set new standards for excellence for the production of therapeutic-grade essential oils in today's modern world.

Gary's long experience as a grower, distiller, researcher, and alternative-care practitioner not only gives him unsurpassed insight into essential oils but also makes him an ideal lecturer and educator on the therapeutic properties of essential oils and their applications. He is sought after by thousands of people to share his knowledge on the powerful potential of essential oils and on how to produce the highest quality therapeutic-grade essential oils.

The dedication to his belief, his *knowing*, brought about the research and discovery that we have compiled into this publication. His tremendous contribution to this new frontier of medicine is immeasurable. The material contained in this book is compiled from his research, lectures, seminars, workshops, and scientific publications as well as from the work of other practitioners and physicians who are at

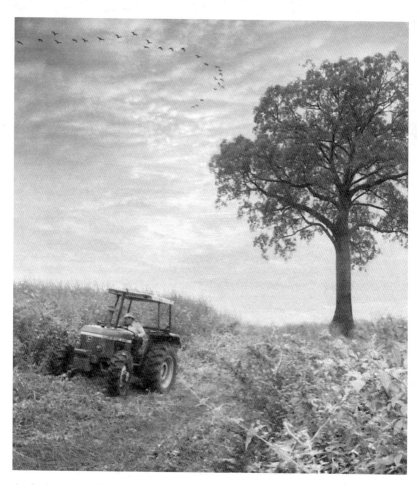

the forefront of understanding the therapeutic and clinical potential of essential oils to maintain physical and emotional wellness as well as aid in alleviating physical, emotional, and spiritual dysfunction.

To these researchers, the publisher is deeply indebted to be able to bring this information to all those in search of natural healing modalities found in the world of essential oils.

Single Oils Directory

Single Oils Directory *(Continued)*

Essential Oil Blends Directory

Personal Usage Directory

Personal Usage Directory *(Continued)*

Personal Usage Directory *(Continued)*

Personal Usage Directory *(Continued)*

Personal Usage Directory *(Continued)*

Chapter 1
Yesterday's Wisdom, Tomorrow's Destiny

Essential Oils—The Missing Link in Modern Medicine

Plants not only play a vital role in the ecological balance of our planet, but they have also been intimately linked to the physical, emotional, and spiritual well-being of mankind since the beginning of time.

The plant kingdom continues to be the subject of an enormous amount of research and discovery. Most often prescription drugs are based on naturally occurring compounds from plants. Each year millions of dollars are allocated to private laboratories and universities that are searching for new therapeutic compounds that lie undiscovered in the bark, roots, flowers, seeds, and foliage of jungle canopies; river bottoms; forests; hillsides; and vast wilderness regions throughout the world.

Essential oils and plant extracts have been woven into history since the beginning of time and are considered by many to be the missing link in modern medicine. They have been used medicinally to kill bacteria, fungi, and viruses and to combat insect, bug, and snake bites in addition to treating all kinds of mysterious maladies. Oils and extracts stimulate tissue and nerve regeneration.

Essential oils also provide exquisite fragrances to balance mood, lift spirits, dispel negative emotions, and create a romantic atmosphere.

Definition of an Essential Oil

An essential oil is that aromatic, volatile liquid that is within many shrubs, flowers, trees, roots, bushes, and seeds and that is usually extracted through steam distillation.

The chemistry of an essential oil is very complex and may consist of hundreds of different and unique chemical compounds. Moreover, essential oils are highly concentrated and far more potent than dried herbs because of the distillation process that makes them so concentrated. It requires a large volume of plant material to produce small amounts of a distilled essential oil. For example, it takes 5,000 pounds of rose petals to produce 1 kilo of rose oil.

Essential oils are also different from vegetable oils such as corn oil, peanut oil, and olive oil. Vegetable oils are greasy and may clog the pores. They also oxidize and become rancid over time and have no antibacterial properties. Most essential oils, on the other hand, do not go rancid and are powerful antimicrobials. Essential oils that are high in plant waxes, such as patchouli, vetiver, and sandalwood, if not distilled properly, could go rancid after time, particularly if exposed to heat for extended periods of time.

Essential oils are substances that definitely deserve the respect of proper education. Users should have a basic knowledge about the safety of the oils, and having a basic understanding of the chemistry of essential oils is very helpful. However, it is difficult to find this knowledge taught in universities or private seminars. Chemistry books are difficult to understand for most people, and they don't usually address the specific chemistry of essential oils. There is very little institutional information, knowledge, and training on essential oils and the scientific approach to their use.

The European communities have tight controls and standards concerning botanical extracts and who may administer them. Only practitioners with proper training and certification can practice in the discipline called "aromatherapy."

In the United States, regulatory agencies have not recognized these disciplines or mandated the type and degree of training required to distribute and use essential oils. This means that in the United States, individuals can call themselves "aromatherapists" after attending brief classes in essential oils and can apply oils to anyone—even though the so-called "aromatherapists" may not have the experience or training to properly understand and use essential oils. This may not only undermine and damage the credibility of the entire discipline of aromatherapy, but it is also dangerous to the patient.

Essential oils are not simple substances. Each oil is a complex structure of hundreds of different chemicals. A single essential oil may contain anywhere from 80 to 300 or more different chemical constituents. An essential oil like lavender is very complex, with many of its constituents occurring in minute quantities—but all contributing to the oil's therapeutic effects to some degree. To understand these constituents and their functions requires years of study.

Even though an essential oil may be labeled as "basil" and have the botanical name *Ocimum basilicum*, it can have widely different therapeutic actions, depending on its chemistry. For example, basil high in linalool or fenchol is primarily used for its antiseptic properties. However, basil high

in methyl chavicol is more anti-inflammatory than antiseptic. A third type of basil high in eugenol has both anti-inflammatory and antiseptic effects.

Additionally, essential oils can be distilled or extracted in different ways that will have dramatic effects on their chemistry and medicinal action. Oils derived from a second or third distillation of the same plant material are usually not as potent as oils extracted during the first distillation. Yet with certain oils, there may be additional chemical constituents that are released only in the second or third distillation.

Oils subjected to high heat and high pressure have a noticeable simpler and inferior profile of chemical constituents, since excessive heat and temperature fracture and break down many of the delicate aromatic compounds within the oil—some of which are responsible for its therapeutic action. In addition, oils that are steam distilled are far different from those that are extracted with solvents.

Of greatest concern is the fact that some oils are adulterated, engineered, or "extended" with the use of synthetic-made compounds that are added to the oil. For example, pure frankincense is often extended with colorless, odorless solvents such as diethylphthalate or dipropylene glycol. The only way to distinguish the "authentic" from the "adulterated" is through analytical testing using gas chromatography, mass spectroscopy, and an optical refractometer.

Unfortunately, a large percentage of essential oils marketed in the United States fall in this adulterated category. When you understand the world of synthetic oils as well as low-grade oils cut with synthetic chemicals, you realize why the vast majority of consumers never know the difference. However, if you do know the smell of the pure oil or the technique for recognizing adulteration through scent, it may be possible to perceive a difference.

Different Schools of Application

Therapeutic treatment using essential oils follows three different models: the English, French, and German.

The English model puts a small amount of an essential oil in a large amount of vegetable oil to massage the body for the purpose of relaxation and relieving stress.

The French model prescribes neat (undiluted) topical application of therapeutic-grade essential oils and/or the ingestion of pure essential oils. Typically, a few drops of an essential oil are added to agave nectar, honey, a small amount of vegetable oil, or put on a piece of bread. Many French practitioners have found that taking the oils internally yields excellent benefits.

The German model focuses on inhalation of essential oils—the true aromatherapy. Research has shown that the effect of fragrance on the sense of smell can exert strong effects on the brain—especially on the hypothalamus (the hormone command center of the body) and limbic system (the seat of emotions). Some essential oils high in sesquiterpenes, such as myrrh, sandalwood, cedarwood, vetiver, and melissa can dramatically increase oxygenation and activity in the brain, which may directly improve the function of many systems of the body.

Together, these three models show the versatility and power of essential oils. By integrating all three models with various methods of application such as Vita Flex, auricular technique, lymphatic massage, and Raindrop Technique, the best possible results may be obtained.

In some cases, inhalation of essential oils might be preferred over topical application, if the goal is to increase growth hormone secretion, promote weight loss, or balance mood and emotions. Sandalwood, peppermint, vetiver, lavender, and white fir oils are effective for inhalation.

In other cases, however, topical application of essential oils would produce better results, particularly in the case of back or muscle injuries or defects. Topically applied, marjoram is excellent for muscles, lemongrass for ligaments, and wintergreen for bones. For indigestion, a drop or two of peppermint oil taken orally or put in a glass of water may be very effective. However, this does not mean that peppermint cannot produce the same results when massaged on the stomach. In some cases, all three methods of application (topical, inhalation, and ingestion) are interchangeable and may produce similar benefits.

The ability of essential oils to act on both the mind and the body is what makes them truly unique among natural therapeutic substances. The fragrance of some essential oils can be very stimulating—both psychologically and physically. The fragrance of other essential oils may be calming and sedating, helping to overcome anxiety or hyperactivity. On a physiological level, essential oils may stimulate immune function and regenerate damaged tissue. Essential oils may also combat infectious disease by killing viruses, bacteria, and other pathogens.

Probably the two most common methods of essential oil application are cold-air diffusing and neat (undiluted) topical application. Other modes of application include incorporating essential oils into the disciplines of reflexology, Vita Flex, and acupressure. Combining these disciplines with essential oils enhances the healing response and often produces amazing results that cannot be achieved by acupuncture or reflexology alone. Just 1–3 drops of an essential oil applied to an acupuncture meridian or Vita Flex point on the hand or foot can produce results within a minute or two.

Several years ago, a professor well known in the field of aromatherapy ridiculed the use of essential oils against disease. However, there are many people who are living proof that essential oils dramatically aided in the recovery of serious illness. Essential oils have been pivotal in helping many people live pain free after years of intense pain. Patients have also witnessed firsthand how essential oils have helped with scoliosis and even restored partial hearing in those who were born deaf and complete hearing with someone who had had some loss of hearing.

For example, a woman from Palisades Park, California, developed scoliosis after surviving polio as a teenager, which was further complicated by a serious fall that dislocated her shoulder. Suffering pain and immobility for 22 years, she had traveled extensively in a fruitless search to locate a practitioner who could permanently reset her shoulder. Upon learning about essential oils, she topically applied the oils of helichrysum and wintergreen, among others, to the shoulder. Within a short time her pain began to diminish and eventually was completely gone, and she was able to raise her arm over her head for the first time in 22 years.

When one sees such dramatic results, it is difficult to discredit the value and the power of essential oils and the potential they hold. One would certainly think that it would be well worth investigating further. It is so sad that many turn away because of traditional beliefs.

Man's First Medicine

From ancient writings and traditions, it seems that aromatics were used for religious rituals, the treatment of illness, and other physical and spiritual needs. Records dating back to 4500 BC describe the use of balsamic substances with aromatic properties for religious rituals and medical applications. Ancient writings tell of scented barks, resins, spices, and aromatic vinegars, wines, and beers that were used in rituals, temples, astrology, embalming, and medicine. The evidence certainly suggests that the people of ancient times had a greater understanding of essential oils than we have today.

The Egyptians were masters in using essential oils and other aromatics in the embalming process. Historical records describe how one of the founders of "pharaonic" medicine was the architect Imhotep, who was the Grand Vizier of King Djoser (2780 - 2720 BC). Imhotep is often given credit for ushering in the use of oils, herbs, and aromatic plants for medicinal purposes. In addition, the Egyptians may have been the first to discover the potential of fragrance. They created various aromatic blends for both personal use and for religious ceremonies.

Many hieroglyphics on the walls of Egyptian temples depict the blending of oils and describe numerous oil recipes. An example of this is the Temple of Edfu, located on the west bank of the Nile River. Over the centuries it was buried beneath sand drifts, which preserved the temple nearly intact. The smaller of two hypostyle halls leads to a small room called a laboratory, where perfumes and ointments were compounded. On the walls are hieroglyphics listing recipes for these aromatic perfumes, including two recipes for kyphi, a blend of incense that contained frankincense, myrrh, honey, raisins soaked in wine, sweet flag, pine resin, and juniper. Another recipe was for "Hekenu" to anoint divine limbs. Similar medicinal formulas and perfume recipes were used by alchemists and high priests to blend aromatic substances for rituals.

Well before the time of Christ, the ancient Egyptians collected essential oils and placed them in alabaster vessels. These vessels were specially carved and shaped for housing scented oils. In 1922, when King Tutankhamen's tomb was opened, some 50 alabaster jars designed to hold 350 liters of oils were discovered. Tomb robbers had stolen nearly all of the precious oils, leaving the heavy jars behind that still contained traces of oil. The robbers literally chose oils over a king's wealth in gold, showing how valuable the essential oils were to them.

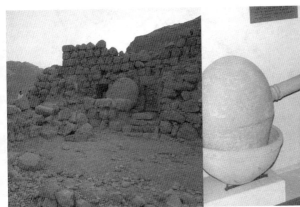

Ancient balsam distillery in Ein Gedi, Israel, in the Judean Deseret, found by D. Gary Young in 1996.

Terra cotta distillery from 350 BC, photographed by D. Gary Young in the museum in Taxila, Pakistan, in 1995

In 1817 the Ebers Papyrus, a medical scroll over 870 feet long, was discovered that dated back to 1500 BC. The scroll included over 800 different herbal prescriptions and remedies. Other scrolls described a high success rate in treating 81 different diseases. Many of the remedies contained myrrh and honey. Myrrh is still recognized for its ability to help with infections of the skin and throat and to regenerate skin tissue. Because of its effectiveness in preventing bacterial growth, myrrh was also used for embalming.

The physicians of Ionia, Attia, and Crete, ancient civilizations based on islands of the Mediterranean Sea, came to the cities of the Nile to increase their knowledge. At this time, the school of Cos was founded and was attended by Hippocrates (460-377 BC), whom the Greeks, with perhaps some exaggeration, named the "Father of Medicine."

The Romans purified their temples and political buildings by diffusing essential oils and also used aromatics in their steam baths to invigorate themselves and ward off disease.

Early History of Essential Oil Extraction

Ancient cultures found that aromatic essences or oils could be extracted from the plant by a variety of methods. One of the oldest and crudest forms of extraction was known as enfleurage. Raw plant material such as stems, foliage, bark, or roots was crushed and mixed with olive oil, animal fat, and some vegetable oils. Cedar bark was stripped from the trunk and branches, ground into a powder, soaked with olive oil, and placed in a wool cloth. The cloth was then heated. The heat pulled the essential oil out of the bark particles into the olive oil, and the wool was pressed to extract the essential oil. Sandalwood oil was also extracted in this fashion.

Enfleurage was also used to extract essential oils from flower petals. In fact, the French word enfleurage means literally "to saturate with the perfume of flowers." For example, petals from roses or jasmine were placed in goose or goat fat. The essential oil droplets were pulled from the petals into the fat and then separated from the

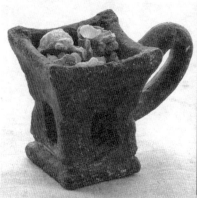
3,500-year-old stone incense burner dug out of the ground in Shabwa, Yemen, in 2009 by D. Gary Young

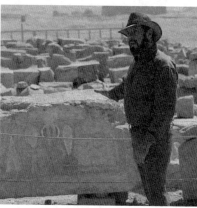
Stones from Queen Hatshepsut's temple in Upper Egypt, with reliefs depicting healing with plants and the lotus oil

fat. This ancient technique was one of the most primitive forms of essential oil extraction.

Other extraction techniques were also used such as:

- Soaking plant parts in boiling water
- Cold-pressing
- Soaking in alcohol
- Steam distillation, meaning that as the steam travels upward, it saturates the plant material, causing the plant membranes containing the oil to break open and release the oil, which then becomes a gas that travels with the steam into the condenser, where it returns to its oily texture and is then separated from the water.

Many ancient cosmetic formulas were created from a base of goat and goose fat and camel milk. Ancient Egyptians made eyeliners, eye shadows, and other cosmetics this way. They also stained their hair and nails with a variety of ointments and perfumes. Fragrance "cones" made of wax and essential oils were worn by women of royalty, who enjoyed the rich scent of the oils as the cones melted with the heat of the day.

In the temples oils were commonly poured into evaporation dishes so that the aroma could fill the chambers associated with sacred rituals and religious rites throughout the day.

Ancient Arabians also developed and refined the process of distillation. They perfected the extraction of rose oil and rose water, which were popular in the Middle East during the Byzantine Empire (330 AD - 1400 AD).

Biblical History of Essential Oils

The Bible contains over 200 references to aromatics, incense, and ointments. Aromatics such as frankincense, myrrh, galbanum, cinnamon, cassia, rosemary, hyssop, and spikenard were used for anointing and healing the sick. In Exodus, the Lord gave the following recipe to Moses for a holy anointing oil:

Myrrh "five hundred shekels" (about 1 gallon)
Cinnamon "two hundred and fifty shekels"
Calamus "two hundred and fifty shekels"
Cassia "five hundred shekels"
Olive Oil "an hin" (about 1 1/3 gallons)

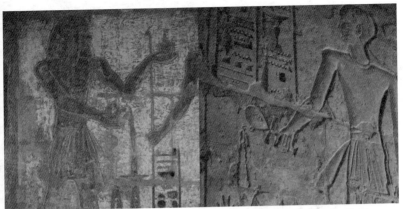

Offering of lotus oil and aloe in the Edfu Temple in Upper Egypt, photographed by D. Gary Young.

Offering of lotus oil, photographed by D. Gary Young.

Psalms 133:2 speaks of the sweetness of brethren dwelling together in unity: "It is like the precious ointment upon the head, that ran down the beard, even Aaron's beard: that went down to the skirts of his garments." Another scripture that refers to anointing and the overflowing abundance of precious oils is Ecclesiastes 9:8: "Let thy garments be always white; and let thy head lack no ointment."

The Bible also lists an incident where an incense offering by Aaron stopped a plague. Numbers 16:46-50 records that Moses instructed Aaron to take a censer, add burning coals and incense, and "go quickly into the congregation to make an atonement for them: for there is a wrath gone out from the Lord; the plague is begun." The Bible records that Aaron stood between the dead and the living, and the plague was stayed. It is significant that according to the biblical and Talmudic recipes for incense, three varieties of cinnamon were involved. Cinnamon is known to be highly antimicrobial, anti-infectious, and antibacterial. The incense ingredient listed as "stacte" is believed to be a sweet, myrrh-related spice, which would make it anti-infectious and antiviral as well.

The New Testament records that wise men presented the Christ child with frankincense and myrrh. There is another precious aromatic, spikenard, described in the anointing of Jesus:

> And being in Bethany in the house of Simon the leper, as he sat at meat, there came a woman having an alabaster box of ointment of spikenard very precious; and she brake the box, and poured it on his head. Mark 14:3.

The anointing of Jesus is also referred to in John 12:3:

> Then took Mary a pound of ointment of spikenard, very costly, and anointed the feet of Jesus, and wiped his feet with her hair: and the house was filled with the odour of the ointment.

See additional biblical references at the end of this chapter.

Other Historical References

Throughout world history, fragrant oils and spices have played a prominent role in everyday life.

Herodotus, the Greek historian who lived from 484 BC to 425 BC, recorded that during the yearly feast of Bel, 1,000 talents' weight of frankincense was offered on the great altar of Bel in Babylon.

The Roman historian Pliny the Elder (AD 23-79) complained that "by our lowest reckoning India, China and the Arabian peninsula take from our empire 100 million sesterces every year, for aromatics."

Diodorus of Sicily lived in the 1st century BC and wrote of the abundance of frankincense in Arabia and how it "suffices for the service and worship of gods all the world over."

Napoleon is reported to have enjoyed cologne water made of neroli and other ingredients so much that he ordered 162 bottles of it.

After conquering Jerusalem, one of the things the Crusaders brought back to Europe was solidified essence of roses.

The 12th-century herbalist Hildegard of Bingen used herbs and oils extensively in healing. This Benedictine nun founded her own convent and was the author of numerous works. Her book, *Physica,* has more than 200 chapters on plants and their uses for healing.

The Rediscovery

The reintroduction of essential oils into modern medicine first began during the late 19th and early 20th centuries.

During World War I, the use of aromatic essences in civilian and military hospitals became widespread. One physician in France, Dr. Moncière, used essential oils extensively for their antibacterial and wound-healing properties and developed several kinds of aromatic ointments.

René-Maurice Gattefossé, PhD, a French cosmetic chemist, is widely regarded as the father of aromatherapy. He and a group of scientists began studying essential oils in 1907.

In his 1937 book, *Aromatherapy*, Dr. Gattefossé told the real story of his now-famous use of lavender essential oil that was used to heal a serious burn. The tale has assumed mythic proportions in essential oil literature. His own words about this accident are even more powerful than what has been told over the years.

Dr. Gattefossé was literally aflame—covered in burning substances—following a laboratory explosion in July 1910. After he extinguished the flames by rolling on a grassy lawn, he wrote that "both my hands were covered with rapidly developing gas gangrene." He further reported that "just one rinse with lavender essence stopped the gasification of the tissue. This treatment was followed by profuse sweating and healing which began the next day."

Robert B. Tisserand, editor of *The International Journal of Aromatherapy*, searched for Dr. Gattefossé's book for 20 years. A copy was located and Tisserand edited the 1995 reprint. Tisserand noted that Dr. Gattefossé's burns "must have been severe to lead to gas gangrene, a very serious infection."

Dr. Gattefossé shared his studies with his colleague and friend Jean Valnet, a medical doctor practicing in Paris. Exhausting his supply of antibiotics as a physician in Tonkin, China, during World War II, Dr. Valnet began using essential oils on patients suffering battlefield injuries. To his surprise, the essential oils showed a powerful effect in fighting infection. He was able to save the lives of many soldiers who might otherwise have died.

Two of Dr. Valnet's students, Dr. Paul Belaiche and Dr. Jean-Claude Lapraz, expanded his work. They clinically investigated the antiviral, antibacterial, antifungal, and antiseptic properties in essential oils.

In 1990, Dr. Daniel Pénoël, a French medical doctor, and Pierre Franchomme, a French

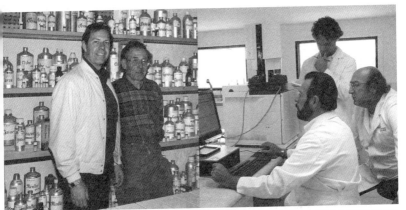

D. Gary Young and Mr. Henri Viaud

Dr. Hervé Casabianca trains Gary and Chris in the laboratory at the Young Living Farm in Ecuador.

biochemist, collaborated together to co-author the first reference book that cataloged the various medical properties of over 270 essential oils and how to use them in a clinical environment. Their work was based on Franchomme's laboratory experience and Pénoël's clinical experience of administering the oils to his patients. The book, published in French, was titled *l'aromathérapie exactement* and became the primary resource for dozens of authors worldwide in writing about the medical benefits of essential oils.

D. Gary Young sought out the best and brightest experts in distillation and chromatographic analysis as he began his essential oil company. He first studied essential oils with Jean-Claude Lapraz in 1985 in Geneva, Switzerland. Then he went to Paris to study with one of Jean Valnet's students, Paul Belaiche, MD. Gary also studied with Daniel Pénoël, co-author of *l'aromathérapie exactement*. In the early '90s he studied with Radwan Farag, PhD, at Cairo University and Professor K. Hüsnü Can Baser at the Andalou University in Eskisehir, Turkey.

Gary Young's training in the art of distillation and essential oil testing began with his lavender partnership with Jean-Noel Landel in Provence, France. Jean-Noel introduced Gary to Henri Viaud, a chemist and distiller of essential oils and author of the 1983 book on quality considerations for essential oils (*Huiles Essentielles—Hydrolats*). Mr. Viaud had his own laboratory and small distiller. Gary was his only student to whom he taught the finer points of distilling.

After studying at the Albert Vieille Laboratory in Grasse, France, in 1994, Gary traveled to Lyon, France, where he studied with the world's foremost authority in chromatography, Hervé Casabianca, PhD. Dr. Casabianca traveled to Young Living laboratories in the U.S. and Ecuador to train staff scientists in gas chromatography/mass spectrometry.

From D. Gary Young to Jean-Claude Lapraz to Jean Valnet to René-Maurice Gattefossé—Gary Young was a pioneer in the world of essential oils, just as they were.

From 1994 to 2014, knowledge and use of es-

Young Living Essential Oils is the World Leader in Essential Oils

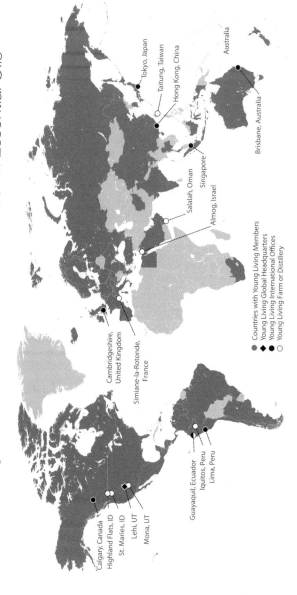

Countries with Young Living Members
Young Living Global Headquarters
Young Living International Offices
Young Living Farm or Distillery

Tokyo, Japan
Taitung, Taiwan
Hong Kong, China
Australia
Brisbane, Australia
Salalah, Oman
Singapore
Almog, Israel
Cambridgeshire, United Kingdom
Simiane-la-Rotonde, France
Calgary, Canada
Highland Flats, ID
St. Maries, ID
Lehi, UT
Mona, UT
Guayaquil, Ecuador
Iquitos, Peru
Lima, Peru

sential oils has spread throughout the world (see map on page 10), making Young Living Essential Oils the World Leader in Essential Oils.*

Health-minded people the world over have learned the value of using high quality natural herbs. Interestingly, most therapeutic herbs can be distilled into an essential oil. The key difference is that of concentration. The essential oil can be from 100 to 10,000 times more concentrated—and therefore more potent—than the herb itself. Even though they are many times more potent than natural herbs, essential oils, unlike prescription drugs, very rarely generate any negative side effects, which carries profound implications for those wanting to maintain or regain their health naturally.

Sometimes the effects of administering essential oils are so dramatic that the patients themselves call it "miraculous." And while no one fully understands yet "why" or "how" essential oils provide such significant benefits, the fact is that they do. With pure essential oils, millions of people can find relief from disease, infections, pain, and even mental difficulties. Their therapeutic potential is enormous and is only just beginning to be tapped.

Because of the research being conducted by many scientists and doctors, the healing power of essential oils is again gaining prominence. Today, it has become evident that we have not yet found permanent solutions for dreaded diseases such as SARS, the Ebola virus, hanta virus, AIDS, HIV, and new strains of tuberculosis and influenza like bird and swine flu.

Essential oils may assume an increasingly important role in combating new mutations of bacteria, viruses, and fungi. More and more researchers are undertaking serious clinical studies on the use of essential oils to combat these types of diseases.

Research conducted at Weber State University in cooperation with D. Gary Young, as well as other documented research, indicates that most viruses, fungi, and bacteria cannot live in the presence of most essential oils, especially those high in phenols, carvacrol, thymol, and terpenes. It may also help us understand why a notorious group of thieves, reputed to be spice traders and perfumers, was protected from the Black Plague as they robbed the bodies of the dead and dying during the 15th century.

A vast body of anecdotal evidence (testimonials) suggests that those who use essential oils are less likely to contract infectious diseases. Moreover, oil users who do contract an infectious illness tend to recover faster than those using antibiotics.

Our modern world has only begun the discovery of the power of God's healing oils—something that the ancient world knew well. Their time was one without laboratories, manufacturing facilities, high technology and equipment, or chemicals. The earth and its healing gifts were the ancient world's medicine—something our modern world should take note of and embrace. Modern medicine is certainly not without its miracles. Millions of lives have been saved in crisis and malfunctions of the body. But the way to live with strength and vitality without pain and disease lies in what God has created, not in what man has altered.

Essential oils are no longer the missing link in modern medicine. Millions of people are applauding their power, and millions more are being introduced and educated to their potential each year. As more and more health practitioners, doctors, scientists, and users of all ages venture into the world of this ancient knowledge, the methods of medicine will take on new dimensions, and exciting discoveries will be made that will benefit mankind today and tomorrow.

Biblical References

Cedarwood

Leviticus 14:51—"And he shall take the cedar wood, and the hyssop, and the scarlet, and the living bird, and dip them in the blood of the slain bird, and in the running water, and sprinkle the house seven times:"

Leviticus 14:52—"And he shall cleanse the house with the blood of the bird, and with the running water, and with the living bird, and with the cedar wood, and with the hyssop, and with the scarlet."

Numbers 19:6—"And the priest shall take cedar wood, and hyssop, and scarlet, and cast *it* into the midst of the burning of the heifer."

Numbers 24:6—"As the valleys are they spread forth, as gardens by the river's side, as the trees of lign aloes which the Lord hath planted, *and* as cedar trees beside the waters."

2 Samuel 5:11—"And Hiram king of Tyre sent messengers to David, and cedar trees, and carpenters, and masons: and they built David an house."

2 Samuel 7:2—"That the king said unto Nathan the prophet, See now, I dwell in an house of cedar, but the ark of God dwelleth within curtains."

2 Samuel 7:7—"In all *the places* wherein I have walked with all the children of Israel spake I a word with any of the tribes of Israel, whom I commanded to feed my people Israel, saying, Why build ye not me an house of cedar?"

1 Kings 4:33—"And he spake of trees, from the cedar tree that *is* in Lebanon even unto the hyssop that springeth out of the wall: he spake also of beasts, and of fowl, and of creeping things, and of fishes."

1 Kings 5:6—"Now therefore command thou that they hew me cedar trees out of Lebanon; and my servants shall be with thy servants: and unto thee will I give hire for thy servants according to all that thou shalt appoint: for thou knowest that *there is* not among us any that can skill to hew timber like unto the Sidonians."

1 Kings 5:8—"And Hiram sent to Solomon, saying, I have considered the things which thou sentest to me for: *and* I will do all thy desire concerning timber of cedar, and concerning timber of fir."

1 Kings 5:10—"So Hiram gave Solomon cedar trees and fir trees *according to* all his desire."

1 Kings 6:9—"So he built the house, and finished it; and covered the house with beams and boards of cedar."

1 Kings 9:11—"(*Now* Hiram the king of Tyre had furnished Solomon with cedar trees and fir trees, and with gold, according to all his desire,) that then king Solomon gave Hiram twenty cities in the land of Galilee."

2 Kings 19:23—"By thy messengers thou hast reproached the Lord, and hast said, With the multitude of my chariots I am come up to the height of the mountains, to the sides of Lebanon, and will cut down the tall cedar trees thereof, *and* the choice fir trees thereof: and I will enter into the lodgings of his borders, *and into* the forest of his Carmel."

1 Chronicles 22:4—"Also cedar trees in abundance: for the Zidonians and they of Tyre brought much cedar wood to David."

2 Chronicles 1:15—"And the king made silver and gold at Jerusalem *as plenteous* as stones, and cedar trees made he as the sycomore trees that *are* in the vale for abundance."

2 Chronicles 2:8—"Send me also cedar trees, fir trees, and algum trees, out of Lebanon: for I know that thy servants can skill to cut timber in Lebanon; and behold, my servants *shall be* with thy servants,"

2 Chronicles 9:27—"And the king made silver in Jerusalem as stones, and cedar trees made he as the sycomore trees that *are* in the low plains in abundance."

Ezra 3:7—"They gave money also unto the masons, and to the carpenters; and meat, and drink, and oil, unto them of Zidon, and to them of Tyre, to bring cedar trees from Lebanon to the sea of Joppa, according to the grant that they had of Cyrus king of Persia."

Isaiah 41:19—"I will plant in the wilderness the cedar, the shittah tree, and the myrtle, and the oil tree; I will set in the desert the fir tree, *and* the pine, and the box tree together:"

Ezekiel 17:3—"And say, Thus saith the Lord God; A great eagle with great wings, longwinged, full of feathers, which had divers colours, came unto Lebanon, and took the highest branch of the cedar:"

Ezekiel 17:22—"Thus saith the Lord God; I will also take of the highest branch of the high cedar, and will set *it*; I will crop off from the top of his young twigs a tender one, and will plant *it* upon an high mountain and eminent:"

Ezekiel 17:23—"In the mountain of the height of Israel will I plant it: and it shall bring forth boughs, and bear fruit, and be a goodly cedar: and under it shall dwell all fowl of every wing; in the shadow of the branches thereof shall they dwell."

Zechariah 11:2—"Howl, fir tree; for the cedar is fallen; because the mighty are spoiled: howl, O ye oaks of Bashan; for the forest of the vintage is come down."

Cinnamon

Revelation 18:13—"And cinnamon, and odours, and ointments, and frankincense, and wine, and oil, and fine flour, and wheat, and beasts, and sheep, and horses, and chariots, and slaves, and souls of men."

Fir

1 Kings 6:15—"And he built the walls of the house within with boards of cedar, both the floor of the house, and the walls of the ceiling: *and* he covered *them* on the inside with wood, and cov-

ered the floor of the house with planks of fir."

1 Kings 6:34—"And the two doors *were of* fir tree: the two leaves of the one door *were* folding, and the two leaves of the other door *were* folding."

1 Kings 9:11—"(*Now* Hiram the king of Tyre had furnished Solomon with cedar trees and fir trees, and with gold, according to all his desire,) that then king Solomon gave Hiram twenty cities in the land of Galilee."

2 Kings 19:23—"By thy messengers thou hast reproached the Lord, and hast said, With the multitude of my chariots I am come up to the height of the mountains, to the sides of Lebanon, and will cut down the tall cedar trees thereof, *and* the choice fir trees thereof: and I will enter into the lodgings of his borders, *and into* the forest of his Carmel."

2 Chronicles 2:8—"Send me also cedar trees, fir trees, and algum trees, out of Lebanon: for I know that thy servants can skill to cut timber in Lebanon; and, behold, my servants *shall be* with thy servants."

2 Chronicles 3:5—"And the greater house he cieled with fir tree, which he overlaid with fine gold, and set thereon palm trees and chains."

Psalms 104:17—"Where the birds make their nests: *as for* the stork, the fir trees *are* her house."

The Song of Solomon 1:17—"The beams of our house *are* cedar, *and* our rafters of fir."

Isaiah 14:8—"Yea, the fir trees rejoice at thee, *and* the cedars of Lebanon, *saying*, Since thou art laid down, no feller is come up against us."

Isaiah 37:24—"By thy servants hast thou reproached the Lord, and hast said, By the multitude of my chariots am I come up to the height of the mountains, to the sides of Lebanon; and I will cut down the tall cedars thereof, *and* the choice fir trees thereof: and I will enter into the height of his border, *and* the forest of his Carmel."

Isaiah 41:19—"I will plant in the wilderness the cedar, the shittah tree, and the myrtle, and the oil tree; I will set in the desert the fir tree, *and* the pine, and the box tree together:"

Isaiah 55:13—"Instead of the thorn shall come up the fir tree, and instead of the brier shall come up the myrtle tree: and it shall be to the Lord for a name, for an everlasting sign [that] shall not be cut off."

Isaiah 60:13—"The glory of Lebanon shall come unto thee, the fir tree, the pine tree, and the box together, to beautify the place of my sanctuary; and I will make the place of my feet glorious."

Ezekiel 27:5—"They have made all thy *ship* boards of fir trees of Senir: they have taken cedars from Lebanon to make masts for thee."

Ezekiel 31:8—"The cedars in the garden of God could not hide him: the fir trees were not like his boughs, and the chestnut trees were not like his branches; nor any tree in the garden of God was like unto him in his beauty."

Hosea 14:8—"Ephraim *shall say,* What have I to do any more with idols? I have heard *him,* and observed him: I *am* like a green fir tree. From me is thy fruit found."

Nahum 2:3—"The shield of his mighty men is made red, the valiant men *are* in scarlet: the chariots *shall be* with flaming torches in the day of his preparation, and the fir trees shall be terribly shaken."

Zechariah 11:2—"Howl, fir tree; for the cedar is fallen; because the mighty are spoiled: howl, O ye oaks of Bashan; for the forest of the vintage is come down."

Frankincense

Leviticus 2:15—"And thou shalt put oil upon it, and lay frankincense thereon: it *is* a meat offering."

Leviticus 2:16—"And the priest shall burn the memorial of it, *part* of the beaten corn thereof, and *part* of the oil thereof, with all the frankincense thereof: *it is* an offering made by fire unto the Lord."

Leviticus 5:11—"But if he be not able to bring two turtledoves, or two young pigeons, then he that sinned shall bring for his offering the tenth part of an ephah of fine flour for a sin offering; he shall put no oil upon it, neither shall he put *any* frankincense thereon: for it *is* a sin offering."

Leviticus 6:15—"And he shall take of it his handful, of the flour of the meat offering, and of the oil thereof, and all the frankincense which *is* upon the meat offering, and shall burn *it* upon the altar *for* a sweet savour, *even* the memorial of it, unto the Lord."

Leviticus 24:7—"And thou shalt put pure frankincense upon *each* row, that it may be on the bread for a memorial, *even* an offering made by fire unto the Lord."

Numbers 5:15—"Then shall the man bring his wife unto the priest, and he shall bring her offering for her, the tenth *part* of an ephah of barley meal; he shall pour no oil upon it, nor put frankincense thereon; for it *is* an offering of jealousy, an offering of memorial, bringing iniquity to remembrance."

1 Chronicles 9:29—"*Some* of them also *were* appointed to oversee the vessels, and all the instruments of the sanctuary, and the fine flour, and the wine, and the oil, and the frankincense, and the spices."

Nehemiah 13:5—"And he had prepared for him a great chamber, where aforetime they laid the meat offerings, the frankincense, and the vessels, and the tithes of the corn, the new wine, and the oil, which was commanded *to be given* to the Levites, and the singers, and the porters; and the offerings of the priests."

Nehemiah 13:9—"Then I commanded, and they cleansed the chambers: and thither brought I again the vessels of the house of God, with the meat offering and the frankincense."

The Song of Solomon 3:6—"Who *is* this that cometh out of the wilderness like pillars of smoke, perfumed with myrrh and frankincense, with all owders of the merchant?"

The Song of Solomon 4:6—"Until the day break, and the shadows flee away, I will get me to the mountain of myrrh, and to the hill of frankincense."

The Song of Solomon 4:14—"Spikenard and saffron; calamus and cinnamon, with all trees of frankincense; myrrh and aloes, with all the chief spices:"

Matthew 2:11—"And when they were come into the house, they saw the young child with Mary his mother, and fell down, and worshiped him: and when they had opened their treasures, they presented unto him gifts; gold, and frankincense, and myrrh."

Revelation 18:13—"And cinnamon, and odours, and ointments, and frankincense, and wine, and oil, and fine flour, and wheat, and beasts, and sheep, and horses, and chariots, and slaves, and souls of men."

Hyssop

Leviticus 14:49—"And he shall take to cleanse the house two birds, and cedar wood, and scarlet, and hyssop:"

Leviticus 14:51—"And he shall take the cedar wood, and the hyssop, and the scarlet, and the living bird, and dip them in the blood of the slain bird, and in the running water, and sprinkle the house seven times:"

Leviticus 14:52—"And he shall cleanse the house with the blood of the bird, and with the running water, and with the living bird, and with the cedar wood, and with the hyssop, and with the scarlet:"

Numbers 19:6—"And the priest shall take cedar wood, and hyssop, and scarlet, and cast it into the midst of the burning of the heifer."

Numbers 19:18—"And a clean person shall take hyssop, and dip it in the water, and sprinkle it upon the tent, and upon all the vessels, and upon the persons that were there, and upon him

that touched a bone, or one slain, or one dead, or a grave:"

1 Kings 4:33—"And he spake of trees, from the cedar tree that is in Lebanon even unto the hyssop that springeth out of the wall: he spake also of beasts, and of fowl, and of creeping things, and of fishes."

Psalms 51:7—"Purge me with hyssop, and I shall be clean: wash me, and I shall be whiter than snow."

John 19:29—"Now there was set a vessel full of vinegar: and they filled a spunge with vinegar, and put it upon hyssop, and put it to his mouth."

Hebrews 9:19—"For when Moses had spoken every precept to all the people according to the law, he took the blood of calves and of goats, with water, and scarlet wool, and hyssop, and sprinkled both the book, and all the people."

Myrrh

Esther 2:12—"Now when every maid's turn was come to go in to king Ahasuerus, after that she had been twelve months, according to the manner of the women, (for so were the days of their purifications accomplished, to wit, six months with oil of myrrh, and six months with sweet odours, and with other things for the purifying of the women;)"

Psalms 45:8—"All thy garments smell of myrrh, and aloes, and cassia, out of the ivory palaces, whereby they have made thee glad."

Proverbs 7:17—"I have perfumed my bed with myrrh, aloes, and cinnamon."

The Song of Solomon 1:13—"A bundle of myrrh is my well-beloved unto me; he shall lie all night betwixt my breasts."

The Song of Solomon 3:6—"Who is this that cometh out of the wilderness like pillars of smoke, perfumed with myrrh and frankincense, with all powders of the merchant?"

The Song of Solomon 4:6—"Until the day break, and the shadows flee away, I will get me to the mountain of myrrh, and to the hill of frankincense."

The Song of Solomon 4:14—"Spikenard and saffron; calamus and cinnamon, with all trees of frankincense; myrrh and aloes, with all the chief spices:"

The Song of Solomon 5:1—"I am come into my garden, my sister, [my] spouse: I have gathered my myrrh with my spice; I have eaten my honeycomb with my honey; I have drunk my wine with my milk: eat, O friends; drink, yea, drink abundantly, O beloved."

The Song of Solomon 5:5—"I rose up to open to my beloved; and my hands dropped *with* myrrh, and my fingers *with* sweet smelling myrrh, upon the handles of the lock."

The Song of Solomon 5:13—"His cheeks *are* as a bed of spices, *as* sweet flowers: his lips *like* lilies, dropping sweet smelling myrrh."

Matthew 2:11—"And when they were come into the house, they saw the young child with Mary his mother, and fell down, and worshiped him: and when they had opened their treasures, they presented unto him gifts; gold, and frankincense, and myrrh."

Mark 15:23—"And they gave him to drink wine mingled with myrrh: but he received *it* not."

John 19:39—"And there came also Nicodemus, which at the first came to Jesus by night, and brought a mixture of myrrh and aloes, about an hundred pound *weight*."

Myrtle

Zechariah 1:8—"I saw by night, and behold a man riding upon a red horse, and he stood among the myrtle trees that *were* in the bottom and behind him *were there* red horses, speckled, and white."

Zechariah 1:10—"And the man that stood among the myrtle trees answered and said, These *are they* whom the Lord hath sent to walk to and fro through the earth."

Zechariah 1:11—"And they answered the angel of the Lord that stood among the myrtle trees, and said, We have walked to and fro through the earth, and, behold, all the earth sitteth still, and is at rest."

Spikenard

The Song of Solomon 4:14—"Spikenard and saffron; calamus and cinnamon, with all trees of frankincense, myrrh and aloes, with all chief spices."

Mark 14:3—"And being in Bethany in the house of Simon the leper, as he sat at meat, there came a woman having an alabaster box of ointment of spikenard very precious; and she brake the box, and poured *it* on his head."

John 12:3—"Then took Mary a pound of ointment of spikenard, very costly, and anointed the feet of Jesus, and wiped his feet with her hair: and the house was filled with the odour of the ointment."

Chapter 2
How Essential Oils Work

Understanding Essential Oil Chemistry

Essential oils are nature's volatile aromatic compounds generated within shrubs, flowers, trees, roots, bushes, and seeds. They are usually extracted through steam distillation, hydrodistillation, or cold-pressed extraction.

The power of an essential oil lies in its constituents and their synergy. **Each** essential oil is composed of 200-500 different bioconstituents, which make them very diverse in their effects. No two oils are alike.

Lavender oil, for example, contains approximately 200 different constituents, of which linalyl acetate, linalool, cis-beta-ocimene, trans-beta-ocimene, and terpinene-4-ol are the major components. Lavender oil has been used for burns, insect bites, headaches, PMS, insomnia, stress, and hair growth. Because essential oils are composites of hundreds of different constituents, each oil can exert many different effects on the body.

Essential oils have a unique ability to penetrate cell membranes and travel throughout the blood and tissues. The unique lipid-soluble structure of essential oils is very similar to the makeup of our cell membranes, and the molecules of essential oils are also relatively small, which enhances their ability to penetrate into the cells. When topically applied to the feet or soft tissue, essential oils can travel throughout the body in a matter of minutes.

Basic Structure of Essential Oil Constituents

The aromatic constituents of essential oils (i.e., terpenes, monoterpenes, phenols, aldehydes, etc.) are constructed from long chains of carbon and hydrogen atoms, which have a predominantly ring-like structure. Links of carbon atoms form the backbone of these chains, with oxygen, hydrogen, nitrogen, sulfur, and other carbon atoms attached at various points of the chain.

Essential oils have different chemistry than fatty oils (also known as fatty acids). In contrast to the simple linear carbon-hydrogen structure of fatty oils, essential oils have a far more complex ring structure and contain sulfur and nitrogen atoms that fatty oils do not have.

The terpenoids found in all essential oils are actually constructed out of the same basic building block—a five-carbon molecule known as isoprene. When two isoprene units link together, they create a monoterpene; when three join, they create a sesquiterpene; and so on.

Essential Oil Constituent Categories

There are 14 categories of essential oil constituents. We will list each category with examples of oils containing such constituents. The information below has been adapted from *The Chemistry of Essential Oils* by David Stewart, PhD,[1] which is highly recommended, and from *l'aromathérapie exactement*[2] by Pierre Franchomme and Daniel Pénoël.

1. **Alkanes:** Few essential oils contain alkanes, and those that do usually contain less than 1 percent. The alkanes undecane, dodecane, and hexadecane are found in ginger oil. Alkane alcohols are found in lemon oil and ginger oil. Rose oil stands alone as an essential oil that contains 11 to 19 percent alkanes, which may be why this exquisite oil exhibits so many unique characteristics.

2. **Phenols:** Common phenols found in essential oils are thymol (thyme and mountain savory) and eugenol (clove, cinnamon, basil, and bay laurel). Phenol is found in very minute quantities (<1 percent) in cassia, cinnamon, and ylang ylang. Phenols are believed to be antiseptic, antimicrobial, and may boost the immune system in various ways. Some phenols are strong and may cause skin irritation.

3. **Monoterpenes:** This class of constituents is the most common and is found in every essential oil. It is estimated that there are 1,000 different monoterpenes found in essential oils. Monoterpenes contain 10 carbons and are characteristically similar to alkanes. Many oils are composed of mostly monoterpenes, including grapefruit and frankincense. They have light fragrances, are supportive, and enhance the therapeutic talents of other constituents. They are commonly the first aroma detected when smelling an essential oil. The monoterpenes α-pinene, d-limonene, l-limonene, sabinene, myrcene, β-phellandrene, camphene, and ocimene are abundant in pine, orange, balsam fir, juniper, frankincense, ginger, spruce, and basil, respectively.

4. **Sesquiterpenes:** There are as many as 3,000 different sesquiterpenes found in essential oils. This class of constituents contains 15 carbons and is characteristically similar to alkanes and monoterpenes. The sesquiterpenes beta-caryophyllene, bisabolen, and guaiene are found in black pepper, myrrh, and patchouli, respectively. Oils with high sesquiterpene content include cedarwood, patchouli, sandalwood, ginger, vetiver, blue cypress, and myrrh. Many sesquiterpenes are specific to one oil only, and most have light aromas, but not all. Caryophyllene, for example, is one exception, that has a strong, woody, spicy aroma and is found in a variety of oils. Sesquiterpenes are soothing to inflamed tissue and can also produce profound effects on emotions and hormonal balance.

Other terpenes:

Diterpenes (20 carbons) are the heaviest molecules found in distilled essential oils. Jasmine absolute contains about 14 percent diterpenes. Therapeutically, diterpenes have some of the same properties as sesquiterpenes and are considered to be expectorants and purgatives.

Triterpenes (30 carbons) and tetraterpenes (40 carbons) are larger molecules than diterpenes and are found mostly in the cold-pressed citrus oils of orange, tangerine, lemon, grapefruit, and lime and also in solvent-extracted oils like jasmine and neroli.

It was once believed that diterpene and triterpene molecules were too large to make it through distillation, but diterpenes like incensole have been documented in essential oils through GC-MS analyses, and triterpenic acids (such as boswellic acids) are detectable in frankincense essential oil through High Performance Liquid Chromatography (HPLC) testing.

5. **Alcohols:** The names of these constituents end in –ol. Borneol is found in lavandin; citronellol is in rose; linalool is in rosewood; α-terpineol and terpinen-4-ol are in mela-

leuca; and lavendulol is in lavender. Alcohols are also found in eucalyptus and fennel oils, as well as many more. Alcohols are energizing, cleansing, antiseptic, antiviral, and have a sweet floral aroma.

6. **Ethers:** This constituent form is not as common in essential oils as others like terpenes, alcohols, or ketones. The names of these constituents end in "-ole," "-cin," or "-ether." Examples of ethers are anethole, in fennel and anise; elemicin, in elemi; estragole, in tarragon; and myristicin, in nutmeg. Ethers are balancing and calming, help release emotions, and have an antidepressant effect.

7. **Aldehydes:** The names of these constituents end in "-al" or "-aldehyde." Benzoic aldehyde is found in onycha; cinnamaldehyde, in cassia; citral, in lemongrass; cuminal, in cumin; neral, in melissa; and phellandral, in eucalyptus dives. The aldehyde octanal is in rose, lavender, and citrus oils. Decanal is found in coriander, lemongrass, and mandarin oils. Aldehydes are antimicrobial, anti-inflammatory, cooling, and have strong aromas. They can also be calming to the nervous system, emotional stress relievers, and blood pressure reducers.

8. **Ketones:** A strong, distinctive odor characterizes ketones. Ketones usually end in "-one." Camphor is found in rosemary; fenchone, in fennel; jasmone, in jasmine; pentanone, in myrrh; piperitone, in peppermint; β-thujone, in Western red cedar; and α-vetivone, in vetiver. Ketones are thought to be calming, with decongesting and analgesic benefits; promote healing (cell regeneration); and cleanse receptor sites.

9. **Carboxylic acids:** These constituents are only minor parts of an essential oil, rarely comprising more than 1-2 percent. They are easy to recognize because they always have the word "acid" in their name. Examples are cinnamic acid, in cinnamon; geranic acid, in geranium; and valerinic acid, in valerian. Carboxylic acids are stimulating and cleansing and are very reactive with other components.

10. **Esters:** Oils composed mainly of esters include birch and wintergreen. The names of esters end in "-ate." Esters usually have a strong sweet aroma. Linalyl acetate is found in bergamot; neryl acetate, in helichrysum; isobutyl angelate, in Roman chamomile; citronellyl formate, in geranium; menthyl acetate, in peppermint; and bornyl acetate, the main constituent in pine, spruce, juniper, and fir. To make an ester, a carboxylic acid and an alcohol are combined. Esters are soothing, balancing, antifungal, and stress and emotional releasing.

11. **Oxides:** These are oxygenated hydrocarbons and are usually derived from terpenes, alcohols, or ketones that have been oxidized. Examples are bisabolol oxide found in German chamomile; pipertone oxide, in peppermint; linalool oxide, in hyssop; rose oxide, in rose; sclareol oxide, in clary sage; and humulene oxide, in clove. These oxides are in very small quantities, but most oils produce the oxide 1,8-cineole, also known as eucalyptol, in varying amounts. This is more abundantly found in eucalyptus (*E. globulus*), rosemary, and thyme. Oils with 1,8-cineole are known for respiratory-decongesting and sinus-clearing benefits.

12. **Lactones:** This constituent group is characterized by tongue-twisting names. Bergaptene is found in fennel essential oil; furanogermacrene, in myrrh; and umbelliferone, in anise. Celery seed is an oil with higher amounts of lactones. Lactones, like ketones, are generally decongesting and expectorant. They generally have mild aromas. They

seem to have antiseptic, antiparasitic, and anti-inflammatory properties, according to Dr. Daniel Pénöel.

13. **Coumarins:** Dr. Stewart notes that coumarins are a subgroup of lactones and are found widely in nature. Because there is a similarity to the name of the blood-thinning drug Coumadin®, he explained that coumarins and Coumadin are *not* similar. One is natural, one synthetic, and they have very different chemical formulas. Coumarins have the fragrance of freshly cut hay or grass. In fact, when you mow your lawn, you are releasing coumarins into the air. They are found in fleabane, bitter orange, lavandin (in very minute quantities), and cassia essential oils. Coumarins are powerful and can have strong therapeutic effects, even in small quantities. Coumarins have antispasmodic, antiviral, antibacterial, and antifungal properties.

14. **Furanoids:** Furanoids or furans are lactones or coumarins with names starting with "furano-" or "furo-" or ending with "furan." Most of the essential oils that contain furans are certain expressed citrus oils. Some essential oils with furanoids are phototoxic (they amplify the effects of the sun) like bergamot, ruta (*graveolens*), grapefruit, and lemon. Other oils containing furanoids, like myrrh, mandarin, sweet orange, and tangerine are not phototoxic. Myrrh is interesting in that it contains more furanoid components than any other essential oil (up to 27 percent), yet it is not phototoxic. Furanoids can have the benefits of lactones or coumarins.

With this brief explanation of constituent chemistry, lavender's components are categorized as esters (linalyl acetate), alcohols (linalool and terpinen-4-ol), and monoterpenes (cis-β-ocimene and trans-β-ocimene).

Sacred frankincense essential oil constituents tell us that it is composed of monoterpenes (α-pinene, limonene, sabinene, myrcene, α-thujene, p-cymene), the sesquiterpene β-caryophyllene, and many more components.

Lemon's constituents can be categorized as monoterpenes (limonene, gamma-terpinene, β-pinene, α-pinene, and sabinene).

The constituents of peppermint are categorized as alcohols (menthol), ketones (menthone), furanoids (menthofuran), monoterpenes (1,8-cineole and pulegone), and esters (menthyl acetate).

These constituents listed are only a small percentage of the total number of constituents present in each essential oil.

Plant Chemotypes and Constituent Variability

A single species of plant can have several different chemotypes (biomolecularly unique variants within one species) based on molecular composition. This means that basil (*Ocimum basilicum*) grown in one area might produce an essential oil with different chemistry than a basil grown in another location. The plant's growing environment, such as soil pH and mineral content, can dramatically affect the plant's ultimate chemistry as well. Different chemotypes of basil are listed below:

- *Ocimum basilicum* CT linalol fenchol (Germany)— antiseptic
- *Ocimum basilicum* CT methyl chavicol (Reunion, Comoro, or Egypt)— anti-inflammatory
- *Ocimum basilicum* CT eugenol (Madagascar)— anti-inflammatory, pain-relieving

Another plant species that occurs in a variety of different chemotypes is rosemary (*Rosmarinus officinalis*).

- *Rosmarinus officinalis* CT camphor is high in camphor, which serves best as a general stimulant and works synergistically with other oils, such as pepper (*Piper nigrum*), and can be a powerful energy stimulant.

- *Rosmarinus officinalis* CT cineole is rich in 1,8-cineole, which is used in other countries for pulmonary congestion and to help with the elimination of toxins from the liver and kidneys. Young Living offers this chemotype of rosemary because of its great value.
- *Rosmarinus officinalis* CT verbenone is high in verbenone and is the most gentle of the rosemary chemotypes. It offers powerful regenerative properties and has outstanding benefits for skin care.

Common thyme (*Thymus vulgaris*) produces several different chemotypes, depending on the conditions of its growth, climate, and altitude. The following are just two chemotypes out of many more.

- *Thymus vulgaris* CT thymol is germicidal and anti-inflammatory.
- *Thymus vulgaris* CT linalool is anti-infectious.

One chemotype of thyme will yield an essential oil with high levels of thymol, depending on the time of year it is distilled. The later it is distilled in the growing season (e.g., mid-summer or fall), the more thymol the oil will contain.

Another example of this variability in chemotype is shown in a Turkish study on Origanum onites.[3] Researchers found that the altitude at which the plants grew affected the morphology of the plant and amount of volatile oil the plant produced. The plant produced more volatile oil the higher the altitude in which it grew. Even on the same mountainside, wildcrafted plants produced varying levels of oil.

Proper cultivation assures that more variable-specific chemotypes, like *Thymus vulgaris* and *Origanum compactum,* will maintain more consistent levels of constituents and oil produced.

Purity and Potency of Essential Oils

One of the factors that determines the purity of an oil is its constituents. These constituents can be affected by a vast number of variables, including the part(s) of the plant from which the oil was produced, soil condition, fertilizer (organic or chemical), geographical region, climate, altitude, harvesting methods, and distillation processes.

The key to producing a therapeutic-grade essential oil is to preserve as many of the delicate aromatic components within the essential oil as possible. Fragile aromatic components are easily destroyed by high temperature and pressure, as well as by contact with reactive metals such as copper or aluminum. This is why all therapeutic-grade essential oils should be distilled in stainless steel cooking chambers at low pressure and low temperature.

The plant material should also be free of herbicides and other agrichemicals. These can react with the essential oil during distillation to produce toxic compounds. Because many pesticides are oil-soluble, they can also mix into the essential oil.

Although chemists have successfully recreated the main constituents and fragrances of some essential oils in the laboratory, these synthetic oils lack therapeutic benefits and may even carry risks. Pure essential oils contain hundreds of different bioconstituents, which lend important therapeutic properties to the oil when combined. Also, many essential oils contain molecules and isomers that are impossible to manufacture in the laboratory.

Today approximately 300 essential oils are distilled or extracted worldwide. Several thousand constituents and aromatic molecules are identified and registered in these 300 essential oils. Ninety-eight percent of essential oil volume produced today is used in the perfume and cosmetic industry. Only about 2 percent of the production volume is for therapeutic and medicinal applications.

Young Living requires all distillers who want to sell to Young Living to submit samples to be analyzed to ensure that all the constituents are present at the right percentage to be therapeutic. You can have pure oils, but if the plants are distilled at the wrong time of day or with incorrect distillation procedures, the constituents that make the oils therapeutic will not be there, and you will not have a therapeutic-grade profile.

In addition, Young Living requires that the farms and the essential oil distillation facilities be subject to site inspection. Of oil samples submitted between May 2007 and October 2011 by distillers wanting to partner with Young Living, over 34 percent did not meet Young Living standards and were rejected.

Because Young Living interacts with the end-users who purchase essential oils, the company is able to monitor human response to and determine the actual therapeutic benefit of various oils, thereby comparing the constituents of different oils to determine their maximum, health-giving potential. Quality and efficacy are moving, evolving targets. No one understands this more than Young Living.

Standards and Testing
Young Living Standards

Over the years, Young Living has bought and compiled an essential oil retention index and mass spectral reference library that contains over 400,000 components. Using this research reference library, Young Living developed its own standards to guarantee the highest possible therapeutic potency for its essential oils.

Young Living's research and quality control laboratories in Utah have four gas chromatograph (GC) instruments, two of which also have a mass spectrometer (GC-MS). The Young Living Ecuador laboratory has a GC-MS. These instruments are the only ones in the world that are matched and calibrated for therapeutic essential oil analysis to the instruments used at the National Center for Scientific Research in France (CNRS: *Centre National de la Recherche Scientifique*) by Dr. Hervé Casabianca.

As a general rule, if one or more marker components in an essential oil fall outside the prescribed percentages, the oil does not meet Young Living pure, therapeutic grade essential oil standards.

A lavender essential oil produced in one region of France might have a slightly different chemistry than that grown in another region and as a result may not meet the standard. It may have excessive camphor levels (1.0 instead of 0.5), a condition that might be caused by distilling lavender that was too green, or the levels of lavandulol may be too low due to certain weather conditions at the time of harvest.

By comparing the gas chromatograph chemistry profile of a lavender essential oil with the Young Living pure, therapeutic-grade standard, one may also distinguish true lavender from various species of lavandin (hybrid lavender). Usually lavandin has high camphor levels, almost no lavandulol, and is easily identified. However, Tasmania produces a lavandin that yields an essential oil with naturally low camphor levels that mimics the composition of true lavender. Only by analyzing the essential oil composition of this Tasmanian lavandin using high resolution gas chromatography and comparing it with the Young Living pure, therapeutic-grade standard for genuine lavender can this hybrid lavender be identified.

Testing Instruments

In the United States, few companies use the proper analytical instruments and methods to properly analyze essential oils. Most labs use equipment best suited for synthetic chemicals—not for natural essential oil analysis.

Young Living Essential Oils uses the proper instruments and has made great effort to calibrate Young Living's GC-MS instruments to the column-wall thickness set by Dr. Casabianca, laboratory director of Natural Product Research, at CNRS labs in France. This ensures identification of more components that otherwise might be missed. In addition to operating its analytical instruments with the same calibration as the CNRS

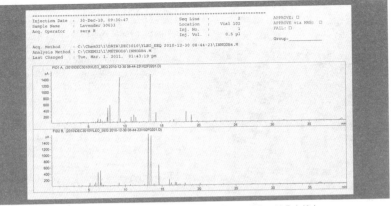

A gas chromatogram for lavender tested at the Young Living analytical laboratory in Spanish Fork, Utah

laboratories, Young Living is continually expanding its analytical component library in order to perform a more thorough compositional analysis.

Gas Chromatography and Mass Spectrometry

Properly analyzing an essential oil by gas chromatography (GC) is a complex undertaking. The injection mixture, capillary column diameter, column length, and oven temperature must fall within certain parameters. GC is the analytical instrumentation used to separate the many natural components biogenerated by the aromatic plant that make up the essential oil. The key components of a GC are the injector, capillary GC column, detector, and oven. A small sample of essential oil is injected into the capillary GC column with a syringe. The capillary GC column is slowly heated within the oven to separate the essential oil components. Finally, the separated components exit the GC column, and the percentage of each component is determined by a Flame Ionization Detector (FID).

Using a longer capillary GC column length increases the separation of each of the components in a complex essential oil. We have found that a 50- or 60-meter-long capillary GC column provides the best separation for essential oil components. Shorter 25- or 30-meter columns provide adequate separation of many components, but they are too short to properly analyze the complex mosaic of natural bioconstituents found in an essential oil. A more detailed analysis of an essential oil can be obtained using a 100-meter-long capillary GC column.

Every capillary GC column has an internal polymer coating (stationary phase) that helps separate the essential oil components. The most common stationary phase for essential oil separations is the polydimethylsiloxane phase that generates a separation based on the boiling points of each essential oil component. In addition, using a "wax-based" stationary phase composed of polyethylene oxide, the GC operator can obtain a separation based on both the boiling points and the polarity of each essential oil component. We use both of these phases simultaneously in one GC to provide two separations from a single injection of

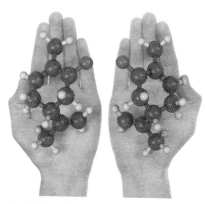

Two chiral forms of the constituent carvone. The left enantiomer is found in dill and caraway, while the form on the right is found in spearmint essential oil.

essential oil. This process allows us to make more certain identification of essential oil components.

Another common analytical instrument for the separation and identification of essential oil components is the GC-MS (gas chromatograph-mass spectrometer). The MS is a special detector that can identify by name each essential oil component from a library of known essential oil components attached to the instrument. The MS identifies the components based on the arrangement of their individual carbon, hydrogen, and oxygen atoms. The GC-MS is used in the first stages of research in order to separate and identify each component of a new essential oil. After the initial research, the GC (with an FID detector) is used for routine quality control to determine percentages of each component in the essential oil.

Chiral GC-MS

While GC-MS is an excellent tool to analyze essential oils, it does have limitations. Sometimes it can be difficult to distinguish between natural and synthetic bioconstituents using GC-MS analysis alone. If synthetic linalyl acetate is added to pure lavender, a GC-MS analysis cannot confidently determine whether that constituent is synthetic or natural, only that it is linalyl acetate. Adding a chiral (pronounced "ky-ral") capillary GC column in the GC-MS can help in distinguishing between synthetic and natural components. Research scientists can use chiral GC-MS to identify whether an essential oil is composed of its natural proportions of chiral components. Some components have what is called chiral polarity. This means they have "left" or "right" versions of the component, called enantiomers.

To see the perfect example of "chirality," bring your hands up, palms facing you. They are mirror images but exact opposites. They are different in that you could not put a right-handed glove on your left hand. The term used to identify rotating to the right is *dextrorotary,* or "*d,*" and rotating to the left, *levorotary,* or "*l.*"

Young Living researchers use a polarimeter to identify the optical rotation of molecules. If the "d" or "l" form deviates from what is listed in a chiral library of left and right enantiomers, the sample will be further analyzed with additional chiral capillary GC column testing or sent to Dr. Casabianca in France. This testing is more detailed and will identify a marker that reveals a synthetic origin. Adulterated or synthetic-based oil would then be rejected.

This complexity is why oils must be analyzed by an analytical chemist specially trained on the interpretation of gas chromatography and mass spectroscopy. The chemist examines the entire essential oil composition to determine its purity, measuring how various components in the oil occur in relation to each other. If some components occur in higher quantities than others, these provide important clues to determine if the oil is adulterated or pure.

Adulteration is such a major concern that each essential oil Young Living offers is tested initially by GC-MS, and every subsequent batch of essential oil is tested, using GC-FID, by Young Living's trained research and quality control scientists. Batches that do not meet established standards are rejected and returned.

Adulteration of essential oils will become more and more common as the supply of top-quality essential oils dwindles and demand continues to increase. Adulteration may occur by diluting the essential oil with fatty lipid oils. This is a common practice by other essential oil companies to increase supply and reduce cost. These adulterated essential oils will jeopardize the integrity of aromatherapy and essential oil use.

Adulterated Oils and Their Dangers

Today much of the lavender oil sold in America is a hybrid called lavandin, grown and distilled throughout the world. Lavandin is often heated to evaporate the camphor, mixed with synthetic linalyl acetate to improve the fragrance, and then sold as lavender oil. Most consumers don't know the difference and are happy to buy it for $7 to $10 per half ounce in various stores and on the Internet. This is one of the reasons why it is important to know about the integrity of the essential oil company or vendor.

Adulterated and mislabeled essential oils may present dangers for consumers. One woman who had heard of the ability of lavender oil to heal burns used "lavender oil" purchased from a local health food store when she spilled boiling water on her arm. But the pain intensified and the burn worsened, so she later complained that lavender oil was worthless for healing burns. When her "lavender" oil was analyzed, it was found to be lavandin, a hybrid of lavender that is biologically different from pure *Lavandula angustifolia*. Lavandin contains higher levels of camphor (7-18 percent) that may burn the skin. In contrast, true lavender contains almost no camphor and has burn-healing agents not found in lavandin.

Jean Valnet, MD, wrote about a similar instance in his book, *The Practice of Aromatherapy*. "A man was being treated for a fistula [an abnormal channel or opening in the skin] of the anus by instillation of pure and natural drops of lavender essence. The patient had begun to recover when he went on a journey, and, discovering he had left his essence at home, bought a fresh supply at a chemist's [drugstore]. Unfortunately this essence was neither natural nor pure: one single installation was followed by a painful inflammation of such severity that the unfortunate person was unable to sit down for more than a fortnight."[4]

In France production of true lavender oil (*Lavandula angustifolia*) dropped from 87 tons in 1967 to only 12 tons in 1998. During this same period, the worldwide demand for lavender oil grew over 100 percent. So where did essential oil marketers obtain enough lavender to meet the demand? They probably used a combination of synthetic and adulterated oils. There are huge chemical companies on the east coast of the U.S. that specialize in creating synthetic chemicals that can mimic every common essential oil. For every kilogram of pure essential oil that is produced, an estimated 10 to 100 kilograms of synthetic oil are created.

Adulterated oils that are mixed with synthetic extenders can be very detrimental, causing rashes, burns, and skin irritations. Common additives such as propylene glycol, DEP, or DOP (solvents that have no smell and increase the volume) can cause allergic reactions, besides being devoid of any therapeutic effects.

Some people assume that because an essential oil is "100 percent pure," it will not burn their skin. This is not true. Some pure essential oils may cause skin irritation if applied undiluted. If straight oregano oil is applied to the skin of some people, it may cause severe reddening. Citrus and spice oils like orange and cinnamon may also produce rashes. Even the terpenes in conifer oils like

Limbic System

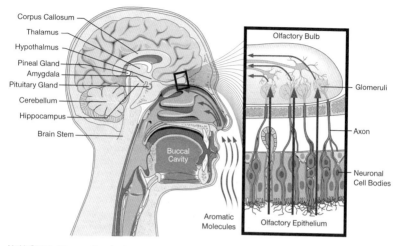

Limbic System—How aromatic molecules influence the emotional center of the brain

pine may cause skin irritation on sensitive people.

Many tourists in Egypt are eager to buy local essential oils, especially lotus oil. Vendors convince the tourists that the oils are 100 percent pure by touching a lighted match to the neck of the oil container to show that the oil is not diluted with alcohol or other petrochemical solvents. However, this test provides no reliable indicator of purity. Many synthetic compounds that are not flammable can be added to an essential oil, including propylene glycol. Furthermore, some natural essential oils high in terpenes can be flammable.

Some researchers feel that because of their complexity, essential oils do not disturb the body's natural balance or homeostasis: if one constituent exerts too strong an effect, another constituent may block or counteract it. However, synthetic chemicals, like pharmaceuticals, usually have only one action and may disrupt the body's homeostasis and cause various adverse side effects.

Powerful Influence of Aromas

The fragrance of an essential oil can directly affect everything from your emotional state to your lifespan. The specific mechanics of the sense of smell are still being explored by scientists but have been described as working like a lock and key or an odor molecule fitting a specific receptor site.

When a fragrance is inhaled, the airborne odor molecules travel up the nostrils to the olfactory epithelium or the center of olfactory sensation. At the olfactory epithelium, which is only about 1 square inch of the nasal cavity, olfactory receptor cells are triggered and send an impulse to the olfactory bulb. Each olfactory receptor type sends an impulse to a particular microregion, or glomerulus, of the olfactory bulb. There are around

2,000 glomeruli in the olfactory bulb, which receive the impulses from the olfactory receptors and allow us to perceive many smells. The olfactory bulb then transmits the impulses to other parts of the brain, including the gustatory center (where the sensation of taste is perceived), the amygdala (where emotional memories are stored), and other parts of the limbic system.

Because the limbic system is directly connected to those parts of the brain that control heart rate, blood pressure, breathing, memory, stress levels, and hormone balance, essential oils can have profound physiological and psychological effects.

Another theory of smell, called the vibration theory, is proposed by an Italian scientist named Luca Turin in a paper published in 1996. He theorizes that rather than the "lock and key" theory of olfaction, it is the vibrational properties of molecules that enable us to distinguish smells. He suggests that the olfactory receptors sense the quantum vibration of each odorants' atoms, which would allow humans to perceive almost limitless numbers of odors, as olfactory receptors are tuned to different frequencies.

While the vibrational theory is still somewhat controversial, Jennifer Brookes, a University College London researcher based at MIT, was lead author on a study that discusses models of receptor selectivity, including those based on shape and other factors like vibrational frequencies.[5] Speaking of Turin's theory, she told the BBC in March 2011, "It's a very interesting idea; there's all sorts of interesting biological physics that implement quantum processes that's cropping up. I believe it's time for the idea to develop and for us to get on with testing it." A colleague of Brookes, A. P. Horsfield, of Imperial College London, was also interviewed by the BBC about the vibrational theory and said, "There's still lots to understand, but the idea that it cannot possibly be right is no longer tenable really. The theory has to at least be considered respectable at this point."[6]

The sense of smell is the only one of the five senses directly linked to the limbic lobe of the brain, the emotional control center. Anxiety, depression, fear, anger, and joy all emanate from this region. The scent of a special fragrance can evoke memories and emotions before we are even consciously aware of it. When smells are concerned, we react first and think later. All other senses (touch, taste, hearing, and sight) are routed through the thalamus, which acts as the switchboard for the brain, passing stimuli onto the cerebral cortex (the conscious thought center) and other parts of the brain.

The limbic lobe (a group of brain structures that includes the hippocampus and amygdala located below the cerebral cortex) can also directly activate the hypothalamus. The hypothalamus is one of the most important parts of the brain. It controls body temperature, hunger, thirst, fatigue, sleep, and circadian cycles. It acts as our hormonal control center and releases hormones that can affect many functions of the body. The production of growth hormones, sex hormones, thyroid hormones, and neurotransmitters such as serotonin are all governed by the hypothalamus.

Essential oils—through their fragrance and unique molecular structure—can directly stimulate the limbic lobe and the hypothalamus, which is responsive to olfactory stimuli. Not only can the inhalation of essential oils be used to combat stress and emotional trauma, but it can also stimulate the production of hormones from the hypothalamus. This results in increased thyroid hormones (our energy hormone) and growth hormones (our youth and longevity hormone).

Essential oils may also be used to reduce appetite and increase satiety through their ability to stimulate the hypothalamus, which governs our feeling of satiety or fullness following meals. In a large clinical study, Alan Hirsch, MD, used fragrances, including peppermint, to trigger weight loss in a large group of patients (over 3,000 individuals) who had previously been unsuccessful in any type of weight-management program.[7] The amount of weight loss among the subjects directly correlated with the frequency of their use of their aroma inhalers. One group in the study lost an average of 4.7 pounds per month over the course of the six months. Hirsch suggests that by inhaling certain aromas, individuals with good olfaction may have induced and sustained weight loss over a 6-month period.

Another double-blind, randomized study by Hirsch documents the ability of aroma to enhance libido and sexual arousal.[8] When 31 male volunteers were subjected to the aromas of 30 different essential oils, each one exhibited a marked increase in arousal, based on measurements of brachial penile index and the measurement of both penile and brachial blood pressures. Among the scents that produced the highest increase in penile blood flow was a combination of lavender and pumpkin fragrances. This study shows that fragrances can enhance sexual arousal by stimulating the limbic system, the emotional center of the brain.

People who have undergone nose surgery or suffer olfactory impairment may find it difficult or impossible to completely detect an odor. These people may not derive the full physiological and emotional benefits of essential oils and their fragrances.

Proper stimulation of the olfactory nerves may offer a powerful and entirely new form of therapy that could be used as an adjunct against many forms of illness. Essential oils, through inhalation, may occupy a key position in this relatively unexplored frontier in medicine.

No one need ever dismiss essential oils as simple perfumes. Now you can understand the complexity and value of each essential oil with its hundreds of different components.

ENDNOTES:

1. Stewart D. *The Chemistry of Essential Oils Made Simple: God's Love Manifest in Molecules.* Care Publications, Marble Hill, MO: 2006.

2. Franchomme P, Pénoël D. *L'aromathérapie exactement.* Roger Jollois, ed., France 31 Août 2003.

3. Gönüz A, Özörgüzü B. An investigation on the morphology, anatomy and ecology of Origanum onites L. Tr. *J. of Botany* 1999 23:19-32.

4. Valnet J. *The Practice of Aromatherapy.* Healing Arts Press, Rochester, VT, 1982, p. 27.

5. Brookes JC, Horsfield AP, Stoneham AM. Odour character differences for enantiomers correlate with molecular flexibility, *J.R. Soc. Interface* (2009) 6, 75-86.

6. Palmer J. Quantum physics explanation for smell gains traction, BBC , March 24, 2011.

7. Hirsch AR, Gomez R. Weight reduction through inhalation of odorants. *J. Neurol. Orthop. Med. Surg.* 1995 16:28-31.

8. Hirsch AR, Gruss JJ. Human male sexual response to olfactory stimuli. *J. Neurol. Orthop. Med. Surg.* 1999 19(1):14-19.

Chapter 3
How to Safely Use Essential Oils

Basic Guidelines for Safe Use

Guidelines are important to follow when using essential oils, especially if you are unfamiliar with the oils and their benefits. Many guidelines are listed below and are elaborated on throughout the chapter. However, no list of do's and don'ts can ever replace common sense. It is foolish to dive headlong into a pond when you do not know the depth of the water. The same is true when using essential oils. Start gradually and patiently find what works best for you and your family members.

Storage

1. Always keep a bottle of a pure vegetable oil (e.g., V-6 Vegetable Oil Complex, olive oil, almond oil, coconut oil, or more fragrant massage oils such as Sensation, Relaxation, Ortho Ease, or Ortho Sport) handy when using essential oils. Vegetable oils will dilute essential oils if the essential oils cause discomfort or skin irritation.

2. Keep bottles of essential oils tightly closed and store them in a cool location away from light. If stored properly, essential oils will maintain their potency for many years.

3. Keep essential oils out of reach of children. Treat the oils as you would any product for therapeutic use. Children love the oils and will often go through an entire bottle in a very short time. They want to give massages and do the same things they see you do.

Usage

4. Essential oils rich in menthol (such as Peppermint) should not be used on the throat or neck area of children under 18 months of age.

5. Angelica, Bergamot, Grapefruit, Lemon, Orange, Tangerine, and other citrus oils are photosensitive and may cause a rash or dark pigmentation on skin exposed to direct sunlight or UV rays within 1–2 days after application.

6. Keep essential oils away from the eye area and never put them directly into ears. Do not handle contact lenses or rub eyes with essential oils on your fingers. Even in minute amounts, many essential oils may damage contacts and will irritate eyes.

7. Pregnant women should consult a health-care professional when starting any type of health program. Oils are safe to use, but one needs to use common sense. Follow the directions and dilute with V-6 Vegetable Oil Complex until you become familiar with the oils you are using.

   Many pregnant women have said that they feel a very positive response from the unborn child when the oils are applied on the skin, but that is each woman's individual experience.

8. Epileptics and those with high blood pressure should consult their health-care professional before using essential oils. Use extra caution with high ketone oils such as Basil, Rosemary, Sage, and Tansy oils.

Essential Oils Certified as GRAS

(Generally Regarded as Safe), or as food additives, by the FDA

Single Oils

Anise	**G F**
Angelica	**G F**
Basil	**G F**
Bergamot	**G F**
Cajuput	**F**
Cardamom	**F**
Carrot Seed	**F**
Cassia	**G F**
Cedarwood	**F**
Celery Seed	**G F**
Cinnamon Bark & Leaf	**G F**
Cistus	**F**
Citronella	**G F**
Citrus Rinds	**G F**
Clary Sage	**G F**
Clove	**G F**
Copaiba	**G F**
Coriander	**G F**
Cumin	**G F**
Dill	**G F**
Eucalyptus Globulus	**G F L**
Elemi	**G F L**
Fennel	**G F**
Frankincense	**G F L**
Galbanum	**G F L**
Geranium	**G F**
German Chamomile	**G F**
Ginger	**G F**
Goldenrod	**G**
Grapefruit	**G F**
Helichrysum	**G F**
Hyssop	**G F**
Idaho Balsam Fir	**F**
Jasmine	**G F**
Juniper	**G F**
Laurus Nobilis	**G F**

Lavender	**G F**
Lavandin	**G F**
Lemon	**G F**
Lemongrass	**G F**
Lime	**G F**
Mandarin	**G F**
Marjoram	**G F**
Melaleuca Alternifolia	**F**
Mountain Savory	**F**
Melissa	**G F**
Myrrh	**G F L**
Myrtle	**G F**
Neroli	**G F**
Nutmeg	**G F**
Onycha *(Styrax benzoin)*	**G F**
Orange	**G F**
Oregano	**G F**
Palmarosa	**G F**
Patchouli	**G F L**
Pepper	**G F**
Peppermint	**G F**
Petitgrain	**G F**
Pine	**G F L**
Roman Chamomile	**G F**
Rose	**G F**
Rosemary	**G F**
Rosewood	**F**
Savory	**G F**
Sage	**G F**
Sandalwood	**G F L**
Spearmint	**G F**
Spikenard	**F**
Spruce	**G F L**
Tangerine	**G F**
Tarragon	**G F**
Thyme	**G F**
Tsuga	**G F L**

Valerian	**G F L**
Vetiver	**G F**
Wintergreen	**F**
Yarrow	**F**
Ylang Ylang	**G F**

Blends

Abundance	**G**
Believe	**F**
Citrus Fresh	**G**
Christmas Spirit	**G**
DiGize	**G**
EndoFlex	**G**
Gratitude	**F**
Joy	**G**
JuvaCleanse	**G**
JuvaFlex	**G**
Longevity	**G**
Thieves	**G**
M-Grain	**G**
Purification	**G**
Relieve It	**G**
Sacred Mountain	**G**
White Angelica	**G**

CODE:

G Generally regarded as safe (GRAS)

F FDA-approved food additive

L Flavoring agent

9. People with allergies should test a small amount of oil on an area of sensitive skin, such as the inside of the upper arm, for 30 minutes before applying the oil on other areas of the body.

10. The bottoms of feet are safe locations to apply essential oils topically.

11. Direct inhalation of essential oils can be a deep and intensive application method, particularly for respiratory congestion and illness. However, this method should not be used more than 10–15 times throughout the day without consulting a health professional. Also, inhalation of essential oils is NOT recommended for those with asthmatic conditions.

12. Before taking GRAS (Generally Regarded As Safe) essential oils internally, test your reactions by diluting 1 drop of essential oil in 1 teaspoon of an oil-soluble liquid like Blue Agave, Yacon Syrup, olive oil, coconut oil, or rice milk. If you intend to consume more than a few drops of diluted essential oil per day, we recommend first consulting a health professional.

13. Be aware that reactions to essential oils, both topically and orally, can be delayed as long as 2–3 days.

14. Add 1–3 drops of undiluted essential oils directly to bath water. If more essential oil is desired, mix the oil first into bath salts or a bath gel base before adding to the bath water. Generally, never use more than 10 drops of essential oils in one bath. When essential oils are put directly into bath water without a dispersing agent, they can cause serious discomfort on sensitive skin because the essential oils tend to float, undiluted, on top of the water.

Chemical Sensitivities and Allergies

Occasionally, individuals beginning to use quality essential oils will suffer rashes or allergic reactions. This may be due to using an undiluted spice, conifer, or citrus oil; or it may be caused by an interaction of the oil with residues of synthetic, petroleum-based, personal-care products that have leached into the skin.

When using essential oils on a daily basis, it is imperative to avoid personal-care products containing ammonium or hydrocarbon-based chemicals. These include quaternary compounds such as quaternariums and polyquaternariums. These chemicals can be fatal if ingested, especially benzalkonium chloride, which, unfortunately, is used in many personal-care products on the market.

Other chemicals such as aluminum compounds, FD&C colors, formaldehyde, all parabens, talc, thimerosal, mercury, and titanium dioxide, just to name a few, are all toxic to the body and should be avoided. These compounds are commonly found in a variety of hand creams, mouthwashes, shampoos, antiperspirants, after-

---

CAUTION: Essential oils may sting if applied in or around the eyes. Some oils may be painful on mucous membranes unless diluted properly. Immediate dilution is strongly recommended if skin becomes painfully irritated or if oil accidentally gets into eyes. Flushing the area with a vegetable oil should minimize discomfort almost immediately.

DO NOT flush with water! Essential oils are oil-soluble, not water-soluble. Water will only spread the oils over a larger surface, possibly worsening the problem. Use V-6 Vegetable Oil Complex, coconut oil, olive oil, or other vegetable oil to flush the essential oils. Keep eyes closed, be patient, and the sting will quickly dissipate.

shave lotions, and hair-care products.

Other compounds that present concerns are sodium lauryl sulfate, propylene glycol—extremely common in everything from toothpaste to shampoo—and aluminum salts found in many deodorants.

Of particular concern are the potentially hazardous preservatives and synthetic fragrances that abound in virtually all modern personal-care products. Some of these include methylene chloride, methyl isobutyl ketone, and methyl ethyl ketone. These are not only toxic, but they can also react with some compounds in natural essential oils. The result can be a severe case of dermatitis or even septicemia (blood poisoning).

A classic case of a synthetic fragrance causing widespread damage occurred in the 1970s. AETT (acetyl ethyl tetramethyl tetralin) appeared in numerous brands of personal-care products throughout the United States. Even after a series of animal studies revealed that it caused significant brain and spinal cord damage, the FDA refused to ban the chemical. Finally, the cosmetic industry voluntarily withdrew AETT after allowing it to be distributed for years.

How many other toxins masquerading as preservatives or fragrances are currently being used in personal-care products?

Many chemicals are easily absorbed through the skin due to its permeability. One study found that 13 percent of BHT (butylated hydroxytoluene) and 49 percent of DDT (a carcinogenic pesticide) can be absorbed into the skin upon topical contact.[1]

Once absorbed, many chemicals can become trapped in the fatty subdermal layers of skin, where they can leach into the bloodstream. They can remain trapped for several months or years until a topical substance like an essential oil starts to move them from their resting place and cause them to come out of the skin in an uncomfortable way. Besides skin irritation, you could experience nausea, headaches, and other slight temporary effects during this detoxifying process. Even in small concentrations, these chemicals and synthetic compounds are toxic and can compromise one's health.

It is all about what chemicals were used, how much, how long, and perhaps the level of toxicity in your body.

Essential oils have been known to digest toxic substances, and so when they come in contact with chemical residue on the skin, the oils start to work against them.

The user may mistakenly assume that the threat of an interaction between oils and synthetic cosmetics used months before is small. However, a case of dermatitis is always a possibility.

Essential oils do not cause skin problems, rashes, or eruptions on the skin; but they may, only indirectly, as they go after the chemicals. Do not make the mistake of blaming the essential oils. Just be glad this chemical residue is coming out of your body.

You can always reduce the amount of oil you are using or stop the use of any oil for a couple of days and then start again slowly. You can also use V-6 Vegetable Oil Complex, other vegetable or massage oils, or natural creams to dilute the oils.

Before You Start

Always skin test an essential oil before using it. Each person's body is different, so apply oils to a small area first. Apply one oil or blend at a time. When layering oils that are new to you, allow enough time (3-5 minutes) for the body to respond before applying a second oil.

Use a small amount when applying essential oils to skin that may carry residue from cosmetics, personal-care products, soaps, and cleansers containing synthetic chemicals. Some of them—especially petroleum-based chemicals—can penetrate and remain in the skin and fatty tissues for days or even weeks after use.

Essential oils may work against such chemicals and toxins built up in the body from chemicals in food, water, and work environment. If you have this kind of an experience using essential oils, it may be wise to reduce or stop using them for a few days and start an internal cleansing program before resuming regular use of essential oils. In addition, double your water intake and keep flushing those toxins out of your body.

You may also want to try the following alternatives to a detoxification program to determine the cause of the problem:

- Dilute 1–3 drops of essential oil in 1/2 teaspoon of V-6 Vegetable Oil Complex, massage oil, or any pure vegetable oil such as almond, coconut, or olive. More dilution may be needed.
- Reduce the number of oils used at any time.
- Use single oils or oil blends one at a time.
- Reduce the amount of oil used.
- Reduce the frequency of application.
- Drink more purified or distilled water.
- Ask your health-care professional to monitor detoxification.
- Test the diluted essential oil on a small patch of skin for 30 minutes. If any redness or irritation results, dilute the area immediately with a pure vegetable or massage oil and then cleanse with soap and water.
- If skin irritation or other uncomfortable side effects persist, discontinue using the oil on that location and apply the oils on the bottoms of the feet.

You may also want to avoid using products that contain the following ingredients to eliminate potential problems:

- Cosmetics, deodorants, and skin-care products containing aluminum, petrochemicals, or other synthetic ingredients
- Perms, hair colors or dyes, hair sprays, or gels containing synthetic chemicals; shampoos, toothpastes, mouthwashes, and soaps containing synthetic chemicals such as sodium laurel sulfate, propylene glycol, or lead acetate
- Garden sprays, paints, detergents, and cleansers containing toxic chemicals and solvents

You can use many essential oils anywhere on the body except on the eyes and in the ears. Other oils may irritate certain sensitive tissues. See recommended dilution rates in the chapters for singles and blends.

Keep "hot" oils such as Oregano, Cinnamon, Thyme, Eucalyptus, Mountain Savory, Lemon, and Orange essential oils or blends such as Thieves, PanAway, Relieve It, and Exodus II out of reach of children. These types of oils should always be diluted for both children and adults.

Children need to be taught how to use the oils so that they understand the safety issue. If a child or infant swallows an essential oil, do the following:

- Seek immediate emergency medical attention, if necessary.
- Give the child milk, cream, yogurt, or another safe, oil-soluble liquid to drink.

NOTE: If your body pH is low, your body will be acidic; therefore, you could also have less of a response or perhaps a minimal negative reaction to the oils.

Topical Application

Many oils are safe to apply directly to the skin. Lavender is safe to use on children without dilution. However, you must be sure the essential oil you are using is not lavandin labeled as lavender or genetically altered lavender. When applying most other essential oils on children, dilute the oils with carrier oil. For dilution, add 15–30 drops of essential oil to 1 oz. of quality carrier oil, as mentioned previously.

Carrier oils such as V-6 Vegetable Oil Complex extend essential oils and provide more efficient use. When massaging, the vegetable oil helps lubricate the skin.

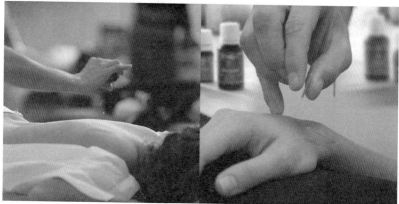

Massage

Acupuncture

When starting an essential oil application, depending on which oil you use, you may want to test for skin sensitivity by applying the oil first to the bottoms of the feet. See the Vita Flex foot charts to identify areas of best application. Start by applying 3–6 drops of a single oil or blend, spreading it over the bottom of each foot.

When applying essential oils to yourself, use 1–2 drops of oil on 2–3 locations 2 times a day. Increase to 4 times a day if needed. Apply the oil and allow it to absorb for 2–3 minutes before applying another oil or before getting dressed to avoid staining clothing.

As a general rule, when applying oils to yourself or another person for the first time, do not apply more than two single oils or blends at one time.

When mixing essential oil blends or diluting essential oils in a carrier oil, it is best to use containers made of glass or earthenware, rather than plastic. Plastic particles can leach into the oil and then into the skin once it is applied.

Before applying oils, wash hands thoroughly with soap and water.

Massage

Start by applying 2 drops of a single oil or blend on the skin and massaging it in. If you are working on a large area, such as the back, mix 1–3 drops of the selected essential oil into 1 teaspoon of pure carrier oil such as V-6 Vegetable Oil Complex, a massage oil, or any other oil of your choice such as jojoba, almond, coconut, olive, and/or grape seed.

Keep in mind that many massage oils such as olive, almond, jojoba, or wheat germ oil may stain some fabrics.

Acupuncture

Licensed acupuncturists can dramatically increase the effectiveness of acupuncture by using essential oils.

To start, place several drops of essential oil into the palm of your hand and dip the acupuncture needle tip into the oil before inserting it into the person. You can premix several oils in your hand if you wish to use more than one oil.

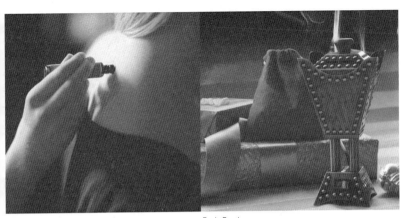

Acupressure

Resin Burning

Acupressure

When performing an acupressure treatment, apply 1–3 drops of essential oil to the acupressure point with your finger. Using an auricular probe with a slender point to dispense oil may enhance the application.

Start by pressing firmly and then releasing. Avoid applying pressure to any particular pressure point too long. You may continue along the acupressure points and meridians or use the reflexology or Vita Flex points as well. Once you have completed small point stimulations, massage the general area with the essential oil.

Warm Compress

For deeper penetration, use a warm compress after applying essential oils. Completely soak the cloth or towel by placing it in comfortably hot water. By the time you wring out the cloth and shake it, it will be a nice, warm temperature to be placed on the location. Then cover the cloth loosely with a dry towel or blanket to seal in the heat. Leave the cloth on for 15-30 minutes. Remove the cloth immediately if there is any discomfort.

Cold Packs

Apply essential oils on the location, followed by cold water or ice packs when treating inflamed or swollen tissues. Frozen packages of peas or corn make excellent ice packs that will mold to the contours of the body part and will not leak. Keep the cold pack on until the swelling diminishes.

For neurological problems, always use cold packs, never hot ones.

Layering

This technique consists of applying multiple oils one at a time. For example, rub Marjoram over a sore muscle, massage it into the tissue gently until the area is dry, and then apply a second oil such as Peppermint until the oil is absorbed and the skin is dry. Then layer on the third oil, such as Basil, and continue massaging.

Making a Compress

- Rub 1–3 drops on the location, diluted or neat, depending on the oil used and the skin sensitivity at that location.
- Cover the location with a hot, damp towel.

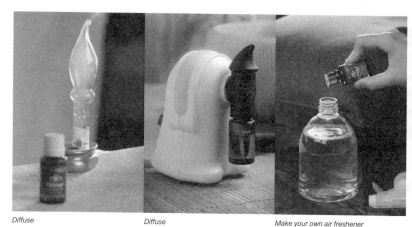

Diffuse

Diffuse

Make your own air freshener

- Cover the moist towel with a dry towel for 10–30 minutes, depending on individual need.

As the oil penetrates the skin, you may experience a warming or even a burning sensation, especially in areas where the greatest benefits occur. If burning becomes uncomfortable, apply V-6 Vegetable Oil Complex, a massage oil, or any pure vegetable oil such as olive, coconut, or almond to the location.

A second type of application is very mild and is suitable for children or those with sensitive skin.

- Place 5-15 drops of essential oil into a basin filled with warm water.
- Water temperature should be approximately 100° F (38° C), unless the patient suffers neurological conditions; in that case, use cool water.
- Vigorously agitate the water and let it stand for 1 minute.
- Place a dry face cloth on top of the water to soak up oils that have floated to the surface.
- Wring out the water and apply the cloth on the location. To seal in the warmth, cover the location with a thick towel for 15–30 minutes.

Bath

Adding essential oils to bath water is challenging because oil does not mix with water. For even dispersion, mix 5–10 drops of essential oil in 1/4 cup of Epsom salts or bath gel base and then put the cup under a running faucet and gradually add water. This method will help the oils disperse in the bath evenly and prevent stronger oils from stinging sensitive areas.

You can also use premixed bath gels and shampoos containing essential oils as a liquid soap in the shower or bath. Lather down with the bath gel, let it soak in, and then rinse. To maximize benefits, leave the soap or shampoo on the skin or scalp for several minutes to allow the essential oils to penetrate.

You can create your own aromatic bath gels by placing 5–15 drops of essential oil in 1/2 oz. of an unscented bath gel base and then add to the bath water as described above.

Shower

Essential oils can be added to Epsom salts and used in the shower. There are special shower heads containing an attached receptacle that can be filled with the essential oil/salts mixture. This allows essential oils to not only make contact with the skin but also diffuses the fragrance of the oils into the air. The shower head receptacle can hold approximately 1/4 to 1/2 cup of bath salts.

Start by adding 5–10 drops of essential oil to 1/4 cup of bath salt. Fill the shower head receptacle with the oil/salt mixture. Make sure neither oils nor salts come in contact with the plastic seal on top of the receptacle. This should provide enough salt material for about 2–3 showers. Some shower heads have a bypass feature that allows the user to switch from aromatic salt water to regular tap water.

How to Enhance the Benefits of Topical Application

The longer essential oils stay in contact with the skin, the more likely they are to be absorbed. The A·R·T Night Reconstructor or A·R·T Day Activator lotions, Sandalwood Moisture Cream, or Boswellia Wrinkle Cream may be layered on top of the essential oils to reduce evaporation of the oils and enhance penetration. This may also help seal and protect cuts and wounds.

Do not use ointments on burns until they are at least three days old; however, LavaDerm Cooling Mist spray may be used immediately to provide comforting relief for minor burns, abrasions, dryness, and other skin irritations.

Diffusing

Diffused oils alter the structure of molecules that create odors, rather than just masking them. They also increase oxygen availability, produce negative ions, and release natural ozone. Many essential oils such as Lemongrass, Orange, Grapefruit, Melaleuca Alternifolia—Tea Tree, Eucalyptus Globulus, Lavender, Frankincense, and Lemon, along with essential oil blends (Purification, Melrose, and Thieves), are extremely effective for eliminating and destroying airborne germs and bacteria.

A cold-air diffuser is designed to atomize a microfine mist of essential oils into the air, where they can remain suspended for several hours. Unlike aroma lamps or candles, a diffuser disperses essential oils without heating or burning, which can render the oil therapeutically less beneficial and even create toxic compounds. Research shows that cold-air diffusing certain oils may:

- Reduce bacteria, fungus, mold, and unpleasant odors
- Relax the body, relieve tension, and clear the mind
- Help with weight management
- Improve concentration, alertness, and mental clarity
- Stimulate neurotransmitters
- Stimulate secretion of endorphins
- Stimulate growth hormone production and receptivity
- Improve the secretion of IgA antibodies that fight candida
- Improve digestive function
- Improve hormonal balance
- Relieve headaches

Guidelines for Diffusing

- Check the viscosity or thickness of the oil you want to diffuse. If the oil has too much natural wax and is too thick, it could plug the diffuser and make cleaning difficult.
- Start by diffusing oils for 15–30 minutes a day. As you become accustomed to the oils and recognize their effects, you may increase the diffusing time to 1–2 hours per day.
- By connecting your diffuser to a timer, you can gain better control over the length and duration of diffusing. For some respiratory conditions, you may diffuse the oils the entire night.
- Do not use more than one blend at a time in a diffuser, as this may alter the smell and the

therapeutic benefit. However, a single oil may be added to a blend when diffusing.

- Place the diffuser high in the room so that the oil mist falls through the air and removes the odor-causing substances.
- If you want to wash the diffuser before using a different oil blend, use Thieves Household Cleaner with warm water or any natural soap and warm water.
- If you do not have a diffuser, you can add several drops of essential oil to a spray bottle with 1 cup purified water and shake. You can use this to mist your entire house, workplace, or car.
- Air Freshener Oil Recipe:
  - 20 drops Lavender
  - 10 drops Lemon
  - 6 drops Bergamot
  - 5 drops Lime
  - 5 drops Grapefruit

Diffuse neat or mix with 1 cup of distilled water in a spray bottle; shake well before spraying.

Other Ways to Diffuse Oils

- Add your favorite essential oils to cedar chips to make your own potpourri.
- Put scented cedar chips in your closets or drawers to deodorize them.
- Sprinkle a few drops of conifer essential oils such as Spruce, Fir (all varieties), Cedar, or Pine onto logs in the fireplace. As the logs burn, they will disperse an evergreen smell. This method has no therapeutic benefit, however.
- Put essential oils on cotton balls or tissues and place them in your car, home, work, or hotel heating or air conditioning vents.
- Put a few drops of oil in a bowl or pan of water and set it on a warm stove.
- On a damp cloth, sprinkle a few drops of one of your purifying essential oils and place the cloth near an intake duct of your heating and cooling system so that the air can carry the aroma throughout your home.

Humidifier and Vaporizer

Essential oils make ideal additions to humidifiers or vaporizers. Always check the viscosity of the oil, because if it is too thick, it could plug the humidifier or make it difficult to clean. The following singles and blends are great to diffuse.

Singles: Idaho Balsam Fir, Frankincense, Sacred Frankincense, Peppermint, Lemon, Eucalyptus Radiata, Melaleuca Alternifolia, Lavender, Ylang Ylang, and many others of your choice

Blends: Purification, Thieves, Raven, Melrose, Joy, RutaVaLa, The Gift, White Angelica, Sacred Mountain, and many others of your choice

---

NOTE: Test the oil before diffusing it in the vaporizer or humidifier; some essential oils may damage the plastic parts of vaporizers.

Other Uses
Direct Inhalation

- Place 2 or more drops into the palm of your left hand and rub clockwise with the flat palm of your right hand. Cup your hands together over your nose and mouth and inhale deeply. (Do not touch your eyes!)
- Add several drops of an essential oil to a bowl of hot (not boiling) water. Inhale the steaming vapors that rise from the bowl. To increase the intensity of the oil vapors inhaled, drape a towel over your head and the bowl before inhaling.
- Apply oils to a cotton ball or tissue (do not use synthetic fibers or fabric) and place it in the air vent of your car.
- Inhale directly.

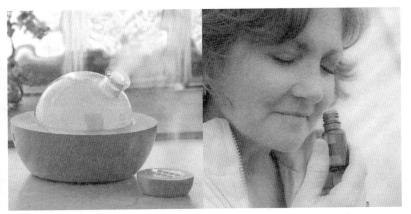

Cold-air diffuser   Direct inhalation

Indirect or Subtle Inhalation
(Wearing as a perfume or cologne)
*   Rub 2 or more drops of oil on your chest, neck, upper sternum, wrists, or under your nose and ears, and enjoy the fragrance throughout the day.
*   There are many necklaces with different types of vessels hanging on them into which you can pour a particular oil to use throughout the day.
*   There are clay-type medallions to hang around your neck or fasten with a clip on your clothing onto which you can put a few oil drops to give off a gentle fragrance the entire day.

Vaginal Retention
For systemic health problems such as Candida or vaginitis, vaginal retention is one of the best ways for the body to absorb essential oils.
*   Mix 20–30 drops of essential oil in 2 tablespoons of carrier oil.
*   Apply this mixture to a tampon (for internal infection) or sanitary pad (for external lesions). Insert the tampon and retain for 8 hours or overnight. Use tampons or sanitary pads made with organic cotton.

Rectal Retention
A retention enema is the most efficient way to deliver essential oils to the urinary tract and reproductive organs. Always use a sterile syringe.
*   Mix 15–20 drops of essential oil in a tablespoon of carrier oil.
*   Place the mixture in a small syringe and inject into the rectum.
*   Retain the mixture through the night (or longer for best results).
*   Clean and disinfect the applicator after each use.

ENDNOTES:
1. Bronaugh RL, et al. Extent of cutaneous metabolism during percutaneous absorption of xenobiotics. *Toxicol. Appl. Pharmacol.* 1989 Jul;99(3):534-43.

Chapter 4
Single Oils

Quality Assurance

This section describes over 80 single essential oils, including botanical information, therapeutic and traditional uses, chemical constituents of each oil, extraction method, cautions, and application instructions.

How to Be Sure Your Essential Oils Are Pure, Therapeutic Grade

How can you be sure that your essential oils are pure, therapeutic grade? Start by asking the following questions from your essential oil supplier:

- Are the fragrances delicate, rich, and organic? Do they "feel" natural? Do the aromas vary from batch to batch as an indication that they are painstakingly distilled in small batches rather than industrially processed on a large scale?
- Does your supplier subject each batch of essential oils through multiple chemical analyses to test for purity and therapeutic quality? Are these tests performed by independent labs?
- Does your supplier grow and distill organically grown herbs?
- Are the distillation facilities part of the farm where the herbs are grown (so oils are freshly distilled), or do herbs wait days to be processed and lose potency?
- Does your supplier use low pressure and low temperature to distill essential oils so as to preserve all of their fragile chemical constituents? Are the distillation cookers fabricated from costly, food-grade stainless steel alloys to reduce the likelihood of the oils chemically reacting with metal?
- Does your supplier personally inspect the fields and distilleries where the herbs are grown and distilled? Do they verify that no synthetic or harmful solvents or chemicals are being used?
- How many years has your supplier been doing all of this?

How to Maximize the Shelf Life of Your Essential Oils

The highest quality essential oils are bottled in dark glass. The reason for this is two-fold. First, glass is more stable than plastic and does not "breathe" the same way plastic does. Second, the darkness of the glass protects the oil from light that may chemically alter or degrade it over time.

After using an essential oil, keep the lid tightly sealed. Bottles that are improperly sealed can result in the loss of some of the lighter, lower-molecular-weight parts of the oil. In addition, over time oxygen in the air reacts with and oxidizes the oil.

Essential oils should be stored away from light, especially sunlight—even if they are already stored in amber glass bottles. The darker the storage conditions, the longer your oil will maintain its original chemistry and quality.

Single Essential Oil Application Codes

(Please see box at bottom page for explanation of codes)

Neat = Straight, undiluted
50-50 = Dilute 50-50

20-80 = Dilute 20-80
PH = Photosensitizing

Amazonian Ylang Ylang.. **50-50**	Clove............................. **20-80**	Geranium........................ **Neat**
Angelica .... **PH 50-50**	Copaiba/Copal .... **Neat**	German Chamomile **PH Neat**
Anise **50-50**	Coriander....................... **50-50**	Ginger............................. **50-50**
Basil **20-80**	Cumin............................. **20-80**	Goldenrod...................... **50-50**
Bergamot.............. **PH 50-50**	Cypress.......................... **50-50**	Grapefruit .... **PH 50-50**
Biblical Sweet Myrrh ...... **Neat**	Davana........................... **50-50**	Helichrysum .... **Neat**
Black Pepper.................. **50-50**	Dill **50-50**	Hinoki........................... **50-50**
Blue Cypress.................. **Neat**	Dorado Azul................... **50-50**	Hong Kuai **50-50**
Blue Tansy .... **Neat**	Douglas Fir **50-50**	Hyssop **50-50**
Calamus **50-50**	Elemi............................. **Neat**	Idaho Balsam Fir **50-50**
Canadian Fleabane **50-50**	Eucalyptus Blue **50-50**	Idaho Blue Spruce **50-50**
Cardamom **50-50**	Eucalyptus Citriodora **50-50**	Idaho Ponderosa Pine **50-50**
Carrot Seed **50-50**	Eucalyptus Dives............ **50-50**	Idaho Tansy................... **Neat**
Cassia **20-80**	Eucalyptus Globulus **50-50**	Ishpingo .... **Neat**
Cedarwood..................... **Neat**	Eucalyptus Polybractea ... **50-50**	Jasmine.......................... **Neat**
Celery Seed **50-50**	Eucalyptus Radiata......... **50-50**	Juniper **50-50**
Cinnamon Bark.............. **20-80**	Eucalyptus Staigeriana **50-50**	Laurus Nobilis............... **50-50**
Cistus .... **Neat**	Fennel **50-50**	Lavandin .... **Neat**
Citronella **50-50**	Frankincense .... **Neat**	Lavender .... **Neat**
Citrus Hystrix .... **PH 50-50**	Frereana Frankincense .... **Neat**	Ledum........................... **Neat**
Clary Sage **50-50**	Galbanum **50-50**	Lemon .... **PH 50-50**

Single Essential Oil Application Codes

Neat = Straight, undiluted
Dilution usually NOT required; suitable for all but the most sensitive skin. Safe for children over 2 years old.

50-50 = Dilute 50-50
Dilution recommended at 50-50 (1 part essential oils to 1 part V-6 Vegetable Oil Complex) for topical and internal use, especially when used on sensitive areas — face, neck, genital area, underarms, etc. Keep out of reach of children.

20-80 = Dilute 20-80
Always dilute 20-80 (1 part essential oils to 4 parts V-6 Vegetable Oil Complex) before applying to the skin or taking internally. Keep out of reach of children.

PH = Photosensitizing
Avoid using on skin exposed to direct sunlight or UV rays (i.e., sunlamps, tanning beds, etc.)

Single Essential Oil Application Codes *(continued)*

(Please see box on next page for explanation of codes)

Neat = Straight, undiluted
50-50 = Dilute 50-50

20-80 = Dilute 20-80
PH = Photosensitizing

Lemongrass **20-80**	Orange .... **PH 50-50**	Spruce **50-50**
Lemon Myrtle **20-80**	Oregano **20-80**	Tangerine .... **PH 50-50**
Lime .... **PH 50-50**	Palmarosa **50-50**	Tarragon.......................... **50-50**
Mandarin .... **PH 50-50**	Palo Santo **50-50**	Thyme............................. **20-80**
Manuka.......................... **Neat**	Patchouli .... **Neat**	Tsuga.............................. **50-50**
Marjoram **50-50**	Peppermint..................... **50-50**	Valerian .... **Neat**
Mastrante **50-50**	Petitgrain .... **Neat**	Vanilla .... **Neat**
Melaleuca Alternifolia **50-50**	Pine................................ **50-50**	Vetiver............................ **Neat**
Melaleuca Cajuput **50-50**	Plectranthus Oregano **50-50**	Vitex **50-50**
Melaleuca Ericifolia........ **50-50**	Ravintsara .... **Neat**	Western Red Cedar **50-50**
Melaleuca Quinquenervia **50-50**	Roman Chamomile........ **Neat**	White Fir **50-50**
Melissa .... **Neat**	Rose .... **Neat**	White Lotus **50-50**
Micromeria **50-50**	Rosemary **50-50**	Wintergreen **50-50**
Mountain Savory............ **20-80**	Rosewood....................... **Neat**	Xiang Mao **50-50**
Mugwort **50-50**	Ruta **50-50**	Yarrow............................ **Neat**
Myrrh............................. **Neat**	Sacred Frankincense .... **Neat**	Ylang Ylang.................... **50-50**
Myrtle **50-50**	Sage................................ **50-50**	Yuzu **50-50**
Neroli .... **Neat**	Sandalwood.................... **Neat**	
Nutmeg.......................... **50-50**	Spanish Sage.................. **50-50**	
Ocotea **50-50**	Spearmint....................... **50-50**	
	Spikenard .... **Neat**	

Store essential oils in a cool location. Excessive heat can derange the molecular structure of the oil the same way ultraviolet light can.

Diluting Essential Oils

Most essential oils require dilution with a vegetable oil when being used either internally or externally. The amount of dilution depends on the essential oil. For example, oregano will require four times as much dilution as that of Roman Chamomile. Vegetable oils such as V-6 Vegetable Oil Complex are specifically formulated to dilute essential oils and have a long shelf life (over two years) without going rancid. For more information on specific usage instructions for each essential oil, please see the "Personal Usage Guide."

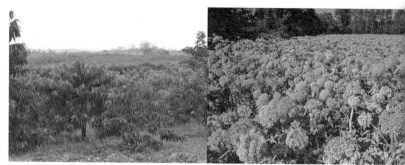

Amazonian Ylang Ylang

Angelica

Single Oils

Amazonian Ylang Ylang
(Cananga odorata Equitoriana)
Botanical Family: Annonaceae
Plant Origin: Ecuador
Extraction Method: Steam distilled from flowers
Key Constituents:
Benzyl Acetate (15-29%)
Germacrene D (10-20%)
Linalool (10-25%)
Benzyl Benzoate (4-12%)
p-Cresyl Methyl Ether (2-10%)
Historical Data: The flowering ylang ylang tree is found in the Philippines, Indonesia, and Madagascar. Gary Young translocated trees to the Young Living Ecuador Farm, where the aromatic flowers bloom every day.
Uses: While renowned for its calming effect, several studies show it brings relief for the depressed and stressed while it increases attentiveness and alertness, causing researchers to say it is "harmonizing."
Fragrant Influence: Balances male-female energies, enhances spiritual attunement, combats anger and low self-esteem, increases focus of thoughts, filters out negative energy, restores confidence and peace
Application: Dilute 1 part essential oil with 1 part V-6 Vegetable Oil Complex or other pure vegetable oil; (1) apply 2-4 drops on location, (2) apply on chakras and/or Vita Flex points, (3) inhale directly, (4) diffuse.
Found In: Oola Balance

Angelica *(Angelica archangelica)*
Botanical Family: Apiaceae
Plant Origin: Belgium, France
Extraction Method: Steam distilled from seed/root
Key Constituents:
Beta-Phellandrene (60-80%)
Limonene (1-4%)
Alpha-Pinene (5-10%)
Historical Data: Known as the "holy spirit root" or the "oil of angels" by the Europeans, angelica's healing powers were so strong that it was believed to be of divine origin. From the time of Paracelsus, it was credited with the ability to protect from the plague. The stems were chewed during the plague of 1660 to prevent infection. When burned, the seeds and roots were thought to purify the air.
Medical Properties: Anticoagulant, relaxant, antispasmodic

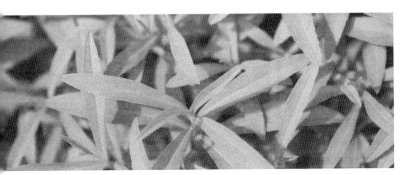
Anise

Uses: Throat/lung infections, indigestion, menstrual problems/PMS, symptoms of dementia

Fragrant Influence: Assists in the release of pent-up negative feelings and restores memories to the point of origin before trauma or anger was experienced

Application: Dilute 1 part essential oil with 1 part V-6 Vegetable Oil Complex or other pure vegetable oil; (1) apply 1-2 drops on location, (2) apply on chakras and/or Vita Flex points, (3) inhale directly, (4) diffuse up to 30 minutes 3 times daily or as needed, (5) dilute as above, put in a capsule, and take up to 3 times daily or as needed as a dietary supplement.
Avoid applying to skin that will be exposed to direct sunlight or UV light within 24 hours.

Found In: Awaken, Forgiveness, Grounding, Harmony, Live with Passion, Oola Balance, Surrender

Anise (Pimpinella anisum)
  Botanical Family: Apiaceae
  Plant Origin: Turkey
  Extraction Method: Steam distilled from the seeds (fruit)

Key Constituents:
  Trans-Anethole (85-95%)
  Methyl Chavicol (2-4%)
ORAC: 333,700 µTE/100g
History: Listed in Dioscorides' *De Materia Medica* (AD 78), Europe's first authoritative guide to medicines, which became the standard reference work for herbal treatments for over 1,700 years.
Medical Properties: Digestive stimulant, anticoagulant, anesthetic/analgesic, antioxidant, diuretic, antitumoral, anti-inflammatory
Uses: Arthritis/rheumatism, cancer
Application: Dilute 1 part essential oil with 1 part V-6 Vegetable Oil Complex or other pure vegetable oil, put in a capsule, and take up to 3 times daily or as needed; (1) dilute 1 part essential oil with 1 part V-6 Vegetable Oil Complex or other pure vegetable oil, then apply on location, (2) apply on chakras and/or Vita Flex points, (3) inhale directly, (4) diffuse up to 30 minutes 3 times daily, or (5) take as a dietary supplement.
Fragrant Influence: Opens emotional blocks and recharges vital energy
Found In: Awaken, ComforTone, Detoxzyme, Digest & Cleanse, DiGize, Dream Catcher,

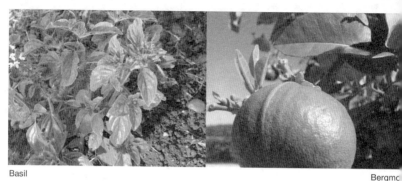

Basil

Bergmc

Essentialzyme, Essentiazymes-4, ICP, JuvaPower, JuvaSpice, ParaFree, Power Meal

Basil *(Ocimum basilicum)*
Botanical Family: Lamiaceae
  Plant Origin: India, Utah, France
  Extraction Method: Steam distilled from leaves, stems, and flowers
  Key Constituents:
    Methylchavicol (estragol) (70-90%)
    Linalol (1-20%)
    1,8-Cineole (Eucalyptol) (1-7%)
  ORAC: 54,000 µTE/100g
  Historical Data: Used extensively in traditional Asian Indian medicine, basil's name is derived from "basileum," the Greek name for king. In the 16th century, the powdered leaves were inhaled to treat migraines and chest infections. The Hindu people put basil sprigs on the chests of the dead to protect them from evil spirits. Italian women wore basil to attract possible suitors. It was listed in Hildegard's Medicine, a compilation of early German medicines by highly regarded Benedictine herbalist Hildegard of Bingen (1098-1179).
  Medical Properties: Powerful antispasmodic, antiviral, antibacterial, anti-inflammatory, muscle relaxant
  Uses: Migraines, throat/lung infections, insect bites
  Fragrant Influence: Fights mental fatigue
  Application: Dilute 1 part essential oil with 4 parts V-6 Vegetable Oil Complex or other pure vegetable oil; (1) apply 2-4 drops on location, temples, neck, (2) apply on chakras and/or Vita Flex points (crown of head, forehead, heart, and navel) or around ear for earache, (3) inhale directly, (4) diffuse, or (5) take as a dietary supplement.
  Cautions: Avoid use if epileptic. Do not pour oil into the ear.
  Found In: Aroma Siez, Clarity, M-Grain

Bergamot *(Citrus aurantium bergamia)*
(also found in literature as *Citrus bergamia*)
  Botanical Family: Rutaceae
  Plant Origin: Italy, Morocco
  Extraction Method: Cold pressed from the rind; also produced by vacuum distillation Furocoumarin-free bergamot oil is specially distilled to minimize the concentration of sun-sensitizing compounds in the oil.
  Key Constituents:
    Limonene (30-45%)
    Linalyl Acetate (22-36%)

Linalol (3-15%)
Gamma-Terpinene (6-10%)
Beta-Pinene (5.5-9.5%)

Historical Data: Christopher Columbus is believed to have brought bergamot to Bergamo in Northern Italy from the Canary Islands. A mainstay in traditional Italian medicine, bergamot has been used in the Middle East for hundreds of years for skin conditions associated with an oily complexion. Bergamot is responsible for the distinctive flavor of the renowned Earl Grey Tea and was used in the first genuine eau de cologne.

Medical Properties: Calming, hormonal support, antibacterial, antidepressant

Uses: Agitation, depression, anxiety, intestinal parasites, insomnia, viral infections (herpes, cold sores)

Fragrant Influence: Relieves anxiety; mood-lifting qualities

Application: Dilute 1 part essential oil with 1 part V-6 Vegetable Oil Complex or other pure vegetable oil; (1) apply 1-2 drops on location, (2) apply on chakras and/or Vita Flex points, (3) inhale directly, (4) diffuse, or (5) take as a dietary supplement.

Caution: Avoid applying to skin that will be exposed to sunlight or UV light within 36 hours.

Found In: A·R·T Renewal Serum, Acceptance, Animal Scents Ointment, AromaGuard Meadow Mist Deodorant, Awaken, Believe, Clarity, Dragon Time Bath & Shower Gel, Dream Catcher, Evening Peace Bath & Shower Gel, Forgiveness, Genesis Hand & Body Lotion, Gentle Baby, Gratitude, Harmony, Humility, Inspiration, Joy, KidScents Lotion, Lady Sclareol, Lavender Conditioner, Lavender-Rosewood Moisturizing Soap, Magnify Your Purpose, Oola Balance, Oola Grow, Phyto Plus, Prenolone Plus Body Cream, Progessence Phyto Plus, Progessence Plus, Relaxation Massage Oil, Rose Ointment, Sandalwood Moisture Cream, Sensation, Sensation Bath & Shower Gel, Sensation Hand & Body Lotion, Sensation Massage Oil, White Angelica, Wolfberry Eye Cream

Biblical Sweet Myrrh
(Commiphora erythraea)

Botanical Family: Burseraceae

Plant Origin: Socotra Island, Yemen

Extraction Method: Steam distilled from resin

Key Constituents:
Trans-Beta-Ocimene (45-65%)
Cis-Alpha-Bisabolene (10-15%)
Alpha-Santalene (12-20%)
Trans-Alpha-Bergamotene (3-8%)
Cis-Alpha-Bergamotene (1-4%)

Historical Data: A close cousin to the more well-known *Commiphora myrrha*, Biblical Sweet Myrrh is also called Opoponax. Used in dozens of perfumes to impart sweet balsamic notes, this myrrh species is found in Chanel's Coco Mademoiselle and Dior's Poison. Like other frankincense species, it is highly anti-inflammatory, an antioxidant, and antimicrobial.

Medical Properties: Analgesic, antioxidant, anti-inflammatory, antimicrobial, antifungal, antiviral

Uses: Arthritis, digestive problems, nerve/muscle pain, fungal infections

Fragrant Influence: Promotes spiritual awareness and is uplifting. It contains sesquiterpenes, which stimulate the limbic system of the brain (the center of memory and emotions) and the hypothalamus, pineal, and pituitary glands. The hypothalamus is the master gland of the human body, producing many vital hormones, including thyroid and growth hormone.

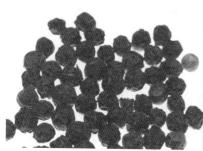
Black Pepper

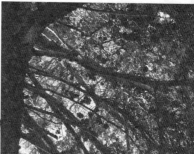
Blue Cypress

Application: (1) Apply 2-4 drops on location, (2) apply on chakras and/or Vita Flex points, (3) inhale directly, (4) diffuse.

Black Pepper *(Piper nigrum)*
Botanical Family: Piperaceae
Plant Origin: Madagascar, Sri Lanka, England, India
Extraction Method: Steam distilled from fruit/berries
Key Constituents:
Beta-Caryophyllene (12-29%)
Limonene (10-17%)
Sabinene (6-15%)
Delta-3-Carene (3-15%)
Alpha-Pinene (3-12%)
Beta-Pinene (5-12%)
ORAC: 79,700 µTE/100g
Historical Data: Used by the Egyptians in mummification, as evidenced by the discovery of black pepper in the nostrils and abdomen of Ramses II. Indian monks ate several black peppercorns a day to give them endurance during their arduous travels. In ancient times pepper was as valuable as gold or silver. When the barbarian Goth tribes of Europe vanquished Rome in 410 AD, they demanded 3,000 pounds of pepper as well as other valuables as a ransom. Traditional Chinese healers used pepper to treat cholera, malaria, and digestive problems.
Medical Properties: Analgesic, stimulates metabolism, antifungal
Uses: Obesity, arthritis, digestive problems, fatigue, nerve/muscle pain, fungal infections, tobacco cessation
Fragrant Influence: Stimulating, energizing, and empowering. A 2002 study found that fragrance inhalation of pepper oil induced a 1.7-fold increase in plasma adrenaline concentration (Haze, et al.).
Application: Dilute 1 part essential oil with 1 part V-6 Vegetable Oil Complex or other pure vegetable oil; (1) apply 2-4 drops on location, (2) apply on chakras and/or Vita Flex points, (3) inhale directly, (4) diffuse, or (5) take as a dietary supplement.
Found In: Awaken, Cel-Lite Magic Massage Oil, Dream Catcher, En-R-Gee, NingXia Nitro, Relieve It

Blue Cypress *(Callitris intratropica)*
Botanical Family: Cupressaceae
Plant Origin: Australia
Extraction Method: Steam distillation from the leaves and wood of the tree

Key Constituents:
  Gamma-Eudesmol (5-12%)
  Guaiol (10-20%)
  Bulnesol (5-11%)
  Dihydrocolumellarin (10-25%)
ORAC: 73,100 µTE/100g
Historical Data: Blue cypress in ancient times was used for incense, perfume, and embalming.
Medical Properties: Anti-inflammatory, antiviral
Uses: Viral infections (herpes simplex, herpes zoster, cold sores, human papilloma virus, etc.)
Application: (1) Apply 2-4 drops on location, dilution not required except for the most sensitive skin, (2) apply on chakras and/or Vita Flex points, (3) inhale directly, or (4) diffuse up to 1 hour 3 times daily.
Found In: Australian Blue, Brain Power, Breathe Again Roll-On, Essential Beauty Serum (Dry Skin), Highest Potential, Oola Grow

Blue Tansy (Tanacetum annuum)
  Botanical Family: Asteraceae or Compositae (daisy)
  Plant Origin: Morocco
  Extraction Method: Steam distilled from flowering plant
  Key Constituents:
    Camphor (10-17%)
    Sabinene (10-17%)
    Beta-Pinene (5-10%)
    Myrcene (7-13%)
    Alpha-Phellandrene (5-10%)
    Para-Cymene (3-8%)
    Chamazulene (3-6%)
  ORAC: 68,800 µTE/100g
  Medical Properties: Anti-inflammatory, analgesic/anesthetic, antifungal, anti-itching, relaxant, hormone-like
  Application: (1) Apply 2-4 drops on location, (2) apply on chakras and/or Vita Flex

points, (3) inhale directly, (4) diffuse up to 1 hour three times daily.
Found In: Acceptance, Australian Blue, Awaken, Dragon Time Bath & Shower Gel, Dream Catcher, Evening Peace Bath & Shower Gel, Highest Potential, JuvaFlex, JuvaTone, KidScents Shampoo, KidScents Tender Tush, Oola Grow, Peace & Calming, Release, SARA, Valor, Valor Moisturizing Soap, Valor Roll-On

Calamus (Acorus calamus)
  Botanical Family: Acoraceae
  Plant Origin: India, Nepal, Brazil
  Extraction Method: Steam extracted from roots
  Key Constituents:
    Cis-Methyl Isoeugenol (13-21%)
    Syobunone (7-16%)
    Acorenone (5-15%)
    Calamuscenone (5-11%)
  Historical Data: Commonly known as sweet flag, this plant may have been the biblical calamus of Exodus 30:23 used in the holy anointing oil. It seems to have originated in India or Arabia but now is found in many places throughout the world. Native Americans used calamus as a medicine and a stimulant, but low doses are also believed to be calming and to induce sleep. The Penobscot people have a tradition that it saved their people from a serious illness.
  Medical Properties: Antibacterial, sedative, carminative, expectorant, antispasmodic, bronchodilator, hepatoprotective
  Uses: Relaxes spasms, lung infections, agitation
  Fragrant Influence: Believed to induce and promote positive thoughts
  Application: Inhale directly, diffuse.
  Caution: Use only oil from the diploid species that does not contain β-asarone.
  Found In: Exodus II

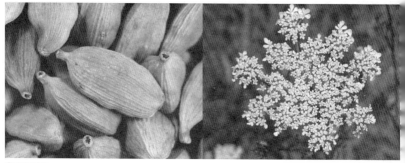

Cardamom

Carrot Seed

Canadian Fleabane *(Conyza canadensis)*
  Botanical Family: Compositae
  Plant Origin: Canada
  Extraction Method: Steam distilled from stems, leaves, and flowers (aerial parts)
  Key Constituents:
    Limonene (60-80%)
    Trans-Alpha-Bergamotene (1-10%)
    Trans-Beta-Ocimene (2-6%)
    Gamma-Curcumene (1-8%)
  ORAC: 26,700 µTE/100g
  Medical Properties: Stimulates liver and pancreas, antiaging (stimulates growth hormone), antirheumatic, antispasmodic, vasodilating, reduces blood pressure, antifungal, antimicrobial
  Uses: Hypertension, hepatitis, accelerated aging
  Application: Dilute 1 part essential oil with 1 part V-6 Vegetable Oil Complex or other pure vegetable oil; (1) apply 2-4 drops on location, (2) apply on chakras and/or Vita Flex points, (3) inhale directly, (4) diffuse, or (5) take as a dietary supplement.
  Found In: CortiStop Women's, EndoGize, Ultra Young Plus

Cardamom *(Elettaria cardamomum)*
  Botanical Family: Zingiberaceae
  Plant Origin: Guatemala, Sri Lanka
  Extraction Method: Steam distilled from seeds
  Key Constituents:
    Alpha-Terpinyl Acetate (45-55%)
    1,8-Cineole (Eucalyptol) (16-36%)
    Linalol (4-7%)
    Linalyl Acetate (3-7%)
  ORAC: 36,500 µTE/100g
  Historical Data: Called "Grains of Paradise" since the Middle Ages, it has been used medicinally by Indian healers for millennia. One of the most prized spices in ancient Greece and Rome, cardamom was cultivated by the king of Babylon around the 7th century BC. It is mentioned in one of the oldest known medical records, the Ebers Papyrus (dating from 16th century BC), an ancient Egyptian list of 877 prescriptions and recipes.
  Medical Properties: Antispasmodic (neuromuscular), expectorant, antiparasitic (worms), antioxidant, antimicrobial
  Uses: Lung/sinus infection, indigestion, senility, headaches

Fragrant Influence: Uplifting, refreshing, and invigorating

Application: (1) Dilute 1 part essential oil with 1 part V-6 Vegetable Oil Complex or other pure vegetable oil, then apply on location, stomach, solar plexus, or thighs; (2) apply on chakras and/or Vita Flex points; (3) inhale directly, (4) diffuse up to 30 minutes 3 times daily, or (5) dilute 1 part essential oil with 1 part V-6 Vegetable Oil Complex or other pure vegetable oil, put 4 drops in a capsule, and take up to 3 times daily as a dietary supplement.

Found In: Clarity, Transformation

Carrot Seed (*Daucus carota*)

Botanical Family: Apiaceae

Plant Origin: France

Extraction Method: Steam distilled from dried seeds

Key Constituents:
Carotol (30-40%)
Alpha-Pinene (12-16%)
Trans-Beta-Caryophyllene (6-10%)
Caryophyllene Oxide (3-5%)

Historical Data: Traditionally used for kidney and digestive disorders and to relieve liver congestion

Medical Properties: Antiparasitic, antiseptic, purgative, diuretic, vasodilatory, antifungal

Uses: Skin conditions (eczema, oily skin, psoriasis, wrinkles), water retention, liver problems

Application: Dilute 1 part essential oil with 1 part V-6 Vegetable Oil Complex or other pure vegetable oil; (1) apply 1-2 drops on location, (2) apply on chakras and/or Vita Flex points, or (3) take as a dietary supplement.

Found In: Animal Scents Ointment, Rose Ointment

Cassia (*Cinnamomum cassia*)

Botanical Family: Lauraceae

Plant Origin: China

Extraction Method: Steam distilled from branches, leaves, and petioles

Note: While its aroma is similar to cinnamon, cassia is chemically and physically quite different.

Key Constituents:
Trans-Cinnamaldehyde (70-88%)
Trans-O-Methoxycinnamaldehyde (3-15%)
Coumarin (1.5-4%)
Cinnamyl Acetate (0-6%)

ORAC: 15,170 µTE/100g

Historical Data: Cassia is rich in biblical history and is mentioned in one of the oldest known medical records, the Ebers Papyrus (dating from 16th century BC), an ancient Egyptian list of 877 prescriptions and recipes.

Medical Properties: Anti-inflammatory (COX-2 inhibitor), antifungal, antibacterial, antiviral, anticoagulant

Uses: Cataracts, fungal infections (ringworm, Candida), atherosclerosis, anxiolytic, diabetes, arteriosclerosis

Application: Dilute 1 part essential oil with 4 parts V-6 Vegetable Oil Complex or other pure vegetable oil; (1) apply 1-2 drops on location, (2) apply on chakras and/or Vita Flex points, (3) diffuse, or (4) take as a dietary supplement.

Caution: May irritate the nasal membranes if inhaled directly from diffuser or bottle

Found In: Exodus II, EndoGize

Bible References:
Exodus 30:23,24,25—"Take thou also unto thee principal spices, of pure myrrh five hundred shekels, and of sweet cinnamon half so much, even two hundred and fifty shekels, and of sweet calamus two hundred and fifty shekels, And of cassia five hundred shekels, after the shekel of the sanctuary,

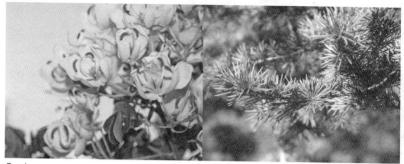
Cassia

Cedarwood

and of oil olive an hin: And thou shalt make
it an oil of holy ointment, an ointment
compound after the art of the apothecary: it
shall be an holy anointing oil."
Psalm 45:8—"All thy garments smell of
myrrh, and aloes, and cassia, out of the ivory
palaces, whereby they have made thee glad."

Cedarwood (*Cedrus atlantica*)

Botanical Family: Pinaceae

Plant Origin: Morocco, USA; *Cedrus atlantica*
is the species most closely related to the
biblical Cedars of Lebanon

Extraction Method: Steam distilled from bark

Key Constituents:
Alpha-Himachalene (10-20%)
Beta-Himachalene (35-55%)
Gamma-Himachalene (8-15%)
Delta-Cadinene (2-6%)

ORAC: 169,000 µTE/100g

Historical Data: Throughout antiquity,
cedarwood has been used in medicines. The
Egyptians used it for embalming the dead. It
was used as both a traditional medicine and
incense in Tibet.

Medical Properties: Combats hair loss
(alopecia areata), antibacterial, lymphatic
stimulant

Uses: Hair loss, arteriosclerosis, ADHD, skin
problems (acne, eczema)

Fragrant Influence: Stimulates the limbic
region of the brain (the center of emotions),
stimulates the pineal gland, which releases
melatonin. Terry Friedmann, MD, found
in clinical tests that this oil may treat ADD
and ADHD (attention deficit disorders) in
children. It is recognized for its calming,
purifying properties.

Application: (1) Apply on location, (2) apply
on chakras and/or Vita Flex points, (3)
inhale directly, (4) diffuse, or (5) take as a
dietary supplement.

Found In: A·R·T Beauty Masque, Australian
Blue, Brain Power, Cel-Lite Magic Massage
Oil, Egyptian Gold, Essential Beauty Serum
(Acne-Prone Skin), Essential Beauty Serum
(Dry Skin), Grounding, Highest Potential,
Inspiration, Into the Future, KidScents Bath
Gel, KidScents Lotion, Live with Passion,
Oola Grow, Peppermint-Cedarwood
Moisturizing Soap, Progessence Plus,
Progessence Phyto Plus, Sacred Mountain,
Sacred Mountain Moisturizing Soap, SARA,
Stress Away, Stress Away Roll-On, Tranquil
Roll-On

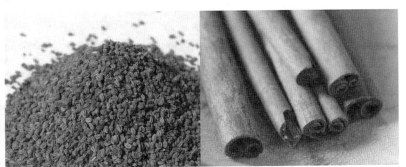

Celery Seed

Cinnamon Bark

Bible References:

Leviticus 14:4—"Then shall the priest command to take for him that is to be cleansed two birds alive and clean, and cedar wood, and scarlet, and hyssop."

Leviticus 14:6—"As for the living bird, he shall take it, and the cedar wood, and the scarlet, and the hyssop, and shall dip them and the living bird in the blood of the bird [that was] killed over the running water."

Leviticus 14:49—"And he shall take to cleanse the house two birds, and cedar wood, and scarlet, and hyssop."

Celery Seed (Apium graveolens)

Botanical Family: Apiaceae

Plant Origin: Europe

Extraction Method: Steam distilled from dried seeds

Key Constituents:

Limonene (60-75%)

Alpha and Beta Selinene (14-20%)

Sednenolide (4-7%)

ORAC: 30,300 µTE/100g

Historical Data: Long recognized as helpful in digestion, liver cleansing, and urinary tract support. It is also said to increase milk flow in nursing mothers.

Medical Properties: Antibacterial, antioxidant, antirheumatic, digestive aid, diuretic, liver protectant

Uses: Arthritis/rheumatism, digestive problems, liver problems/hepatitis

Application: (1) Dilute 1 part essential oil with 2 parts V-6 Vegetable Oil Complex or other pure vegetable oil and apply 1-2 drops on location, (2) apply on chakras and or Vita Flex points, (3) diffuse up to 1 hour 3 times daily, (4) inhale directly, or (5) dilute 2 drops with V-6 Vegetable Oil Complex or other pure vegetable oil, put in a capsule, and take up to 3 times daily.

Found In: GLF, JuvaCleanse

Cinnamon Bark (Cinnamomum zeylanicum) (Syn. C. verum)

Botanical Family: Lauraceae

Plant Origin: Sri Lanka, Madagascar, Ceylon

Extraction Method: Steam distilled from bark

Key Constituents:

Trans-Cinnamaldehyde (50-75%)

Eugenol (4-7%)

Beta-Caryophyllene (3-8%)

Linalol (3-9%)

ORAC: 10,340 µTE/100g

History: Listed in Dioscorides' *De Materia Medica* (AD 78), Europe's first authoritative

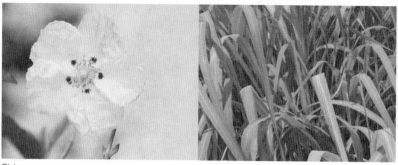

Cistus

CItronella

guide to medicines, which became the standard reference work for herbal treatments for over 1,700 years.

Medical Properties: Anti-inflammatory (COX-2 inhibitor), powerfully antibacterial, antiviral, antifungal, anticoagulant, circulatory stimulant, stomach protectant (ulcers), antiparasitic (worms)

Uses: Cardiovascular disease, infectious diseases, viral infections (herpes, etc.), digestive complaints, ulcers, and warts

Fragrant Influence: Thought to attract wealth

Application: Dilute 1 part essential oil with 4 parts V-6 Vegetable Oil Complex or other pure vegetable oil; (1) apply 1-2 drops on location, (2) apply on chakras and/or Vita Flex points, (3) diffuse, or (4) take as a dietary supplement.

Caution: May irritate the nasal membranes if inhaled directly from diffuser or bottle

Found In: Abundance, Christmas Spirit, Cinnamint Lip Balm, Egyptian Gold, Exodus II, Gathering, Highest Potential, Inner Defense, KidScents Slique Toothpaste, Magnify Your Purpose, Mineral Essence, Oola Grow, Slique Bars, Thieves, Thieves AromaBright Toothpaste, Thieves Cleansing Soap, Thieves Dental Floss, Thieves Dentarome Plus Toothpaste, Thieves Dentarome Ultra Toothpaste, Thieves Foaming Hand Soap, Thieves Fresh Essence Plus Mouthwash, Thieves Household Cleaner, Thieves Lozenges (Hard, Soft), Thieves Spray, Thieves Waterless Hand Purifier, Thieves Wipes

Bible References:

Exodus 30:23—"Take thou also unto thee principal spices, of pure myrrh five hundred shekels, and of sweet cinnamon half so much, even two hundred and fifty shekels, and of sweet calamus two hundred and fifty shekels..."

Proverbs 7:17—"I have perfumed my bed with myrrh, aloes, and cinnamon."

The Song of Solomon 4:14—"Spikenard and saffron; calamus and cinnamon, with all trees of frankincense; myrrh and aloes, with all the chief spices:"

Cistus *(Cistus ladanifer)*
(also known as *Labdanum*)

Botanical Family: Cistaceae

Plant Origin: Spain

Extraction Method: Steam distilled from leaves and branches

Key Constituents:
Alpha-Pinene (40-60%)

Camphene (2-5%)
Bornyl Acetate (3-6%)
Trans-Pinocarveol (3-6%)
ORAC: 3,860 µTE/100g
Historical Data: Cistus is also known as "rock rose" and has been studied for its effects on the regeneration of cells.
Medical Properties: Antiviral, antibacterial, antihemorrhagic, anti-inflammatory, supports sympathetic nervous system, immune stimulant
Uses: Hemorrhages, arthritis
Fragrant Influence: Calming to the nerves, elevates the emotions
Application: (1) Apply 2-4 drops on location, (2) apply on chakras and/or Vita Flex points, (3) inhale directly, (4) diffuse, or (5) take 4 drops as dietary supplement.
Found In: ImmuPower, KidScents Tender Tush, Oola Balance, The Gift

Citronella (Cymbopogon nardus)
Botanical Family: Poaceae
Plant Origin: Sri Lanka
Extraction Method: Steam distilled from aerial parts and leaves
Key Constituents:
Geraniol (18-30%)
Limonene (5-10%)
Trans-Methyl Isoeugenol (4-10%)
Geranyl Acetate (5-10%)
Borneol (3-8%)
ORAC: 312,000 µTE/100g
Historical Data: Used by various cultures to treat intestinal parasites, menstrual problems, and as a stimulant. Historically used to sanitize and deodorize surfaces. Enhanced insect repelling properties when combined with cedarwood.
Medical Properties: Powerful antioxidant, antibacterial, antifungal, insect repellent, anti-inflammatory, antispasmodic, antiparasitic (worms), relaxant
Uses: Respiratory infections, muscle/nerve pain, digestive/intestinal problems, anxiety, skin problems (acne, eczema, oily skin), skin-penetration enhancer
Fragrant Influence: Refreshing and uplifting
Application: (1) Dilute 1 part essential oil with 1 part V-6 Vegetable Oil Complex or other pure vegetable oil, then apply on location, (2) apply on chakras and/or Vita Flex points, (3) inhale directly, (4) diffuse up to 30 minutes 3 times daily, or dilute 1 part essential oil with 1 part V-6 Vegetable Oil Complex or other pure vegetable oil, put in a capsule, and take up to 3 times daily or as needed as a dietary supplement.
Found In: Animal Scents Shampoo, Purification

Citrus Hystrix/Combava (Citrus hystrix)
(also known as Kaffir lime)
Botanical Family: Rutaceae
Plant Origin: Indochina, Malaysia
Extraction Method: Steam distilled from leaves
Key Constituents:
Citronnellal (65-80%)
Linalol (3-6%)
Citronnellol (2-5%)
Isopulegol (2-4%)
ORAC: 69,200 µTE/100g
Historical Data: Used as a flavorant and as a nausea, fainting, and headache treatment. Also used for stomach aches and dyspepsia.
Medical Properties: Anti-inflammatory, antimicrobial, antidepressant, relaxant, antitumoral, antioxidant, rich in citronellal, which possesses calmative properties
Uses: Stress, anxiety, trauma
Application: (1) Dilute 1 part essential oil with 1 part V-6 Vegetable Oil Complex or other pure vegetable oil, then apply on

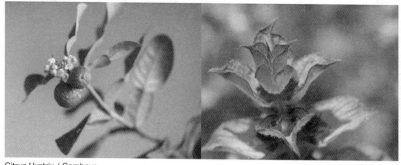

Citrus Hystrix / Combava

Clary Sage

location, (2) apply on chakras and/or Vita Flex points, (3) inhale directly, (4) diffuse up to 30 minutes 3 times daily, or (5) take as a dietary supplement.
Found In: Trauma Life

Clary Sage *(Salvia sclarea)*
Botanical Family: Lamiaceae
Plant Origin: Utah, France
Extraction Method: Steam distilled from flowering plant
Key Constituents:
Linalyl Acetate (56-78%)
Linalol (7-24%)
Germacrene D (2-12%)
Sclareol (.4-3%)
ORAC: 221,000 µTE/100g
Historical Data: Clary sage seeds were historically used by soaking the seeds and using the mucilage as an eye-wash and to draw thorns or splinters from the skin. It was also used to treat skin infections, soothe and calm the skin, acne, digestive disorders, and women's ailments. Aromatically, clary sage was used to enhance the immune system, calm digestive disorders, reduce inflammation such as eczema, calm muscle spasms, and for respiratory conditions.

Medical Properties: Anticoagulant, antioxidant, antidiabetic, estrogen-like, antifungal, antispasmodic, relaxant, cholesterol-reducing, antitumoral, anesthetic
Uses: Leukemia, menstrual discomforts/PMS, hormonal imbalance, insomnia, circulatory problems, high cholesterol, insect repellant
Fragrant Influence: Enhances one's ability to dream and is very calming and stress relieving
Application: Dilute 1 part essential oil with 1 part V-6 Vegetable Oil Complex or other pure vegetable oil; (1) apply on location, feet, ankles, wrists, (2) apply on chakras and/or Vita Flex points, (3) inhale directly, (4) diffuse, (5) take as a dietary supplement, or (6) rub 6-8 drops on lower back during PMS.
Found In: Cel-Lite Magic Massage Oil, CortiStop Women's, Dragon Time, Dragon Time Bath & Shower Gel, Dragon Time Massage Oil, EndoGize, Estro, Evening Peace Bath & Shower Gel, FemiGen, Into the Future, Lady Sclareol, Lavender Conditioner, Lavender Shampoo, Live with Passion, Oola Grow, Prenolone Plus Body Cream, SclarEssence, Transformation

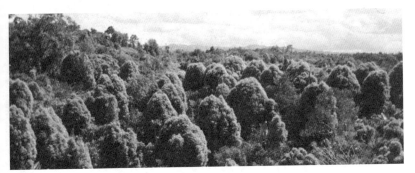
Clove

Clove *(Syzygium aromaticum)*
  Botanical Family: Myrtaceae
  Plant Origin: Madagascar, Spice Islands
  Extraction Method: Steam distilled from
    flower bud and stem
  Key Constituents:
    Eugenol (75-87%)
    Eugenol Acetate (8-15%)
    Beta-Carophyllene (2-7%)
  ORAC: 1,078,700 µTE/100g
  Historical Data: The people on the island of
    Ternate were free from epidemics until the
    16th century, when Dutch conquerors
    destroyed the clove trees that flourished on
    the islands. Many of the islanders died from
    the epidemics that followed.
    Cloves were reputed to be part of the
    "Marseilles Vinegar" or "Four Thieves
    Vinegar" that bandits who robbed the dead
    and dying used to protect themselves during
    the 15th century plague.
    Clove was listed in Hildegard's *Medicine,*
    a compilation of early German medicines
    by highly regarded Benedictine herbalist
    Hildegard of Bingen (1098-1179).
    Healers in China and India have used clove
    buds since ancient times as part of their
    treatments.

Eugenol, clove's principal constituent, was
used in the dental industry for years to
numb gums.
  Medical Properties: Antiaging, antitumoral,
    antimicrobial, antifungal, antiviral,
    analgesic/anesthetic, antioxidant,
    anticoagulant, anti-inflammatory, stomach
    protectant (ulcers), antiparasitic (worms),
    anticonvulsant, bone preserving
  Uses: Antiaging, cardiovascular disease,
    diabetes, arthritis/rheumatism, hepatitis,
    intestinal parasites/infections, for numbing
    all types of pain, throat/sinus/lung
    infections, cataracts, ulcers, lice, toothache,
    acne
  Fragrant Influence: A mental stimulant;
    encourages sleep, stimulates dreams, and
    creates a sense of protection and courage
  Application: Dilute 1 part essential oil with 4
    parts V-6 Vegetable Oil Complex or other
    pure vegetable oil; (1) apply 2-4 drops
    on location, gums, or mouth; (2) apply
    on chakras and/or Vita Flex points; (3)
    diffuse; or (4) take as a dietary supplement.
    For tickling cough, put a drop on back of
    tongue.
  Caution: Anticoagulant properties can be
    enhanced when combined with Warfarin,
    aspirin, etc.

57

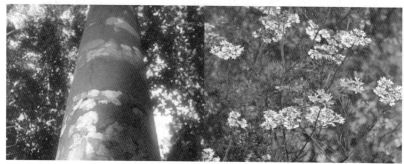

Copaiba

Coriander

Found In: Abundance, AromaGuard Meadow Mist Deodorant, AromaGuard Mountain Mint Deodorant, BLM, Deep Relief Roll-On, En-R-Gee, Essential Beauty Serum (Dry Skin), Essentialzyme, Essentialzymes-4, ImmuPower, Inner Defense, K&B, KidScents Slique Toothpaste, Longevity, Longevity Softgels, Melrose, OmegaGize³, PanAway, ParaFree, Progessence Phyto Plus, Progessence Plus, Thieves, Thieves AromaBright Toothpaste, Thieves Cleansing Soap, Thieves Dental Floss, Thieves Dentarome Plus Toothpaste, Thieves Dentarome Ultra Toothpaste, Thieves Foaming Hand Soap, Thieves Fresh Essence Plus Mouthwash, Thieves Household Cleaner, Thieves Lozenges (Hard, Soft), Thieves Spray, Thieves Waterless Hand Purifier, Thieves Wipes

Copaiba (Copal) *(Copaifera reticulata, C. langsdorfii, or multijuga)*

Botanical Family: Fabaceae

Plant Origin: Brazil

Extraction Method: Steam distilled (vacuum distilled) from gum resin exudate from tapped trees

Chemical Constituents:
Alpha-Copaene (2-5%)

Alpha-Humulene (6-10%)
Beta-Caryophyllene (39-72%)
Delta-Cadinene (2-3%)
Delta-Elemene (2-3%)
Gamma-Elemene (1-8%)
Germacrene D (4-6%)
Trans-Alpha-Bergamotene (3-11%)

Note: The word "Copal" is derived from the Spanish word for incense (copelli) and can refer to any number of different resinous gums or exudates from trees in Malaysia and South America. Copals are known as black *(Protium copal)*, white *(blanco)* *(Bursera bipinnata)*, gold *(oro)* *(H. courbaril)*, and Brazilian *(Copaifera langsdorfii or reticulata)*. Only the Brazilian copal or copaiba has a GRAS distinction in the U.S. and has the most published research on its anti-inflammatory effects.

Historical Data: Healers and *curanderos* in the Amazon use copaiba resin for all types of pain and inflammatory disorders, both internal (stomach ulcers and cancer) and external (skin disorders and insect bites). In Peruvian traditional medicine, three or four drops of the resin are mixed with a spoonful of honey and taken as a natural sore throat remedy. It is also employed in Peruvian and Brazilian herbal medicine systems as an anti-inflammatory and antiseptic for the urinary tract (cystitis, bladder, and kidney disorders) and in the treatment of urinary problems, stomach ulcers, syphilis, tetanus, bronchitis, and tuberculosis.

In Brazilian herbal medicine, the resin is highly regarded as a strong antiseptic and expectorant for the respiratory tract (including bronchitis and sinusitis) and as an antiseptic gargle. It is a popular home remedy in Brazil for sore throats and tonsillitis (1/2 teaspoon of resin is added to warm water).

Medical Properties: Anti-inflammatory (powerful), neuroprotective, antimicrobial, anxiolytic, mucolytic, antiulcer, anticancer, antiseptic, kidney stone preventative

Uses: Pain relief (strong anti-inflammatory), arthritis, rheumatism, cancer, skin disorders (psoriasis), insect bites, stomach distress, urinary disorders, sore throat, anxiety

Application: Diffuse, inhale directly, or apply topically. Add to food or soy or rice milk as a dietary supplement.

Safety Data: Approved as a food additive in the U.S.

Found in: A·R·T Beauty Masque, Breathe Again Roll-On, Copaiba Vanilla Moisturizing Conditioner, Copaiba Vanilla Moisturizing Shampoo, Deep Relief Roll-On, Progessence Phyto Plus, Progessence Plus, Stress Away, Stress Away Roll-On

Coriander *(Coriandrum sativum)*
  Botanical Family: Apiaceae
  Plant Origin: Russia
  Extraction Method: Steam distilled from seeds (fruit)
  Chemical Constituents:
    Linalol (65-78%)
    Alpha-Pinene (3-7%)
    Camphor (4-6%)
    Gamma-Terpinene (2-7%)
    Limonene (2-5%)
    Geranyl Acetate (1-3.5%)
    Geraniol (0.5-3%)
  ORAC: 298,300 µTE/100g
  Historical Data: Coriander seeds were found in the ancient Egyptian tomb of Ramses II. This oil has been researched at Cairo University for its effects in lowering glucose and insulin levels and supporting pancreatic function. It has also been studied for its effects in strengthening the pancreas.
  Medical Properties: Anti-inflammatory, antioxidant, sedative, analgesic, antimicrobial, antifungal, liver protectant
  Uses: Diabetes, arthritis, intestinal problems, skin conditions
  Fragrant Influence: Soothing and calming
  Application: Dilute 1 part essential oil with 1 part V-6 Vegetable Oil Complex or other pure vegetable oil; (1) apply 2-4 drops on location, (2) apply on chakras and/or Vita Flex points, (3) inhale directly, (4) diffuse, or (5) take as a dietary supplement.
  Found In: A·R·T Renewal Serum, Acceptance, Animal Scents Ointment, AromaGuard Meadow Mist Deodorant, Awaken, Believe, Clarity, Dragon Time Bath & Shower Gel, Evening Peace Bath & Shower Gel, Forgiveness, Genesis Hand & Body Lotion, Gentle Baby, Gratitude, Harmony, Humility, Inspiration, Joy, KidScents Lotion, Lady Sclareol, Lavender-Rosewood Moisturizing Soap, Magnify Your Purpose, Oola Balance, Oola Grow, Relaxation Massage Oil, Rose Ointment, Sandalwood Moisture Cream, Sensation, Sensation Bath & Shower Gel, Sensation Hand & Body Lotion, Sensation Massage Oil, Wolfberry Eye Cream

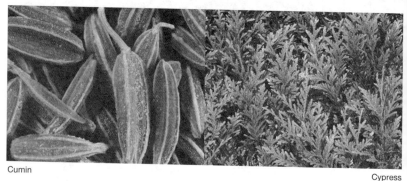

Cumin

Cypress

Cumin *(Cuminum cyminum)*
  Botanical Family: Apiaceae
  Plant Origin: Egypt
  Extraction Method: Steam distilled from seeds
  Key Constituents:
    Cuminaldehyde (16-22%)
    Gamma-Terpinene (16-22%)
    Beta-Pinene (12-18%)
    Para-Mentha-1,3 + 1,4-dien-7-al (25-35%)
    Para-Cymene (3-8%)
  ORAC: 82,400 µTE/100g
  Historical Data: The Hebrews used cumin as
    an antiseptic for circumcision. In ancient
    Egypt, cumin was used for cooking and
    mummification.
  Medical Properties: Antitumoral, anti-
    inflammatory, antioxidant, antiviral,
    antifungal, antimicrobial, digestive aid, liver
    protectant, immune stimulant
  Uses: Cancer, infectious disease, digestive
    problems
  Application: (1) Dilute 1 drop with 4 drops
    vegetable oil, test on small area of skin or the
    underside of arm, then apply; (2) apply on
    chakras and/or Vita Flex points; (3) inhale
    directly; (4) diffuse up to 10 minutes 3 times
    daily; or dilute 1 part essential oil with 4
    parts V-6 Vegetable Oil Complex or other
    pure vegetable oil, put in a capsule, and take
    1 daily or as directed by a health professional.
  Cautions: Dilute before applying to skin.
    Avoid direct sunlight or UV rays for up to
    12 hours after applying.
  Found In: Detoxzyme, ImmuPower, ParaFree,
    Protec

Cypress *(Cupressus sempervirens)*
  Botanical Family: Cupressaceae
  Plant Origin: France, Spain
  Extraction Method: Steam distilled from
    branches
  Key Constituents:
    Alpha-Pinene (40-65%)
    Beta-Pinene (0.5-3%)
    Delta-3-Carene (12-25%)
    Limonene (1.8-5%)
    Cedrol (0.8-7%)
    Myrcene (1-3.5%)
  ORAC: 24,300 µTE/100g
  Historical Data: The Phoenicians and Cretans
    used cypress for building ships and bows,
    while the Egyptians made sarcophagi from
    the wood. The Greeks used cypress to
    carve statues of their gods. The Greek word
    "sempervivens," from which the botanical
    name is derived, means "live forever." The

tree shares its name with the island of Cypress, where it is used for worship. Cypress wood is noted for its durability as it was used most famously for the original doors of St. Peter's Basilica at the Vatican that legends say lasted over 1,000 years.

Medical Properties: Improves circulation; is anti-infectious, antispasmodic, and an antioxidant; discourages fluid retention; improves respiration; promotes liver health

Uses: Diabetes, circulatory disorders, grounding, stabilizing

Fragrant Influence: Eases the feeling of loss and creates a sense of security and grounding. Also helps heal emotional trauma, calms, soothes anger, and helps life flow better. Can help soothe irritating coughs and minor chest discomfort.

Application: Dilute 1 part essential oil with 1 part V-6 Vegetable Oil Complex or other pure vegetable oil; (1) apply 2-4 drops on location, massaging toward center of body, (2) apply on chakras and/or Vita Flex points, (3) inhale directly, (4) diffuse, or (5) take as a dietary supplement.

Found In: Aroma Life, Aroma Siez, Cel-Lite Magic Massage Oil, R.C.

Bible Reference:
Isaiah 44:14—"He heweth him down cedars, and taketh the cypress and the oak, which he strengtheneth for himself among the trees of the forest: he planteth an ash, and the rain doth nourish it."

Davana (*Artemisia pallens*)
Botanical Family: Asteraceae
Extraction Method: Steam distilled from flowers and leaves
Key Constituents:
Davanone 1-2 (40-60%)
Davana Ether 1-3 (5-10%)
Ethyl Cinnamate (1-6%)
Bicyclogermacrene (5-14%)

Historical Data: Grows in the same areas of India as sandalwood. Has been used in India for diabetes, digestive problems (expels parasites), fighting infections, and calming anger. It has been recommended as an aphrodisiac and is often used in perfumery. It has a very rich, concentrated aroma and is usually used only in very small quantities. It should always be diluted because it is high in ketones. The aroma tends to develop differently, depending on the individual chemistry of the person wearing the oil.

Medical Properties: Anti-infectious, antiviral, aphrodisiac, anthelmintic, calmative, analgesic, anti-inflammatory

Uses: Skin infections, headaches, emotional stress, worm infestations, sugar metabolism

Application: Dilute at least 50-50 with V-6 Vegetable Oil Complex and apply 1-2 drops on location or apply on chakras/Vitaflex points. Davana is usually used as a complement in very small amounts in essential oil blends.

Found In: A·R·T Creme Masque, Lavender Bath & Shower Gel, Trauma Life

Dill (*Anethum graveolens*)
Botanical Family: Apiaceae
Plant Origin: Austria, Hungary
Extraction Method: Steam distilled from whole plant
Key Constituents:
Carvone (30-45%)
Limonene (15-25%)
Alpha- and Beta-Phellandrene (20-35%)
ORAC: 35,600 µTE/100g
Historical Data: The dill plant is mentioned in the Papyrus of Ebers from Egypt (1550 BC). Roman gladiators rubbed their skin with dill before each match. Listed in Dioscorides'

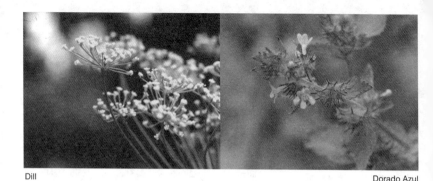

Dill

Dorado Azul

De Materia Medica (AD 78), Europe's first authoritative guide to medicines, which became the standard reference work for herbal treatments for over 1,700 years. It was listed in Hildegard's *Medicine,* a compilation of early German medicines by highly regarded Benedictine herbalist Hildegard of Bingen (1098-1179).

Medical Properties: Antidiabetic, antispasmodic, antifungal, antibacterial, expectorant, pancreatic stimulant, insulin/ blood sugar regulator

Uses: Diabetes, digestive problems, liver deficiencies

Fragrant Influence: Calms the autonomic nervous system and, when diffused with Roman Chamomile, combats ADHD.

Application: Dilute 1 part essential oil with 1 part V-6 Vegetable Oil Complex or other pure vegetable oil; (1) apply 2-4 drops on location or abdomen, (2) apply on chakras and/or Vita Flex points, (3) inhale directly, (4) diffuse, or (5) take as a dietary supplement.

Dorado Azul *(Hyptis suaveolens)*
  Botanical Family: Lamiaceae
  Plant Origin: Ecuador
  Extraction Method: Steam distilled from stems/leaves/flowers (aerial parts)
  Key Constituents:
    Alpha-Fenchol (4-12%)
    Beta-Pinene (7-12%)
    Bicyclogermacrene (4-8%)
    1,8-Cineole (Eucalyptol) (23-46%)
    Limonene (3-7%)
    Sabinene (7-18%)

Historical Data: Until about 2006, Dorado Azul was recognized in Ecuador as only a weed. It did not even have a botanical name until Gary Young distilled and analyzed it for the first time and gave it its identity. It has a red liquid when distilled.

Medical Properties: Anti-inflammatory, antioxidant, antimicrobial, antiseptic, antihyperglycemic, gastroprotective, liver protectant, respiratory stimulant

Uses: Colds, coughs, flu, bronchitis, asthma, allergic reactions that cause constriction and compromised breathing, any compromise

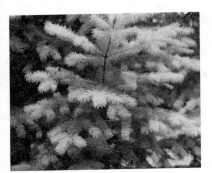
Douglas Fir

to the respiratory tract, hormone balancer, diabetes, vascular dilator, circulatory stimulant, arthritic and rheumatoid-type pain, reducing candida and other intestinal tract problems, digestion, hygienic action for the mouth, enhances mood

Application: Dilute 1 part essential oil with 1 part V-6 Vegetable Oil Complex or other pure vegetable oil; (1) apply 2-4 drops on location or abdomen, (2) apply on chakras and/or Vita Flex points, (3) inhale directly, (4) diffuse up to 30 minutes 3 times daily, or (5) take as a dietary supplement: 1-10 drops in a capsule or 1-2 drops under the tongue or add to drinking water.

Found In: Common Sense

Douglas Fir *(Pseudotsuga menziesii)*

Botanical Family: Pinaceae

Plant Origin: Idaho

Extraction Method: Steam distilled from wood/bark/twigs/needles

Key Constituents:
Alpha-Pinene (25-40%)
Beta-Pinene (7-15%)
Limonene (6-11%)
Bornyl Acetate (8-15%)

ORAC: 69,000 µTE/100g

Medical Properties: Antitumoral, antioxidant, antifungal, pain relieving

Uses: Respiratory/sinus infections

Application: Dilute 1 part essential oil with 1 part V-6 Vegetable Oil Complex or other pure vegetable oil; (1) apply 2-4 drops on location, (2) apply on chakras and/or Vita Flex points, (3) inhale directly, or (4) diffuse.

Found In: Regenolone Moisturizing Cream

Elemi *(Canarium luzonicum)*

Botanical Family: Burseraceae

Plant Origin: Philippines

Extraction Method: Steam distilled from the gum/resin of the tree

Key Constituents:
Limonene (40-72%)
Alpha-Phellandrene (10-24%)
Sabinene (3-8%)
Elemol (1-25%)

Historical Data: Elemi has been used in Europe for hundreds of years in salves for skin and is included in celebrated healing ointments such as *baum paralytique*. Used by a 17th century physician, J. J. Wecker on the battle wounds of soldiers, elemi belongs to the same botanical family as frankincense *(Boswellia carterii)* and myrrh *(Commiphora myrrha)*. The Egyptians used elemi for embalming, and subsequent cultures (particularly in Europe) used it for skin care and for reducing fine lines, wrinkles, and improving skin tone.

Medical Properties: Antispasmodic, anti-inflammatory, antimicrobial, antiseptic, anticancer

Uses: Muscle/nerve pain, skin problems (scars, acne, wrinkles)

Fragrant Influence: Its spicy, incense-like fragrance is very conducive toward meditation. Can be grounding and used to clear the mind.

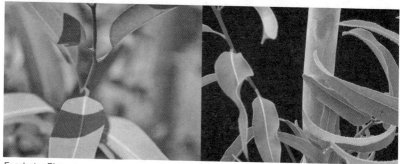

Eucalyptus Blue

Eucalyptus Citriodora

Application: (1) Apply 2-4 drops on location, (2) apply on chakras and/or Vita Flex points, (3) inhale directly, (4) diffuse, or (5) use as a dietary supplement: put one drop in a capsule and take, or put 1 drop in 4 fl. oz. of liquid (rice milk, etc.).

Found In: Ortho Sport Massage Oil

Eucalyptus Blue *(Eucalyptus bicostata)*

Botanical Family: Myrtaceae

Plant Origin: Ecuador

Extraction Method: Steam distilled from the leaves

Key Constituents:

1,8-Cineole (Eucalyptol) (40-80%)

Alpha-pinene (10-30%)

Aromadendrene (≤ 7%)

Limonene (4-8%)

Historical Data: Eucalyptus blue is grown and distilled on Young Living's farm in Ecuador. It is called blue gum, a tree that has been crossbred over 250 years in the wilds of the Andean Mountains in Ecuador and is a cross between *Eucalyptus citriodora* and *Eucalyptus globulus*. The native people of Ecuador have used the disinfecting leaves to cover wounds and to repel insects.

Although it contains a high percentage of eucalyptol, because of its balanced chemical constituents within the eucalyptus, it is the only eucalyptus that has been found in the world today that does not cause an allergic reaction in people who have allergies to eucalyptol. Eucalyptus Blue is preferred over many of the eucalyptus species, simply because of its well-balanced chemistry and its non-allergen effect for all types of respiratory conditions. In a recent study of eight eucalyptus species, *Eucalyptus bicostata* had the best antiviral activity. It is a great companion to Dorado Azul.

Medical Properties: Expectorant, diaphoretic, insecticidal, oestrogenic, antifungal, antiviral, antibacterial

Uses: Supports respiratory function to promote normal breathing, relieves sore muscles, calming, invigorating

Fragrant Influence: Has a fresh, balanced, invigorating aroma

Application: Dilute 1 part essential oil with 1 part V-6 Vegetable Oil Complex or other pure vegetable oil; (1) apply 2-4 drops on location or abdomen, (2) apply on chakras and/or Vita Flex points, (3) inhale directly, (4) diffuse in diffuser or humidifier

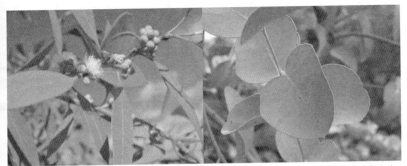

Eucalyptus Dives

Eucalyptus Globulus

Cautions: Do not use Eucalyptus Blue as a dietary supplement. Large amounts of any eucalyptus oil may be toxic. Keep out of reach of children.

Found In: Breathe Again Roll-On

Eucalyptus Citriodora
(Eucalyptus citriodora)

Botanical Family: Myrtaceae

Plant Origin: China

Extraction Method: Steam distilled from leaves

Key Constituents:
Citronellal (75-85%)
Neo-Isopulegol + Isopulegol (0-10%)

ORAC: 83,000 µTE/100g

Historical Data: Traditionally used to perfume linen closets and as an insect repellent

Medical Properties: Analgesic, antiviral, antibacterial, antifungal, anticancer, liver protectant, expectorant, insecticidal

Uses: Fungal infections (ringworm, Candida), respiratory infections, viral infections (herpes, shingles)

Application: Dilute 1 part essential oil with 1 part V-6 Vegetable Oil Complex or other pure vegetable oil, (1) apply 2-4 drops on location, (2) apply on chakras and/or Vita Flex points, (3) inhale directly, or (4) diffuse up to 30 minutes 3 times daily.

Found In: R.C.

Eucalyptus Dives *(Eucalyptus dives)*

Botanical Family: Myrtaceae

Plant Origin: Australia

Extraction Method: Steam distilled from leaves

Key Constituents:
Alpha- and Beta-Phellandrene (23-30%)
Piperitone (35-45%)
Para-Cymene (6-10%)
Alpha-Thujene (2-6%)
Terpinen-4-ol (3-6%)

Medical Properties: Mucolytic, diuretic, antibacterial

Uses: Hypertension, throat/lung/sinus infections

Fragrant Influence: Has a fresh, invigorating aroma that helps clear sinus and bronchi

Application: Dilute 1 part essential oil with 1 part V-6 Vegetable Oil Complex or other pure vegetable oil; (1) apply 2-4 drops on location, (2) apply on chakras and/or Vita Flex points, or (3) diffuse.

Eucalyptus Globulus
(Eucalyptus globulus)

Botanical Family: Myrtaceae

Plant Origin: China

Extraction Method: Steam distilled from leaves

Key Constituents:

1,8-Cineole (Eucalyptol) (70-90%)

Alpha-Pinene (1-5%)

Limonene (6-9%)

Para-Cymene (1-5%)

ORAC: 2,400 µTE/100g

Historical Data: For centuries, Australian Aborigines used the disinfecting leaves to cover wounds. Shown by laboratory tests to be a powerful antimicrobial agent, *E. globulus* contains a high percentage of eucalyptol (a key ingredient in many antiseptic mouth rinses). It is often used for the respiratory system. Eucalyptus has also been investigated for its powerful insect repellent effects (Trigg, 1996). Eucalyptus trees have been planted throughout parts of North Africa to successfully block the spread of malaria. According to Jean Valnet, MD, a solution of 2 percent eucalyptus oil sprayed on the skin will kill 70 percent of ambient staph bacteria. Some doctors still use solutions of eucalyptus oil in surgical dressings.

Medical Properties: Expectorant, mucolytic, antimicrobial, antibacterial, antifungal, antiviral, antiaging, antiulcer, antidiabetic

Uses: Respiratory/sinus infections, decongestant, rheumatism/arthritis, soothe sore muscles

Fragrant Influence: Promotes health, well-being, purification, and healing

Application: Dilute 1 part essential oil with 1 part V-6 Vegetable Oil Complex or other pure vegetable oil; (1) apply 2-4 drops on location, (2) apply on chakras and/or Vita Flex points, (3) inhale directly, (4) diffuse, or (5) take as a dietary supplement.

Found In: Breathe Again Roll-On, Ortho Ease Massage Oil, Ortho Sport Massage Oil, R.C., Thieves Dentarome Ultra Toothpaste

Eucalyptus Polybractea
(Eucalyptus polybractea)

Botanical Family: Myrtaceae

Plant Origin: Australia

Extraction Method: Steam distilled from leaves

Key Constituents:

1,8-Cineole (Eucalyptol) (85-95%)

Limonene (≤ 2%)

Para-Cymene (1-5%)

Alpha-Pinene (1-3%)

Medical Properties: antiviral, antibacterial, anti-inflammatory, expectorant, mucolytic, insect repellent

Uses: Acne, urinary tract/bladder infections, viral infections (herpes)

Application: Dilute 1 part essential oil with 1 part V-6 Vegetable Oil Complex or other pure vegetable oil; (1) apply 2-4 drops on location, (2) apply on chakras and/or Vita Flex points, (3) diffuse or put in humidifier, or (4) take as a dietary supplement.

Eucalyptus Radiata *(Eucalyptus radiata)*

Botanical Family: Myrtaceae

Plant Origin: Australia

Extraction Method: Steam distilled from leaves

Key Constituents:

1,8-Cineole (Eucalyptol) (60-75%)

Alpha Terpineol (5-10%)

Limonene (4-8%)

Alpha Pinene (2-6%)

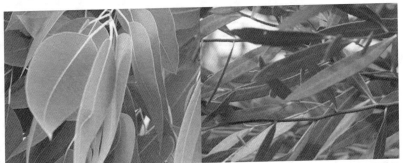

Eucalyptus Polybractea

Eucalyptus Radiata

Historical Data: This eucalyptus species has been treasured in folk medicine. A 2011 study conducted at Heidelberg University found that *Eucalyptus radiata* has the second highest abundance of 1,8 cineole after *E. globulus*.

Medical Properties: Antibacterial, antiviral, expectorant, anti-inflammatory

Uses: Respiratory/sinus infections, viral infections, fights herpes simplex when combined with bergamot

Application: Dilute 1 part essential oil with 1 part V-6 Vegetable Oil Complex or other pure vegetable oil; (1) apply 2-4 drops on location, (2) apply on chakras and/or Vita Flex points, (3) inhale directly, (4) diffuse or put in humidifier.

Found In: AromaGuard Mountain Mint Deodorant, Breathe Again Roll-On, Inner Defense, KidScents Slique Toothpaste, Ortho Ease Massage Oil, Raven, R.C., Thieves, Thieves AromaBright Toothpaste, Thieves Cleansing Soap, Thieves Dental Floss, Thieves Dentarome Plus Toothpaste, Thieves Dentarome Ultra Toothpaste, Thieves Foaming Hand Soap, Thieves Fresh Essence Plus Mouthwash, Thieves Household Cleaner, Thieves Lozenges (Hard, Soft), Thieves Spray, Thieves Waterless Hand Purifier, Thieves Wipes

Eucalyptus Staigeriana
(Eucalyptus staigeriana)

Botanical Family: Myrtaceae

Plant Origin: Australia, Brazil

Extraction Method: Steam distilled from leaves

Key Constituents:
Alpha-Phellandrene (4-7%)
Limonene (4-10%)
1,8 Cineole (Eucalyptol) (15-35%)
Neral (7-15%)
Geranial (10-20%)

Historical Data: This gentle eucalyptus species was valued by Australian Aborigines as a general cure-all. By 1788 it was introduced in Europe, where it was valued for treating respiratory conditions and for colic.
Recent research documents staigeriana as a powerful antiparasitic as well as being highly antimicrobial.

Medical Properties: Antibacterial, diuretic, decongestant, expectorant, antiparasitic

Uses: Helps wounds, burns, and insect bites

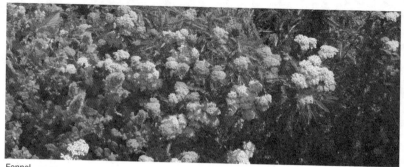

Fennel

heal; suppresses coughs; relieves muscle aches

Fragrant Influences: Eucalyptus Staigeriana, also known as lemon iron bark, has a lemon-scented aroma, without the medicine-like scent of other eucalyptus oils. It can be used on people with sensitive skin.

Application: Dilute 1 part essential oil with 1 part V-6 Vegetable Oil Complex or other pure vegetable oil; (1) apply 2-4 drops on location, (2) apply on chakras and/or Vita Flex points, (3) inhale directly, (4) diffuse or put in humidifier.

Found In: Breathe Again Roll-On, Essential Beauty Serum (Acne-Prone Skin)

Fennel *(Foeniculum vulgare)*

Botanical Family: Apiaceae

Plant Origin: Hungary

Extraction Method: Steam distilled from the crushed seeds (fruit)

Key Constituents:
Trans-Anethole (60-80%)
Fenchone (8-20%)
Alpha-Pinene (1-8%)
Methyl Chavicol (2-6%)

ORAC: 238,400 µTE/100g

Historical Data: Fennel was believed to ward off evil spirits and to protect against spells cast by witches during medieval times. Sprigs were hung over doors to fend off evil phantasms. For hundreds of years, fennel seeds have been used as a digestive aid and to balance menstrual cycles. It is mentioned in one of the oldest known medical records, the Ebers Papyrus (dating from 16th century BC), an ancient Egyptian list of 877 prescriptions and recipes. It was listed in Hildegard's *Medicine*, a compilation of early German medicines by highly regarded Benedictine herbalist Hildegard of Bingen (1098-1179).

Medical Properties: Antidiabetic, anti-inflammatory, antitumoral, estrogen-like, digestive aid, antiparasitic (worms), antiseptic, antispasmodic, analgesic, increases metabolism

Uses: Diabetes, cancer, obesity, arthritis/rheumatism, urinary tract infection, fluid retention, intestinal parasites, menstrual problems/PMS, digestive problems

Application: Dilute 1 part essential oil with 1 part V-6 Vegetable Oil Complex or other pure vegetable oil; (1) apply 2-4 drops on location, (2) apply on chakras and/or Vita Flex points, (3) inhale directly, (4) diffuse, or (5) take as a dietary supplement.

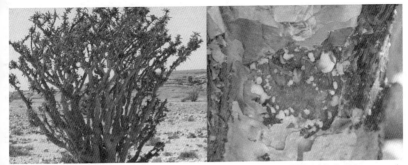

Frankincense (Boswellia carteri)

Milky white frankincense resin

Caution: Avoid using if epileptic

Found In: Allerzyme, CortiStop Women's, Detoxzyme, Digest & Cleanse, DiGize, Dragon Time, Dragon Time Bath & Shower Gel, Dragon Time Massage Oil, Essentialzyme, Essentialzymes-4, Estro, FemiGen, ICP, JuvaFlex, JuvaPower, JuvaSpice, K&B, Mister, ParaFree, Power Meal, Prenolone Plus Body Cream, Prostate Health, SclarEssence

Frankincense (Boswellia carterii)
  Botanical Family: Burseraceae
  Plant Origin: Somalia/Yemen
  Extraction Method: Steam distilled from gum/resin
  Key Constituents:
   Alpha-Pinene (30-65%)
   Limonene (8-20%)
   Sabinene (1-8%)
   Myrcene (1-14%)
   Beta-Caryophyllene (1-5%)
   Alpha-Thujene (1-15%)
   Incensole
  ORAC: 630 µTE/100g
  Historical Data: Also known as "olibanum," the name frankincense is derived from the Medieval French word for "real incense."

Frankincense is considered the "holy anointing oil" in the Middle East and has been used in religious ceremonies for thousands of years. It was well known during the time of Christ for its anointing and healing powers and was one of the gifts given to Christ at His birth. "Used to treat every conceivable ill known to man," frankincense was valued more than gold during ancient times, and only those with great wealth and abundance possessed it. It is mentioned in one of the oldest known medical records, Ebers Papyrus (dating from 16th century BC), an ancient Egyptian list of 877 prescriptions and recipes.

Medical Properties: Antitumoral, immuno-stimulant, antidepressant, muscle relaxing

Uses: Depression, cancer, respiratory infections, inflammation, immune-stimulating

Fragrant Influence: Increases spiritual awareness, promotes meditation, improves attitude, and uplifts spirits

Application: (1) Apply 2-4 drops on location, (2) apply on chakras and/or Vita Flex points, (3) inhale directly, (4) diffuse, (5) when using as a dietary supplement, dilute 1 drop of frankincense in 4 drops V-6 or olive oil, put in a capsule, and take 1 capsule before each meal or as desired.

Found In: Abundance, Acceptance, A·R·T Day Activator, A·R·T Gentle Foaming Cleanser, A·R·T Night Reconstructor, A·R·T Purifying Toner, Awaken, Believe, Boswellia Wrinkle Cream, Brain Power, ClaraDerm, Common Sense, CortiStop Women's, Egyptian Gold, Exodus II, Forgiveness, Gathering, Gratitude, Harmony, Highest Potential, Humility, ImmuPower, Inspiration, Into the Future, KidScents Tender Tush, Longevity, Longevity Softgels, Oola Balance, Oola Grow, Protec, 3 Wise Men, Transformation, Trauma Life, Valor, Valor Moisturizing Soap, Valor Roll-On, Wolfberry Eye Cream

Bible References:

The Bible contains over 52 references to frankincense, considering that "incense" is often translated from the Hebrew and Greek as "frankincense" and is referring to the same resin.

Exodus 30:34—"And the Lord said unto Moses, Take unto thee sweet spices, stacte, and onycha, and galbanum; these sweet spices with pure frankincense: of each shall there be a like weight:"

Leviticus 2:1—"And when any will offer a meat offering unto the Lord, his offering shall be of fine flour; and he shall pour oil upon it, and put frankincense thereon:"

Leviticus 2:2—"And he shall bring it to Aaron's sons the priests: and he shall take thereout his handful of the flour thereof, and of the oil thereof, with all the frankincense thereof; and the priest shall burn the memorial of it upon the altar, to be an offering made by fire, of a sweet savour unto the Lord:"

Frereana Frankincense
(Boswellia frereana)

Botanical Family: Burseraceae

Plant Origin: Somalia

Extraction Method: Steam distilled from gum/resin

Key Constituents:
Alpha-Thujene (23-45%)
Alpha-Pinene (5-9%)
Sabinene (1-8%)
Para-Cymene (10-20%)
Terpinen-4-ol (2-9%)

Historical Data: This species of frankincense is native to northern Somalia where the locals call it "Maydi" and the "King of Frankincense." Frereana incense has been a part of Eastern Orthodox and Catholic worship for hundreds of years.

Since *Boswellia carterii* also grows in Somalia, it is hard to explain why frereana has such a unique chemical composition, so different from *B. carterii* and other frankincense species. As shown by Frank and Unger, as well as EJ Blain, frereana contains no boswellic acids. S. Hamm reports that frereana "is devoid of diterpenes of the incensole family."

There are unique constituents of frereana found in no other frankincense that have mostly been overlooked by researchers. Two frereana studies in 2010 and 2006 reported strong anti-inflammatory activity. Sadly, some trusting purchasers have received an amalgamation of cheaper frankincense resins rather than pure *Boswellia frereana*.

Political conditions in Somalia make it essential for a "feet on the ground" presence in order to secure contracts to obtain pure, high quality frereana resin. For this reason Gary Young personally visited Somalia in November 2013 to contract with local clans of harvesters.

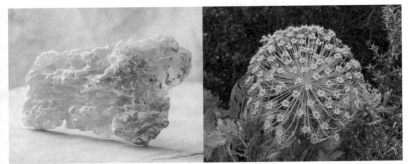

Frereana Frankincense

Galbanum

Medical Properties: Anti-inflammatory

Uses: Arthritis/rheumatism

Fragrant Influence: Frereana's more lemony scent is uplifting and cheering.

Application: (1) Apply 2-4 drops on location, (2) apply on chakras and/or Vita Flex points, (3) inhale directly, (4) diffuse, (5) when using as a dietary supplement, dilute 1 drop of frankincense in 4 drops V-6 or olive oil, put in a capsule, and take 1 capsule before each meal or as desired.

Found In: Slique Gum

Galbanum (Ferula gummosa)

Botanical Family: Apiaceae

Plant Origin: Iran

Extraction Method: Steam distilled from gum/resin derived from stems and branches

Key Constituents:
Alpha-Pinene (5-21%)
Beta-Pinene (40-70%)
Delta-3-Carene (2-16%)
Myrcene (2.5-3.5%)
Sabinene (0.3-3%)

ORAC: 26,200 µTE/100g

Historical Data: Mentioned in Egyptian papyri and the Old Testament (Exodus 30:34), it was esteemed for its medicinal and spiritual properties. Dioscorides, an ancient Roman historian, records that galbanum was used for its antispasmodic, diuretic, and pain-relieving properties.

Medical Properties: Antiseptic, analgesic, light antispasmodic, anti-inflammatory, circulatory stimulant, anticonvulsant

Uses: Digestive problems (diarrhea), nervous tension, rheumatism, skin conditions (scar tissue, wrinkles)

Fragrant Influence: Harmonic and balancing, amplifies spiritual awareness and meditation. When combined with Frankincense or Sandalwood, the frequency rises dramatically.

Application: Dilute 1 part Galbanum with 1 part vegetable oil; (1) apply 2-4 drops on location, (2) apply on chakras and/or Vita Flex points, (3) inhale directly, (4) diffuse up to 1 hour 3 times daily, or, (5) put in a capsule, and take up to 3 times daily or as needed as a dietary supplement.

Found In: Exodus II, Gathering, Gratitude, Highest Potential, Oola Balance, Oola Grow, The Gift

Bible Reference:
Exodus 30:34—"And the Lord said unto Moses, Take unto thee sweet spices, stacte,

71

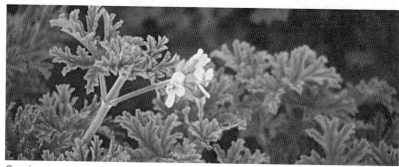
Geranium

and onycha, and galbanum; these sweet spices with pure frankincense: of each shall there be a like weight:"

Geranium *(Pelargonium graveolens)*
Botanical Family: Geraniaceae
Plant Origin: Egypt, India
Extraction Method: Steam distilled from the flowers and leaves
Key Constituents:
Citronellol (25-36%)
Geraniol (10-18%)
Citronellyl Formate (5-8%)
Linalol (4-8%)
Historical Data: Geranium has been used for centuries for regenerating and healing skin conditions.
Medical Properties: Antispasmodic, antioxidant, antitumoral, anti-inflammatory, anticancer, hemostatic (stops bleeding), antibacterial, antifungal, improves blood flow, liver and pancreas stimulant, dilates bile ducts for liver detoxification, helps cleanse oily skin; revitalizes skin cells
Uses: Hepatitis/fatty liver (Jean Valnet, MD), skin conditions (dermatitis, eczema, psoriasis, acne, vitiligo), fungal infections (ringworm), viral infections (herpes, shingles), hormone imbalances, circulatory problems (improves blood flow), menstrual problems/PMS
Fragrant Influence: Helps release negative memories and eases nervous tension; balances the emotions, lifts the spirit, and fosters peace, well-being, and hope
Application: (1) Apply 2-4 drops on location, (2) apply on chakras and/or Vita Flex points, (3) inhale directly, (4) diffuse, or (5) when using as a dietary supplement, dilute 1 drop of geranium in 4 drops V-6 or olive oil, put in a capsule, and take 1 capsule before each meal or as desired.
Found In: A·R·T Creme Masque, A·R·T Renewal Serum, Acceptance, Animal Scents Ointment, Animal Scents Shampoo, AromaGuard Meadow Mist Deodorant, Awaken, Believe, Boswellia Wrinkle Cream, Clarity, Copaiba Vanilla Moisturizing Conditioner, Copaiba Vanilla Moisturizing Shampoo, Dragon Time Bath & Shower Gel, EndoFlex, Envision, Evening Peace Bath & Shower Gel, Forgiveness, Gathering, Genesis Hand & Body Lotion, Gentle Baby, Gratitude, Harmony, Highest Potential, Humility, Inspiration, Joy, JuvaFlex, JuvaTone, K&B, KidScents Bath Gel,

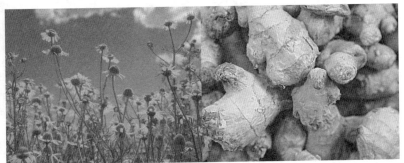

German Chamomile

Ginger

KidScents Lotion, Lady Sclareol, Lavender-Rosewood Moisturizing Soap, Magnify Your Purpose, Melaleuca-Geranium Moisturizing Soap, Oola Balance, Oola Grow, Prenolone Plus Body Cream, Prostate Health, Relaxation, Relaxation Massage Oil, Release, SARA, Sandalwood Moisture Cream, Sensation, Sensation Bath & Shower Gel, Sensation Hand & Body Lotion, Trauma Life, White Angelica, Wolfberry Eye Cream

German Chamomile *(Matricaria recutita)*
  Botanical Family: Asteraceae
  Plant Origin: Utah, Idaho, Egypt, Hungary
  Extraction Method: Steam distilled from flowers
  Key Constituents:
    Chamazulene (2-5%)
    Bisabolol Oxide A (32-42%)
    Trans-Beta-Farnesene (18-26%)
    Bisbolol Oxide B (3-6%)
    Bisbolone Oxide A (3-6%)
    Cis Spiro Ether (4-8%)
  ORAC: 218,600 µTE/100g
  Historical Data: Listed in Dioscorides' *De Materia Medica* (AD 78), Europe's first authoritative guide to medicines, which became the standard reference work for herbal treatments for over 1,700 years.
  Medical Properties: Powerful antioxidant, inhibits lipid peroxidation, antitumoral, anti-inflammatory, relaxant, anesthetic; promotes digestion, liver, and gallbladder health.
  Uses: Hepatitis/fatty liver, arteriosclerosis, insomnia, nervous tension, arthritis, carpal tunnel syndrome, skin problems such as acne, eczema, scar tissue
  Fragrant Influence: Dispels anger, stabilizes emotions, and helps release emotions linked to the past. Soothes and clears the mind.
  Application: (1) Apply 2-4 drops on location, (2) apply on chakras and/or Vita Flex points, (3) inhale directly, (4) diffuse up to 1 hour 3 times daily, or (5) put 2 drops in a capsule, take 3 times daily or as needed.
  Found In: A·R·T Day Activator, A·R·T Night Reconstructor, ComforTone, EndoFlex, JuvaTone, OmegaGize[3], Surrender

Ginger *(Zingiber officinale)*
  Botanical Family: Zingiberaceae
  Plant Origin: India, China
  Extraction Method: Steam distilled from rhizomes/root

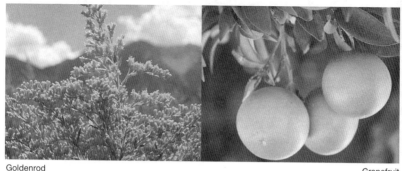

Goldenrod

Grapefruit

Key Constituents:
Zingiberene (30-40%)
Beta-Sesquiphellandrene (8-19%)
1,8-Cineole (Eucalyptol) + Beta-
Phellandrene (4-10%)
AR Curcumene (5-10%)
Camphene (5-9%)

ORAC: 99,300 µTE/100g

Historical Data: Traditionally used to combat nausea. Women in the West African country of Senegal weave belts of ginger root to restore their mates' sexual potency.

Medical Properties: Anti-inflammatory, anticoagulant, digestive aid, anesthetic, expectorant, antifungal

Uses: Rheumatism/arthritis, digestive disorders, respiratory infections/congestion, muscular aches/pains, nausea

Fragrant Influence: Gentle, stimulating, endowing physical energy, courage

Application: Dilute 1 part essential oil with 1 part V-6 Vegetable Oil Complex or other pure vegetable oil; (1) apply 2-4 drops on location, (2) apply on chakras and/or Vita Flex points, (3) inhale directly, (4) diffuse, or (5) take as a dietary supplement.

Caution: Anticoagulant properties can be enhanced when combined with Warfarin, aspirin, etc.

Found In: Abundance, Allerzyme, Comfor-Tone, DiGize, Digest & Cleanse, EndoGize, Essentialzymes-4, ICP, Live with Passion, Magnify Your Purpose, Ultra Young Plus

Goldenrod *(Solidago canadensis)*
Botanical Family: Asteraceae
Plant Origin: Canada
Extraction Method: Steam distilled from flowering tops

Key Constituents:
Alpha-Pinene (10-24%)
Germacrene D (15-37%)
Myrcene (4-10%)
Sabinene (5-18%)
Limonene (10-20%)

ORAC: 61,900 µTE/100g

Historical Data: The genus name, *Solidago*, comes from the Latin solide, which means "to make whole." During the Boston Tea Party, when English tea was dumped into Boston Harbor, colonists drank goldenrod tea instead, which gave it the nickname "Liberty Tea."

Medical Properties: Diuretic, anti-inflammatory, antihypertensive, liver stimulant

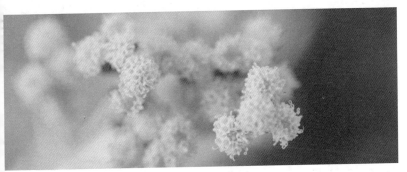

Helichrysum

Uses: Hypertension, liver congestion, hepatitis/fatty liver, circulatory conditions, urinary tract/bladder conditions

Application: Dilute 1 part essential oil with 1 part V-6 Vegetable Oil Complex or other pure vegetable oil; (1) apply 2-4 drops on location or compress, (2) apply on chakras and/or Vita Flex points, (3) inhale directly, (4) diffuse, or (5) take as a dietary supplement.

Found In: Common Sense

Grapefruit (Citrus paradisi)

Botanical Family: Rutaceae

Plant Origin: South Africa and California. (Grapefruit is a hybrid between *Citrus maxima* and *Citrus sinensis*.)

Extraction Method: Cold pressed from rind

Key Constituents:
Limonene (88-95%)
Myrcene (1-4%)

ORAC: 22,600 µTE/100g

Medical Properties: Antitumoral, metabolic stimulant, antiseptic, detoxifying, diuretic, fat-dissolving, cleansing for kidneys, lymphatic and vascular system; antidepressant, rich in limonene, which has been extensively studied in over 50 clinical studies for its ability to combat tumor growth

Uses: Alzheimer's, fluid retention, depression, obesity, liver disorders, anxiety, cellulite

Fragrant Influence: Refreshing and uplifting. A Mie University study found that citrus fragrances boosted immunity, induced relaxation, and reduced depression (Komori, et al., 1995).

Application: Dilute 1 part essential oil with 1 part V-6 Vegetable Oil Complex or other pure vegetable oil; (1) apply 2-4 drops on location, (2) apply on chakras and/or Vita Flex points, (3) inhale directly, (4) diffuse, or (5) take as a dietary supplement.

Caution: Avoid applying to skin that will be exposed to sunlight or UV light within 24 hours.

Found In: Cel-Lite Magic Massage Oil, Citrus Fresh, GLF, Grapefruit Lip Balm, KidScents Slique Toothpaste, Power Meal, Slique Essence, Super C

Helichrysum (Helichrysum italicum)

Botanical Family: Asteraceae

Plant Origin: Yugoslavia, Corsica, Croatia, Spain

Extraction Method: Steam distilled from flower

Key Constituents:

Neryl Acetate (3-35%)
Gamma-Curcumene (10-28%)
Alpha-Pinene (15-32%)
Beta-Caryophyllene (2-9%)
Beta-Selinene (4-8%)

ORAC: 1,700 µTE/100g

Medical Properties: Anticoagulant, anesthetic, antispasmodic, antiviral, liver protectant/detoxifier/stimulant, chelates chemicals and toxins, regenerates nerves

Uses: Herpes virus, arteriosclerosis, atherosclerosis, hypertension, blood clots, liver disorders, circulatory disorders, skin conditions (eczema, psoriasis scar tissue, varicose veins)

Fragrant Influence: Uplifting to the subconscious

Application: (1) Apply 2-4 drops on location, temple, forehead, back of neck, or outside of ear, (2) apply on chakras and/or Vita Flex points, (3) inhale directly, (4) diffuse, or (5) take as a dietary supplement.

Caution: Anticoagulant properties can be enhanced when combined with Warfarin, aspirin, etc.

Found In: Aroma Life, Awaken, Brain Power, ClaraDerm, Deep Relief Roll-On, Forgiveness, GLF, JuvaCleanse, JuvaFlex, Live with Passion, M-Grain, PanAway, Trauma Life

Hinoki (*Chamaecyparis obtusa*)

Botanical Family: Cupressaceae

Plant Origin: Southern Japan

Extraction Method: Steam distilled from sustainably harvested, culled wood

Key Constituents:
Alpha-Pinene (35-60%)
Gamma-Cadinene (3-8%)
Delta-Cadinene (7-14%)
Tau-Cadinol (7-15%)
Tau-Muurolol (6-12%)

Historical Data: Hinoki wood has been used to construct many holy temples in Japan, including Horyuji Temple and Osaka Castle, and is said to be the "tree where God stayed." Hinoki wood is resistant to decay and carries a symbolic reputation of being immortal.

Medical Properties: Contains tau-muurolene, a powerful antifungal compound; reduces agitation and hyperactivity

Uses: Antibacterial, antiviral, antidepressant, anti-inflammatory, astringent, odor eliminator, promotes hair growth, stimulates digestion, relieves pain

Fragrant Influence: Calming and centering

Application: (1) Dilute with carrier oil 1:1 and apply 2-4 drops to desired location, temple, forehead, back of neck, or outside of ear, (2) diffuse up to 30 minutes 3 times daily

Hong Kuai (*Chamaecyparis formosensis*)

Botanical Family: Cupressaceae

Plant Origin: Taiwan

Extraction Method: Steam distilled from sustainably harvested, culled wood

Key Constituents:
Alpha-Pinene (4-6%)
Myrtenal (3-7%)
Myrtenol (11-18%)
Myrtanol (13-19%)
Delta-Cadinene (7-10%)
Alpha-Elemol (1-4%)
Tau-Muurolol (3-6%)

Historical Data: Hong Kuai trees grow up to 55-60 meters tall in high altitude areas of Taiwan and can live over 1,000 years. The wood of these trees is highly resistant to decay and valued for building temples. The highly scented oil was known for supporting respiratory health.

Medical Properties: Antifungal, anticancer,

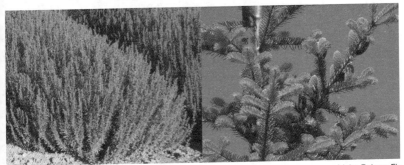

Hyssop

Idaho Balsam Fir

immune support

Uses: Fungal infections (ringworm), cancer, respiratory problems

Fragrant Influence: Calming and centering

Application: (1) Dilute with carrier oil 1:1 and apply 2-4 drops to desired location, temple, forehead, back of neck, or outside of ear, (2) diffuse up to 30 minutes 3 times daily

Hyssop *(Hyssopus officinalis)*

Botanical Family: Lamiaceae

Plant Origin: France, Hungary, Utah

Extraction Method: Steam distilled from stems and leaves

Key Constituents:

Beta-Pinene (13.5-23%)

Sabinene (2-3%)

Pinocamphone (5.5-17.5%)

Iso-Pinochamphone (34.5-50%)

Gemacrene D (2-3%)

Limonene (1-4%)

ORAC: 20,900 µTE/100g

Historical Data: While there is some uncertainty that *Hyssopus officinalis* is the same species of plant as the hyssop referred to in the Bible, there is no question that *H. officinalis* has been used medicinally for almost a millennium for its antiseptic properties. It has also been used for opening the respiratory system.

Medical Properties: Mucolytic, decongestant, anti-inflammatory, regulates lipid metabolism, antiviral, antibacterial, and antiparasitic

Uses: Respiratory infections/congestion, parasites (expelling worms), viral infections, and circulatory disorders

Fragrant Influence: Stimulates creativity and meditation

Application: Dilute 1 part essential oil with 1 part V-6 Vegetable Oil Complex or other pure vegetable oil; (1) apply 2-4 drops on location, (2) apply on chakras and/or Vita Flex points, (3) inhale directly, (4) diffuse, or (5) take as a dietary supplement.

Caution: Avoid use if epileptic.

Found In: Awaken, Egyptian Gold, Exodus II, GLF, Harmony, ImmuPower, Oola Balance, Relieve It, White Angelica

Bible References:

Exodus 12:22— "And ye shall take a bunch of hyssop, and dip it in the blood that is in the bason, and strike the lintel and the two side posts with the blood that is in the bason; and none of you shall go out at the door of his house until the morning."

Leviticus 14:4—"Then shall the priest command to take for him that is to be cleansed two birds alive and clean, and cedar wood, and scarlet, and hyssop:"

Leviticus 14:6—"As for the living bird, he shall take it, and the cedar wood, and the scarlet, and the hyssop, and shall dip them and the living bird in the blood of the bird that was killed over the running water:"

Idaho Balsam Fir (Abies balsamea)

Botanical Family: Pinaceae

Plant Origin: Highland Flats in Naples, Idaho

Extraction Method: Steam distilled from leaves (needles) and branches

Key Constituents:

Alpha-Pinene (6-9%)

Beta-Pinene (14-24%)

Camphene (10-15%)

Limonene (1-5%)

ORAC: 20,500 µTE/100g

Historical Data: The fir tree—a tree commonly used as a Christmas tree today—has been prized through the ages for its medicinal effects and ability to heal respiratory conditions and muscular and rheumatic pain.

Medical Properties: Anticoagulant, antibacterial, anti-inflammatory, antitumoral

Uses: Throat/lung/sinus infections, fatigue, arthritis/rheumatism, urinary tract infections, scoliosis/lumbago/sciatica

Fragrant Influence: Grounding, stimulating to the mind, and relaxing to the body

Application: Dilute 1 part essential oil with 1 part V-6 Vegetable Oil Complex or other pure vegetable oil; (1) apply 2-4 drops on location or use neat in Raindrop Technique,

(2) apply on chakras and/or Vita Flex points, (3) inhale directly, (4) diffuse, or (5) take as a dietary supplement.

Found In: Animal Scents Ointment, Believe, BLM, Deep Relief Roll-On, En-R-Gee, Egyptian Gold, Gratitude, Oola Balance, Sacred Mountain, Sacred Mountain Moisturizing Bar Soap, Slique Slim Caps, The Gift, Transformation

Bible References:

2 Samuel 6:5—"And David and all the house of Israel played before the Lord on all manner of [instruments made of] fir wood, even on harps, and on psalteries, and on timbrels, and on cornets, and on cymbals."

1 Kings 5:8—"And Hiram sent to Solomon, saying, I have considered the things which thou sentest to me for: [and] I will do all thy desire concerning timber of cedar, and concerning timber of fir."

1 Kings 5:10—"So Hiram gave Solomon cedar trees and fir trees [according to] all his desire."

Idaho Blue Spruce (Picea pungens)

Botanical Family: Pinaceae

Plant Origin: Idaho

Extraction Method: Steam distilled from all tree parts

Key Constituents:

Alpha-Pinene (15-40%)

Camphene (6-8%)

Beta-Pinene (6-11%)

Myrcene (3-7%)

Limonene (18-25%)

Bornyl Acetate (3-10%)

ORAC: 575 µTE/g

Historical Data: Northwestern Native Americans considered the Idaho blue spruce to be a sacred tree and used it for smudging/purification rites. Spruce leaves, inner bark, gum, and twigs have been

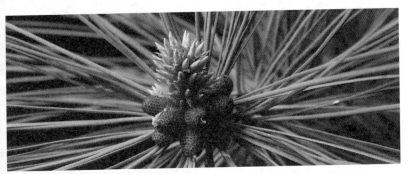
Idaho Ponderosa Pine

used historically by Native Americans for a variety of functions. Leaves were used as inhalants, fumigators, and revivers. The inner bark of the spruce was used for lung and throat troubles, inward troubles, in a poultice applied to wounds and for cuts and swelling, as a medicinal salt, applied to areas of inflammation, and in an antiscorbutic drink for scurvy and colds. Spruce gum was also used for calking canoes. Various parts of the tree were also combined and used for stomach troubles, scabs, sores, as a salve for cuts and wounds, and in a tea for scurvy and cough remedy.

Medical Properties: Antinociceptive (analgesic; reduces sensitivity to pain), antioxidative, antibacterial, relaxant, possibly anticancerous

Uses: Antibacterial, pain relief, insecticide, antioxidant, expectorant, induces relaxation, nAChR (nicotinic acetylcholine receptor) inhibitor, prevents oxidation of LDL, GABAa agonist, antimicrobial

Fragrant Influence: Releases emotional blocks, bringing about a feeling of balance and grounding

Application: (1) Apply 2-4 drops directly to desired area; no dilution required, (2) apply on chakras and/or Vita Flex points, (3) inhale directly, (4) diffuse for 1 hour 3 times daily, or (5) take 2 drops in a capsule daily as a dietary supplement.

Found In: Believe, Transformation

Idaho Ponderosa Pine *(Pinus ponderosa)*
Botanical Family: Pinus
Plant Origin: Idaho
Extraction Method: Steam distilled from all tree parts
Key Constituents:
Delta-3-Carene (35-50%)
Beta-Pinene (16-30%)
Alpha-Pinene (7-10%)
Limonene (5-8%)

Historical Data: This large pine tree is native to western North America but grows throughout the temperate world. The official state tree of Montana, the ponderosa pine gains its fragrant scent from an abundance of terpenes, including Delta-3-Carene, Beta-Pinene, Alpha-Pinene, and Limonene listed above. A measurement by Ascending the Giants in 2011 landed a ponderosa pine in the record books as the tallest known pine (268.29 feet tall). Native Americans used the ponderosa pine to reduce coughs and fevers, while the pitch was used as an ointment for skin conditions. In sweat lodges, the tree boughs were used for muscular pain, and the pollen and needles were used in healing ceremonies.

Medical Properties: Antimicrobial, antifungal

Uses: Respiratory ailments, arthritis, rheumatism

Fragrant Influence: Relaxing, calming, and restorative; also emotionally uplifting

Application: (1) Apply 2-4 drops on location, (2) apply on chakras and/or Vita Flex points, (3) inhale directly, (4) diffuse.

Cautions: (1) Do not take if pregnant or planning on becoming pregnant. (2) Not for dietary use. (3) Not for use on children.

Idaho Tansy (*Tanacetum vulgare*)

Botanical Family: Asteraceae

Plant Origin: Idaho

Extraction Method: Steam distilled from leaves and stems

Key Constituents:
Beta-Thujone (65-80%)
Camphor (3-8%)
Sabinene (1-4%)
Germacrene D (3-7%)

Historical Data: This antimicrobial oil has been used extensively as an insect repellent. According to F. Joseph Montagna's herbal desk reference, it may tone the entire system (Montagna, 1990).

Medical Properties: Analgesic, antioxidant, antiviral, anticoagulant, immune stimulant, insect repellent

Uses: Arteriosclerosis, hypertension, arthritis/rheumatism

Application: Dilute 1 part essential oil with 1 part V-6 Vegetable Oil Complex or other pure vegetable oil; (1) apply 2-4 drops on location, (2) apply on chakras and/or Vita Flex points, (3) inhale directly, or (4) diffuse.

Caution: Do not use if pregnant.

Found In: ImmuPower, Into the Future, Lady Sclareol, Oola Grow, ParaFree

Ishpingo (*Ocotea quixos*)

Botanical Family: Lauraceae

Plant Origin: Ecuador

Extraction Method: Steam distillation from flower/fruit

Key Constituents:
Trans-Cinnamaldehyde (10-3%)
Methyl Cinnamate (7-25%)
Cinnamyl Acetate (5-18%)
Alpha-Pinene (3-9%)

Historical Data: Ocotea is distilled from the flower and fruit of a tree found in the Amazon wilderness on the ranges of the west side of the Andes Mountains. It is commonly referred to by the native people throughout Ecuador as false canilla or false cinnamon. The tree grows to a very large size, reaching up to 48 inches in diameter and over 60 feet tall, making a large canopy top. Historical usage of ocotea dates back more than 500 years, when it was used to aromatize sweets and cakes. Of 79 octotea species' studies on PubMed, only two refer to the properties of ocotea essential oil distilled from flowers or fruit rather than the leaves and bark of the tree.

Medical Properties: Antimicrobial, antioxidant, antifungal

Found In: Chocolessence

Jasmine (*Jasminum officinale*)

Botanical Family: Oleaceae

Plant Origin: India

Extraction Method: Absolute extraction from flower. Jasmine is actually an "essence" not an essential oil. The flowers must be picked at night to maximize fragrance.

Note: One pound of jasmine oil requires

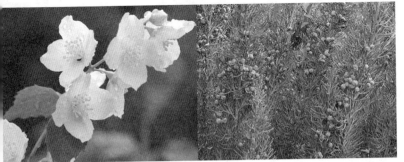

Jasmine

Juniper

about 1,000 pounds of jasmine or 3.6 million fresh, unpacked blossoms. The blossoms must be collected before sunrise, or much of the fragrance will have evaporated. The quality of the blossoms may also be compromised if they are crushed. A single pound of pure jasmine oil may cost between $1,200 and $4,500. In contrast, synthetic jasmine oils can be obtained for $3.50 per pound, but they do not possess the therapeutic qualities as the pure oil.

Key Constituents:
Benzyl Acetate (18-28%)
Benzyl Benzoate (14-21%)
Linalol (3-8%)
Phytol (6-12%)
Isophytol (3-7%)
Squalene (3-7%)

Historical Data: Nicknamed as the "queen of the night" and "moonlight of the grove." For centuries, women have treasured jasmine for its beautiful, seductive fragrance.

Medical Properties: Uplifting, antidepressant, stimulating, antibacterial, antiviral

Uses: Anxiety, depression, menstrual problems/PMS, skin problems (eczema, wrinkles, greasy), frigidity

Fragrant Influence: Uplifting, counteracts hopelessness, nervous exhaustion, anxiety, depression, indifference, and listlessness.

Application: (1) Apply 2-4 drops on location, (2) apply on chakras and/or Vita Flex points, (3) inhale directly, or (4) diffuse.

Found In: A·R·T Creme Masque, A·R·T Renewal Serum, Awaken, Clarity, Dragon Time, Dragon Time Bath & Shower Gel, Dragon Time Massage Oil, Evening Peace Bath & Shower Gel, Forgiveness, Genesis Hand & Body Lotion, Gentle Baby, Harmony, Highest Potential, Inner Child, Into the Future, Joy, Lady Sclareol, Lavender Conditioner, Lavender Shampoo, Live with Passion, Oola Balance, Oola Grow, Sensation, Sensation Hand & Body Lotion, Sensation Massage Oil, Sensation Bath & Shower Gel, The Gift

Juniper *(Juniperus osteosperma and J. scopulorum)*

Botanical Family: Cupressaceae

Plant Origin: Utah

Extraction Method: Steam distilled from stems/leaves/flowers (aerial parts)

Key Constituents:
Alpha-Pinene (20-40%)
Sabinene (3-18%)

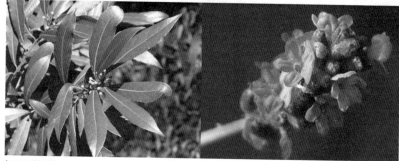

Laurus Nobilis

Lavandin

Myrcene (1-6%)
Camphor (10-18%)
Limonene (3-8%)
Bornyl Acetate (12-20%)
Terpinen-4-ol (3-8%)

ORAC: 250 µTE/100g

Historical Data: Bundles of juniper berries were hung over doorways to ward off witches during medieval times. Juniper has been used for centuries as a diuretic. Until recently, French hospital wards burned sprigs of juniper and rosemary to protect from infection.

Medical Properties: Antiseptic, digestive cleanser/stimulant, purifying, detoxifying, increases circulation through the kidneys and promotes excretion of toxins, promotes nerve regeneration

Uses: Skin conditions (acne, eczema), liver problems, urinary/bladder infections, fluid retention

Fragrant Influence: Evokes feelings of health, love, and peace and may help to elevate one's spiritual awareness

Application: Dilute 1 part essential oil with 1 part V-6 Vegetable Oil Complex or other pure vegetable oil; (1) apply 2-4 drops on location, (2) apply on chakras and/or Vita Flex points, (3) inhale directly, (4) diffuse, or (5) take as a dietary supplement.

Found In: Allerzyme, Awaken, Cel-Lite Magic Massage Oil, DiGize, Dream Catcher, En-R-Gee, Grounding, Hope, Into the Future, K&B, Morning Start Bath & Shower Gel, Morning Start Moisturizing Soap, Oola Grow, Ortho Ease Massage Oil, 3 Wise Men

Bible Reference:
Job 30:4—"Who cut up mallows by the bushes, and juniper roots for their meat."

Laurus Nobilis (*Laurus nobilis*)
(Also known as Bay Laurel)

Botanical Family: Lauraceae

Plant Origin: Croatia

Extraction Method: Steam distilled from leaves and twigs

Key Constituents:
1,8-Cineole (Eucalyptol) (40-50%)
Alpha-Terpenyl Acetate (7-14%)
Alpha-Pinene (4-8%)
Beta-Pinene (3-6%)
Sabinene (6-11%)
Linalol (2-7%)

ORAC: 98,900 µTE/100g

Historical Data: Both the leaves and the black berries were used to alleviate indigestion and loss of appetite. During the Middle Ages, laurus nobilis was used for angina, migraine, heart palpitations, and liver and spleen complaints.

Medical Properties: Antimicrobial, expectorant, mucolytic, antibacterial (staph, strep, *E. coli*), antifungal (Candida), anticoagulant, anticonvulsant

Uses: Nerve regeneration, arthritis (rheumatoid), oral infections (gingivitis), respiratory infections, viral infections

Application: Dilute 1 part essential oil with 1 part V-6 Vegetable Oil Complex or other pure vegetable oil; (1) apply 2-4 drops on location or abdomen, (2) apply on chakras and/or Vita Flex points, (3) inhale directly, (4) diffuse, or (5) take as a dietary supplement.

Found In: Breathe Again Roll-On, ParaFree

Lavandin *(Lavandula x hybrida)*

Botanical Family: Lamiaceae

Plant Origin: France

Extraction Method: Steam distilled from the flowering top

Key Constituents:
Linalyl acetate (25-38%)
Linalol (24-37%)
Camphor (6-8.5%)
1,8-Cineole (Eucalyptol) (4-8%)
Borneol (1.5-3.5%)
Terpinen-4-ol (1.5-5%)
Lavandulyl Acetate (1.5-3.5%)

Historical Data: Also known as *Lavandula x intermedia*, lavandin is a hybrid plant developed by crossing true lavender with spike lavender or aspic *(Lavandula latifolia)*. It has been used to sterilize the animal cages in veterinary clinics and hospitals throughout Europe.

Medical Properties: Antibacterial, antifungal

Uses: Lavandin is a stronger antiseptic than lavender *(Lavandula angustifolia)*. Its greater penetrating qualities make it well suited to help with respiratory, circulatory, and muscular conditions. However, its camphor content invalidates its use to soothe burns.

Fragrant Influence: Similar calming effects as lavender

Application: (1) Apply 2-4 drops on location, (2) apply on chakras and/or Vita Flex points, (3) inhale directly, or (4) diffuse.

Caution: Avoid using for burns; instead, use pure lavender *(Lavandula angustifolia)*.

Found In: Animal Scents Shampoo, Purification, Release

Lavender *(Lavandula angustifolia)*

Botanical Family: Lamiaceae

Plant Origin: Utah, Idaho, France

Extraction Method: Steam distilled from flowering top

Key Constituents:
Linalyl Acetate (21-47%)
Linalol (23-46%)
Cis-Beta-Ocimene (1-8%)
Trans-Beta-Ocimene (1-5%)
Terpinen-4-ol (1-8%)

ORAC: 360 µTE/100g

Historical Data: The French scientist René Gattefossé was the first to discover lavender's ability to promote tissue regeneration and speed wound healing when he severely burned his arm in a laboratory explosion. Today, lavender is one of the few essential oils to still be listed in the British Pharmacopoeia.

Medical Properties: Antiseptic, antifungal, analgesic, antitumoral, anticonvulsant, vasodilating, relaxant, anti-inflammatory, reduces blood fat/cholesterol, combats excess sebum on skin

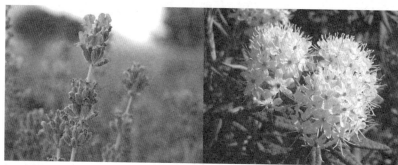

Lavender

Ledum

Uses: Respiratory infections, high blood pressure, arteriosclerosis, menstrual problems/PMS, skin conditions (perineal repair, acne, eczema, psoriasis, scarring, stretch marks), burns, hair loss, insomnia, nervous tension

Fragrant Influence: Calming, relaxing, and balancing, both physically and emotionally. Lavender has been documented to improve concentration and mental acuity. University of Miami researchers found that inhalation of lavender oil increased beta waves in the brain, suggesting heightened relaxation. It also reduced depression and improved cognitive performance (Diego MA, et al., 1998). A 2001 Osaka Kyoiku University study found that lavender reduced mental stress and increased alertness (Motomura, 2001).

Application: (1) Apply 2-4 drops on location, (2) apply on chakras and/or Vita Flex points, (3) inhale directly, (4) diffuse, or (5) take as a dietary supplement.

Caution: True lavender is often adulterated with hybrid lavender (lavandin), synthetic linalol and linalyl acetate, or synthetic fragrance chemicals like ethyl vanillin.

Found In: A·R·T Beauty Masque, A·R·T Gentle Foaming Cleanser, A·R·T Purifying Toner, AromaGuard Meadow Mist Deodorant, Aroma Siez, Awaken, Brain Power, ClaraDerm, Copaiba Vanilla Moisturizing Conditioner, Copaiba Vanilla Moisturizing Shampoo, Dragon Time, Dragon Time Bath & Shower Gel, Dragon Time Massage Oil, Egyptian Gold, Envision, Essential Beauty Serum (Dry Skin), Estro, Forgiveness, Gathering, Gentle Baby, Harmony, Highest Potential, KidScents Tender Tush, LavaDerm Cooling Mist, Lavender Bath & Shower Gel, Lavender Conditioner, Lavender Foaming Hand Soap, Lavender Hand & Body Lotion, Lavender Lip Balm, Lavender Mint Daily Conditioner, Lavender Mint Daily Shampoo, Lavender-Rosewood Moisturizing Soap, Lavender Shampoo, M-Grain, Mister, Motivation, Oola Balance, Oola Grow, Orange Blossom Facial Wash, Prostate Health, R.C., Relaxation Massage Oil, RutaVaLa, RutaVaLa Roll-On, Sandalwood Moisture Cream, SARA, Sleep Essence, Stress Away, Stress Away Roll-On, Surrender, Tranquil Roll-On, Trauma Life, Wolfberry Eye Cream

Ledum *(Ledum groenlandicum)*

Botanical Family: Ericaceae

Plant Origin: North America (Canada)

Extraction Method: Steam distilled from flowering tops

Key Constituents:

Limonene (10-40%)

Cis-Para-Mentha-1(7),8-dien-8-ol (1-12%)

Trans-Para-Mentha-1(7),8-dien-8-ol (2-8%)

Alpha-Selinene (4-20%)

Trans-Para-Mentha-1,3,8-Triene (2-7%)

Historical Data: Known colloquially as "Labrador tea," ledum is a strongly aromatic herb that has been used for centuries in folk medicine. The native people of Eastern Canada used this herb for tea, as a general tonic, and to treat a variety of kidney-related problems. Ledum has helped protect the native people of North America against scurvy for more than 5,000 years. The Cree used it for fevers and colds.

Medical Properties: Anti-inflammatory, antitumoral, antibacterial, diuretic, liver-protectant

Uses: Liver problems/hepatitis/fatty liver, obesity, water retention

Application: (1) Apply 2-4 drops on location, (2) apply on chakras and/or Vita Flex points, (3) inhale directly, (4) diffuse, or (5) take as a dietary supplement.

Found In: GLF, JuvaCleanse

Lemon *(Citrus limon)*

Botanical Family: Rutaceae

Plant Origin: California, Italy

Extraction Method: Cold pressed from rind. It takes 3,000 lemons to produce 1 kilo of oil.

Key Constituents:

Limonene (59-73%)

Gamma-Terpinene (6-12%)

Beta-Pinene (7-16%)

Alpha-Pinene (1.5-3%)

Sabinene (1.5-3%)

ORAC: 660 µTE/100g

Historical Data: Lemon oil has been widely used in skin care to cleanse skin, reduce wrinkles, and combat acne. Lemon peel was used as an antiseptic, carminative, diuretic, eupeptic, a vascular stimulant and protector, and as a vitaminic (Arias, et al., 2005). It is also used as a flavorant, for cleaning, cooking, and to treat scurvy and a variety of other ailments.

Medical Properties: Antitumoral, antiseptic, improves microcirculation, immune stimulant (may increase white blood cells), improves memory, relaxation; rich in limonene, which has been extensively studied in over 50 clinical studies for its ability to combat tumor growth

Uses: Circulatory problems, arteriosclerosis, obesity, parasites, urinary tract infections, varicose veins, anxiety, hypertension, digestive problems, acne

Fragrant Influence: It promotes clarity of thought and purpose with a fragrance that is invigorating, enhancing, and warming. A Mie University study found that citrus fragrances boosted immunity, induced relaxation, and reduced depression (Komori, et al., 1995).

Application: Dilute 1 part essential oil with 1 part V-6 Vegetable Oil Complex or other pure vegetable oil; (1) apply 2-4 drops on location, (2) apply on chakras and/or Vita Flex points, (3) inhale directly, (4) diffuse, or (5) take as a dietary supplement.

Caution: Avoid applying to skin that will be exposed to sunlight or UV light within 24 hours.

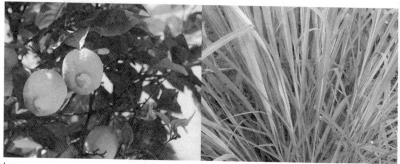

Lemon

Lemongrass

Found In: A·R·T Gentle Foaming Cleanser, A·R·T Purifying Toner, AlkaLime, Animal Scents Shampoo, AromaGuard Meadow Mist Deodorant, AromaGuard Mountain Mint Deodorant, Awaken, Citrus Fresh, Clarity, Digest & Cleanse, Deep Relief Roll-On, Dragon Time Bath & Shower Gel, Evening Peace Bath & Shower Gel, Forgiveness, Genesis Hand & Body Lotion, Gentle Baby, Harmony, Inner Defense, Joy, JuvaTone, KidScents Bath Gel, KidScents Shampoo, KidScents Slique Toothpaste, Lavender Bath & Shower Gel, Lavender Conditioner, Lavender Foaming Hand Soap, Lavender Hand & Body Lotion, Lavender Shampoo, Lemon-Sandalwood Cleansing Soap, Master Formula HERS, Master Formula HIS, MegaCal, Mineral Essence, MultiGreens, NingXia Red, Oola Balance, Orange Blossom Facial Wash, Power Meal, Raven, Sensation Hand & Body Lotion, Slique Essence, Super C, Surrender, Thieves, Thieves AromaBright Toothpaste, Thieves Cleansing Bar Soap, Thieves Dental Floss, Thieves Dentarome Plus Toothpaste, Thieves Dentarome Ultra Toothpaste, Thieves Foaming Hand Soap, Thieves Fresh Essence Plus Mouthwash, Thieves Household Cleaner, Thieves Lozenges (Hard, Soft), Thieves Spray, Thieves Waterless Hand Purifier, Thieves Wipes, Transformation

Lemongrass *(Cymbopogon flexuosus)*
Botanical Family: Poaceae
Plant Origin: India, Guatemala
Extraction Method: Steam distilled from herb/grass
Key Constituents:
Geranial (35-47%)
Geraniol (1.5-8%)
Neral (25-35%)
Geranyl Acetate (1-6%)
ORAC: 1,780 µTE/100g
Historical Data: Lemongrass is used for purification and digestion. Historically it was used for hypertension, inflammation, as a sedative, and for treatment of fevers and digestion. In a 2008 study, 91 single essential oils were tested against MRSA (Methicillin-resistant *Staphylococcus aureus*) and lemongrass. The study found that "Remarkably, lemongrass essential oil completely inhibited all MRSA growth on the plate" (Chao S, et al., 2008).

Medical Properties: Antifungal, antibacterial, antiparasitic, anti-inflammatory, regenerates connective tissues and ligaments, dilates blood vessels, improves circulation, promotes lymph flow, anticancerous. Several research articles document strong antifungal and antibacterial properties of lemongrass.

Uses: Bladder infection, respiratory/sinus infection, digestive problems, parasites, torn ligaments/muscles, fluid retention, varicose veins, Salmonella, *Candida albicans*

Fragrant Influence: Promotes psychic awareness and purification

Application: Dilute 1 part essential oil with 4 parts V-6 Vegetable Oil Complex or other pure vegetable oil; (1) apply 1-2 drops on location, (2) apply on chakras and/or Vita Flex points, (3) inhale directly, (4) diffuse, or (5) take as a dietary supplement.

Found In: DiGize, En-R-Gee, Essentialzymes-4, ICP, Inner Child, Inner Defense, Morning Start Bath & Shower Gel, Morning Start Moisturizing Soap, MultiGreens, Ortho Ease Massage Oil, Ortho Sport Massage Oil, Purification, Slique Slim Caps, Super C, SuperCal

Lemon Myrtle (*Backhousia citriodora*)

Botanical Family: Myrtaceae

Plant Origin: Australia

Extraction Method: Steam distilled from leaves

Key Constituents:
 Geranial (45-60%)
 Neral (30-45%)

ORAC: 2368 μmole TE/gram

Historical Data: The aboriginal people of Australia valued lemon myrtle's flavor in cooking, calling it "bush food." It is also known as the "queen of lemon herbs." Lemon myrtle can replace lemon in milk-based foods, as it does not have lemon's curdling problems. Lemon myrtle was also widely used as a healing plant. It is the highest natural source of the constituent citral. Since citral, consisting of isomers geranial and neral, has a strong and sweet lemon scent, lemon myrtle continues to be valued in perfumery. It is used in health care and cleaning products such as soaps, shampoos, and lotions. Lemon myrtle is cultivated in Queensland and the north coast of New South Wales, Australia.

Medical Properties: Antiseptic, antimicrobial, antifungal, anti-inflammatory, central nervous system stimulant

USES: Weight loss, respiratory/sinus infection, treatment of MCV in children

Fragrant Influences: Uplifting and invigorating, lemon myrtle's fresh and sweet lemon scent encourages follow-through with goals.

Application: Dilute 1 part essential oil with 4 parts V-6 Vegetable Oil Complex or other pure vegetable oil; (1) apply 1-2 drops on location, (2) apply on chakras and/or Vita Flex points, (3) inhale directly, (4) diffuse.

Found In: Slique Slim Caps

Lime (*Citrus latifolia* or *C. aurantifolia* Swingle)

Botanical Family: Rutaceae

Plant Origin: *C. latifolia:* Mexico, *C. aurantifolia* Swingle: Southeast Asia

Extraction Method: Cold expression from the rind of the unripe fruit

Key Constituents:
 Limonene (42-50%)
 Gamma-Terpinene (8-11%)
 Beta-Pinene (18-24%)

ORAC: 26,200 μTE/100g

Historical Data: Primarily used in skin care and in supporting and strengthening the respiratory and immune systems

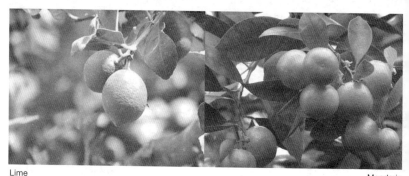

Lime

Mandarin

Medical Properties: Antirheumatic, antiviral, antibacterial

Uses: Skin conditions (acne, herpes), insect bites, respiratory problems, decongests the lymphatic system, weight loss

Application: (1) dilute 1 part essential oil with 1 part V-6 Vegetable Oil Complex or other pure vegetable oil, then apply on location, (2) apply on chakras and/or Vita Flex points, (3) inhale directly, (4) diffuse up to 30 minutes 3 times daily, or (5) dilute 1 part essential oil with 1 part V-6 Vegetable Oil Complex or other pure vegetable oil, put in a capsule, and take up to 3 times daily or as needed as a dietary supplement.

Caution: Avoid applying to skin that will be exposed to sunlight or UV light within 48 hours.

Found In: A·R·T Beauty Masque, AlkaLime, Common Sense, Copaiba Vanilla Moisturizing Conditioner, Copaiba Vanilla Moisturizing Shampoo, Stress Away, Stress Away Roll-On

Mandarin (*Citrus reticulata*)
  Botanical Family: Rutaceae
  Plant Origin: Madagascar, Italy
  Extraction Method: Cold pressed from rind
  Key Constituents:
    Limonene (65-75%)
    Gamma-Terpinene (16-22%)
    Alpha-Pinene (2-3%)
    Beta-Pinene (1.2-2%)
    Myrcene (1.5-2%)
  ORAC: 26,500 µTE/100g
  Historical Data: This fruit was traditionally given to Imperial Chinese officials named the Mandarins.

  Medical Properties: Light antispasmodic, digestive tonic (digestoid), antifungal, and stimulates gallbladder; rich in limonene, which has been extensively studied in over 50 clinical studies for its ability to combat tumor growth

  Uses: Digestive problems, fluid retention, insomnia, anxiety, intestinal problems, skin problems (congested and oily skin, scars, acne), stretch marks (when combined with either Jasmine, Lavender, Sandalwood, and/or Frankincense)

  Fragrant Influence: Appeasing, gentle, promotes happiness. A Mie University

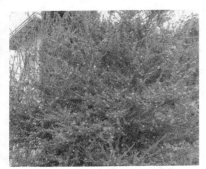
Manuka

study found that citrus fragrances boosted immunity, induced relaxation, and reduced depression (Komori, et al., 1995).

Application: Dilute 1 part essential oil with 1 part V-6 Vegetable Oil Complex or other pure vegetable oil; (1) apply 2-4 drops on location, (2) apply on chakras and/or Vita Flex points, (3) inhale directly, (4) diffuse, or (5) take as a dietary supplement.

Caution: Avoid applying to skin that will be exposed to sunlight or UV light within 24 hours.

Found In: Awaken, Citrus Fresh, Dragon Time Bath & Shower Gel, Joy

Manuka *(Leptospermum scoparium)*
Botanical Family: Myrtaceae
Plant Origin: New Zealand and Australia
Extraction Method: Steam distillation of chopped leaves and small stems
Key Constituents:
Leptospermone (16-19%)
Trans-Calamenene (12-16%)
Flavesone (2-8%)
Isoleptospermone (4-7%)
Alpha-Copaene (3-6%)
Cadena-3,5-diene (3-7%)
Alpha-Selinene (2-5%)

ORAC: 106,200 µTE/100g

Historical data: Similar to tea tree oil but warmer, richer, and milder, manuka oil has long been used in treatment of skin, foot, and hair problems. Like tea tree oil, it is antibacterial, antiviral, and antifungal, so it can help in eliminating a wide variety of problems. Some research suggests that manuka is more potent in fighting bacteria and fungi than tea tree oil. "Manuka" is the Maori name for the bushy tree from which the oil is produced.

Medical Properties: Antibacterial, antifungal, anti-inflammatory, anti-acne. Although research is ongoing, many believe manuka has potential in fighting antibiotic-resistant organisms, such as MRSA. A leading German aromatherapist reports that the manuka aroma is psychologically very beneficial for people who suffer from stress and anxiety. Its skin-healing properties are exceptional.

Uses: Skin infections, acne, bedsores, mild sunburn, fungal infections, itching, respiratory infections, sore throats, pain relief in muscles and joints, athletes foot and ringworm, dandruff, body odor, cold sores, dermatitis, rhinitis, tonsillitis, stress relief, sleep aid

Application: Apply 2-4 drops on affected area 1-3 times daily

Found In: Essential Beauty Serum (Acne-Prone Skin)

Marjoram *(Origanum majorana)*
Botanical Family: Lamiaceae
Plant Origin: France, Egypt
Extraction Method: Steam distilled from leaves
Key Constituents:
Terpinen-4-ol (20-33%)
Gamma-Terpinene (10-17%)

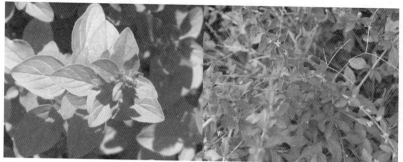

Marjoram

Mastrante

Linalol + Cis-4-Thujanol (4-26%)
Alpha-Terpinene (6-10%)
Alpha-Terpineol (2-7%)
Sabinene (4-9%)

ORAC: 130,900 µTE/100g

Historical Data: Marjoram was known as the "herb of happiness" to the Romans and "joy of the mountains" to the Greeks. It was believed to increase longevity. Listed in Dioscorides' *De Materia Medica* (AD 78), Europe's first authoritative guide to medicines, which became the standard reference work for herbal treatments for over 1,700 years. It was listed in Hildegard's *Medicine,* a compilation of early German medicines by highly regarded Benedictine herbalist Hildegard of Bingen (1098-1179).

Medical Properties: Its muscle-soothing properties help relieve body and joint discomfort. May also help soothe the digestive tract and is a general relaxant. Antibacterial, antifungal, vasodilator, lowers blood pressure, promotes intestinal peristalsis, expectorant, mucolytic.

Uses: Arthritis/rheumatism, muscle/nerve pain, headaches, circulatory disorders, respiratory infections, menstrual problems/PMS, fungal infections, ringworm, shingles, sores, spasms, and fluid retention

Fragrant Influence: Assists in calming the nerves

Application: Dilute 1 part essential oil with 1 part V-6 Vegetable Oil Complex or other pure vegetable oil; (1) apply 2-4 drops on location, (2) apply on chakras and/or Vita Flex points, (3) inhale directly, (4) diffuse, or (5) take as a dietary supplement.

Found In: Aroma Life, Aroma Siez, Dragon Time, Dragon Time Bath & Shower Gel, M-Grain, Ortho Ease Massage Oil, R.C., SuperCal

Mastrante *(Lippia alba)*

Botanical Family: Verbenaceae

Plant Origin: Ecuador

Extraction Method: Steam distilled from leaves

Key Constituents:
Carvone (35-50%)
Limonene (20-30%)
Germacrene D (10-17%)
Alpha-Bourbonene (1-3%)
Camphor (0.5-2%)

Historical Data: The plant Mastrante *(Lippia alba)* was given its botanical name by the Scottish botanist Philip Miller (1691-1771)

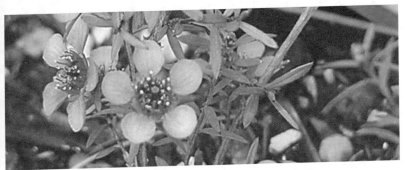
Melaleuca Alternifolia

and the British plant taxonomist N.E. Brown (1849-1934). As a result, in the scientific literature it is listed as: *"Lippia alba* (Miller or Mill.) N.E. Brown." In Brazil, it is called *"erva cidreira do campo,"* which means "lemon balm of the field." The aromatic shrub grows in southern Texas, Mexico, the Caribbean, and Central and South America. The leaves of Mastrante are used to flavor foods, most notably molé sauces from Oaxaca, Mexico. In folk medicine it is known as a sedative, an antidepressant, and has pain-relieving properties.

Medical Properties: Antioxidant, analgesic, antibacterial, antiviral, antifungal, antispasmodic

Uses: Anticandida agent, coughs, bronchitis, migraine headaches in women, as a vasorelaxant for heart disease

Fragrant Influence: This earthy aroma is grounding and calming.

Application: Dilute 1 part essential oil with 1 part V-6 Vegetable Oil Complex or other pure vegetable oil; (1) apply 2-4 drops on location, (2) apply on chakras and/or Vita Flex points, (3) inhale directly, or (4) diffuse.

Melaleuca Alternifolia
(Melaleuca alternifolia)

Botanical Family: Myrtaceae

Plant Origin: Australia, France

Extraction Method: Steam distilled from leaves

Key Constituents:
Terpinen-4-ol (30-45%)
Gamma-Terpinene (10-28%)
Alpha-Terpinene (5-13%)
1,8-Cineole (Eucalyptol) (0-15%)
Alpha-Terpineol (1.5-8%)
Para-Cymene (0.5-12%)
Limonene (0.5-4%)
Aromadendrene (trace-7%)
Delta-Cadinene (trace-8%)
Alpha-Pinene (1-6%)

Historical Data: Highly regarded as an antimicrobial and antiseptic essential oil. It has high levels of terpinen-4-ol.

Medical Properties: Powerful antibacterial, antifungal, antiviral, antiparasitic, anti-inflammatory action

Uses: Fungal infections (Candida, ringworm), sinus/lung infections, tooth/gum disease, water retention/hypertension, skin conditions (acne, sores)

Fragrant Influence: Promotes cleansing and purity

Application: Dilute 1 part essential oil with 1 part V-6 Vegetable Oil Complex or other pure vegetable oil; (1) apply 2-4 drops on location, (2) apply on chakras and/or Vita Flex points, (3) inhale directly, or (4) diffuse.

Found In: Animal Scents Ointment, AromaGuard Meadow Mist Deodorant, ClaraDerm, Essential Beauty Serum (Acne-Prone Skin), Melaleuca-Geranium Moisturizing Soap, Melrose, ParaFree, Purification, Rehemogen, Rose Ointment

Melaleuca Cajuput (Var. Cajeput)
(Melaleuca leucadendron)

Botanical Family: Myrtaceae

Plant Origin: Australia

Extraction Method: Steam distilled from leaves

Key Constituents:
1,8-Cineole (Eucalyptol) (50-65%)
Alpha-Terpineol (7-13%)
Limonene (3-8%)
Alpha-Pinene (1-3%)

ORAC: 37,600 µTE/100g

Historical Data: Traditionally used in Malaysia and other Indonesian islands for respiratory/throat infections, headaches, rheumatism, toothache, skin conditions, and sore muscles. Cajuput derives its name from the Malaysian word for white tree.

Medical Properties: Antibacterial, antiparasitic, antispasmodic, anti-inflammatory, analgesic

Uses: Throat/lung/sinus infections, urinary tract infections, coughs, intestinal problems

Application: (1) Dilute 1 drop essential oil with 1 drop V-6 Vegetable Oil Complex or other pure vegetable oil and apply on location, (2) apply on chakras and/or Vita Flex points, (3) inhale directly, (4) diffuse up to 30 minutes 3 times daily, or (5) dilute 1 part essential oil with 1 part V-6 Vegetable Oil Complex or other pure vegetable oil, put in a capsule, and take up to 3 times daily or as needed as a dietary supplement.

Caution: Do not use synthetic cajuput, as it could cause further blistering and skin eruption.

Melaleuca Ericifolia *(Melaleuca ericifolia)*

Botanical Family: Myrtaceae

Plant Origin: Australia

Extraction Method: Steam distilled from leaves and branches

Key Constituents:
Alpha-Pinene (5-10%)
1,8-Cineole + Beta-Phellandrene (18-28%)
Alpha-Terpineol (1-5%)
Para-Cymene (1-6%)
Linalol (34-45%)
Aromadendrene (2-6%)

ORAC: 61,100 µTE/100g

Medical Properties: Powerful antibacterial, antifungal, antiviral, antiparasitic, anti-inflammatory

Uses: Herpes virus, respiratory/sinus infections

Application: Dilute 1 part essential oil with 1 part V-6 Vegetable Oil Complex or other pure vegetable oil; (1) apply 2-4 drops on location, temples, wrists, throat, face, or chest, (2) apply on chakras and/or Vita Flex points, (3) inhale directly, (4) diffuse, or (5) take as a dietary supplement.

Found In: Melaleuca-Geranium Moisturizing Soap

Melaleuca Quinquenervia
(Melaleuca quinquenervia)
(also found in literature as Niaouli)

Botanical Family: Myrtaceae

Plant Origin: Australia, New Caledonia

Extraction Method: Steam distilled from leaves and twigs

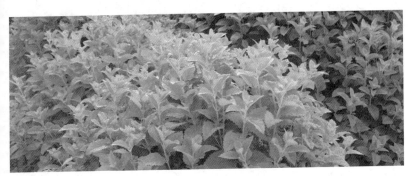
Melissa

Key Constituents:
1,8-Cineole (Eucalyptol) (55-75%)
Alpha-Pinene (5-12%)
Limonene (1-9%)
Beta-Pinene (1-5%)
Viridiflorol (2-6%)

ORAC: 18,600 μTE/100g

Medical Properties: Male hormone-like, anti-inflammatory, antibacterial, antiviral, and antiparasitic (amoeba and parasites in the blood), vasodilating, skin penetration enhancer (hormones)

Uses: Hypertension, urinary tract/bladder infections, respiratory/sinus infections, allergies

Application: Dilute 1 part essential oil with 1 part V-6 Vegetable Oil Complex or other pure vegetable oil; (1) apply 2-4 drops on location, (2) apply on chakras and/or Vita Flex points, (3) inhale directly, or (4) diffuse.

Found In: AromaGuard Meadow Mist Deodorant, Melrose

Melissa (Melissa officinalis)
(Also known as lemon balm)
  Botanical Family: Lamiaceae
  Plant Origin: Utah, Idaho, France

Extraction Method: Steam distilled from aerial parts before flowering

Key Constituents:
Geranial (25-35%)
Neral (18-28%)
Beta-Caryophyllene (12-19%)

ORAC: 134,300 μTE/100g

Historical Data: Anciently, melissa was used for nervous disorders and many different ailments dealing with the heart or the emotions. It was also used to promote fertility. Melissa was the main ingredient in Carmelite water, distilled in France since 1611 by the Carmelite monks.

Medical Properties: Anti-inflammatory, antiviral, relaxant, hypotensive, anti-oxidative, antitumoral

Uses: Viral infections (herpes, etc.), depression, anxiety, insomnia

Fragrant Influence: Brings out gentle characteristics within people. It is calming and uplifting and balances emotions. It removes emotional blocks and instills a positive outlook on life.

Application: (1) Apply 2-4 drops directly to affected area as needed; dilution not required except for extremely sensitive skin, (2) apply on chakras and/or Vita Flex

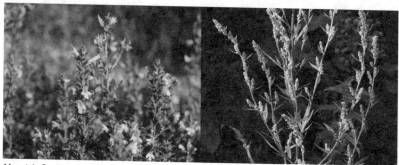

Mountain Savory

Mugwort

points, (3) inhale directly, (4) diffuse up to 1 hour 3 times daily or (5) put 2 drops of Melissa in a capsule, take as dietary supplement 3 times daily or as needed.

Found In: A·R·T Gentle Foaming Cleanser, A·R·T Purifying Toner, Awaken, Brain Power, Forgiveness, Hope, Humility, Live with Passion, MultiGreens, White Angelica

Micromeria *(Micromeria fruticosa)*
Botanical Family: Lamiaceae
Plant Origin: Israel
Extraction Method: Steam distilled from leaf, stem, and flower
Key Constituents:
Pulegone (50-65%)
Menthol (7-12%)
Beta-Caryophyllene (3-9%)
Isopulegol (3-6%)
Menthone (1-5%)
Neomenthol (1-5%)
Historical Data: Micromeria is found in Israel and in the eastern Mediterranean. It is known in folk medicine as having anti-inflammatory properties and for digestive support.
Medical Properties: Anti-inflammatory, gastroprotective

Uses: Stomach upsets
Fragrant Influence: Revitalizes and refreshes the mind
Application: Dilute 1 part essential oil with 2 parts V-6 Vegetable Oil Complex or other pure vegetable oil; (1) apply 2-4 drops on location, (2) apply on chakras and/or Vita Flex points.
Caution: Contains high levels of pulegone. Do not use if pregnant or trying to conceive.

Mountain Savory *(Satureja montana)*
Botanical Family: Lamiaceae
Plant Origin: France
Extraction Method: Steam distilled from flowering plant
Key Constituents:
Carvacrol (22-35%)
Thymol (14-24%)
Gamma-Terpinene (8-15%)
Carvacrol Methyl Ether (4-9%)
Beta-Caryophyllene (3-7%)
ORAC: 11,300 µTE/100g
Historical Data: Mountain savory has been used historically as a general tonic for the body.
Medical Properties: Strong antibacterial, antifungal, antiviral, antiparasitic, immune

stimulant, anti-inflammatory action

Uses: Viral infections (herpes, HIV, etc.), scoliosis/lumbago/back problems

Fragrant Influence: Revitalizes and stimulates the nervous system. It is a powerful energizer and motivator.

Application: Dilute 1 part essential oil with 4 parts V-6 Vegetable Oil Complex or other pure vegetable oil; (1) apply 2-4 drops on location, (2) apply on chakras and/or Vita Flex points, (3) diffuse, or (4) take as a dietary supplement.

Found In: ImmuPower, Surrender

Mugwort (Artemisia vulgaris)

Botanical Family: Asteraceae

Plant Origin: Canada

Extraction Method: Steam distilled from leaves and roots

Key Constituents:
Sabinene (6-14%)
Myrcene (20-30%)
Linalol (6-18%)
Beta-Thujone (2-19%)
Trans-Beta-Caryophyllene (2-12%)

Historical Data: Used by Chinese in moxibustion (an indirect heat treatment). Was worn to protect against evil spirits in 14th century England. Introduced by the Portuguese to the French in the 1800s, where it became known as a cure for blindness and other diseases. Has been placed under pillows to produce vivid dreams.

Medical Properties: Antibacterial, antifungal, antiparasitic, gastrointestinal regulator

Uses: Intestinal complaints, worm infestations, headaches, muscle spasms, circulatory problems, menstrual problems/PMS, dysentery, gout

Application: Dilute 1 part essential oil with 1 part V-6 Vegetable Oil Complex or other pure vegetable oil; (1) apply 1-2 drops on location, (2) apply on chakras and/or Vita Flex points, (3) diffuse, or (4) take as a dietary supplement.

Found In: ComforTone, Inspiration

Myrrh (Commiphora myrrha)

Botanical Family: Burseraceae

Plant Origin: Somalia

Extraction Method: Steam distilled from gum/resin

Key Constituents:
Lindestrene (7-16%)
Curzerene (9-32%)
Furanoendesma-1,3-diene (25-50%)
2-Methoxy Furanogermacrene (1-10%)
Beta-Elemene (1-9%)

ORAC: 379,800 µTE/100g

Historical Data: It is mentioned in one of the oldest known medical records, the Ebers Papyrus (dating from 16th century BC), an ancient Egyptian list of 877 prescriptions and recipes. The Arabian people used myrrh for many skin conditions such as chapped and cracked skin and wrinkles. It was listed in Hildegard's *Medicine*, a compilation of early German medicines by highly regarded Benedictine herbalist Hildegard of Bingen (1098-1179).

Medical Properties: Powerful antioxidant, antitumoral, anti-inflammatory, antibacterial, antiviral, antiparasitic, analgesic/anesthetic

Uses: Diabetes, cancer, hepatitis, fungal infections (Candida, ringworm), tooth/gum infections, skin conditions (eczema, chapped, cracked, wrinkles, stretch marks)

Fragrant Influence: Promotes spiritual awareness and is uplifting. It contains sesquiterpenes, which stimulate the limbic system of the brain (the center of memory and emotions) and the

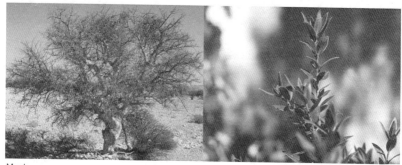

Myrrh

Myrtle

hypothalamus, pineal, and pituitary glands. The hypothalamus is the master gland of the human body, producing many vital hormones, including thyroid and growth hormone.

Application: (1) Apply 2-4 drops on location, (2) apply on chakras and/or Vita Flex points, (3) inhale directly, (4) diffuse, or (5) take as a dietary supplement.

Found In: Abundance, Animal Scents Ointment, Boswellia Wrinkle Cream, ClaraDerm, Egyptian Gold, EndoGize, Essential Beauty Serum (Dry Skin), Exodus II, Gratitude, Hope, Humility, Lavender Bath & Shower Gel, Lavender Foaming Hand Soap, Lavender Hand & Body Lotion, Oola Balance, Protec, Rose Ointment, Sandalwood Moisture Cream, The Gift, 3 Wise Men, Thyromin, White Angelica

Bible References:

Genesis 37:25—"And they sat down to eat bread: and they lifted up their eyes and looked, and behold, a company of Ishmeelites came from Gilead with their camels bearing spicery and balm and myrrh, going to carry it down to Egypt."

Genesis 43:11—"And their father Israel said unto them, If it must be so now, do this; take of the best fruits in the land in your vessels, and carry down the man a present, a little balm, and a little honey, spices, and myrrh, nuts, and almonds:"

Exodus 30:23—"Take thou also unto thee principal spices, of pure myrrh five hundred shekels, and of sweet cinnamon half so much, even two hundred and fifty shekels, and of sweet calamus two hundred and fifty shekels,"

Myrtle (Myrtus communis)

Botanical Family: Myrtaceae

Plant Origin: Tunisia, Morocco

Extraction Method: Steam distilled from leaves

Key Constituents:

Alpha-Pinene (15-60%)

1,8-Cineole (Eucalyptol) (15-40%)

Limonene (4-18%)

Myrtenyl Acetate (trace-20%)

ORAC: 25,400 µTE/100g

Historical Data: Myrtle has been researched by Dr. Daniel Pénoël for normalizing hormonal imbalances of the thyroid and ovaries, as well as balancing the hypothyroid. It has also been researched for its soothing effects on the respiratory system.

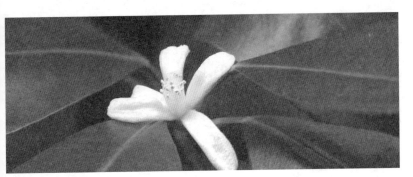
Neroli

Medical Properties: Antimutagenic, liver stimulant, prostate and thyroid stimulant, sinus/lung decongestant, antispasmodic, antihyperglycemic, anti-inflammatory, antinociceptive

Uses: Thyroid problems, throat/lung/sinus infections, prostate problems, skin irritations (acne, blemishes, bruises, oily skin, psoriasis, etc.), muscle spasms

Fragrant Influence: Elevating and euphoric

Application: Dilute 1 part essential oil with 1 part V-6 Vegetable Oil Complex or other pure vegetable oil; (1) apply 2-4 drops on location, (2) apply on chakras and/or Vita Flex points, (3) inhale directly, (4) diffuse or put in humidifier, or (5) take as a dietary supplement.

Found In: Breathe Again Roll-On, EndoFlex, Inspiration, JuvaTone, Mister, Prostate Health, Purification, R.C., SuperCal, Thyromin

Bible References:
Nehemiah 8:15—"And that they should publish and proclaim in all their cities, and in Jerusalem, saying, Go forth unto the mount, and fetch olive branches, and pine branches, and myrtle branches, and palm branches, and branches of thick trees, to make booths, as it is written."

Isaiah 41:19—"I will plant in the wilderness the cedar, the shittah tree, and the myrtle, and the oil tree; I will set in the desert the fir tree, and the pine, and the box tree together:"

Isaiah 55:13—"Instead of the thorn shall come up the fir tree, and instead of the brier shall come up the myrtle tree: and it shall be to the Lord for a name, for an everlasting sign that shall not be cut off."

Neroli (Citrus aurantium)

Botanical Family: Rutaceae

Plant Origin: Tunisia

Extraction Method: Absolute extraction from flowers of the bitter orange tree

Key Constituents:
Linalol (28-44%)
Limonene (9-18%)
Beta-Pinene (7-17%)
Linalyl Acetate (3-15%)
Trans-Ocimene (3-8%)
Alpha-Terpineol (2-5.5%)
Trans-Nerolidol (1-5%)
Myrcene (1-4%)

Historical Data: Highly regarded by the ancient Egyptians for its ability to heal the

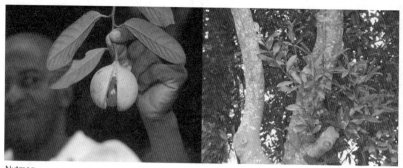

Nutmeg

Ocotea

mind, body, and spirit.

Medical Properties: Antiparasitic, digestive tonic, antidepressive, hypotensive (lowers blood pressure)

Uses: Hypertension, anxiety, depression, hysteria, insomnia, skin conditions (scars, stretch marks, thread veins, wrinkles)

Fragrant Influence: A natural relaxant used to treat depression and anxiety. It strengthens and stabilizes the emotions and uplifts and inspires the hopeless, encouraging confidence, courage, joy, peace, and sensuality. It brings everything into focus at the moment.

Application: Dietary Supplement: Dilution not required except for the most sensitive skin; (1) apply 2-4 drops on location, (2) apply on chakras and/or Vita Flex points, (3) inhale directly, (4) diffuse up to 1 hour 3 times daily, or (5) dilute 1 part essential oil with 1 part V-6 Vegetable Oil Complex or other pure vegetable oil, put in a capsule, and take up to 3 times daily or as needed.

Found In: Acceptance, Awaken, Humility, Inner Child, Live with Passion, Oola Grow, Present Time

Nutmeg (*Myristica fragrans*)

Botanical Family: Myristicaceae

Plant Origin: Tunisia, Indonesia

Extraction Method: Steam distilled from fruits and seeds

Key Constituents:
Sabinene (14-29%)
Beta-Pinene (13-18%)
Alpha-Pinene (15-28%)
Limonene (2-7%)
Gamma-Terpinene (2-6%)
Terpinene-4-ol (2-6%)
Myristicine (5-12%)

ORAC: 158,100 µTE/100g

Historical Data: It was listed in Hildegard's *Medicine,* a compilation of early German medicines by highly regarded Benedictine herbalist Hildegard of Bingen (1098-1179).

Medical Properties: Anti-inflammatory, anticoagulant, antiseptic, antiparasitic, analgesic, liver protectant, stomach protectant (ulcers), circulatory stimulant, adrenal stimulant, muscle relaxing, increases production of growth hormone/melatonin

Uses: Rheumatism/arthritis, cardiovascular disease, hypertension, hepatitis, ulcers, digestive disorders, antiparasitic, nerve pain, fatigue/exhaustion, neuropathy

Application: Dilute 1 part essential oil with 2 parts V-6 Vegetable Oil Complex or other pure vegetable oil; (1) apply 1-2 drops on location, (2) apply on chakras and/or Vita Flex points, (3) inhale directly, (4) diffuse, or (5) take as a dietary supplement.

Found In: EndoFlex, En-R-Gee, Magnify Your Purpose, NingXia Nitro, ParaFree, Power Meal

Ocotea *(Ocotea quixos)*

Botanical Family: Lauraceae

Plant Origin: Ecuador, Central and South America

Extraction Method: Steam distilled from the leaves

Key Constituents:
Beta-Caryophyllene (10-35%)
Cinnamyl Acetate (1-24%)
Methyl Cinnamate (4-24%)
Alpha-Humulene (1-17%)
Trans-Cinnamaldehyde (trace-12%)

Historical Data: Ocotea is distilled from a tree found in the Amazon wilderness, on the ranges of the west side of the Andes Mountains. It is commonly referred to by the native people throughout Ecuador as false canilla or false cinnamon. The tree grows to a very large size, reaching up to 48 inches in diameter and over 60 feet tall, making a large canopy top. Historical usage of ocotea dates back more than 500 years, when it was used to aromatize sweets and cakes.

Medical Properties: Antifungal, disinfectant, anti-inflammatory

Uses: Hypertension, high blood pressure, anxiety, internal irritation, may lower insulin needs for diabetics and reduce blood sugar fluctuations, infection, digestive support

Fragrant Influence: Has a complex aroma, which may increase feelings of fullness;

related to the cinnamon species but has an aroma that is different from any common cinnamon

Application: Dilute 1 part essential oil with 2 parts V-6 Vegetable Oil Complex or other pure vegetable oil; (1) apply 1-2 drops on location (test on a small, inconspicuous area of skin to observe sensitivity), (2) apply on chakras and/or Vita Flex points, (3) inhale directly, (4) diffuse, or (5) put in a capsule and take 1 daily or as directed by a health professional.

Found In: A·R·T Beauty Masque, A·R·T Creme Masque, Common Sense, KidScents Slique Toothpaste, Oola Balance, Slique Essence, Slique Tea, Stress Away, Stress Away Roll-On, Thieves AromaBright Toothpaste, Transformation

Orange *(Citrus sinensis)*

Botanical Family: Rutaceae

Plant Origin: USA, South Africa, Italy, China

Extraction Method: Cold pressed from rind

Key Constituents:
Limonene (85-96%)
Myrcene (0.5-3%)

ORAC: 1,890 µTE/100g

Medical Properties: Antitumoral, relaxant, anticoagulant, circulatory stimulant. Rich in limonene, which has been extensively studied in over 50 clinical studies for its ability to combat tumor growth.

Uses: Arteriosclerosis, hypertension, cancer, insomnia, and complexion (dull and oily), fluid retention, wrinkles

Fragrant Influence: Uplifting and antidepressant. A Mie University study found that citrus fragrances boosted immunity, induced relaxation, and reduced depression (Komori, et al., 1995).

Application: Dilute 1 part essential oil with 1 part V-6 Vegetable Oil Complex or other

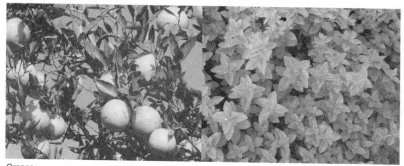

Orange

Oregano

pure vegetable oil; (1) apply 2-4 drops on location, (2) apply on chakras and/or Vita Flex points, (3) inhale directly, (4) diffuse, or (5) take as a dietary supplement.

Caution: Avoid applying to skin that will be exposed to sunlight or UV light within 24 hours.

Found In: Abundance, Awaken, Balance Complete, Christmas Spirit, Cinnamint Lip Balm, Citrus Fresh, Envision, Harmony, ImmuPro, Inner Child, Into the Future, Lady Sclareol, Longevity, Longevity Softgels, NingXia Red, Oola Balance, Oola Grow, Peace & Calming, Power Meal, Pure Protein Complete, SARA, Slique Bars, Super C, Super C Chewable, Thieves Foaming Hand Soap, Thieves Lozenges (Soft)

Oregano *(Origanum vulgare)*

Botanical Family: Lamiaceae

Plant Origin: USA, France, Germany, Turkey

Extraction Method: Steam distilled from leaves

Key Constituents:
Carvacrol (60-75%)
Gamma-Terpinene (3.5-8.5%)
Para-Cymene (5.5-9%)
Beta-Caryophyllene (2-5%)
Myrcene (1-3%)
Thymol (0-5%)

ORAC: 15,300 µTE/100g

Historical Data: Listed in Hildegard's *Medicine,* a compilation of early German medicines by highly regarded Benedictine herbalist Hildegard of Bingen (1098-1179).

Medical Properties: Antiaging, powerful anti-viral, antibacterial, antifungal, antiparasitic, anti-inflammatory, antioxidant, immune stimulant, antinociceptive, radioprotective, liver protectant

Uses: Arthritis, rheumatism, respiratory infectious diseases, infections, tuberculosis, digestive problems

Fragrant Influence: Creates a feeling of security.

Application: Dilute 1 part essential oil with 4 parts V-6 Vegetable Oil Complex or other pure vegetable oil; (1) apply 1-2 drops on location (or neat as in Raindrop Technique), (2) apply on chakras and/or Vita Flex points, (3) diffuse, or (4) take as a dietary supplement.

Caution: High in phenols, Oregano may irritate the nasal membranes or skin if

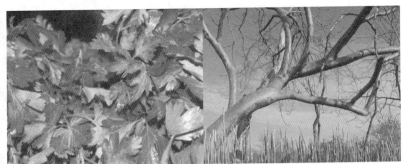

Palmarosa

Palo Santo

inhaled directly from diffuser or bottle or applied neat.

Found In: ImmuPower, Inner Defense, Ortho Sport Massage Oil, Regenolone Moisturizing Cream

Palmarosa *(Cymbopogon martini)*

Botanical Family: Poaceae

Plant Origin: India

Extraction Method: Steam distilled from leaves

Key Constituents:
Geraniol (70-85%)
Geranyl Acetate (6-10%)
Linalol (3-7%)

ORAC: 127,800 µTE/100g

Historical Data: A relative of lemongrass, palmarosa was used in temple incense by the ancient Egyptians.

Medical Properties: Antibacterial, antifungal, antiviral, supports heart and nervous system, reduces blood sugar fluctuations, stimulates new skin cell growth, regulates sebum production in skin

Uses: Fungal infections/Candida, neuroprotective, cardiovascular/circulatory diseases, digestive problems, skin problems (acne, eczema)

Fragrant Influence: Creates a feeling of security. It also helps to reduce stress and tension and promotes recovery from nervous exhaustion.

Application: Dilute 1 part essential oil with 1 part V-6 Vegetable Oil Complex or other pure vegetable oil, put in a capsule, and take up to 3 times daily; (1) apply 2-4 drops on location, dilution not required except for the most sensitive skin, (2) apply on chakras and/or Vita Flex points, (3) inhale directly, (4) diffuse up to 1 hour 3 times daily, or (5) take as a dietary supplement.

Found In: Animal Scents Ointment, Awaken, Clarity, Dragon Time Bath & Shower Gel, Evening Peace Bath & Shower Gel, Forgiveness, Genesis Hand & Body Lotion, Gentle Baby, Harmony, Joy, Oola Balance, Rose Ointment, Sensation Hand & Body Lotion

Palo Santo *(Bursera graveolens)*

Botanical Family: Burseraceae

Plant Origin: Ecuador

Extraction Method: Steam distilled from the sawdust of the dead bark, wood, and branches

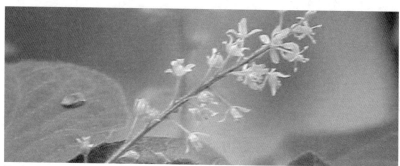
Patchouli

Key Constitutents:
>Limonene (45-80%)
>Alpha-Terpineol (4-18%)
>Para-Cymene (1-6%)
>Carvone (0.5-6%)
>Beta-Bisabolene (0.5-7)
>Fonenol (0.5-4%)
>**Note:** Constituents can vary depending on whether the wood is harvested from coastal or inland areas and if the trunk is red or white.

Historical Data: Palo Santo comes from the same botanical family as Frankincense, although it is found in South America. Like Frankincense, Palo Santo is known as a spiritual oil, with a deep-rooted tradition in which it was used by the Incas to purify and cleanse the air of negative energies and for good luck. It is used in South America to repel mosquitoes, for fevers, infections, and skin diseases. It is currently used by shamans of the Andes in curing ceremonies. Even its Spanish name reflects how highly this oil was regarded: *palo santo* means "holy or sacred wood."

Medical Properties: Anticancerous, antiblastic, anti-inflammatory, antibacterial, antifungal, antiviral

Uses: Inflammation, regrowth of knee cartilage, joints, arthritis, rheumatism, gout, respiratory problems, reduces airborne contaminants when diffused

Applications: Dilute 1 part essential oil with 1 part V-6 Vegetable Oil Complex or other pure vegetable oil; (1) apply 2-4 drops on location, (2) apply on chakras and/or Vita Flex points, (3) inhale directly, (4) diffuse, or (5) take as a dietary supplement 10-15 drops in a capsule 1 or 2 times a day, 1-6 drops under the tongue, or in a glass of water.

Cautions: If pregnant or under a doctor's care, consult your physician. Should not be used on children under 18 months old.

Found In: Deep Relief Roll-On, Transformation

Patchouli *(Pogostemon cablin)*
>**Botanical Family:** Lamiaceae
>**Plant Origin:** Indonesia
>**Extraction Method:** Steam distilled from flowers
>**Key Constituents:**
>>Patchoulol (27-35%)
>>Bulnesene (13-21%)
>>Alpha-Guaiene (11-16%)

Beta-Patchoulene (1.8-3.5%)
Beta-Caryophyllene (2-5%)
Pogostol (1-2.5%)
Norpatchoulenol (0.35-1%)
Copaene (trace-1%)

ORAC: 49,400 µTE/100g

Medical Properties: Relaxant, antitumoral, digestive aid that combats nausea, anti-inflammatory, antimicrobial, antifungal, insecticidal, prevents wrinkles and chapped skin, relieves itching

Uses: Hypertension, inflammatory bowel disease, skin conditions (eczema, acne), fluid retention, Listeria infection, insect repellent

Application: (1) Apply 2-4 drops on location, (2) apply on chakras and/or Vita Flex points, (3) inhale directly, (4) diffuse, or (5) take as a dietary supplement.

Fragrant Influence: A relaxant that clarifies thoughts, allowing the discarding of jealousies, obsessions, and insecurities.

Found In: Abundance, Allerzyme, Animal Scents Ointment, DiGize, Live with Passion, Magnify Your Purpose, Orange Blossom Facial Wash, Peace & Calming, Rose Ointment

Peppermint *(Mentha piperita)*
Botanical Family: Lamiaceae
Plant Origin: North America, Mediterranean area, Great Britain
Extraction Method: Steam distilled from leaves and stems
Key Constituents:
Menthol (25-50%)
Menthone (12-44%)
Menthofuran (0.5-5%)
1.8-Cineole (Eucalyptol) (1-8%)
Isomenthone (1-7%)
Neomenthol (1.5-7%)
Pulegone (0.5-3%)
Menthyl Acetate (1-18%)

ORAC: 37,300 µTE/100g

Historical Data: Peppermint is one of the oldest and most highly regarded herbs for soothing digestion. Jean Valnet, MD, studied peppermint's effect on the liver and respiratory systems. Alan Hirsch, MD, studied peppermint's ability to directly affect the brain's satiety center (the ventromedial nucleus of the hypothalamus), which triggers a sensation of fullness after meals. A highly regarded digestive stimulant.

Medical Properties: Anti-inflammatory, antitumoral, antiparasitic (worms), antibacterial, antiviral, antifungal, gallbladder/digestive stimulant, pain relieving, curbs appetite

Uses: Rheumatism/arthritis, respiratory infections (pneumonia, tuberculosis, etc.), obesity, viral infections (herpes simplex, herpes zoster, cold sores, human papilloma virus, etc.), fungal infections/Candida, digestive problems, headaches, nausea, skin conditions (itchy skin, varicose veins, eczema, psoriasis, dermatitis), scoliosis/lumbago/back problems

Fragrant Influence: Purifying and stimulating to the conscious mind. Research indicates that peppermint aroma, inhaled during mental tasks, may help attention, performance, and focus (Barker, et al., 2003). Peppermint may also be an effective appetite suppressant when inhaled (Hirsch and Gomez, 1995). University of Kiel researchers found that peppermint lessened headache pain in a double-blind, placebo-controlled, cross-over study.

Application: Dilute 1 part essential oil with 2 parts V-6 Vegetable Oil Complex or other pure vegetable oil; (1) apply 1-2 drops on location, abdomen, and/or temples; (2) apply on chakras and/or Vita Flex points; (3) inhale directly; (4) diffuse; or (5) take as a dietary supplement.

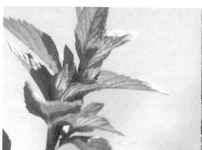
Peppermint

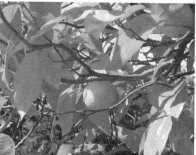
Petitgrain

To improve concentration, alertness, and memory, place 1-2 drops on the tongue. Inhale 5-10 times a day to curb appetite.

Cautions: Avoid contact with eyes, mucus membranes, sensitive skin, or fresh wounds or burns. Do not apply on infants younger than 18 months of age.

Found In: Allerzyme, Aroma Siez, AromaGuard Mountain Mint Deodorant, BLM, Breathe Again Roll-On, Chocolessence, Cinnamint Lip Balm, Clarity, ComforTone, CortiStop Women's, Deep Relief Roll-On, DiGize, Digest & Cleanse, Einkorn Nuggets, Essentialzyme, Essentialzymes-4, KidScents Mightyzyme, Lavender Mint Daily Conditioner, Lavender Mint Daily Shampoo, M-Grain, Mineral Essence, Mister, Morning Start Bath & Shower Gel, Morning Start Moisturizing Soap, NingXia Nitro, Ortho Ease Massage Oil, Ortho Sport Massage Oil, PanAway, Peppermint-Cedarwood Moisturizing Soap, Progessence Phyto Plus, Progessence Plus, Prostate Health, R.C., Raven, Regenolone Moisturizing Cream, Relaxation Massage Oil, Relieve It, Satin Facial Scrub Mint, SclarEssence, Slique Gum, Thieves AromaBright Toothpaste, Thieves Dental Floss, Thieves Dentarome Plus Toothpaste, Thieves Dentarome Ultra Toothpaste, Thieves Fresh Essence Plus Mouthwash, Thieves Lozenges (Hard, Soft), Thieves Waterless Hand Purifier, Thyromin, Transformation

Petitgrain *(Citrus sinensis)*
(Syn. Citrus aurantium amara)

Botanical Family: Rutaceae

Plant Origin: Paraguay

Extraction Method: Steam distilled from leaves and twigs

Key Constituents:
Linalyl Acetate (40-55%)
Linalol (15-30%)
Alpha-Terpineol (3.5-7.5%)
Geranyl Acetate (2-5%)
Geraniol (2-4.5%)

ORAC: 73,600 µTE/100g

Historical Data: Petitgrain derives its name from the extraction of the oil, which at one time was from the green, unripe oranges when they were still about the size of a cherry.

Medical Properties: Antispasmodic, anti-inflammatory, relaxant, reestablishes nerve equilibrium

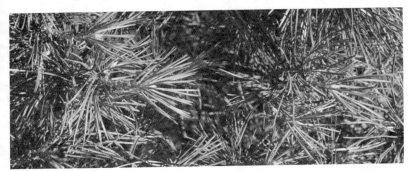
Pine

Uses: Insomnia, anxiety, muscle spasms, skin conditions, antitumoral

Fragrant Influence: Uplifting and refreshing to the senses; clears confusion, reduces mental fatigue and depression; stimulates the mind and improves memory.

Application: (1) Apply 2 drops on location, dilution not required except for the most sensitive skin; (2) apply on chakras and/or Vita Flex points; (3) inhale directly; or (4) diffuse up to 1 hour 3 times daily; (5) take as a dietary supplement.

Pine *(Pinus sylvestris)*
Botanical Family: Pinaceae (pine)
Plant Origin: Austria, USA, Canada
Extraction Method: Steam distilled from needles
Key Constituents:
Alpha-Pinene (55-70%)
Beta-Pinene (3-8%)
Limonene (5-10%)
Delta-3-Carene (6-12%)
Historical Data: Pine was first investigated by Hippocrates, the father of Western medicine, for its benefits to the respiratory system. In 1990, Dr. Pénoël and Dr. Franchomme described pine oil's antiseptic

properties in their medical textbook. Pine is used in massage for stressed muscles and joints. It shares many of the same properties as *Eucalyptus globulus*, and the action of both oils is enhanced when blended. Native Americans stuffed mattresses with pine needles to repel lice and fleas. It was used to treat lung infections and even added to baths to revitalize those suffering from mental or emotional fatigue.

Medical Properties: Hormone-like, antidiabetic, cortisone-like, antiseptic, lymphatic stimulant

Uses: Throat/lung/sinus infections, rheumatism/arthritis, skin parasites, urinary tract infection

Fragrant Influence: Relieves anxiety and revitalizes mind, body, and spirit. It also has an empowering, yet grounding fragrance.

Application: Dilute 1 part essential oil with 1 part V-6 Vegetable Oil Complex or other pure vegetable oil; (1) apply 2-4 drops on location, (2) apply on chakras and/or Vita Flex points, (3) inhale directly, or (4) diffuse.

Caution: Beware of pine oils adulterated with turpentine, a low-cost, but potentially hazardous, filler.

Found In: Grounding, R.C.

Bible References:

Nehemiah 8:15—"And that they should publish and proclaim in all their cities, and in Jerusalem, saying, Go forth unto the mount, and fetch olive branches, and pine branches, and myrtle branches, and palm branches, and branches of thick trees, to make booths, as it is written."

Isaiah 41:19—"I will plant in the wilderness the cedar, the shittah tree, and the myrtle, and the oil tree; I will set in the desert the fir tree, and the pine, and the box tree together:"

Isaiah 60:13—"The glory of Lebanon shall come unto thee, the fir tree, the pine tree, and the box together, to beautify the place of my sanctuary; and I will make the place of my feet glorious."

Plectranthus Oregano
(Plectranthus amboinicus)

Botanical Family: Lamiaceae

Plant Origin: Ecuador

Extraction Method: Steam distilled from leaves

Key Constituents:

Para-Cymene (14-27%)

Gamma-Terpinene (16-24%)

Carvacrol (25-45%)

Beta-Caryophyllene (4-11%)

Alpha-Bergamotene (2-6%)

Historical Data: The leaves of this plant have been used in traditional medicine for coughs, sore throats, and for nasal congestion. Also used for infections and for rheumatism, Plectranthus Oregano's flavor makes it popular for cooking, especially in soups.

Medical Properties: Antitumoral, antibacterial, antioxidant, analgesic, anti-inflammatory, antihyperlipodemic, liver protectant

Uses: Infections, cancer, arthritis, diabetes, rheumatism

Application: Dilute 1 part essential oil with 4 parts V-6 Vegetable Oil Complex or other pure vegetable oil; (1) apply 2-4 drops on location, (2) apply on chakras and/or Vita Flex points, (3) inhale directly, or (4) diffuse.

Ravintsara *(Cinnamomum camphora)*

Botanical Family: Lauraceae

Plant Origin: Madagascar

Extraction Method: Steam distilled from branches and leaves

Key Constituents:

1,8-Cineole (Eucalyptol) (50-65%)

Sabinene (9-16%)

Alpha-Terpineol (5-10%)

Alpha-Pinene (4-6%)

ORAC: 890 µTE/100g

Historical Data: Ravintsara is referred to by the people of Madagascar as "the oil that heals." It is antimicrobial and supporting to the nerves and respiratory system. It is also known to be clarifying, stimulating, and purifying. It also helps to clear brain fog and strengthen motivation.

Medical Properties: Antitumoral, antiviral, antibacterial

Uses: Herpes virus/viral infections (including colds, respiratory infections), throat/lung infections, hepatitis, shingles, pneumonia

Application: (1) Apply 2-4 drops on location, (2) apply on chakras and/or Vita Flex points, (3) inhale directly, or (4) diffuse.

Found In: ImmuPower, Raven

Roman Chamomile *(Anthemis nobilis)*

Botanical Family: Asteraceae

Plant Origin: Utah, France

Extraction Method: Steam distilled from flowering top

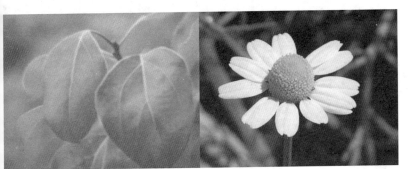

Ravintsara

Roman Chamomile

Key Constituents:
  Isobutyl Angelate + Isamyl Methacrylate (30-45%)
  Isoamyl Angelate (12-22%)
  Methyl Allyl Angelate (6-10%)
  Isobutyl n-butyrate (2-9%)
  2-Methyl Butyl Angelate (3-7%)

ORAC: 240 µTE/100g

Historical Data: Used in Europe for skin regeneration. For centuries, mothers have used chamomile to calm crying children, combat digestive and liver ailments, and relieve toothaches.

Medical Properties: Relaxant, antispasmodic, anti-inflammatory, antiparasitic, antibacterial, anesthetic

Uses: Relieves restlessness, anxiety, ADHD, depression, insomnia, skin conditions (acne, dermatitis, eczema)

Fragrant Influence: Because it is calming and relaxing, it can combat depression, insomnia, and stress. It minimizes anxiety, irritability, and nervousness. It may also dispel anger, stabilize the emotions, and help to release emotions that are linked to the past.

Application: (1) Apply 2-4 drops on location, ankles, or wrists; (2) apply on chakras and/or Vita Flex points; (3) inhale directly; (4) diffuse; or (5) take as a dietary supplement.

Found In: A·R·T Creme Masque, Awaken, ClaraDerm, Clarity, Dragon Time Bath & Shower Gel, Evening Peace Bath & Shower Gel, Forgiveness, Genesis Hand & Body Lotion, Gentle Baby, Harmony, Joy, JuvaFlex, K&B, KidScents Tender Tush, M-Grain, Motivation, Oola Balance, Oola Grow, Rehemogen, Satin Facial Scrub, Sensation Hand & Body Lotion, Surrender, Tranquil Roll-On, Wolfberry Eye Cream

Rose (*Rosa damascena*)

Botanical Family: Rosaceae

Plant Origin: Bulgaria, Turkey

Extraction Method: Therapeutic-grade oil is steam distilled from flowers (a two-part process).

Note: The Bulgarian *Rosa damascena* (high in citronellol) is very different from Morrocan *Rosa centifolia* (high in phenyl ethanol). They have different colors, aromas, and therapeutic actions.

Key Constituents:
  Citronellol (24-50%)
  Geraniol (10-22%)

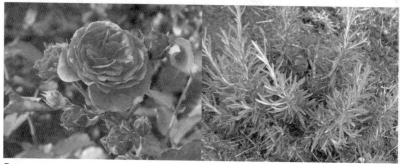

Rose

Rosemary

Nerol (5-12%)

Beta-Phenylethyl Alcohol (0.5-5%)

ORAC: 160,400 µTE/100g

Historical Data: Rose has been used for the skin for thousands of years. The Arab physician, Avicenna, was responsible for first distilling rose oil, eventually authoring an entire book on the healing attributes of the rose water derived from the distillation of rose. Throughout much of ancient history, the oil was produced by enfleurage, a process of pressing the petals along with a vegetable oil to extract the essence. Today, however, almost all rose oils are solvent extracted.

Medical Properties: Anti-inflammatory, anti-HIV, antioxidant, anxiolytic, hepatoprotective, relaxant, reduces scarring, antiulcer, immunomodulating, cancer chemopreventive, DNA damage prevention

Uses: Hypertension, heart strengthening, anxiety, viral infections (herpes simplex), skin conditions (scarring, wrinkles, acne), ulcers

Fragrant Influence: Its beautiful fragrance is intoxicating and aphrodisiac-like. It helps bring balance and harmony, allowing one to overcome insecurities. The effect of rose on the heart brings good cheer with calming and a lightness of spirit.

Application: (1) Apply 2-4 drops on location, (2) apply on chakras and/or Vita Flex points, (3) inhale directly, (4) diffuse, or (5) take as a dietary supplement.

Found In: Awaken, Egyptian Gold, Envision, Forgiveness, Gathering, Gentle Baby, Harmony, Highest Potential, Humility, Joy, Oola Balance, Oola Grow, Rose Ointment, SARA, Trauma Life, White Angelica

Rosemary *(Rosmarinus officinalis CT Cineole)*

Botanical Family: Lamiaceae

Plant Origin: Tunisia, Morocco, Spain

Extraction Method: Steam distilled from leaves

Key Constituents:

1,8-Cineole (Eucalyptol) (38-55%)

Camphor (5-15%)

Alpha-Pinene (9-14%)

Beta-Pinene (4-9%)

Camphene (2.5-6%)

Borneol (1.5-5%)

Limonene (1-4%)

ORAC: 330 µTE/100g

Historical Data: Rosemary was part of the "Marseilles Vinegar" or "Four Thieves Vinegar" that bandits who robbed the dead and dying used to protect themselves during the 15th century plague. The name of the oil is derived from the Latin words for dew of the sea (ros + marinus). According to folklore history, rosemary originally had white flowers; however, they turned red after the Virgin Mary laid her cloak on the bush. Since the time of ancient Greece (about 1,000 BC), rosemary was burned as incense. Later cultures believed that it warded off devils, a practice that eventually became adopted by the sick, who then burned rosemary to protect against infection. It was listed in Hildegard's *Medicine,* a compilation of early German medicines by highly regarded Benedictine herbalist Hildegard of Bingen (1098-1179). Until recently, French hospitals used rosemary to disinfect the air.

Medical Properties: Liver-protecting, anti-inflammatory, antitumoral, antifungal, antibacterial, anticancer, antidepressant, hypertension moderator (high blood pressure), enhances mental clarity/concentration

Uses: Infectious disease, liver conditions/hepatitis, throat/lung infections, hair loss (alopecia areata), acne, impaired memory/Alzheimer's, weight loss

Fragrant Influence: Helps overcome mental fatigue and improves mental clarity and focus. University of Miami scientists found that inhaling rosemary boosted alertness, eased anxiety, and amplified analytic and mental ability.

Application: Dilute 1 part essential oil with 1 part V-6 Vegetable Oil Complex or other pure vegetable oil; (1) apply 2-4 drops on location, (2) apply on chakras and/or Vita Flex points, (3) inhale directly, (4) diffuse, or (5) take as a dietary supplement.

Cautions: Do not use on children under 4 years of age. Do not use Rosemary for high blood pressure if already taking ACE inhibitor prescription drugs.

Found In: AromaGuard Meadow Mist Deodorant, AromaGuard Mountain Mint Deodorant, Clarity, ComforTone, En-R-Gee, Essentialzyme-4, ICP, Inner Defense, JuvaFlex, JuvaTone, KidScents Slique Toothpaste, Melrose, Morning Start Bath & Shower Gel, Morning Start Moisturizing Bar Soap, MultiGreens, Orange Blossom Facial Wash, Purification, Rehemogen, Sandalwood Moisture Cream, Satin Facial Scrub, Thieves, Thieves AromaBright Toothpaste, Thieves Cleansing Soap, Thieves Dental Floss, Thieves Dentarome Plus Toothpaste, Thieves Dentarome Ultra Toothpaste, Thieves Foaming Hand Soap, Thieves Fresh Essence Plus Mouthwash, Thieves Household Cleaner, Thieves Lozenges (Hard, Soft), Thieves Spray, Thieves Waterless Hand Purifier, Thieves Wipes, Transformation

Rosewood (Aniba rosaeodora)

Botanical Family: Lauraceae

Plant Origin: Brazil

Extraction Method: Steam distilled from wood

Key Constituents:
Linalol (70-90%)
Alpha-Terpineol (2-7%)
Alpha-Copaene (trace-3%)
1,8-Cineole (Eucalyptol) (trace-3%)
Geraniol (0.5-2.5%)

ORAC: 113,200 µTE/100g

Medical Properties: Antibacterial, antiviral, antiparasitic, antifungal, antimutagenic, anxiolytic, improves skin elasticity.

Uses: Fungal infections/Candida, skin conditions (eczema, psoriasis)

Fragrant Influence: Empowering and emotionally stabilizing

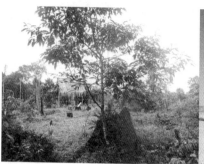
Rosewood

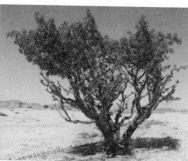
Sacred Frankincense (Boswellia sacra)

Application: (1) Apply 2-4 drops on location, (2) apply on chakras and/or Vita Flex points, (3) inhale directly, (4) diffuse, or (5) take as a dietary supplement.

Found In: Gentle Baby, KidScents Tender Tush, Lavender-Rosewood Moisturizing Soap, Oola Grow, Progessence Phyto Plus, Progessence Plus, Valor, Valor Moisturizing Soap, Valor Roll-On, White Angelica

Ruta (Ruta graveolens)

Botanical Family: Rutaceae

Plant Origin: Ecuador

Extraction Method: Steam distilled from aerial parts of the herb

Key Constituents:
2-Nonanone (40-53%)
2-Undecanone (35-48%)
2-Nonyl Acetate (0.5-2%)
Geijerene (1-3%)
2-Decanone (1-3%)

Historical Data: Commonly known as rue. In traditional medicine it was used as a magic herb and as a protection against evil. It was used to treat nervous afflictions, digestive problems, hysterics, and as an abortifacient. Formerly used to treat menstrual disorders and hysteria. Anecdotal reports suggest it

has sleep-inducing properties.

Medical Properties: Anti-inflammatory, anti-diabetic, antimicrobial, hypotensive, anxiolytic, sleep promoting

Uses: Hysteria, stress, nervousness, digestion

Fragrant Influence: Calming and relaxing

Application: (1) Apply 2-4 drops on location, (2) apply on chakras and/or Vita Flex points, (3) inhale directly, (4) diffuse.

Caution: Avoid applying to skin that will be exposed to sunlight or UV light within 12 hours.

Found In: Common Sense, RutaVaLa, RutaVaLa Roll-On, SleepEssence

Sacred Frankincense (Boswellia sacra)

Botanical Family: Burseraceae

Plant Origin: Oman

Extraction Method: Steam distilled from gum/resin

Key Constituents:
Alpha-pinene (53-90%)
Camphene (1-4%)
Sabinene (1-7%)
Para-cymene (0.4-4%)
Limonene (2-7.5%)

Historical Data: Young Living's Sacred Frankincense oil is the first Omani

Frankincense to be available to those outside of Saudi royals or the privileged of Oman. It is regarded the world over as the rarest, most sought-after aromatic in existence.

After 15 years of research, 15 trips to Oman, and numerous meetings and negotiations with Omani officials, Gary Young was granted the first export permit in the modern history of Oman for the release and export of the oil and permission to build a Young Living distillery in the country and to export the resulting essential oil out of Oman. Gary Young was on-site to supervise the building of Young Living's Omani distillery, and Young Living has contracted with local harvesters to secure our supply of Omani resin. This marks the first time any Westerners have been able to experience the unique spiritual properties of Sacred Frankincense essential oil.

Omani Frankincense is highly regarded as the Frankincense of the ancients and the traditional spiritual oil of biblical times. Historically, it is believed that this beautiful, white hojari resin produced the Frankincense that was taken to the Christ Child. Science continues to document the oil's immense healing properties, which users of this oil already know.

Medical Properties: Frankincense has been tested as an anticancer agent (Ni, et al., 2012; Suhail, et al., 2011). Therapeutic-grade Frankincense oil contains boswellic acids, which are potent anti-inflammatory agents against rheumatoid arthritis and osteoporosis.

Traditional Uses: It supports skin health and treats stomach disorders, ulcers, cancer, dental and gum diseases, bad blood, infections, mental disorders, and insect bites. It is calming, meditative, relaxing, and promotes higher states of spiritual awareness and higher levels of consciousness and sensitivity.

Application: Dilution is not required except for the most sensitive skin; (1) apply 2-4 drops on location, (2) chakras and/or Vita Flex points, (3) inhale directly, (4) diffuse up to 1 hour 3 times daily, or (5) take as a dietary supplement; put 2 drops in a capsule and take 3 times daily or as needed or put 1-2 drops in water and drink.

Found In: Oola Balance, The Gift, Progessence Phyto Plus, Progessence Plus, Transformation

Complement To: *Boswellia carterii*, traditional frankincense

Sage *(Salvia officinalis)*

Botanical Family: Lamiaceae

Plant Origin: Spain, Croatia, France

Extraction Method: Steam distilled from leaves

Key Constituents:
Alpha-Thujone (18-43%)
Beta-Thujone (3-8.5%)
1,8-Cineole (Eucalyptol) (5.5-13%)
Camphor (4.5-24.5%)
Camphene (1.5-7%)
Alpha-Pinene (1-6.5%)
Alpha-Humulene (trace-12%)

ORAC: 14,800 µTE/100g

Historical Data: Known as "herba sacra" or sacred herb by the ancient Romans, sage's name, *Salvia,* is derived from the word for "salvation." Sage has been used in Europe for oral infections and skin conditions. It has been recognized for its benefits of strengthening the vital centers and supporting metabolism.

Medical Properties: Antibacterial, antifungal, antioxidant, antitumoral, anti-inflammatory, anxiolytic, hormone regulating, estrogen-like, antiviral, circulatory stimulant, gallbladder stimulant

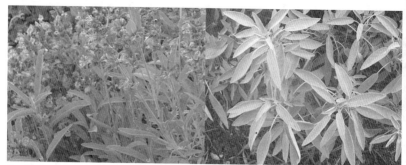

Sage

Spanish Sage

Uses: Menstrual problems/PMS, estrogen, progesterone, and testosterone deficiencies, liver problems

Fragrant Influence: Mentally stimulating, anxiety-reducing, and helps combat despair and mental fatigue. Sage strengthens the vital centers of the body, balancing the pelvic chakra, where negative emotions from denial and abuse are stored.

Application: Dilute 1 part essential oil with 1 part V-6 Vegetable Oil Complex or other pure vegetable oil; (1) apply 2-4 drops on location, (2) apply on chakras and/or Vita Flex points, (3) inhale directly, (4) diffuse, or (5) take as a dietary supplement.

Cautions: Avoid if epileptic. Avoid use on persons with high blood pressure.

Found In: Dragon Time Bath & Shower Gel, Dragon Time Massage Oil, EndoFlex, Envision, FemiGen, K&B, Magnify Your Purpose, Mister, Prenolone Plus Body Cream, Protec

Sandalwood *(Santalum album)*
Botanical Family: Santalaceae
Plant Origin: India
Extraction Method: Steam distilled from wood

Key Constituents:
Alpha-Santalol (41-55%)
Beta-Santalol (16-24%)
ORAC: 160 µTE/100g
Historical Data: Used for centuries in Ayurvedic medicine for skin revitalization, yoga, and meditation. Listed in Dioscorides' *De Materia Medica* (AD 78), Europe's first authoritative guide to medicines, which became the standard reference work for herbal treatments for over 1,700 years. Research at Brigham Young University in Provo, Utah, documented its ability to inhibit several types of cancerous cells (Stevens).

Medical Properties: Antitumoral, antibacterial, antiviral, immune stimulant

Uses: Cancer, viral infections (herpes simplex, herpes zoster, cold sores, human papilloma virus, etc.), skin conditions (acne, wrinkles, scars, etc.)

Fragrant Influence: Enhances deep sleep, may help remove negative programming from the cells. It is high in sesquiterpenes that stimulate the pineal gland and the limbic region of the brain, the center of emotions. The pineal gland is responsible for releasing melatonin, a powerful immune stimulant and antitumoral agent. Can be grounding and stabilizing.

Application: (1) Apply 2-4 drops on location, (2) apply on chakras and/or Vita Flex points, (3) inhale directly, (4) diffuse, or (5) take as a dietary supplement.

Found In: Acceptance, A·R·T Day Activator, A·R·T Gentle Foaming Cleanser, A·R·T Night Reconstructor, A·R·T Purifying Toner, Awaken, Boswellia Wrinkle Cream, Brain Power, Dream Catcher, Essential Beauty Serum (Dry Skin), Evening Peace Bath & Shower Gel, Forgiveness, Gathering, Harmony, Highest Potential, Inner Child, Inspiration, KidScents Tender Tush, Lady Sclareol, Lemon-Sandalwood Cleansing Soap, Live with Passion, Magnify Your Purpose, Oola Balance, Oola Grow, Release, Sandalwood Moisture Cream, 3 Wise Men, Transformation, Trauma Life, Ultra Young Plus, White Angelica

Spanish Sage *(Salvia lavandulifolia)*
(Also referred to as Sage Lavender)

Botanical Family: Lamiaceae

Plant Origin: Central Europe and Asia Minor, esp. Spain

Extraction Method: Steam distilled from the leaves

Key Constituents:
1,8-cineole (Eucalyptol) (10-30%)
Alpha-Pinene (4-11%)
Limonene (2-6%)
Camphor (11-36%)
Linalol (0.3-4%)
Alpha-Terpinyl Acetate (0.5-9%)
Linalyl Acetate (0.1-5%)

Historical Data: The sage plant has been highly praised throughout history for its powers of longevity and healing. Pliny the Elder said that sage (called "salvia" by the Romans) was used as a local anesthetic for the skin and as a diuretic, in addition to other uses. It was considered a sacred herb to the Romans and was harvested by a person wearing a white tunic, who had well-washed, bare feet.

During the Middle Ages, the plant was prized throughout Europe because of its exceptional healing effects and was used in a mixture with other herbs designed to ward off the plague. In Spain, Spanish sage is used in cooking. It has a stronger aroma and flavor than common sage (*S. officinalis*).

Medical Properties: Antiseptic, astringent, chemopreventive, expectorant, reduces mucous, reduces fevers, purifies the blood, eliminates toxins, aids digestion, lowers blood sugar levels without affecting insulin levels, acts as a tonic to improve general health

Uses: Age-related memory loss, cuts, acne, arthritis, dandruff, colds, flu, eczema, hair loss, sweating, anxiety, headaches, asthma, laryngitis, coughs, muscular aches and pains, depression, epilepsy, soothing agent, menstrual disorders, digestive disorders. In food it is used as a spice; in manufacturing it is used as a fragrance component in soaps and cosmetics

Fragrant Influence: Camphoraceous, herbaceous, similar to rosemary

Application: Dilute 1 part essential oil with 1 part V-6 Vegetable Oil Complex or other pure vegetable oil; (1) apply 2-4 drops on location, (2) apply on chakras and/or Vita Flex points, (3) inhale directly, (4) diffuse, or (5) take as a dietary supplement.

Cautions: Avoid if epileptic. Avoid use on persons with high blood pressure.

Found In: Awaken, Harmony, Lady Sclareol, Oola Balance, SclarEssence

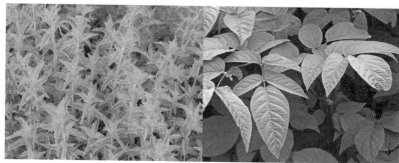

Spearmint

Spikenard

Spearmint *(Mentha spicata)*
  Botanical Family: Lamiaceae
  Plant Origin: Utah, China
  Extraction Method: Steam distilled from
    leaves
  Key Constituents:
    Carvone (45-80%)
    Limonene (10-30%)
    Cis-Dihydrocarvone (1-8%)
  ORAC: 540 µTE/100g
  Medical Properties: Increases metabolism,
    antibacterial, antispasmodic, anti-
    inflammatory, antiseptic, mucolytic,
    gallbladder stimulant, digestive aid,
    antitumor
  Uses: Obesity, intestinal/digestive disorders,
    nausea, hepatitis
  Fragrant Influence: Opens and releases
    emotional blocks and brings about a feeling
    of balance and a lasting sense of well-being
  Application: Dilute 1 part essential oil with 2
    parts V-6 Vegetable Oil Complex or other
    pure vegetable oil; (1) apply 2-4 drops on
    location, (2) apply on chakras and/or Vita
    Flex points, (3) inhale directly, (4) diffuse,
    or (5) take as a dietary supplement.
  Found In: Cinnamint Lip Balm, Citrus
    Fresh, Einkorn Nuggets, EndoFlex, GLF,

KidScents Slique Toothpaste, Lavender
Mint Daily Conditioner, Lavender
Mint Daily Shampoo, NingXia Nitro,
OmegaGize³, Relaxation Massage Oil,
Slique Essence, Slique Gum, Thieves
AromaBright Toothpaste, Thieves Fresh
Essence Plus Mouthwash, Thyromin

Spikenard *(Nardostachys jatamansi)*
  Botanical Family: Valerianaceae
  Plant Origin: India
  Extraction Method: Steam distilled from
    roots
  Key Constituents:
    Calarene (10-35%)
    Beta-Maaliene (4-13%)
    Alpha-Copaene (5-14%)
    Aristolene (2-9%)
    Seychellene (1-5%)
    Patchouli Alcohol (2-7%)
    9-Aristolen-1-ol (1-5%)
  ORAC: 54,800 µTE/100g
  Historical Data: Highly regarded in India as
    a medicinal herb. It was the one of the most
    precious oils in ancient times, used only by
    priests, kings, or high initiates. References in
    the New Testament describe how Mary of
    Bethany used spikenard oil to anoint the feet

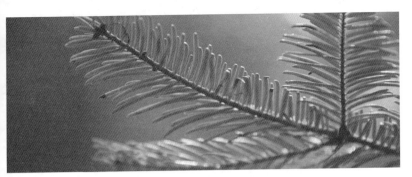
Spruce

of Jesus before the Last Supper (John 12:3).

Medical Properties: Antibacterial, antifungal, anti-inflammatory, antioxidant, relaxant, immune stimulant

Uses: Insomnia, menstrual problems/PMS, heart arrhythmias, nervous tension

Fragrant Influence: Relaxing, soothing, helps nourish and regenerate the skin

Application: (1) Apply 2-4 drops on location, (2) apply on chakras and/or Vita Flex points, (3) inhale directly, (4) diffuse, or (5) take as a dietary supplement.

Found In: Animal Scents Shampoo, Egyptian Gold, Exodus II, Humility, Inspiration, LavaDerm Cooling Mist, Oola Balance, The Gift

Bible References:

The Song of Solomon 1:12—"While the king sitteth at his table, my spikenard sendeth forth the smell thereof."

The Song of Solomon 4:13—"Thy plants are an orchard of pomegranates, with pleasant fruits; camphire, with spikenard,"

The Song of Solomon 4:14—"Spikenard and saffron; calamus and cinnamon, with all trees of frankincense; myrrh and aloes, with all the chief spices:"

Spruce (*Picea mariana*)

Botanical Family: Pinaceae

Plant Origin: Canada

Extraction Method: Steam distilled from branches, needles, and twigs

Key Constituents:

Bornyl Acetate (24-35%)

Camphene (14-26%)

Alpha-Pinene (12-19%)

Beta-Pinene (2-10%)

Delta-3-Carene (4-10%)

Limonene (3-6%)

Myrcene (1-5%)

Santene (1-5%)

Tricyclene (1-4%)

Historical Data: The Lakota Indians used spruce to strengthen their ability to communicate with the Great Spirit. Traditionally, it was believed to possess the frequency of prosperity.

Medical Properties: Antispasmodic, antiparasitic, antiseptic, anti-inflammatory, hormone-like, cortisone-like, immune stimulant, antidiabetic

Uses: Arthritis/rheumatism, fungal infections (Candida), sinus/respiratory infections, sciatica/lumbago

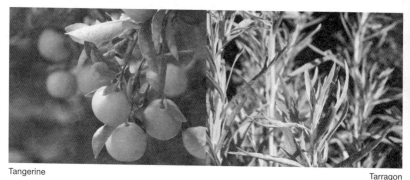

Tangerine

Tarragon

Fragrant Influence: Releases emotional blocks, bringing about a feeling of balance and grounding

Application: Dilute 1 part essential oil with 1 part V-6 Vegetable Oil Complex or other pure vegetable oil; (1) apply 2-4 drops on location, (2) apply on chakras and/or Vita Flex points, (3) inhale directly, (4) diffuse, or (5) take as a dietary supplement

Found In: Abundance, Awaken, Christmas Spirit, Envision, Gathering, Grounding, Harmony, Highest Potential, Hope, Inner Child, Inspiration, Motivation, Oola Balance, Oola Grow, Present Time, R.C., Relieve It, Sacred Mountain, Sacred Mountain Moisturizing Soap, Surrender, 3 Wise Men, Trauma Life, Valor, Valor Moisturizing Soap, Valor Roll-On, White Angelica

Tangerine (*Citrus reticulata*)
  Botanical Family: Rutaceae
  Plant Origin: Brazil
  Extraction Method: Cold pressed from rind
  Key Constituents:
    Limonene (90-97%)
    Gamma-Terpinene (0.3-3%)
    Myrcene (1-3%)

Medical Properties: Antitumoral, relaxant, antispasmodic, digestive aid, and circulatory enhancer; rich in limonene, which has been extensively studied in over 50 clinical studies for its ability to combat tumor growth.

Uses: Obesity, anxiety, insomnia, irritability, lung health, learning and memory support, Alzheimer's, liver problems, digestive problems, parasites, fluid retention

Fragrant Influence: Promotes happiness, calming, helps with anxiety and nervousness. A Mie University study found that citrus fragrances boosted immunity, induced relaxation, and reduced depression (Komori, et al., 1995).

Application: Dilute 1 part essential oil with 1 part V-6 Vegetable Oil Complex or other pure vegetable oil; (1) apply 2-4 drops on location, (2) apply on chakras and/or Vita Flex points, (3) inhale directly, (4) diffuse, or (5) take as a dietary supplement.

Caution: Avoid applying to skin that will be exposed to sunlight or UV light within 24 hours.

Found In: Awaken, Citrus Fresh, ComforTone, Dream Catcher, Inner Child, Joy, KidScents Shampoo, KidScents

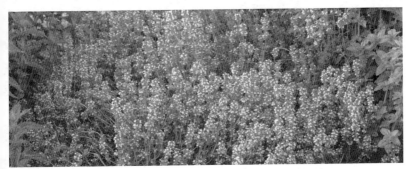
Thyme

Slique Toothpaste, NingXia Red, Peace
& Calming, Relaxation Massage Oil,
SleepEssence, Slique Essence, Super C

Tarragon (*Artemisia dracunculus*)
  Botanical Family: Asteraceae
  Plant Origin: Italy
  Extraction Method: Steam distilled from
  leaves
  Key Constituents:
    Methyl Chavicol (Estragole) (68-80%)
    Trans-Beta-Ocimene (6-12%)
    Cis-Beta-Ocimene (6-12%)
    Limonene (2-6%)
  ORAC: 37,900 µTE/100g
  Medical Properties: Antispasmodic,
  antibacterial, anti-inflammatory,
  antiparasitic, digestive aid, anticonvulsant,
  enhances insulin sensitivity
  Uses: Intestinal disorders, urinary tract
  infection, nausea, menstrual problems/PMS
  Fragrant Influence: May help alleviate deep
  depression
  Application: Dilute 1 part essential oil with 1
  part V-6 Vegetable Oil Complex or other pure
  vegetable oil; (1) apply 2-4 drops on location,
  (2) apply on chakras and/or Vita Flex points,
  or (3) take as a dietary supplement.

Caution: Avoid use if epileptic.
Found In: Allerzyme, ComforTone, DiGize,
  Essentialzyme, Essentialzymes-4, ICP

Thyme (*Thymus vulgaris*)
  Botanical Family: Lamiaceae
  Plant Origin: Mediterranean area
  Extraction Method: Steam distilled from
  leaves, stems, flowers
  Key Constituents:
    Thymol (37-55%)
    Para-cymene (14-28%)
    Gamma-Terpinene (4-11%)
    Linalol (3-6.5%)
    Carvacrol (0.5-5.5%)
    Myrcene (1-2.8%)
  ORAC: 15,960 µTE/100g
  Historical Data: Also known as Red Thyme.
  It is mentioned in one of the oldest known
  medical records, the Ebers Papyrus (dating
  from 16th century BC), an ancient Egyptian
  list of 877 prescriptions and recipes. The
  Egyptians used thyme for embalming.
  Listed in Dioscorides' *De Materia Medica*
  (AD 78), Europe's first authoritative guide
  to medicines, which became the standard
  reference work for herbal treatments for over
  1,700 years.

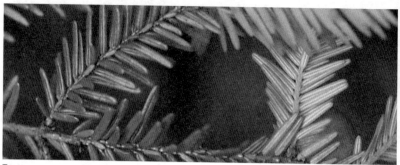
Tsuga

Thyme was listed in Hildegard's *Medicine,* a compilation of early German medicines by highly regarded Benedictine herbalist Hildegard of Bingen (1098-1179).

Medical Properties: Antiaging, antioxidant, anti-inflammatory, antispasmodic, highly antimicrobial, antifungal, antiviral, antiparasitic. A solution of thyme's most active ingredient, thymol, is used in many over-the-counter products such as mouthwash and vapor rubs because of its purifying agents.

Uses: Infectious diseases, cardiovascular disease, Alzheimer's disease, hepatitis

Fragrant Influence: It may be beneficial in helping to overcome fatigue and exhaustion after illness.

Application: Dilute 1 part essential oil with 4 parts V-6 Vegetable Oil Complex or other pure vegetable oil; (1) apply 1-2 drops on location, (2) apply on chakras and/or Vita Flex points, (3) diffuse, or (4) take as a dietary supplement.

Caution: May irritate the nasal membranes or skin if inhaled directly from diffuser or bottle or applied neat.

Found In: Essential Beauty Serum (Acne-Prone Skin), Inner Defense, Longevity, Longevity Softgels, Ortho Ease Massage Oil, Ortho Sport Massage Oil, ParaFree, Rehemogen, Thieves Dentarome Ultra Toothpaste

Tsuga *(Tsuga canadensis)*

Botanical Family: Pinaceae

Plant Origin: Canada

Extraction Method: Steam distilled from needles and twigs of the conifer tree commercially known as eastern hemlock

Key Constituents:
Alpha-Pinene (18-25%)
Beta-Pinene (1-3%)
Camphene (13-17%)
Limonene (3-5%)
Bornyl Acetate (27-40%)
Tricyclene (5-7%)
Myrcene (2-5%)

ORAC: 7,100 µTE/100g

Medical Properties: Analgesic, antirheumatic, blood cleanser, stimulant, cell regenerating

Uses: Respiratory conditions, kidney/urinary infections, skin conditions, venereal diseases

Application: Dilute 1 part essential oil with 1 part V-6 Vegetable Oil Complex or other pure vegetable oil; (1) apply 2-4 drops on location, (2) apply on chakras and/or Vita Flex points, (3) inhale directly, (4) diffuse

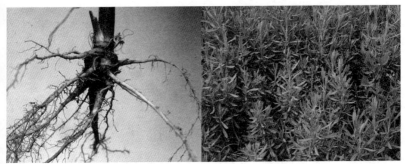

Valerian

Vanilla

Valerian *(Valeriana officinalis)*
  Botanical Family: Valerianaceae
  Plant Origin: Belgium, Croatia
  Extraction Method: Steam distilled from root
  Key Constituents:
    Bornyl Acetate (35-43%)
    Camphene (22-31%)
    Alpha-Pinene (5-8%)
    Beta-Pinene (3-6%)
    Limonene (1-3%)
    Valerenal (2-8%)
    Myrtenyl Acetate (2-5%)
  ORAC: 6,200 µTE/100g
  Historical Data: During the last three decades, valerian has been clinically investigated for its tranquilizing properties. Researchers have pinpointed the sesquiterpenes valerenic acid and valerone as the active constituents that exert a calming effect on the central nervous system. The German Commission E has pronounced valerian to be an effective treatment for restlessness and for sleep disturbances resulting from nervous conditions.
  Medical Properties: Sedative and tranquilizing to the central nervous system, antispasmodic
  Uses: Insomnia, anxiety, dysmenorrhea
  Fragrant Influence: Calming, relaxing, grounding, emotionally balancing
  Application: (1) Apply 2-4 drops on location, (2) apply on chakras and/or Vita Flex points, (3) inhale directly, (4) diffuse, or (5) take as a dietary supplement.
  Found In: RutaVaLa, RutaVaLa Roll-On, SleepEssence, Trauma Life

Vanilla *(Vanilla planifolia)*
  Botanical Family: Orchidaceae
  Plant Origin: Brazil
  Extraction Method: Proprietary vacuum distillation
  Key Constituents:
    Vanillin (85-95%)
  Historical Data: Vanilla essential oil, created for the first time by Young Living Essential Oils, is the highest known oil in vanillin, which is similar in chemical structure to the aromatic compound eugenol, found in cloves. Recent tests conducted at independent laboratories found that the vanilla content of this vanilla oil is over 10 times higher than commercially available super-concentrated vanilla extracts. The same way that eugenol in clove oil numbs dental tissue, vanillin numbs stress and food cravings.

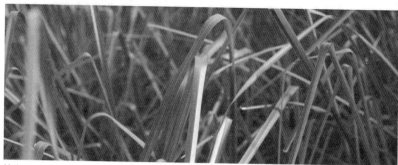
Vetiver

The importance of vanillin is now being investigated by scientists who are researching the ways in which activating vanilloid-type brain receptors can enhance well-being and combat depression.

Medical Properties: Mood elevating; weakens or numbs stress and food cravings

Uses: Appetite control, depression

Fragrant Influence: Uplifts mood through vanilloid receptor action in brain

Application: (1) Apply 2-4 drops on location, (2) apply on chakras and/or Vita Flex points, (3) inhale directly, (4) diffuse, (5) take as a dietary supplement

Found In: A·R·T Beauty Masque, A·R·T Creme Masque, Chocolessence, Copaiba Vanilla Moisturizing Conditioner, Copaiba Vanilla Moisturizing Shampoo, NingXia Nitro, Slique Bars, Slique Tea, Slique Tea (International), Stress Away, Stress Away Roll-On

Vetiver *(Vetiveria zizanioides)*
Botanical Family: Poaceae
Plant Origin: Haiti, Ecuador
Extraction Method: Steam distilled from root
Key Constituents:
Isovalencenol (1-16%)
Khusimol (7-21%)
Alpha-Vetivone (2-7%)
Beta-Vetivone (4-14%)
Beta-Vetivenene (1-8%)
ORAC: 74,300 µTE/100g

Historical Data: It is well known for its anti-inflammatory properties and is traditionally used for arthritic symptoms.

Medical Properties: Antiseptic, antispasmodic, relaxant, circulatory stimulant

Uses: ADHD, anxiety, rheumatism/arthritis, depression (including postpartum), insomnia, skin care (oily, aging, acne, wrinkles)

Fragrant Influence: Psychologically grounding, calming, and stabilizing. It helps us cope with stress and recover from emotional trauma. Terry Friedmann, MD, found in preliminary clinical tests that vetiver may be successful in the treatment of ADD and ADHD (attention deficit disorders) in children (Friedmann 2002).

Application: (1) Apply 2-4 drops on location, (2) apply on chakras and/or Vita Flex points, (3) inhale directly, (4) diffuse, (5) take as a dietary supplement, or (6) gargle with mouthwash.

Found In: A·R·T Creme Masque, Deep Relief Roll-On, Inspiration, Lady Sclareol, Melaleuca-Geranium Moisturizing Soap,

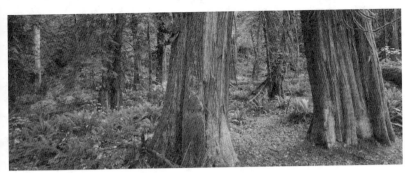
Western Red Cedar

Ortho Ease Massage Oil, Ortho Sport Massage Oil, ParaFree, SleepEssence, Thieves Fresh Essence Plus Mouthwash

Vitex (Vitex agnus-castus)
Botanical Family: Lamiaceae
Plant Origin: Italy, Croatia
Extraction Method: Steam distilled from leaves, berries, and stems
Key Constituents:
Alpha-Pinene (4-10%)
Sabinene (20-35%)
1,8-Cineole (Eucalyptol) (18-30%)
Terpinyl Acetate (2-7%)
Beta-Caryophyllene (3-9%)
Beta-Farnesene (4-9%)
Historical Data: Commonly referred to as the chaste tree, vitex has been used medicinally for over 2,000 years for a variety of health problems. It has been used for hundreds of years in Europe for female reproductive system disorders. It is well-tolerated and effective for symptoms of premenstrual syndrome. The essential oil is more effective than the water or hydroalcoholic extracts, according to recent patient research. Through its action on the anterior pituitary, vitex acts to reduce estrogen and increase progesterone production. In moderating prolactin (luteotropic hormone) levels, vitex reduces symptoms of PMS (Milewicz, et al.) The European Commission E has approved the use of chaste tree fruit for premenstrual complaints, irregularities of the menstrual cycle, and for lactation insufficiency. Chaste tree use may interfere with oral contraceptives, hormone replacement therapy or medication, and neuroleptic medications.
Medical Properties: Antibacterial, anti-inflammatory, cancer chemoprevention, estrogenic, hormone-like activity
Uses: Inflammation, female reproductive system conditions (PMS, irregularities, menopause, mastalgia, etc.)
Application: (1) Apply 2-4 drops on location, (2) apply on chakras and/or Vita Flex points, (3) inhale directly, (4) diffuse.
Found In: Progessence Phyto Plus

Western Red Cedar (Thuja plicata)
Botanical Family: Cupressaceae
Plant Origin: Utah, Idaho, Canada
Extraction Method: Steam distilled from needles and branches
Key Constituents:
Alpha-Thujone (60-80%)

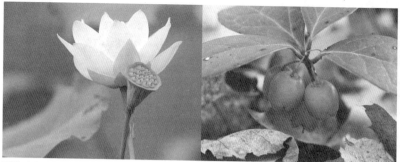

White Lotus

Wintergreen

Beta-Thujone (4-7%)
Alpha-Pinene (2-20%)
Sabinene (2-4%)

Historical Data: This oil is different from Canadian Red Cedar, which is distilled from the bark of the same plant, *Thuja plicata*. This oil is not red in color, because it is derived from needles and branches.

Medical Properties: Antiseptic, antimicrobial

Uses: Throat/lung infections, urinary tract infections

Application: Dilute 1 part essential oil with 1 part V-6 Vegetable Oil Complex or other pure vegetable oil; (1) apply 1-2 drops on location, (2) apply on chakras and/or Vita Flex points, (3) inhale directly, (4) diffuse, (5) add to woodchips and place in closets and dressers to repel insects.

Found In: KidScents Lotion

White Fir (Abies concolor)

Botanical Family: Pinaceae

Plant Origin: Idaho

Extraction Method: Steam distilled from wood/bark/twigs/needles

Key Constituents:
Alpha-Pinene (8-12%)
Beta-Pinene (20-30%)

Camphene (7-15%)
Bornyl Acetate (11-16%)
Delta-Cadinene (2-7%)

ORAC: 47,900 µTE/100g

Medical Properties: Antitumoral, anticancerous, antioxidant, pain relieving

Uses: Respiratory infections, antifungal

Application: Dilute 1 part essential oil with 1 part V-6 Vegetable Oil Complex or other pure vegetable oil; (1) apply 2-4 drops on location, (2) apply on chakras and/or Vita Flex points, (3) inhale directly, or (4) diffuse.

Found In: AromaGuard Mountain Mint Deodorant, Australian Blue, Grounding, Highest Potential, Into the Future, Oola Grow

White Lotus (Nymphaea lotus)

Botanical Family: Nymphaeaceae

Plant Origin: Egypt

Extraction Method: Steam distilled from the flowers

Key Constituents:
Tetradecene (7-9%)
Pentadecane (8-11%)
Heptadecadiene (9-11%)
Pentadecene (6-9%)
Octadecene (7-10%)

Ethyl-9-Hexadecenoate (9-12%)
Ethyl Hexadecanoate (17-22%)
Ethyl Linoleate (8-11%)
Historical Data: In ancient Egypt the lotus was used widely as a religious and ceremonial icon. In 400 AD, the Christian church of Ephesus designated Mary as "The Bearer of God." The numerous churches dedicated to Mary that were built thereafter incorporated the image of the lotus, including one image of lotus leaves, flowers, and fruits surrounding a golden cross.
Medical Properties: Anticancerous, anti-inflammatory, immune supporting
Traditional Uses: White lotus was traditionally used by the Egyptians for spiritual, emotional, and physical application. Research in China found that white lotus contains anticancerous and strong immune supporting properties.
Other Uses: Inflamed eyes, jaundice, kidneys, liver spots, menstruation (promotes), palpitations, rheumatism, sciatica, sprains, sunburn, toothaches, tuberculosis, vomiting
Fragrant Influence: Stimulates a positive attitude and a general feeling of well-being
Found In: Into the Future, Oola Grow, SARA

Wintergreen (Gaultheria procumbens)
Botanical Family: Ericaceae
Plant Origin: China, North America
Extraction Method: Steam distilled from leaves and bark
Key Constituent:
Methyl Salicylate (90+%)
ORAC: 101,800 µTE/100g
Historical Data: Leaves have been chewed to increase respiratory capacity by Native Americans when running long distances and performing difficult labor. Settlers in early America had their children chew the leaves for several weeks each spring to prevent tooth decay. Wintergreen was used as a substitute for black tea during the Revolutionary War.
Medical Properties: Anticoagulant, antispasmodic, highly anti-inflammatory, vasodilator, analgesic/anesthetic, reduces blood pressure and all types of pain. Methyl salicylate, the principal constituent of wintergreen oil, has been incorporated into numerous liniments and ointments for musculoskeletal problems. The oil is also used as a flavoring agent in candies and chewing gums.
Uses: Arthritis/rheumatism, muscle/nerve pain, hypertension, arteriosclerosis, hepatitis/fatty liver
Fragrant Influence: It stimulates and increases awareness in all levels of the sensory system.
Application: Dilute 1 part essential oil with 2 parts V-6 Vegetable Oil Complex or other pure vegetable oil; (1) apply 1-2 drops on location, (2) apply on chakras and/or Vita Flex points, (3) inhale directly, (4) diffuse, or (5) take as a dietary supplement.
Cautions: Avoid use if epileptic. Anticoagulant properties can be enhanced when used with Warfarin or aspirin.
Found In: BLM, Deep Relief Roll-On, Ortho Ease Massage Oil, Ortho Sport Massage Oil, PanAway, Raven, Regenolone Moisturizing Cream, SuperCal, Thieves Dentarome Ultra Toothpaste

Xiang Mao (Cymbopogon citratus)
Botanical Family: Poaceae
Plant Origin: Taiwan
Extraction Method: Steam distilled from grasses
Key Constituents:
Limonene (3-7%)
Citronellal (40-50%)
Citronellol (11-16%)
Geraniol (15-18%)
Germacrene-D (1-3%)

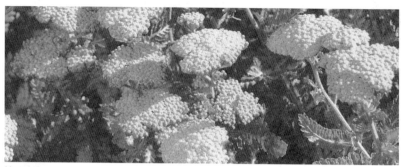
Yarrow

Alpha-Elemol (1-2%)

Historical Data: This aromatic grass is sometimes called red lemongrass and has been used in folk medicine as a calming agent. It was also used to keep air in the home fresh.

Medical Properties: Chemopreventive, antimicrobial, anxiolytic, renal protective, gastroprotective, antifungal, antiparasitic, cholesterol reducer

Uses: Bladder infection, respiratory/sinus infection, digestive problems, parasites, torn ligaments/muscles, fluid retention, varicose veins, Salmonella, *Candida albicans*

Fragrant Influence: Like its close cousin, *Cymbopogon flexuosus,* this lemongrass species sharpens awareness and is a purifier

Application: Dilute 1 part essential oil with 4 parts V-6 Vegetable Oil Complex or other pure vegetable oil; (1) apply 1-2 drops on location, (2) apply on chakras and/or Vita Flex points, (3) inhale directly, (4) diffuse

Yarrow *(Achillea millefolium)*
  Botanical Family: Asteraceae
  Plant Origin: North America, Europe, Asia
  Extraction Method: Steam distilled from flowers, leaves, and stems

Key Constituents:
  Chamazulene (5-18%)
  Trans-Beta-Caryophyllene (5-13%)
  Germacrene D (8-25%)
  Sabinene (5-15%)
  Beta-Pinene (4-10%)
  1,8-Cineole (Eucalyptol) (2-10%)
ORAC: 55,900 µTE/100g
Historical Data: The Greek Achilles, hero of the Trojan War, was said to have used the yarrow herb to help cure the injury to his Achilles tendon. Yarrow was considered sacred by the Chinese, who recognized the harmony of the Yin and Yang energies within it. It has been said that the fragrance of yarrow makes possible the meeting of heaven and earth. Yarrow was used by Germanic tribes for the treatment of battle wounds.
Medical Properties: Anti-inflammatory, hormone-like, combats scarring, supports prostate
Uses: Prostate problems, menstrual problems/PMS, varicose veins
Fragrant Influence: Balancing highs and lows, both external and internal, yarrow simultaneously inspires and grounds us. Useful during meditation and supportive to intuitive energies. Reduces confusion and

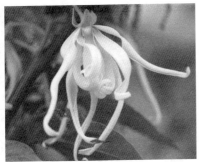
Ylang Ylang

ambivalence.

Application: (1) Apply 2-4 drops on location, dilution not required except for the most sensitive skin; (2) apply on chakras and/or Vita Flex points; (3) inhale directly; (4) diffuse up to 1 hour 3 times daily; or (5) put 2 drops in a capsule and take 3 times daily or as needed.

Found In: Dragon Time, Dragon Time Massage Oil, Mister, Prenolone Plus Body Cream

Ylang Ylang *(Cananga odorata)*

Botanical Family: Annonaceae

Plant Origin: Madagascar, Ecuador

Extraction Method: Steam distilled from flowers. Flowers are picked early in the morning to maximize oil yield. The highest quality oil is drawn from the first distillation and is known as ylang ylang complete.

Key Constituents:
Germacrene D (14-27%)
(E,E)-Alpha-Farnesene (5-23%)
Benzyl Acetate (1-15%)
Geranyl Acetate (2-11%)
Beta-Caryophyllene (2-19%)
Benzyl Benzoate (4-8%)
Linalol (2-16%)
Para-Cresyl Methyl Ether (0.5-9%)
Methyl Benzoate (1-5%)
Benzyl Salicyclate (1-5%)

ORAC: 130,000 µTE/100g

Historical Data: Ylang ylang means "flower of flowers." The flowers have been used to cover the beds of newlywed couples on their wedding night. Traditionally used in hair formulas to promote thick, shiny, lustrous hair.

Medical Properties: Antispasmodic, vasodilating, antidiabetic, anti-inflammatory, antiparasitic, regulates heartbeat

Uses: Cardiac arrhythmia, cardiac problems, anxiety, hypertension, depression, hair loss, intestinal problems

Fragrant Influence: Balances male-female energies, enhances spiritual attunement, combats anger, combats low self-esteem, increases focus of thoughts, filters out negative energy, restores confidence and peace

Application: Dilute 1 part essential oil with 1 part V-6 Vegetable Oil Complex or other pure vegetable oil; (1) apply 2-4 drops on location, (2) apply on chakras and/or Vita Flex points, (3) inhale directly, (4) diffuse, or (5) take as a dietary supplement.

Caution: Use sparingly if you have low blood pressure.

Found In: A·R·T Creme Masque, A·R·T Renewal Serum, Acceptance, Animal Scents Ointment, Aroma Life, AromaGuard Meadow Mist Deodorant, Australian Blue, Awaken, Believe, Boswellia Wrinkle Cream, Clarity, Common Sense, Dragon Time Bath & Shower Gel, Dragon Time Massage Oil, Dream Catcher, Evening Peace Bath & Shower Gel, FemiGen, Forgiveness, Gathering, Genesis Hand & Body Lotion, Gentle Baby, Gratitude, Grounding, Harmony, Highest Potential, Humility, Inner Child, Inspiration, Into the Future, Joy, KidScents Lotion, Lady Sclareol, Lavender-Rosewood Moisturizing Soap, Magnify Your Purpose, Motivation, Oola Grow, Peace & Calming, Prenolone Plus Body Cream, Present Time, Relaxation Massage Oil, Release, Rose Ointment, Sacred Mountain, Sacred Mountain Moisturizing Soap, Sandalwood Moisture Cream, SARA, Sensation, Sensation Bath & Shower Gel, Sensation Hand & Body Lotion, Sensation Massage Oil, White Angelica, Wolfberry Eye Cream

Yuzu *(Citrus junos)*

Botanical Family: Rutaceae

Plant Origin: China

Extraction Method: Cold-pressed from rind

Key Constituents:

Limonene (60-85%)

Beta-Phellandrene (1-5%)

Gamma-Terpinene (5-15%)

Linalool (0.5-3%)

ORAC: 620 µmole TE/gram

Historical Data: Thought to be a hybrid between Ichang papeda and Satsuma mandarin. Commonly used in cooking and for enhancing flavors due to the fragrant rind. There are a few reports on the use of yuzu essential oil for cosmetics and aromatherapy.

Medical Properties: Anti-inflammatory, anticancer, antidiabetic, asthma

Uses: Flavorant, inflammation, brain protection, stress

Fragrant Influence: High levels of limonene positively affect mood and heighten senses.

Application: (1) Apply 2-4 drops on location, (2) apply on chakras and/or Vita Flex points, (3) inhale directly, (4) diffuse, or (5) take as a dietary supplement

Caution: Avoid applying to skin that will be exposed to sunlight or UV light within 24 hours.

Found In: NingXia Red

Chapter 5

Oil Blends

Formulating Essential Oil Blends

This section describes specific blends that were formulated after years of research for both physical and emotional health. Each of these blends is formulated to maximize the synergistic effect between various oil chemistries and harmonic frequencies. When chemistry and frequency coincide, noticeable physical, spiritual, and emotional benefits can be attained.

Remember that some essential oils may be irritating to those with sensitive skin, and remember to avoid getting them in your eyes. In case you accidentally do get oil in an eye, dilute it quickly with a few drops of V-6 Vegetable Oil Complex, olive oil, or any other vegetable oil that is readily available, and call your doctor if necessary. Do not use water to rinse the eye, as water drives the oil into the tissues and creates more burning and pain.

All essential oils should be stored in a cool, dark place to preserve their fragile constituents that may dissipate over time or be damaged by harmful sunlight.

Essential Oil Blends

Abundance™

This blend exemplifies the true power of synergy: Together, all of its component oils are magnified in vibration, creating the law of attraction and the energy and frequency of prosperity and plentitude.

Ingredients:

Orange *(Citrus sinensis)* brings joy, security, peace, and happiness to those who possess it.

Frankincense *(Boswellia carterii)* was valued more than gold during ancient times, and only those with great wealth and abundance possessed it. It is considered a holy anointing oil in the Middle East and has been used in religious ceremonies for thousands of years. Frankincense contains sesquiterpenes, which stimulate and elevate the mind, overcoming stress and despair.

Patchouli *(Pogostemon cablin)* is used by East Indians to fragrance their clothing and homes to attract the good things of life. Legends say that Patchouli represented money, and those who possessed it were considered wealthy. It is also relaxing and helps clarify thoughts.

Clove *(Syzygium aromaticum)* is an oil from the Orient associated with great abundance, and those who possessed it were considered wealthy.

Ginger *(Zingiber officinale)* was highly prized in ancient times and amplifies the law of attraction.

Essential Oil Blend Application Codes

Neat = Straight, undiluted
Dilution usually NOT required; suitable for all but the most sensitive skin. Safe for children over 2 years old.

50-50 = Dilute 50-50
Dilution recommended at 50-50 (1 part essential oils to 1 part V-6 Vegetable Oil Complex) for topical and internal use, especially when used on sensitive areas — face, neck, genital area, underarms, etc. Keep out of reach of children.

20-80 = Dilute 20-80
Always dilute 20-80 (1 part essential oils to 4 parts V-6 Vegetable Oil Complex) before applying to the skin or taking internally. Keep out of reach of children.

PH = Photosensitizing
Avoid using on skin exposed to direct sunlight or UV rays (i.e., sunlamps, tanning beds, etc.).

Abundance	50-50	GLF
Acceptance	Neat	Gratitude
Aroma Life	Neat	Grounding
Aroma Siez	50-50	Harmony
Australian Blue	Neat	Highest Potential
Awaken	Neat	Hope
Believe	50-50	Humility
Brain Power	Neat	ImmuPower
Breathe Again Roll-On	Neat	Inner Child
Christmas Spirit	50-50	Inspiration
Citrus Fresh	50-50	Into The Future
Clarity	50-50	Joy
Common Sense	Neat	JuvaCleanse
Deep Relief Roll-On	Neat	JuvaFlex
DiGize	20-80	Lady Sclareol
Dragon Time	50-50	Live with Passion
Dream Catcher	50-50	Longevity
Egyptian Gold	50-50	Magnify Your Purpose
EndoFlex	50-50	Melrose
En-R-Gee	50-50	M-Grain
Envision	Neat	Mister
Evergreen Essence	50-50	Motivation
Exodus II	20-80	Oola Balance
Forgiveness	Neat	Oola Grow
Gathering	50-50	PanAway
Gentle Baby	50-50	Peace & Calming

Abundance 50-50
Acceptance .... **Neat**
Aroma Life .... **Neat**
Aroma Siez 50-50
Australian Blue .... **Neat**
Awaken .... **Neat**
Believe 50-50
Brain Power .... **Neat**
Breathe Again Roll-On....**Neat**
Christmas Spirit 50-50
Citrus Fresh 50-50
Clarity 50-50
Common Sense .... **Neat**
Deep Relief Roll-On ....**Neat**
DiGize **20-80**
Dragon Time................ 50-50
Dream Catcher 50-50
Egyptian Gold...............50-50
EndoFlex....................... 50-50
En-R-Gee 50-50
Envision .... **Neat**
Evergreen Essence..........50-50
Exodus II...................... **20-80**
Forgiveness .... **Neat**
Gathering...................... 50-50
Gentle Baby 50-50

GLF **20-80**
Gratitude...................... 50-50
Grounding 50-50
Harmony...................... 50-50
Highest Potential.......... 50-50
Hope.............................**Neat**
Humility .... **Neat**
ImmuPower **20-80**
Inner Child 50-50
Inspiration...................... **Neat**
Into The Future............. **Neat**
Joy...................... **PH. 50-50**
JuvaCleanse .... **Neat**
JuvaFlex......................... **Neat**
Lady Sclareol ....**Neat**
Live with Passion.......... 50-50
Longevity **20-80**
Magnify Your Purpose ... 50-50
Melrose 50-50
M-Grain........................ 50-50
Mister .... **Neat**
Motivation .... **Neat**
Oola Balance.................50-50
Oola Grow 50-50
PanAway 50-50
Peace & Calming .... **Neat**

Present Time .... **Neat**
Purification 50-50
Raven 50-50
R.C. 50-50
Release .... **Neat**
Relieve It 50-50
RutaVaLa .... **PH. 50-50**
RutaVaLa Roll-On ....**Neat**
Sacred Mountain 50-50
SARA .... **Neat**
SclarEssence 50-50
Sensation....................... **Neat**
Slique Essence ....**Neat**
Stress Away....................**Neat**
Stress Away Roll-On........**Neat**
Surrender 50-50
The Gift .... **Neat**
Thieves **20-80**
3 Wise Men.................... **Neat**
Tranquil Roll-On .... **Neat**
Transformation..... **PH..50-50**
Trauma Life................... **Neat**
Valor .... **Neat**
Valor Roll-On .... **Neat**
White Angelica..... **PH... Neat**

Myrrh *(Commiphora myrrha)* possesses the frequency of wealth, according to legends, and is referenced throughout the Old and New Testaments, *"A bundle of myrrh is my well-beloved unto me . . . "* (Song of Solomon 1:13). It was also part of a formula the Lord gave to Moses (Exodus 30:22-27). It was used traditionally in the royal palaces by the queens during pregnancy and birthing. Conferring a sense of dignity and stateliness, myrrh is a kingly oil.

Cinnamon Bark *(Cinnamomum zeylanicum)* is the oil of wealth from the Orient and part of the formula the Lord gave to Moses (Exodus 30:22-27). It was regarded by the emperors of China and India to have great value; their riches were measured by the amount of oil they possessed.

Spruce *(Picea mariana)* was traditionally believed to possess the frequency of prosperity. It helps relieve emotional blocks, bringing about a sense of balance.

Applications:

- For topical use, dilute 1 part Abundance with 1 part V-6 Vegetable Oil Complex. Apply 1-2 drops on location.
- Diffuse, directly inhale, or add 2-4 drops to bath water.
- Apply 1 to 2 drops over heart or on wrists, neck, and temples.
- Put 2 drops on a wet cloth and put in clothes dryer; however, it may stain white fabrics.
- Put 4-8 drops on cotton balls or tissues and put in or on vents.
- For aromatic use, diffuse up to 30-45 minutes daily. Avoid contact with eyes.
- Use Release first to release emotions that prevent us from receiving abundance. Follow with one or several blends such as Acceptance, Believe, Envision, Into the Future, The Gift, Joy, Magnify Your Purpose, Motivation, or Valor.

Acceptance™

Acceptance stimulates the mind, compelling us to open and accept new things, people, or relationships in life, allowing one to reach a higher potential. It also helps us to overcome procrastination and denial.

Ingredients:

Almond oil *(Prunus dulcis)* is used in this blend as a carrier oil. It is sweet to the taste and offers a rich source of vitamin E. In the ancient Ayurveda system of health care native to India, the almond is considered a nutrient for the brain and nervous system.

Coriander *(Coriandrum sativum)* has long been revered as a home remedy for relieving feelings of nausea, aiding digestion, and supporting healthy immune function.

Geranium *(Pelargonium graveolens)* assists in balancing hormones. It is antispasmodic, relaxant, anti-inflammatory, antibacterial, antifungal, and stimulates the liver and pancreas.

Bergamot *(Citrus bergamia)* (furocoumarin-free) is simultaneously uplifting and calming, with a unique ability to relieve anxiety, stress, and tension.

Frankincense *(Boswellia carterii)* is considered a holy anointing oil and has been used in religious ceremonies for thousands of years. It stimulates the limbic part of the brain, which elevates the mind, helping to overcome stress and despair. It is used in European medicine to combat depression.

Sandalwood *(Santalum album)* is high in sesquiterpene compounds, which stimulate the pineal gland and the limbic region of the brain, the center of emotions and memory. Used traditionally in yoga and meditation. May help remove negative programming in the cells.

Blue Tansy *(Tanacetum annuum)* helps cleanse the liver and lymphatic system, helping to overcome anger and negative emotions. Promotes a feeling of self-control.

Neroli *(Citrus sinensis)* was used by the ancient Egyptians for healing the mind, body, and spirit. It is stabilizing and strengthening to the emotions, promoting peace, confidence, and awareness. It brings everything into focus.

Ylang Ylang *(Cananga odorata)* promotes relaxation, balances male and female energies, restores confidence and equilibrium, and alleviates insomnia.

Applications:
- Diffuse or add 1-2 drops to bath water.
- Apply over heart and thymus, on wrists, behind ears, on neck and temples.

Aroma Life™

Aroma Life improves cardiovascular, lymphatic, and circulatory systems; lowers high blood pressure; and reduces stress.

Ingredients:

Sesame seed oil *(Sesamum indicum)* is used as a cosmetic carrier oil and is reputed to penetrate the skin easily. It is an antioxidant rich in vitamin E and has been associated with lowering cholesterol levels. It contains magnesium, copper, calcium, iron, zinc, and vitamin B6. Copper provides relief for rheumatoid arthritis. Magnesium supports vascular and respiratory health. Calcium helps prevent colon cancer, osteoporosis, migraine, and PMS. Zinc promotes bone health.

Cypress *(Cupressus sempervirens)* improves circulation and lymphatic drainage. It reduces edema and water retention and strengthens the vascular system.

Marjoram *(Origanum majorana)* helps regenerate smooth muscle tissue and assists in relieving muscle spasms. It calms nervous tension and has diuretic-like action.

Ylang Ylang *(Cananga odorata)* is used traditionally to balance heart function and to treat tachycardia (rapid heartbeat) and high blood pressure. It also combats insomnia.

Helichrysum *(Helichrysum italicum)* improves circulation and reduces blood viscosity. It is anticoagulant, regulates cholesterol, stimulates liver cell function, and reduces plaque deposits from the veins and arteries.

Applications:
- For topical use, apply 4 drops on the heart, abdomen, or in conjunction with Raindrop Technique as needed.
- Diffuse, directly inhale, or add 2-4 drops to bath water.
- Apply 1 to 2 drops over heart and along spine from first to fourth thoracic vertebrae (which correspond to the cardiopulmonary nerves).
- Dilute 1:15 with vegetable oil for a full-body massage.

Aroma Siez™

Aroma Siez is an advanced complex of anti-inflammatory, muscle-relaxing essential oils that promote circulation and relieve headaches and tight, inflamed, aching muscles resulting from injury, fatigue, or stress.

Ingredients:

Basil *(Ocimum basilicum)* combats muscle spasms and inflammation. It is relaxing to both striated and smooth muscles (involuntary muscles such as those found in the heart and digestive system).

Marjoram *(Origanum majorana)* helps regenerate smooth muscle tissue and assists in relieving spasms; reduces the pain of sprains, bruises, and migraine headaches; and calms the nerves. It is antibacterial and antiseptic.

Lavender *(Lavandula angustifolia)* relieves muscle spasms, sprains, pains, headaches, inflammation, anxiety, burns, and skin conditions (psoriasis), preventing scarring and stretch marks. It is hypotensive, anti-infectious, and anticoagulant. It is also calming and uplifting.

Peppermint (*Mentha piperita*) has powerful, pain-blocking, anti-inflammatory, and antispasmodic properties. A 2013 study conducted at the South African Tshwane University in Pretoria found that the main constituent of peppermint, menthol, not only is a highly effective skin penetrator but has analgesic effects (Kamatou GP, et al., 2013).

Cypress (*Cupressus sempervirens*) is antibacterial, antimicrobial, antiseptic, and improves circulation and lymphatic drainage. It reduces edema and water retention and strengthens the vascular system.

Applications:

- For topical use, dilute 1 drop of Aroma Siez with 1 drop of V-6 Vegetable Oil Complex or olive oil and apply to affected area as needed.
- Apply on location to sore muscles, ligaments, or areas of poor circulation.
- Use with Raindrop Technique.

Caution: Possible skin sensitivity.

Australian Blue™

This blend includes a rare Australian aromatic called blue cypress, a part of the aboriginal pharmacopoeia for thousands of years. It is distilled from the wood of *Callitris intratropica*, the northern cypress pine, which has antiviral properties. Its aromatic influence uplifts and inspires while simultaneously grounds and stabilizes.

Ingredients:

Blue Cypress (*Callitris intratropica*) contains guaiol and guaiazulene, strong anti-inflammatory and antiviral compounds. Oral traditions indicate that the aboriginal

Tiwi people of Northern Australia used resins from the bark of the blue cypress as a skin wash for sores and cuts. It is also used to relieve pain and repel insects.

Ylang Ylang (*Cananga odorata*) promotes relaxation and balances male and female energies. It also restores confidence and equilibrium.

Cedarwood (*Cedrus atlantica*) is high in sesquiterpenes, which stimulate the limbic part of the brain, the center of emotions and memory. It stimulates the pineal gland, which releases melatonin that improves mental awareness and memory. Cedarwood is also very grounding emotionally.

Blue Tansy (*Tanacetum annuum*) is anti-inflammatory and combats anger and negative emotions, promoting a feeling of self-control.

White Fir (*Abies concolor*) is antimicrobial, antiseptic, antiarthritic, and stimulating. It supports the body and reduces the symptoms of arthritis, rheumatism, bronchitis, coughs, and sinusitis. It creates a feeling of grounding, anchoring, and empowering.

Applications:

- Diffuse, directly inhale, or add 2-4 drops to bath water.
- Apply 1 to 2 drops on wrists, neck, temples, or foot Vita Flex points.
- Dilute 1:15 with vegetable oil for a full-body massage.
- It may also be diffused for 30 minutes or up to 1 hour 3-4 times daily.

Awaken™

Five specific blends combine to awaken and enhance inner self-awareness that strengthens the desire to reach one's highest potential. It stimulates right brain creativity, amplifying the function of the pineal and pituitary glands in balancing the energy centers of the body and helps us identify our true desires and how best to pursue them.

Ingredients:

Fractionated (virgin) coconut oil *(Cocos nucifera)* has been processed or "fractioned" to create a strong shelf life. With its antiseptic and disinfectant properties, it gives a strong, stabilizing foundation to the formulation.

Joy produces an uplifting, magnetic energy that brings joy to the heart. It inspires romance and helps overcome grief and depression.

Forgiveness helps release negative memories, enabling one to move past emotional barriers and achieve higher awareness. It invites one to forgive and let go.

Present Time has an empowering fragrance, which gives a feeling of being "in the moment." One can go forward and progress only when in the present time.

Dream Catcher helps open the mind and enhance dreams and visualization, promoting greater potential for realizing your dreams and staying on your path. It also protects from negative dreams that might cloud your vision.

Harmony promotes physical and emotional healing by bringing about a harmonic balance to the energy centers of the body. It reduces stress and creates a feeling of well-being.

Applications:

- Diffuse, directly inhale, or add 2-4 drops to bath water.
- Apply 1 to 2 drops over heart, on wrists, neck, temples, forehead, or foot Vita Flex points.
- Dilute 1:15 with vegetable oil for a full-body massage.
- Put 2 drops on a wet cloth and put in clothes dryer.

- Put 4-8 drops on cotton balls or tissues and put in or on vents.
- For clearing allergies, rub over sternum.

Caution: Possible sun sensitivity.

Believe™

Believe helps release the unlimited potential everyone possesses. It restores feelings of hope, making it possible to more fully experience health, happiness, and vitality.

Ingredients:

Idaho Balsam Fir *(Abies balsamea)* opens emotional blocks and recharges vital energy. It gives a feeling of strength and inner peace.

Coriander *(Coriandrum sativum)* has long been revered as a home remedy for relieving feelings of nausea, aiding digestion, and supporting healthy immune function.

Bergamot *(Citrus bergamia)* (furocoumarin-free) is simultaneously uplifting and calming, with a unique ability to relieve anxiety, stress, and tension.

Frankincense *(Boswellia carterii)* is considered a holy anointing oil in the Middle East and has been used in religious ceremonies for thousands of years. It stimulates the limbic part of the brain, elevating the mind and helping to overcome stress and despair. It is used in European medicine to combat depression.

Idaho Blue Spruce *(Picea pungens)* has an aroma that is grounding, stimulating to the mind, and relaxing to the body.

Ylang Ylang *(Cananga odorata)* promotes relaxation, balances male and female energies, restores confidence and equilibrium, and alleviates insomnia.

Geranium *(Pelargonium graveolens)* assists in balancing hormones. It is antispasmodic, relaxant, anti-inflammatory, antibacterial, antifungal, and stimulates the liver and pancreas.

Applications:

- Dilute 1 part essential oil to 1 part V-6 Vegetable Oil Complex.
- Directly inhale or add 2-4 drops to bath water.
- Apply 1 to 2 drops over heart, on wrists, neck, temples, forehead, or foot Vita Flex points.
- Dilute 1:15 with vegetable oil for a full-body massage.
- Put 2 drops on a wet cloth and put in clothes dryer.
- Put 4-8 drops on cotton balls or tissues and place in or on vents.
- It may also be diffused 30 to 60 minutes according to one's desire and how one feels.

Caution: Possible skin sensitivity.

Brain Power™

Brain Power promotes deep concentration and channels physical energy into mental energy. It also increases mental potential and clarity, and long-term use may retard the aging process. Many of the oils in this blend are high in sesquiterpene compounds that increase activity in the pineal, pituitary, and hypothalamus glands and thereby increase output of growth hormone and melatonin.

The oils also help dissolve petrochemicals that congest the receptor sites, clearing the "brain fog" that people experience due to exposure to synthetic petrochemicals in food, skin, hair-care products, and air.

Ingredients:

Sandalwood (*Santalum album*) is high in sesquiterpene compounds, which stimulate the pineal gland and the limbic region of the brain, the center of our emotions and memory. It is used traditionally in yoga and meditation.

Cedarwood (*Cedrus atlantica*) is high in sesquiterpenes, which can stimulate the limbic part of the brain, the center of emotions and memory. It stimulates the pineal gland, which releases melatonin, thereby improving thoughts, cognition, and memory.

Frankincense (*Boswellia carterii*) stimulates the limbic part of the brain, which elevates the mind, helping to overcome stress and despair. It is used in European medicine to combat depression.

Melissa (*Melissa officinalis*) stimulates the limbic part of the brain, the emotional center of memories. It removes emotional blocks and instills a positive outlook on life.

Blue Cypress (*Callitris intratropica*) improves circulation and increases the flow of oxygen to the brain, stimulating the amygdala, pineal gland, pituitary gland, and hypothalamus.

Lavender (*Lavandula angustifolia*) has been documented to improve concentration and mental acuity.

Japanese researchers at Yamanashi Prefectural University tested lavender aroma for concentration in the late afternoon, when work concentration was at its lowest. Of three groups of young men tested in the 2005 study (control group, jasmine group, and lavender group), the lavender group had significantly higher concentration levels than the other two groups (Sakamoto R, et al., 2005).

A study at Kyushu University in Japan in 2008 corroborated this finding after tests of lavender outperformed a control group and helped to maintain sustained attention during a long-term vigilance task (Shimizu K, et al., 2008).

Helichrysum (*Helichrysum italicum*) helps improve circulation and stimulate optimum nerve function. Enhances awareness and cognition and helps release feelings of anger, which allows one to gain focus and concentration.

Applications:

- Diffuse, directly inhale, or add 2-4 drops to bath water.
- Apply 1 to 2 drops on back of neck, throat, temples, or under nose.
- Apply 1 or 2 drops with a finger on insides of cheeks in mouth.
- Put 2 drops on a wet cloth and put in clothes dryer.
- Put 4-8 drops on cotton balls or tissues and put in or on vents.

Caution: Possible skin sensitivity.

Breathe Again™ Roll-On

This supercharged version of the R.C. blend is packaged in a convenient dispenser for easy use when air pollution makes it difficult to breathe or throat and nasal congestion strike. Contains four different eucalyptus oils and five additional essential oils, all known for their ability to relax airways, make breathing easier, and reduce coughing. In addition, these oils have anti-inflammatory characteristics.

Ingredients:

Fractionated (virgin) coconut oil *(Cocos nucifera)* has been processed or "fractioned" to create a strong shelf life. With its antiseptic and disinfectant properties, it gives a strong, stabilizing foundation to the delicate roll-on formulation.

Eucalyptus Staigeriana *(E. staigeriana),* known as Lemon Iron Bark or Lemon-scented Ironbark, has a lemon-scented aroma. It is antiviral, antiseptic, an expectorant, anti-inflammatory, and a digestive stimulant. It may be used on people with sensitive skin.

Eucalyptus Globulus *(E. globulus)* is fantastic on the skin for burns, blisters, wounds, insect bites, lice, and skin infections, as well as in combating the effects of colds and

the flu. It has the highest antiseptic cineole content and therefore is one of the strongest antiseptics among the eucalyptus varieties. Eucalyptus also has a history of soothing sore muscles and joints.

Laurus Nobilis (bay laurel) *(Laurus nobilis)* is anti-infectious, antibacterial, antiviral, antifungal, antiparasitic, antiseptic, and antinausea. In India, it is used as a sedative for whooping cough and toothaches. It can help relieve symptoms of bronchitis, skin disease, cholera, and diarrhea. It has also been used as a circulatory stimulant.

Rose hip seed oil *(Rosa rubiginosa)* is the best oil available for anti-aging and skin rejuvenation. It contains linolenic acids, oleic acid, and palmitic acid, which are important nutrients for the skin, regenerating tissue, reducing scar tissue, and minimizing wrinkles.

It also contains vitamins A and E and essential fatty acids, which help delay the effects of aging skin and increase collagen for greater elasticity. This oil assists with cell regeneration, further promoting healthy skin.

Peppermint *(Mentha piperita)* is a powerful anti-inflammatory and antiseptic for the respiratory system. It is used to treat bronchitis and pneumonia. High in menthol and menthone, it helps suppress coughs and clears lung and nasal congestion.

Eucalyptus Radiata *(E. radiata)* is commonly known as "narrow-leaved peppermint" and contains a high percentage of cineole (also known as eucalyptol). It is less harsh than other eucalyptus oils. It is popularly used to relieve colds and congestion and is more pleasant to inhale and less likely to irritate the skin. It can also be used on sore muscles and joints and is antiseptic. It has a crisp, clean, camphorous aroma with hints of citrus.

Copaiba (*Copaifera reticulata/langsdorfii*) is commonly used in anti-inflammatory recipes used traditionally for medicine by Shamans in the Amazon. It can also be effective in reducing muscle spasms.

Myrtle (*Myrtus communis*) is a wonderfully mild and gentle respiratory treatment, sometimes recommended for treating asthma attacks and respiratory problems with children.

Myrtle has a mildly sedative action that can make it useful in treating insomnia and nervous conditions. It is nonirritating and nonsensitizing, which makes it an appropriate oil to use with children and the elderly in cases of respiratory afflictions, chronic lung conditions, colds, infections, etc.

Blue Cypress (*Callitris intratropica*) improves circulation and increases the flow of oxygen to the brain, stimulating the amygdala, pineal gland, pituitary gland, and hypothalamus.

Eucalyptus Blue (*Eucalyptus bicostata*) can be used to combat the effects of colds and flu and has a fresh, camphorous aroma with a hint of peppermint.

Applications:

- Apply to throat, neck, or chest every 15-30 minutes for up to four applications for relief of symptoms related to colds, coughs, or sinus/lung congestion.

Chivalry

Harkening back to stories of gallant knights of old, Chivalry instills respect, honor, and integrity. It empowers you to higher ideals and instills courage.

Ingredients:

Valor balances energies to instill courage, confidence, and self-esteem. It helps the body self-correct its balance and alignment.

Ylang Ylang (*Cananga odorata*) promotes relaxation, balances male and female energies, restores confidence and equilibrium, and alleviates insomnia.

Joy produces an uplifting, magnetic energy that brings joy and happiness to the heart. It inspires romance and helps overcome grief and depression.

Harmony promotes physical and emotional healing by bringing about a harmonic balance to the energy centers of the body. It reduces stress and creates a feeling of well-being.

Gratitude fosters humility, strength, and open-mindedness.

Rose (*Rosa damascena*) has the highest frequency among essential oils. It creates a sense of balance, harmony, and well-being and elevates the mind. It creates a magnetic energy that attracts love and brings joy to the heart.

Geranium (*Pelargonium graveolens*) assists in balancing hormones. It is antispasmodic, relaxant, anti-inflammatory, antibacterial, antifungal, and stimulates the liver and pancreas.

Applications:

- For topical use, dilute 1:15 with V-6 Vegetable Oil Complex for a full-body massage. Apply 1-2 drops on location.
- Diffuse, directly inhale, or add 2-4 drops to bath water.
- Apply 1 to 2 drops over heart or on wrists, neck, temples, or foot VitaFlex points.
- Put 2 drops on a wet cloth and put in clothes dryer.
- Put 4-8 drops on cotton balls or tissues and put in or on vents.

Caution: Possible sun/skin sensitivity.

Christmas Spirit™

A purifying blend of evergreen, citrus, and spice, reminiscent of winter holidays, and brings joy, peace, happiness, and security.

Ingredients:

Orange *(Citrus sinensis)* is elevating to the mind and body, bringing security, joy, and peace.

Cinnamon Bark *(Cinnamomum zeylanicum)* is the oil of wealth from the Orient and part of the formula the Lord gave to Moses (Exodus 30:22-27).

Emperors of China and India measured their wealth partly by the amount of cinnamon they possessed. Traditionally, it was thought to have a frequency that attracted wealth and abundance.

It is highly antiviral, antifungal, and antibacterial. It brings back memories of wassail, home-cooked food, and fond memories of the holidays.

Spruce *(Picea mariana)* helps the respiratory and nervous systems. It is anti-infectious, antiseptic, and anti-inflammatory. Its aromatic influences help to open and release emotional blocks, bringing about feelings of balance and grounding.

Traditionally, spruce oil was believed to possess the frequency of prosperity. This oil brings memories of Christmas trees and makes the whole house feel more like home during the holidays.

Applications:

- Dilute 1 part essential oil to 1 part V-6 Vegetable Oil Complex.
- Diffuse, inhale directly, or add 2-4 drops to bath water.
- Apply 1 to 2 drops over heart, on wrists, neck, temples, or foot Vita Flex points.
- Dilute 1:15 with vegetable oil for a full-body massage.
- Put 2 drops on a wet cloth and put in clothes dryer.
- Put 4-8 drops on cotton balls or tissues and put in or on vents. Add to cedar chips for dresser drawers.
- Add a few drops to the wood before putting it in the fireplace.
- Splash a few drops on your paper vacuum cleaner bag for an uplifting and happy feeling while cleaning the house.

Caution: Possible sun/skin sensitivity.

Citrus Fresh™

Citrus Fresh stimulates the right brain to amplify creativity and well-being, eradicate anxiety, and works well as an air purifier. When diffused, it adds a clean, fresh scent to any environment.

Ingredients:

Orange *(Citrus sinensis)* is elevating to the mind and body, bringing security, joy, and peace. It is high in limonene, which prevents DNA damage, and has anticoagulant properties.

Tangerine *(Citrus reticulata)* contains esters and aldehydes that are sedating and calming, combating anxiety and nervousness. It is high in limonene, which prevents DNA damage.

Grapefruit *(Citrus paradisi)* is decongesting and fat-dissolving. It is high in limonene, which prevents DNA damage, and has anticoagulant properties. This aroma can be very calming and can bring a sense of wholeness.

Lemon *(Citrus limon)* has an extremely cleansing smell. This oil helps purify and uplift.

Mandarin *(Citrus reticulata)* has sedative and slightly hypnotic properties that combat insomnia, stress, and irritability. It is high in limonene, which prevents DNA damage. It also has anticoagulant properties.

Spearmint *(Mentha spicata)* oil helps support the respiratory, glandular, and nervous systems. With its hormone-like activity, it helps open and release emotional blocks and brings about a feeling of balance. It is antispasmodic, anti-infectious, antiparasitic, antiseptic, and anti-inflammatory. It has also been used to increase metabolism to burn fat.

Applications:

- Dilute 1 part essential oil to 1 part vegetable oil.
- A favorite for diffusing, directly inhaling, or adding 2-4 drops to bath water.
- Apply 1 to 2 drops on edge of ears, wrists, neck, temples, or foot VitaFlex points.
- Dilute 1:15 with vegetable oil for a full-body massage.
- Put 2 drops on a wet cloth and put in clothes dryer.
- Put 4-8 drops on cotton balls or tissues and put in or on vents.
- It can also be ingested.

Caution: Possible sun/skin sensitivity.

Clarity™

Promotes a clear mind and amplifies mental alertness and vitality. It increases energy when overly tired and brings greater focus to the spirit and mind.

Ingredients:

Basil *(Ocimum basilicum)* alleviates mental fatigue and muscle spasms.

Cardamom *(Elettaria cardamomum)* is uplifting, refreshing, and invigorating. It may be beneficial for clearing confusion. In a study done by Dember, et al., 1995, Cardamom was found to enhance performance accuracy.

Rosemary *(Rosmarinus officinalis CT cineol)* helps overcome mental fatigue, stimulates memory, and opens the conscious mind. University of Miami scientists found that inhaling Rosemary boosted alertness, eased anxiety, and amplified analytic and mental ability.

Peppermint *(Mentha piperita)* stimulates the mind and sense awareness. Dr. William N. Dember of the University of Cincinnati found that inhaling Peppermint oil increased mental accuracy by 28 percent.

Coriander *(Coriandrum sativum)* has long been revered as a home remedy for relieving feelings of nausea, aiding digestion, and supporting healthy immune function.

Geranium *(Pelargonium graveolens)* is antispasmodic, relaxant, anti-inflammatory, and uplifting.

Bergamot *(Citrus bergamia)* (furocoumarin-free) is simultaneously uplifting and calming, with a unique ability to relieve anxiety, stress, and tension.

Lemon *(Citrus limon)* is stimulating and invigorating. A recent Brazilian university study found that lemon essential oil had sedative, anxiolytic, and antidepressant effects (LM Lopes C, et al., 2011).

Ylang Ylang *(Cananga odorata)* promotes relaxation, balances male and female energies, restores confidence and equilibrium, and alleviates insomnia.

Jasmine *(Jasminum officinale)* stimulates the mind and improves concentration.

Roman Chamomile *(Anthemis nobilis)* combats restlessness, tension, and insomnia. It purges toxins from the liver, where anger is stored. It also clears mental blocks.

Palmarosa *(Cymbopogon martinii)* is stimulating and revitalizing and enhances both the nervous and cardiovascular system.

Applications:

- Dilute 1 part essential oil to 1 part V-6 Vegetable Oil Complex.
- Diffuse, directly inhale, or add 2-4 drops to bath water.

- Apply 1 to 2 drops on edge of ears, wrists, neck, forehead, temples, or VitaFlex points on the foot (brain and large toe).
- Clarity works well with Brain Power, Palo Santo, Lemon, or Peppermint to enhance its effects.

Caution: Possible sun/skin sensitivity.

Common Sense™

Common sense is a proprietary blend of pure Young Living essential oils especially formulated by D. Gary Young to increase mental acuity, helping to improve decision-making abilities and strengthen every-day thinking skills.

Ingredients:

Frankincense (*Boswellia carterii*) stimulates the limbic part of the brain, which elevates the mind, helping to overcome stress and despair. It is used in European medicine to combat depression.

Ylang Ylang (*Cananga odorata*) is relaxing and helps release feelings of anger, tension, and irritability. It also restores confidence and equilibrium.

Ocotea (*Octotea quixos*) has high levels of alpha-humulene to balance the body's response to stress and difficult situations.

Goldenrod (*Solidago canadensis*) supports the circulatory system, urinary tract, and liver function. It has relaxing and calming effects. The genus name Solidago, comes from the Latin word solide, which means "to make whole."

Ruta (*Ruta graveolens*) is farmed, harvested, and distilled at the Young Living farm in Ecuador. It relaxes the mind and body, calms nervousness, and rebalances energy.

Dorado Azul (*Hyptis suaveolens*) has a rich, herbaceous scent that is rich in eucalyptol and beta-pinene. It strengthens the lungs, promoting calm, easy breathing.

Lime (*Citrus aurantifolia*) creates a feeling of

happiness that counteracts negativity.

Applications:

- Diffuse up to 30 minutes 3 times daily or wear as a perfume.

Deep Relief Roll-On™

This convenient roll-on relieves muscle soreness and tension, soothes sore joints and ligaments, helps calm stressed nerves, and reduces inflammation. This powerful blend contains nine essential oils, most of which are known for their anti-inflammatory and pain-relieving characteristics.

This highly portable roll-on with its no-mess application is easy to carry in your pocket, purse, brief case, etc. It also passes through airport security for "easy breathing" while flying high.

Ingredients:

Peppermint (*Mentha piperita*) has been found to relieve surface pain and tension of the neck and head. It is also a highly regarded herb for soothing stomach discomfort.

Fractionated (virgin) coconut oil (*Cocos nucifera*) has been processed or "fractioned" to create a strong shelf life. With its antiseptic and disinfectant properties, it gives a strong, stabilizing foundation to the delicate roll-on formulation.

Lemon (*Citrus limon*) is stimulating and invigorating. A recent Brazilian university study found that lemon essential oil had sedative, anxiolytic, and antidepressant effects (LM Lopes C, et al., 2011).

Idaho Balsam Fir (*Abies balsamea*) has been prized through the ages for its medicinal effects and its ability to soothe muscular and rheumatic pain. Like other conifer oils, its aroma is grounding, stimulating to the mind, and relaxing to the body.

Clove (*Syzygium aromaticum*) has been used for decades as a natural anesthetic in dentistry. It was one of the ingredients in the original "Four Thieves Vinegar" that protected bandits who robbed the dead and dying during the 15th century plague. It has been shown to be extremely antioxidant as well as analgesic, anesthetic, and anti-inflammatory.

Copaiba (*Copaifera reticulata/langsdorfii*) is commonly used for anti-inflammatory recipes used traditionally by the tribal chiefs in the Amazon. It can also be effective in reducing muscle spasms.

Wintergreen (*Gaultheria procumbens*) is anti-inflammatory and antispasmodic. It is analgesic and reduces all types of pain.

Helichrysum (*Helichrysum italicum*) has been extensively studied in Europe for its unusual abilities to improve circulation, regenerate tissue, and relieve pain.

Vetiver (*Vetiveria zizanioides*) is well known for its anti-inflammatory properties and is traditionally used to relieve symptoms of arthritis.

Palo Santo (*Bursera graveolens*), harvested in Ecuador, is similar to frankincense and has traditionally been used to purify and cleanse the spirit from negative energies.

Applications:

- Apply generously on location every 15 minutes for up to four applications.
- For head tension, apply over temples and on forehead.

  Cautions: Keep out of reach of children. Do not ingest this blend. If pregnant, nursing, taking medication, or have a medical condition, consult a health-care professional prior to use.

DiGize™

This blend relieves digestive problems, including indigestion, heartburn, gas, and bloating. It helps fight Candida as it kills and digests parasite infestation.

Ingredients:

Tarragon (*Artemisia dracunculus*) is antiseptic and combats intestinal parasites and urinary tract infection. It is antispasmodic, anti-inflammatory, anti-infectious, and prevents fermentation.

Ginger (*Zingiber officinale*) has been traditionally used to combat nausea and gastrointestinal fermentation. It is antispasmodic, antiseptic, and helps to calm and alleviate indigestion.

Peppermint (*Mentha piperita*) is one of the most highly regarded herbs for improving digestion and combating parasites. It relaxes the smooth muscles of the intestinal tract and promotes peristalsis. It kills bacteria, yeasts, fungi, and mold.

Juniper (*Juniperus osteosperma* and *J. scopulorum*) works as a powerful detoxifier and cleanser and amplifies kidney function.

Fennel (*Foeniculum vulgare*) is antiseptic and stimulating to the gastrointestinal system. It is antispasmodic, antiseptic, and used for flatulence and nausea. It promotes digestion and prevents fermentation.

Anise (*Pimpinella anisum*) is antispasmodic, antiseptic, stimulates and increases bile flow, and helps calm and relieve spastic colitis, indigestion, and intestinal pain.

Patchouli (*Pogostemon cablin*) is a powerful digestive aid that alleviates nausea. Its antimicrobial and anti-inflammatory properties help reduce fluid retention.

Lemongrass (*Cymbopogon flexuosus*) has been documented to have powerful antifungal properties. It is vasodilating, anti-inflammatory, and improves digestion.

Applications:

- Dilute 1 part essential oil to 4 parts V-6 Vegetable Oil Complex or other vegetable oil of choice.
- Massage or use as a compress on the stomach.

- Apply to Vita Flex points on feet and ankles for stomach and intestinal relief.
- For internal use, dilute as directed above and take 1 capsule before each meal or as desired.

Caution: Possible sun sensitivity.

Dragon Time™

This blend relieves PMS symptoms and menstrual discomforts, including cramping and irregular periods. It helps balance emotions, alleviating mood swings and headaches caused by hormonal imbalance.

Ingredients:

Fennel *(Foeniculum vulgare)* is antiseptic and antispasmodic and has estrogen-like and hormone-like activities.

Clary sage *(Salvia sclarea)* supports the body's production of scleral, important for balancing hormones. It contains natural sclareol, a phytoestrogen that mimics estrogen function. It helps with menstrual cramps, PMS, circulatory problems, and hormone balancing.

Marjoram *(Origanum majorana)* relieves muscle spasms and calms nerves. It relieves menopausal symptoms as well as painful periods.

Lavender *(Lavandula angustifolia)* is a relaxant that relieves anxiety, headaches, and PMS symptoms.

Yarrow *(Achillea millefolium)* balances hormones and reduces inflammation.

Jasmine *(Jasminum officinale)* is used for muscle spasms, frigidity, depression, and nervous exhaustion and helps brings out feminine attributes.

Applications:

- Dilute 1 part essential oil to 1 part vegetable oil.

- Diffuse, directly inhale, or add 2-4 drops to bath water.
- Apply 1 to 2 drops on wrists, neck, temples, or foot Vita Flex points.
- Dilute 1:15 with vegetable oil for a full-body massage.
- Apply with a hot compress or directly over lower abdomen, across lower back, or on location of pain.
- May also be used on both sides of ankles and feet.

Caution: Possible sun sensitivity.

Dream Catcher™

This blend stimulates the emotional centers of the brain, awakening creative thoughts and enhancing dreams and visualizations, promoting greater potential for realizing your dreams and staying on your path. It also protects from negative thoughts and dreams that might cloud your vision.

Ingredients:

Sandalwood *(Santalum album)* is high in sesquiterpene compounds, which stimulate the pineal gland and the limbic region of the brain, the center of our emotions and memory. It has been used traditionally in yoga and meditation. It also promotes and enhances deep sleep.

Tangerine *(Citrus reticulata)* combats anxiety, nervousness, and depression. A 1995 Mie University study found that the application of citrus fragrance to depressive patients made it possible to markedly reduce doses of antidepressants (Komori T, et al., 1995). Citrus fragrances boost immunity and are extremely uplifting and calming.

Ylang Ylang *(Cananga odorata)* promotes relaxation, balances male and female energies, restores confidence and equilibrium, and alleviates insomnia.

Black Pepper *(Piper nigrum)* stimulates the endocrine system and increases energy.

Bergamot *(Citrus bergamia)* (furocoumarin-free) is simultaneously uplifting and calming, with a unique ability to relieve anxiety, stress, and tension.

Juniper *(Juniperus osteosperma* and *J. scopulorum)* elevates spiritual awareness to create feelings of love and peace. Juniper has also been used to cleanse the spirit.

Anise *(Pimpinella anisum)* has a sedative effect, slowing down circulation, respiration, and nervous response. It is found effective in sedating nervous afflictions, hyper reactions, and convulsions.

Blue Tansy *(Tanacetum annuum)* helps to overcome anger and negative emotions, promoting a feeling of self-control.

Applications:
- Dilute 1 part essential oil to 1 part V-6 Vegetable Oil Complex.
- Diffuse up to 1 hour 3 times daily.
- Directly inhale (most effective before and during sleep) or add 2-4 drops to bath water.
- Apply on forehead, ears, throat, eyebrows, base of neck, and under nose.
- Use during meditation, in saunas, or just before sleeping.
- For topical use, dilute 1 drop with V-6 Vegetable Oil Complex or oil of choice and apply as needed.

Cautions: Possible sun/skin sensitivity. Avoid direct sunlight or UV rays for 12 hours after applying product.

Note: If unpleasant dreams occur, continue to use, since subconscious memories and thoughts will still need to be resolved. Hold on to your dreams and visualize the problems being solved. It may be helpful to write the dreams down upon arising.

Egyptian Gold™

This is a very unique blend that combines the most valuable essences of the Middle East and Central Europe. It offers a truly enchanting aromatic effect that stimulates the central nervous system and the immune and respiratory systems.

Ingredients:

Frankincense *(Boswellia carterii)* is considered a holy anointing oil in the Middle East. It stimulates the hypothalamus to amplify immunity.

In ancient times, it was well known for its healing powers and was reportedly used to treat every conceivable ill. It was considered to be a gift of the highest caliber during the time of Christ.

Lavender *(Lavandula angustifolia)* is relaxing and grounding. University of Miami researchers found that inhalation of Lavender oil increased beta waves in the brain, suggesting heightened relaxation. It also reduced depression and improved cognitive performance (Diego MA, et al., 1998).

Idaho Balsam Fir *(Abies balsamea)* has been researched for its ability to kill airborne germs and bacteria. As a confer oil, it creates a feeling of grounding, anchoring, and empowering.

Myrrh *(Commiphora myrrha)* is an antimicrobial and antimutagenic oil. It is referenced in the Bible, *"A bundle of myrrh is my well-beloved unto me . . ."* (Song of Solomon 1:13). Its high levels of sesquiterpenes stimulate the hypothalamus and the pituitary and amplify immune response. It possesses the frequency of wealth, according to legends of antiquity.

Spikenard *(Nardostachys jatamansi)* was used by Mary of Bethany to anoint the feet of Jesus. It strengthens immunity and hypothalamus function.

Hyssop *(Hyssopus officinalis)* is anti-inflammatory, antiparasitic, anti-infectious, and a decongestant and works well for opening up the respiratory system.

Cedarwood *(Cedrus atlantica)* is high in sesquiterpenes, which can stimulate the limbic part of the brain, the center of emotions and memory. It stimulates the pineal gland, which releases melatonin, thereby improving thoughts, cognition, and memory.

Rose *(Rosa damascena)* has the highest frequency among essential oils. It creates a sense of balance, harmony, and well-being and elevates the mind. It creates a magnetic energy that attracts love and brings joy to the heart.

Cinnamon Bark *(Cinnamomum zeylanicum)* is part of the formula the Lord gave to Moses (Exodus 30:22-27). It is antibacterial, antiparasitic, antiviral, and antifungal.

Applications:

- This is a blend for dietary, topical, or aromatic use.
- When using as a supplement, dilute 1 drop of essential oil with 4 drops of V-6 Vegetable Oil Complex or oil of choice and put in a capsule. Then take 1 capsule before each meal or as desired.
- Diffuse, directly inhale, or add 2-4 drops to bath water.
- Apply 1 to 2 drops over heart, on wrists, neck, temples, or foot Vita Flex points.
- Dilute 1:15 with vegetable oil for a full-body massage.
- Put 2 drops on a wet cloth and put in clothes dryer.
- Put 4-8 drops on cotton balls or tissues and place in or on vents.

Caution: Possible sun sensitivity.

EndoFlex™

This blend amplifies metabolism and vitality and creates hormonal balance.

Ingredients:

Sesame seed oil *(Sesamum indicum)* is used as a cosmetic carrier oil and is reputed to penetrate the skin easily. It is an antioxidant rich in vitamin E.

Spearmint *(Mentha spicata)* is used to increase metabolism to burn fat. With its hormone-like activity, it supports the nervous and glandular systems. Spearmint is antispasmodic, antiseptic, anti-inflammatory, and also highly invigorating and stimulating.

Sage *(Salvia officinalis)* strengthens the vital energy centers of the body. The Lakota Indians used sage for purifying, healing, and dispelling negative emotions.

Geranium *(Pelargonium graveolens)* assists in balancing hormones. It is antispasmodic, relaxant, anti-inflammatory, antibacterial, antifungal, and stimulates the liver and pancreas.

Myrtle *(Myrtus communis)* helps normalize hormonal imbalances of the thyroid and ovaries.

German Chamomile *(Matricaria recutita)* is highly anti-inflammatory and liver-protecting.

Nutmeg *(Myristica fragrans)* supports the adrenal glands for increased energy. It is powerfully stimulating and energizing.

Applications:

- Diffuse up to 30 minutes 3 times daily, directly inhale, or add 2-4 drops to bath water
- Apply over lower back, thyroid, kidneys, liver, feet, glandular areas, and foot Vita Flex points for these organs.
- For use as a dietary supplement, dilute with 1 drop of V-6 Vegetable Oil Complex, put in a capsule, and take up to 3 times daily or

as needed.

- For topical use dilute 1 drop of EndoFlex with 1 drop of V-6 Vegetable Oil Complex. Apply to affected area as needed.

En-R-Gee™

This blend increases vitality, circulation, and alertness.

Ingredients:

Rosemary *(Rosmarinus officinalis* CT cineol) helps overcome mental fatigue, stimulates memory, and opens the conscious mind. University of Miami scientists found that inhaling rosemary boosted alertness, eased anxiety, and amplified analytic and mental ability.

Juniper *(Juniperus osteosperma* and *J. scopulorum)* detoxifies, cleanses, improves nerve and kidney function, and elevates spiritual awareness.

Lemongrass *(Cymbopogon flexuosus)* increases blood circulation and vasodilation.

Nutmeg *(Myristica fragrans)* supports the adrenal glands for increased energy. It is powerfully stimulating and energizing.

Idaho Balsam Fir *(Abies balsamea)* is stimulating and calming at the same time and empowers and motivates one to go forward and achieve goals.

Clove *(Syzygium aromaticum)* is a powerful, general stimulant with its antioxidant properties.

Black pepper *(Piper nigrum)* stimulates the endocrine system and increases energy in all systems of the body.

Applications:

- Dilute 1 part essential oil to 2 parts V-6 Vegetable Oil Complex.
- Diffuse, directly inhale, or add 2-4 drops

to bath water. It may also be used with Raindrop Technique.

- For topical use, dilute as indicated above and apply on desired location or on temples, back of neck, forehead, chakra, and Vita Flex points.
- Diffuse for 15-20 minutes several times daily as desired.
- Rub En-R-Gee on feet and Awaken on temples for intensified effect.

Cautions: Possible skin sensitivity. Avoid contact with mucous membranes or sensitive skin. Not intended for use on children.

Envision™

This blend renews focus and stimulates creative and intuitive abilities needed to achieve goals and dreams. It helps to reawaken internal drive and independence and to overcome fears and emotional blocks.

Ingredients:

Spruce *(Picea mariana)* helps to open and release emotional blocks, bringing about a feeling of balance and grounding. Traditionally, spruce oil was believed to possess the frequency of prosperity.

Geranium *(Pelargonium graveolens)* helps release negative memories, thereby opening and elevating the mind.

Orange *(Citrus sinensis)* is elevating to the mind and body. A Brazilian university evaluated the potential anxiolytic effect of *Citrus sinensis* essential oil and found in a placebo-controlled study that the aroma of sweet orange oil was acutely anxiolytic, giving support to its calming use as a tranquilizer by aromatherapists (Goes TC, et al., 2012).

Lavender *(Lavandula angustifolia)* has been documented to improve concentration and mental acuity.

University of Miami researchers found that inhalation of lavender oil increased beta waves in the brain, suggesting heightened relaxation. It also reduced depression and improved cognitive performance (Diego MA, et al., 1998).

Japanese researchers at Yamanashi Prefectural University tested lavender aroma for concentration in the late afternoon, when work concentration was at its lowest. Of three groups of young men tested in the study (control group, jasmine group, and lavender group), the lavender group had significantly higher concentration levels than the other two groups (Sakamoto R, et al., 2005).

Sage *(Salvia officinalis)* strengthens the vital centers of the body. The Lakota Indians used sage for purifying, healing, and dispelling negative emotions. It was known as a sacred herb by the Romans.

Rose *(Rosa damascena)* possesses the highest frequency of the oils. It creates a sense of balance, harmony, and well-being and elevates the mind. Rose creates a magnetic energy that attracts love and brings joy to the heart.

Applications:

- Diffuse, directly inhale, or add 2-4 drops to bath water.
- Apply 1 to 2 drops on forehead, edge of ears, wrists, neck, temples, or foot Vita Flex points.
- Put 2 drops on a wet cloth and put in clothes dryer.
- Put 4-8 drops on cotton balls or tissues and put in or on vents.

Evergreen Essence™

Evergreen Essence™ essential oil blend has a refreshing, crisp scent that is invigorating and emotionally strengthening. With an arrangement of popular evergreen trees, the scents of pine, fir, and spruce complement one another and may assist in the release of occasional emotional blocks.* Refreshing to the senses, Evergreen Essence may bring a feeling of balance, peace, and security. The relaxing scent may also help clear the mind for a calming sense of meditation and reflection.

Ingredients:

The evergreen trees that are used in this refreshing blend are Idaho Blue Spruce, Idaho Ponderosa Pine, Scotch Pine, Red Fir, Western Red Cedar, White Fir, Black Pine, Pinyon Pine, and Lodgepole Pine.

Applications:

- Dilute 1 part essential oil to 1 part V-6 Vegetable Oil Complex.
- Diffuse, inhale directly, or add 2-4 drops to bath water.
- Apply 1-2 drops over heart, on wrists, neck, temples, or foot Vita Flex points.
- Dilute 1:15 with vegetable oil for a full-body massage.
- Put 2 drops on a wet cloth and put in clothes dryer.
- Put 4-8 drops on cotton balls or tissues and put in or on vents.
- Add to cedar chips for dresser drawers.
- Add a few drops to the wood before putting it in the fireplace.
- Splash a few drops on your paper vacuum cleaner bag for an uplifting and happy feeling while cleaning the house.

Exodus II™

Some researchers believe that these aromatics were used by Aaron, the brother of Moses, to protect the Israelites from a plague. Modern science shows that these oils contain immune-stimulating and antimicrobial compounds. Because of the complex chemistry of essential oils, it is very difficult for viruses and bacteria to mutate and acquire resistance to them.

Ingredients:

Olive oil (*Olea europaea*) is an ancient beauty secret discovered over 5,000 years ago. It promotes a smooth complexion with youthful elasticity; conditions dry, brittle nails; and makes the hair shine with vibrancy.

The Egyptians, Greeks, and Romans were all enamored with this prized oil as they enjoyed its radiant, youthful benefits. Olive oil preserves the taste, aroma, vitamins, and properties of the olive fruit, and in ancient times it was considered a magical source for the fountain of youth, wealth, and power.

Myrrh (*Commiphora myrrha*) is antimicrobial and antimutagenic. It is referenced in the Bible, "*A bundle of myrrh is my well-beloved unto me . . .*" (Song of Solomon 1:13). Its levels of sesquiterpenes stimulate the hypothalamus and pituitary and amplify immune response.

Cassia (*Cinnamomum cassia*) is anti-infectious, antibacterial, and anticoagulant. It was part of the formula the Lord gave to Moses for the holy anointing oil (Exodus 30:22-27).

Cinnamon Bark (*Cinnamomum zeylanicum*) is part of the formula the Lord gave to Moses (Exodus 30:22-27). It is antibacterial, antiparasitic, antiviral, and antifungal.

Calamus (*Acorus calamus*) is part of the formula the Lord gave to Moses (Exodus 30:22-27). It is antispasmodic, anti-inflammatory, and helps to alleviate gastrointestinal disturbances.

Hyssop (*Hyssopus officinalis*) is anti-inflammatory, antiparasitic, anti-infectious, and decongestant.

Galbanum (*Ferula gummosa*) has been prized for healing since biblical times. Exodus 30:34 states, "And the Lord said unto Moses, Take unto thee sweet spices, stacte, and onycha, and galbanum; sweet spices with pure frankincense:"

Spikenard (*Nardostachys jatamansi*) was used by Mary of Bethany to anoint the feet of Jesus. It strengthens immunity and hypothalamus function.

Frankincense (*Boswellia carterii*) is considered a holy anointing oil in the Middle East. It stimulates the hypothalamus to amplify immunity.

Applications:

- Diffuse, directly inhale, or add 2-4 drops to bath water.
- Apply 1 to 2 drops on ears, wrists, foot Vita Flex points, or along spine Raindrop Technique-style.
- For topical use, dilute 1 drop of Exodus II with 4 drops of V-6 Vegetable Oil Complex or oil of choice, and test for sensitivity on the underside of the arm.
- Apply to affected area as needed.
- Diffuse 10 to 15 minutes every 2-3 hours or as desired.

Cautions: Possible skin sensitivity. Not intended for children under 12 years of age, unless directed by a health professional.

Forgiveness™

This blend helps to release hurt feelings and negative emotions. It also helps release negative memories, allowing one to move past emotional barriers and attain higher awareness, assisting the person to forgive and let go.

Ingredients:

Sesame seed oil (*Sesamum indicum*) is used as a cosmetic carrier oil and is reputed to penetrate the skin easily. It is an antioxidant rich in vitamin E.

Melissa (*Melissa officinalis*) brings out gentleness. It is calming and balancing to the emotions, affecting the limbic part of the brain, the emotional center of memories. It helps alleviate depression, hypertension, and anxiety.

Geranium *(Pelargonium graveolens)* assists in balancing hormones, with antidepressant, uplifting, and tension-relieving properties.

Frankincense *(Boswellia carterii)* is considered a holy anointing oil in the Middle East and has been used in religious ceremonies for thousands of years. It stimulates the limbic part of the brain, elevating the mind, and helping to overcome stress and despair. It is used in European medicine to combat depression.

Sandalwood *(Santalum album)* is high in sesquiterpene compounds, which stimulate the pineal gland and the limbic region of the brain, the center of emotions and memory. It is used traditionally in yoga and meditation and may help remove negative programming in the cells.

Coriander *(Coriandrum sativum)* has long been revered as a home remedy for relieving feelings of nausea, aiding digestion, and supporting healthy immune function.

Angelica *(Angelica archangelica)* helps to calm emotions and bring memories back to the point of origin before trauma or anger was experienced, helping to let go of negative feelings.

Lavender *(Lavandula angustifolia)* has been documented to improve concentration and mental acuity.

Japanese researchers at Yamanashi Prefectural University tested lavender aroma for concentration in the late afternoon, when work concentration was at its lowest. Of three groups of young men tested in the 2005 study (control group, jasmine group, and lavender group), the lavender group had significantly higher concentration levels than the other two groups (Sakamoto R, et al., 2005).

A study at Kyushu University in Japan in 2008 corroborated this finding after tests of lavender outperformed a control group and helped to maintain sustained attention during a long-term vigilance task (Shimizu K, et al., 2008).

Bergamot *(Citrus bergamia)* (furocoumarin-free) is simultaneously uplifting and calming, with a unique ability to relieve anxiety, stress, and tension.

Lemon *(Citrus limon)* is stimulating and invigorating, promoting a deep sense of well-being. A recent Brazilian university study found that lemon essential oil had sedative, anxiolytic, and antidepressant effects (LM Lopes C, et al., 2011).

Ylang Ylang *(Cananga odorata)* promotes relaxation, balances male and female energies, restores confidence and equilibrium, and alleviates insomnia.

Jasmine *(Jasminum officinale)* has therapeutic effects, both emotional and physical. It is uplifting, antidepressant, and counteracts indifference, frigidity, and hopelessness.

Helichrysum *(Helichrysum italicum)* helps release feelings of anger, promoting forgiveness.

Roman Chamomile *(Anthemis nobilis)* combats restlessness, tension, and opens mental blocks. It purges toxins from the liver, where anger is stored.

Palmarosa *(Cymbopogon martinii)* is stimulating and revitalizing, enhancing both the nervous and cardiovascular system, and creates a feeling of security.

Rose *(Rosa damascena)* has the highest frequency among essential oils. It creates a sense of balance, harmony, and well-being and elevates the mind. It creates a magnetic energy that attracts love and brings joy to the heart.

Applications:

- Diffuse, directly inhale, or add 2-4 drops to bath water.
- Apply 1 to 2 drops behind ears, on wrists, neck, temples, navel, solar plexus, or heart.
- Dilute 1:15 with vegetable oil for a full-body massage.
- Put 4-8 drops on cotton balls or tissues and put in or on vents.

Cautions: Possible sun/skin sensitivity. Avoid contact with eyes.

Gathering™

This blend is created to help us overcome the bombardment of chaotic energy that alters our focus and takes us off our path toward higher achievements. Galbanum, a favorite oil of Moses, has a strong effect when blended with Frankincense and Sandalwood in gathering our emotional and spiritual thoughts, helping us to achieve our potential. These oils help increase the oxygen around the pineal and pituitary gland, bringing greater harmonic frequency to receive the communication we desire.

This blend helps bring people together on a physical, emotional, and spiritual level for greater focus and clarity. It helps one stay focused, grounded, and clear in gathering one's potential for self-improvement.

Ingredients:

Lavender (*Lavandula angustifolia*) has been documented to improve concentration and mental acuity.

Japanese researchers at Yamanashi Prefectural University tested lavender aroma for concentration in the late afternoon, when work concentration was at its lowest. Of three groups of young men tested in the 2005 study (control group, jasmine group,

and lavender group), the lavender group had significantly higher concentration levels than the other two groups (Sakamoto R, et al., 2005).

A study at Kyushu University in Japan corroborated this finding after tests of lavender outperformed a control group and helped to maintain sustained attention during a long-term vigilance task (Shimizu K, et al., 2008).

Geranium (*Pelargonium graveolens*) stimulates nerves and assists in balancing hormones. Its aromatic influence helps release negative memories, thereby opening and elevating the mind.

Galbanum (*Ferula gummosa*) was used for both medicinal and spiritual purposes. When combined with frankincense and sandalwood, its frequency increases dramatically. ("And the Lord said unto Moses, Take unto thee sweet spices, stacte, and onycha, and galbanum; sweet spices with pure frankincense:" Exodus 30:34).

Frankincense (*Boswellia carterii*) is considered a holy anointing oil in the Middle East and has been used in religious ceremonies for thousands of years.

It stimulates the limbic part of the brain, elevating the mind and helping to overcome stress and despair. It is used in European medicine to combat depression. It helps connect us with our greater powers.

Sandalwood (*Santalum album*) is high in sesquiterpene compounds, which stimulate the pineal gland and the limbic region of the brain, the center of emotions and memory. It is used traditionally in yoga and meditation and is very grounding and stabilizing.

Ylang Ylang (*Cananga odorata*) increases relaxation and balances male and female energies. It also restores confidence, equilibrium, and balance.

Spruce (*Picea mariana*) helps to open and release emotional blocks, creating a feeling of balance and grounding. Traditionally, Spruce oil was believed to possess the frequency of prosperity.

Cinnamon Bark (*Cinnamomum zeylanicum*) is the oil of wealth from the Orient and part of the formula the Lord gave to Moses (Exodus 30:22-27). It has been traditionally used to help one release malice or spite.

Rose (*Rosa damascena*) has the highest frequency among essential oils. It creates a sense of balance, harmony, and well-being and elevates the mind. It creates a magnetic energy that attracts love and brings joy to the heart.

Applications:

- Dilute 1 part essential oil to 1 part V-6 Vegetable Oil Complex.
- Diffuse, directly inhale, or add 2-4 drops to bath water.
- Apply 1 to 2 drops on edge of ears, wrists, neck, or temples.
- It may also be applied along the spine in a Raindrop Technique-style.
- Dilute 1:15 with V-6 Vegetable Oil Complex for a full-body massage.
- Put 2 drops on a wet cloth and put in clothes dryer.
- Put 4-8 drops on cotton balls or tissues and put in or on vents.
- Use Forgiveness on the navel, The Gift and Sacred Mountain on the crown (to clear negative attitudes), Valor on the crown or feet, 3 Wise Men on the crown, Clarity on the temples, and Dream Catcher on the forehead, ears, throat, eyebrows, base of neck, and under the nose.

Caution: Possible skin sensitivity.

Gentle Baby™

This blend is comforting, soothing, relaxing, and beneficial for reducing stress during pregnancy. It helps reduce stretch marks and scar tissue, rejuvenates the skin, improves elasticity, and reduces wrinkles.

It is particularly soothing to babies with dry, chapped skin and diaper rash. Skin issues improve when using Gentle Baby with Rose Ointment on the top of it. It is calming and brings a feeling of peace for tiny babies, children, and adults.

Ingredients:

Geranium (*Pelargonium graveolens*) has been used for centuries for skin care. It revitalizes tissue and nerves and has relaxing, anti-inflammatory, anti-infectious effects.

Rosewood (*Aniba rosaeodora*) is high in linalool, which has a relaxing, empowering, and uplifting effect. It is also very grounding and strengthening.

Coriander (*Coriandrum sativum*) has long been revered as a home remedy for relieving feelings of nausea, aiding digestion, and supporting healthy immune function.

Palmarosa (*Cymbopogon martinii*) combats candida, rashes, scaly, and flaky skin. It stimulates new cell growth, as it moisturizes and promotes healing. It is antimicrobial and helps reduce tension and recovery from nervous exhaustion.

Lavender (*Lavandula angustifolia*) is known as the universal oil. It is beneficial for skin conditions such as burns, rashes, and psoriasis and prevents scarring and stretch marks. It is relaxing, grounding, and combats depression.

Ylang Ylang (*Cananga odorata*) increases relaxation and balances male and female energies. It also restores confidence and equilibrium.

Roman Chamomile (*Anthemis nobilis*) combats restlessness, insomnia, muscle tension, and inflammation.

Lemon *(Citrus limon)* A Brazilian university study found that lemon essential oil had sedative, anxiolytic, and antidepressant effects (LM Lopes C, et al., 2011).

Jasmine *(Jasminum officinale)* is beneficial for dry, greasy, irritated, or sensitive skin. It also brings out femininity and helps with depression and nervous exhaustion.

Rose *(Rosa damascena)* oil has been used to beautify the skin for thousands of years. It reduces scarring and promotes elasticity for healthy skin.

Applications:
- Dilute 1 part essential oil to 1 part V-6 Vegetable Oil Complex.
- Diffuse or apply on location for dry, chapped skin or diaper rash.
- Apply over mother's abdomen, on feet, lower back, face, and neck areas.
- Dilute with vegetable oil for body massage and for applying on baby's skin.
- **For Pregnancy and Delivery:** Use for massage throughout entire pregnancy for relieving stress and anxiety, creating serenity, and preventing scarring. Massage on the perineum to help it stretch for easier birthing.

Caution: Possible sun sensitivity.

GLF™

The initials of this essential oil blend stand for Gallbladder and Liver Flush. It is formulated with oils that help to cleanse and restore liver and gallbladder function when taken in capsules as a dietary supplement.

Ingredients:

Ledum *(Ledum groenlandicum)* strengthens the liver and improves bile function.

Helichrysum *(Helichrysum italicum)* stimulates liver cell function and removes plaque from veins and arteries.

Celery Seed *(Apium graveolens)* is a powerful liver cleanser.

Grapefruit *(Citrus paradisi)* is decongesting and fat-dissolving. It is high in limonene, which prevents DNA damage, and has anticoagulant properties.

Hyssop *(hyssopus officinalis)* is a decongestant that is also anti-inflammatory, antiparasitic, and anti-infectious. It cleans the gallbladder and dissolves stones.

Spearmint *(Mentha spicata)* is antispasmodic, anti-infectious, antiparasitic, antiseptic, and anti-inflammatory. It has also been used to increase metabolism for fat burning.

Applications:
- Make a mixture diluted 80/20 with V-6 Vegetable Oil Complex and take 1-3 capsules daily to support a detoxification and cleansing routine focused on the liver and gallbladder.

Gratitude™

This delightful blend is designed to elevate, soothe, and bring relief to the body while helping to foster a grateful attitude. It is also nourishing and supportive to the skin. The New Testament tells us that on one occasion, Christ healed 10 lepers (Luke 17:12-19), but only one returned to express his thanks. This blend embodies the spirit of that grateful leper.

Ingredients:

Idaho Balsam Fir *(Abies balsamea)* opens emotional blocks and recharges vital energy.

Frankincense *(Boswellia carterii)* is considered a holy anointing oil in the Middle East and has been used in religious ceremonies for thousands of years.

It stimulates the limbic part of the brain, elevating the mind and helping to overcome stress and despair. It is used in European medicine to combat depression.

Coriander *(Coriandrum sativum)* has long

been revered as a home remedy for relieving feelings of nausea, aiding digestion, and supporting healthy immune function.

Myrrh (*Commiphora myrrha*) is referenced throughout the Old and New Testaments, constituting a part of a holy anointing formula given to Moses (Exodus 30:22-27). It has one of the highest levels of sesquiterpenes, a class of compounds that can stimulate the hypothalamus, pituitary, and amygdala, the control center for emotions and hormone release in the brain. It possesses the frequency of wealth, according to legends.

Ylang Ylang (*Cananga odorata*) promotes relaxation, balances male and female energies, restores confidence and equilibrium, and alleviates insomnia.

Galbanum (*Ferula gummosa*) was used for both medicinal and spiritual purposes. It is antimicrobial and supporting to the body. When combined with Frankincense and Sandalwood, its frequency increases dramatically ("And the Lord said unto Moses, Take unto thee sweet spices, stacte, and onycha, and galbanum; sweet spices with pure frankincense:" Exodus 30:34).

Bergamot (*Citrus bergamia*) (furocoumarin-free) is simultaneously uplifting and calming, with a unique ability to relieve anxiety, stress, and tension

Geranium (*Pelargonium graveolens*) assists in balancing hormones. It is antispasmodic, relaxant, anti-inflammatory, antibacterial, antifungal, and stimulates the liver and pancreas.

Applications:
- Diffuse, directly inhale, or add 2-4 drops to bath water.
- Apply 1 to 2 drops behind ears, over heart, on wrists, base of neck, temples, or base of spine.

- Put 4-8 drops on cotton balls or tissues and put in or on vents.

Caution: Possible skin sensitivity.

Grounding™

This blend creates a feeling of solidarity and balance. It stabilizes and grounds us in order to cope constructively with reality. When we're hurting emotionally, we resort to avoidance. When this happens, it is easy to make poor choices that lead to unhealthy relationships and unwise business decisions. We seek to escape because we do not have anchoring or awareness to know how to deal with our emotions.

Ingredients:

White Fir (*Abies concolor*) creates a feeling of grounding, anchoring, and empowering.

Spruce (*Picea mariana*) helps to open and release emotional blocks, creating a feeling of balance and grounding.

Ylang Ylang (*Cananga odorata*) increases relaxation, balances male and female energies, and restores confidence and equilibrium.

Pine (*Pinus sylvestris*) helps reduce stress, relieve anxiety, and energize the entire body. It has a grounding, yet empowering aromatic effect.

Cedarwood (*Cedrus atlantica*) is high in sesquiterpenes, which can stimulate the limbic part of the brain, the center of emotions and memory.
It stimulates the pineal gland, which releases melatonin, thereby improving thoughts, cognition, and memory. Cedarwood has been used for stabilizing and grounding oneself.

Angelica (*Angelica archangelica*) helps to bring memories back to the point of origin before trauma or anger was experienced, helping us to release negative feelings.

Juniper *(Juniperus osteosperma* and *J. scopulorum)* elevates spiritual awareness, creating feelings of love and peace.

Applications:

- Dilute 1 part essential oil to 1 part V-6 Vegetable Oil Complex.
- Diffuse, inhale directly, or add 2-4 drops to bath water.
- Apply 1 to 2 drops behind ears, on wrists, base of neck, temples, or base of spine.
- Put 4-8 drops on cotton balls or tissues and put in or on vents.

Caution: Possible sun/skin sensitivity.

Harmony™

This blend promotes physical and emotional healing by creating a harmonic balance for the energy centers of the body. It brings us into harmony with all things, people, and cycles of life. It is beneficial in reducing stress, amplifying well-being, and dissipating feelings of discord. It is also uplifting and elevating the mind, creating a positive attitude.

Ingredients:

Sandalwood *(Santalum album)* is high in sesquiterpenes, which stimulate the pineal gland and the limbic region of the brain, the center of our emotions. It is used traditionally in yoga and meditation and may help remove negative programming in the cells.

Lavender *(Lavandula angustifolia)* is relaxing and calming and helps to overcome insomnia, headaches, and anxiety. It promotes a feeling of overall well-being.

Ylang Ylang *(Cananga odorata)* promotes relaxation, balances male and female energies, restores confidence and equilibrium, and alleviates insomnia.

Frankincense *(Boswellia carterii)* stimulates the limbic part of the brain, elevating the mind and helping to overcome stress and despair. It has an ancient history for its uses

in religious rituals and is used for meditation and prayer. In European medicine, it is known to alleviate depression.

Orange *(Citrus sinensis)* is elevating to the mind and body. A Brazilian university evaluated the potential anxiolytic effect of *Citrus sinensis* essential oil and found in a placebo-controlled study that the aroma of sweet orange oil was acutely anxiolytic, giving support to its calming use as a tranquilizer by aromatherapists (Goes TC, et al., 2012).

Angelica *(Angelica archangelica)* helps to bring memories back to the point of origin before trauma or anger was experienced, helping us to release negative feelings.

Geranium *(Pelargonium graveolens)* stimulates nerves and assists in balancing hormones. Its aromatic influence helps release negative memories, thereby opening and elevating the mind. It purges toxins from the liver, where anger is stored.

Hyssop *(Hyssopus officinalis)* is very balancing for emotions and can be spiritually uplifting.

Spanish Sage *(Salvia lavandulifolia)* is high in limonene, which prevents DNA damage.

Spruce *(Picea mariana)* helps to open and release emotional blocks, creating a feeling of balance and grounding. Traditionally, spruce oil was believed to possess the frequency of prosperity.

Coriander *(Coriandrum sativum)* has long been revered as a home remedy for relieving feelings of nausea, aiding digestion, and supporting healthy immune function.

Bergamot *(Citrus bergamia)* (furocoumarin-free) is simultaneously uplifting and calming, with a unique ability to relieve anxiety, stress, and tension.

Lemon *(Citrus limon)* is stimulating and invigorating, promoting a deep sense of well-being. A Brazilian university study found that lemon essential oil had sedative, anxiolytic, and antidepressant effects (LM Lopes C, et al., 2011).

Jasmine *(Jasminum officinale)* is uplifting and relieves anxiety and hopelessness. It also helps with nervous exhaustion and frigidity.

Roman Chamomile *(Anthemis nobilis)* combats restlessness, tension, and insomnia and purges toxins from the liver, where anger is stored.

Palmarosa *(Cymbopogon martinii)* is stimulating and revitalizing, enhancing both the nervous and cardiovascular systems.

Rose *(Rosa damascena)* has the highest frequency among essential oils. It creates a sense of balance, harmony, and well-being and also elevates the mind. Its magnetic energy attracts pure love and brings joy to the heart.

Applications:
- Dilute 1 part essential oil to 1 part vegetable oil.
- Diffuse, directly inhale, or add 2-4 drops to bath water.
- Dilute 1:15 with V-6 Vegetable Oil Complex for a full-body massage.
- Put 4-8 drops on cotton balls or tissues and put in or on vents.
- Add 2 drops to a wet cloth and put in clothes dryer.
- For topical use, apply 1-2 drops on edge of ears, wrists, neck, temples, over heart, on chakra, and on Vita Flex points.
- Directly inhale as needed or diffuse for 20-30 minutes daily.

Caution: Possible sun/skin sensitivity.

Highest Potential™

This blend combines powerful emotional blends with the most exotic essential oils of Jasmine and Ylang Ylang and the potent biblical oils of Frankincense, Galbanum, Cedarwood, and Sandalwood found in Gathering.

It elevates the mind as you gather your thoughts and mental energy to achieve your highest potential. This blend harmonizes several grounding, calming, inspiring, and empowering essential oils into one intoxicating blend.

Biochemist R. W. Moncrieff wrote that Ylang Ylang "soothes and inhibits anger born of frustration," which removes road-blocks and opening new vistas. The uplifting fragrance of Jasmine spurs creativity, while the Lavender in Gathering clears the thought processes for focused intentions.

Ingredients:

Australian Blue uplifts and inspires, while it grounds and stabilizes at the same time for strength and stability while we are working toward our goals.

Gathering collects our emotional and spiritual thoughts and helps overcome the bombardment of chaotic energy that alters our focus and takes us off our path toward higher achievements.

Jasmine *(Jasminum officinale)* is exhilarating to the mind and emotions, helping to unlock past blocks and release the mental blocks of frigidity and hopelessness.

Ylang Ylang *(Cananga odorata)* increases relaxation, balances male and female energies, and restores confidence and equilibrium.

Applications:
- Dilute 1 part essential oil to 1 part vegetable oil.
- Diffuse, directly inhale, or add 2-4 drops to bath water.
- Apply 2-4 drops on edge of ears, wrists, neck, or temples.
- Put 2 drops on a wet cloth and put in clothes dryer.
- Put 4-8 drops on cotton balls or tissues and put in or on vents.

Caution: Possible skin sensitivity.

Hope™

Hope is essential for moving forward in life. Hopelessness can cause a loss of vision, goals, and dreams. This blend helps you to reconnect with a feeling of strength and grounding, restoring hope for tomorrow. It has helped many overcome suicidal depression.

Ingredients:

Almond oil *(Prunus dulcis)* is used in this blend as a carrier oil.
In the ancient Ayurveda system of health care native to India, the almond is considered a nutrient for the brain and nervous system.

Melissa *(Melissa officinalis)* brings out gentleness as it calms and balances the emotions that come from the limbic part of the brain, the emotional center of memories. It helps to remove emotional blocks and instills a positive outlook on life.

Juniper *(Juniperus osteosperma and J. scopulorum)* elevates spiritual awareness and creates feelings of love and peace.

Myrrh *(Commiphora myrrha)* is referenced throughout the Old and New Testaments and constitutes a part of a holy anointing formula given to Moses (Exodus 30:22-27). It contains sesquiterpenes, a class of compounds that stimulate the hypothalamus, pituitary, and amygdala, the control center for emotions and hormone release in the brain. It also possesses the frequency of wealth, according to legends.

Spruce *(Picea mariana)* opens and releases emotional blocks, creating a feeling of balance and grounding. Traditionally, it was believed to possess the frequency of prosperity.

Applications:

- Diffuse, directly inhale, or add 2-4 drops to bath water.
- Put 4-8 drops on cotton balls or tissues and put in or on vents.
- For topical use, apply 2-4 drops on edge of ears, wrists, neck, temples, over heart, on chakra, and on Vita Flex points.
- For aromatic use directly inhale as needed or diffuse or humidify for 30-35 minutes daily.

Caution: Possible skin sensitivity.

Humility™

Having humility and forgiveness helps us to heal ourselves and our earth (Chronicles 7:14). Humility is an integral ingredient in obtaining forgiveness and is needed for a closer relationship with God. Through the frequency and fragrance of this blend, you may arrive at a place where healing can begin.

Ingredients:

Fractionated (virgin) coconut oil *(Cocos nucifera)* has been processed or "fractioned" to create a strong shelf life. With its antiseptic and disinfectant properties, it gives a strong, stabilizing foundation to the formulation.

Coriander *(Coriandrum sativum)* has long been revered as a home remedy for relieving feelings of nausea, aiding digestion, and supporting healthy immune function.

Ylang Ylang *(Cananga odorata)* promotes relaxation, balances male and female energies, restores confidence and equilibrium, and alleviates insomnia.

Bergamot *(Citrus bergamia)* (furocoumarin-free) is simultaneously uplifting and calming, with a unique ability to relieve anxiety, stress, and tension.

Geranium *(Pelargonium graveolens)* assists in balancing hormones. It is antispasmodic, relaxant, anti-inflammatory, antibacterial, antifungal, and stimulates the liver and pancreas.

Melissa *(Melissa officinalis)* was anciently used for nervous disorders and to relieve anxiety and depression. It brings out gentleness and is calming and balancing to the emotions that affect the limbic part of the brain, the emotional center of memories.

Frankincense (*Boswellia carterii*) is considered a holy anointing oil in the Middle East and has been used in religious ceremonies for thousands of years.
It stimulates the limbic part of the brain, elevating the mind and helping to overcome stress and despair.

Myrrh (*Commiphora myrrha*) is referenced throughout the Bible and was part of a holy anointing formula given to Moses (Exodus 30:22-27). It is high in sesquiterpenes, a class of compounds that can stimulate the hypothalamus, pituitary, and amygdala, the control center for emotions and hormone release in the brain.

Spikenard (*Nardostachys jatamansi*) was highly prized at the time of Christ and was used by Mary of Bethany to anoint the feet of Jesus. It stimulates the limbic part of the brain, tapping emotional memories. It can be relaxing and help with nervous tension.

Neroli (*Citrus sinensis*) was used by the ancient Egyptians for healing the mind, body, and spirit. It is stabilizing and strengthening to the emotions, promoting peace, confidence, and awareness. It brings everything into focus and is also used for depression and anxiety.

Rose (*Rosa damascena*) possesses the highest frequency of the oils. It creates a sense of balance, harmony, and well-being and elevates the mind.

Applications:
- Diffuse, directly inhale, or add 2-4 drops to bath water.
- Apply 1 to 2 drops over heart, on neck, forehead, or temples.
- Put 2 drops on a wet cloth and put in clothes dryer.
- Put 4-8 drops on cotton balls or tissues and put in or on vents.

ImmuPower™
This blend strengthens immunity and DNA repair in the cells. It is strongly antiseptic and anti-infectious.

Ingredients:

Hyssop (*Hyssopus officinalis*) is anti-inflammatory, antiviral, antiparasitic, mucolytic, decongestant, and anti-infectious.

Mountain Savory (*Satureja montana*) is immune stimulating, antiviral, antibacterial, antifungal, and antiparasitic. It is excellent for HIV, herpes, etc., and back ailments such as lumbago, scoliosis, etc.

Cistus (*Cistus ladanifer*) enhances immunity and immune cell regeneration. It is anti-infectious, antiviral, and antibacterial.

Ravintsara (*Cinnamomum camphora*) is referred to by the people of Madagascar as the oil that heals. It is antiseptic, anti-infectious, antiviral, antibacterial, and antifungal.

Frankincense (*Boswellia carterii*) stimulates the hypothalamus and pituitary to amplify immunity.

Oregano (*Origanum vulgare*) is one of the most powerful antimicrobial essential oils. Oregano is antiviral, antibacterial, antifungal, and antiparasitic.

Clove (*Syzygium aromaticum*) is one of the most powerful antioxidants of all essential oils and prevents cellular DNA damage. It is also strongly antimicrobial, antiseptic, antiviral, anti-inflammatory, and antifungal.

Cumin (*Cuminum cyminum*) amplifies immunity and DNA repair. It is antiseptic, antibacterial, and anti-inflammatory.

Idaho Tansy (*Tanacetum vulgare*) is antiviral, anti-infectious, antibacterial, and fights colds, flu, and infections. According to E.

Joseph Montagna's *Herbal Desk Reference*, tansy tones the entire body.

Applications:

- Diffuse, humidify, directly inhale, or add 2-4 drops to bath water.
- Apply around navel, chest, temples, wrists, under nose, or on Vita Flex points on the bottoms of feet.
- Use with Raindrop Technique.
- Dilute 1:15 with vegetable oils for body massage.
- Put 4-8 drops on cotton balls or tissues and put in or on vents.
- For topical use, dilute 1 drop of ImmuPower with 4 drops of V-6 Vegetable Oil Complex or oil of choice. Then apply to affected area as needed.
- For aromatic use diffuse up to 30 minutes 3 times daily.
- Alternate the diffused oils with Thieves and Exodus II. To enhance effects, add Melissa, Palo Santo, Clove, Cistus, or Dorado Azul.

Cautions: Possible skin sensitivity. Test for sensitivity by putting a drop of oil on the underside of arm after diluting. These oils need to be well-diluted before using on children.

Inner Child™

When children have been abused, they become disconnected from their inner child, or identity, which causes confusion. This fractures the personality and creates problems that tend to surface in the early- to mid-adult years, often mislabeled as a mid-life crisis. This fragrance stimulates memory response and helps one reconnect with the inner-self or identity. This is one of the first steps to finding emotional balance.

Ingredients:

Orange (*Citrus sinensis*) is elevating to the mind and body and brings joy and peace. A Brazilian university evaluated the potential anxiolytic effect of *Citrus sinensis* essential oil and found in a placebo-controlled study that the aroma of sweet orange oil was acutely anxiolytic, giving support to its calming use as a tranquilizer by aromatherapists (Goes TC, et al., 2012).

Tangerine (*Citrus reticulata*) contains esters and aldehydes that are sedating and calming, helping to combat anxiety and nervousness.

Ylang Ylang (*Cananga odorata*) increases relaxation and balances male and female energies, restoring confidence and equilibrium. It combats anger and low self-esteem and filters out negative energy.

Jasmine (*Jasminum officinale*) stimulates the mind and improves concentration. It is also an antidepressant and uplifts while relieving indifference and listlessness.

Sandalwood (*Santalum album*) is high in sesquiterpene compounds, which stimulate the pineal gland and the limbic region of the brain, the center of emotions and memory. It is used traditionally in yoga and meditation and may help remove negative programming.

Lemongrass (*Cymbopogon flexuosus*) increases blood circulation and promotes awareness as it uplifts and purifies the spirit.

Spruce (*Picea mariana*) opens and releases emotional blocks, fostering a sense of balance and grounding. Traditionally, it was believed to possess the frequency of prosperity.

Neroli (*Citrus sinensis*) was used by the ancient Egyptians for healing the mind, body, and spirit. It is stabilizing and strengthening to the emotions, promoting peace, confidence, and awareness. It uplifts the spirit, encourages true joy, and helps with insomnia.

Applications:

- Dilute 1 part essential oil to 1 part V-6 Vegetable Oil Complex.

- Diffuse, directly inhale, or add 2-4 drops to bath water.
- Apply 1 to 2 drops on edge of ears, wrists, neck, or temples.
- Dilute 1:15 with vegetable oil for body massage.
- Add 2 drops to a wet cloth and put in clothes dryer.
- Put 4-8 drops on cotton balls or tissues and put in or on vents.

Caution: Possible sun sensitivity.

Inspiration™

This blend is formulated to help find a calm space in our minds and bring us closer to that creative center where our higher intuition operates. These oils were traditionally used by the Native Americans to enhance spirituality, prayer, and inner awareness.

Ingredients:

Cedarwood *(Cedrus atlantica)* is high in sesquiterpenes, which can stimulate the limbic part of the brain, the center of emotions and memory. It stimulates the pineal gland, which releases melatonin, thereby improving thoughts, cognition, and memory. Cedarwood is also very grounding and centering.

Spruce *(Picea mariana)* opens and releases emotional blocks, fostering a sense of balance and grounding. Traditionally, it was believed to possess the frequency of prosperity.

Myrtle *(Myrtus communis)* is energizing, inspiring, elevating, and euphoric.

Coriander *(Coriandrum sativum)* has long been revered as a home remedy for relieving feelings of nausea, aiding digestion, and supporting healthy immune function.

Sandalwood *(Santalum album)* is extremely high in sesquiterpene compounds, which stimulate the pineal gland and the limbic region of the brain, the center of emotions and memory. It is used traditionally in yoga and meditation and may help remove negative programming from the cells.

Frankincense *(Boswellia carterii)* stimulates the limbic part of the brain, elevating the mind and helping to overcome stress and despair. It is used in European medicine to combat depression.

Frankincense contains sesquiterpenes, which stimulate the limbic system of the brain (the center of memory and emotions) and the hypothalamus, pineal, and pituitary glands. The hypothalamus is the master gland of the human body, producing many vital hormones, including thyroid and growth hormone.

Bergamot *(Citrus bergamia)* (furocoumarin-free) is simultaneously uplifting and calming, with a unique ability to relieve anxiety, stress, and tension.

Spikenard *(Nardostachys jatamansi)* was highly prized at the time of Christ and was used by Mary of Bethany to anoint the feet of Jesus. It stimulates the limbic part of the brain, tapping emotional memories. It can be relaxing and help with nervous tension.

Vetiver *(Vetiveria zizanioides)* is psychologically grounding and stabilizing. It has been shown to help with concentration and coping with stress and insomnia.

Ylang Ylang *(Cananga odorata)* promotes relaxation, balances male and female energies, restores confidence and equilibrium, and alleviates insomnia.

Geranium *(Pelargonium graveolens)* assists in balancing hormones. It is antispasmodic, relaxant, anti-inflammatory, antibacterial, antifungal, and stimulates the liver and pancreas.

Applications:

- Diffuse, directly inhale, or add 2-4 drops to bath water.
- Apply 1 to 2 drops on edge of ears, wrists, neck, temples, forehead, crown of head,

bottoms of feet, or along spine.

- Add 2 drops to a wet cloth and put in clothes dryer.
- Put 4-8 drops on cotton balls or tissues and put in or on vents.

Caution: Possible skin sensitivity.

Into the Future™

This blend helps one leave the past behind in order to progress with vision and excitement. So many times we find ourselves settling for mediocrity and sacrificing our own potential and success because of fear of the unknown and the future. This blend inspires determination and a pioneering spirit and creates a strong emotional feeling of being able to reach one's potential.

Ingredients:

Almond oil *(Prunus dulcis)* is used in this blend as a carrier oil.
   In the ancient Ayurveda system of health care native to India, the almond is considered a nutrient for the brain and nervous system.

Clary Sage *(Salvia sclarea)* enhances circulation and hormonal balance.

Ylang Ylang *(Cananga odorata)* increases relaxation, balances male and female energies, and restores confidence and equilibrium.

White Fir *(Abies concolor)* creates a feeling of grounding, anchoring, and empowering.

Idaho Tansy *(Tanacetum vulgare)* is antiviral, anti-infectious, antibacterial, and fights colds, flu, and infections. According to E. Joseph Montagna's PDR on herbal formulas, tansy helps combat skin problems and strengthens the kidneys, heart, joints, and digestive system.[5]

Frankincense *(Boswellia carterii)* is considered a holy anointing oil in the Middle East and has been used in religious ceremonies for thousands of years.

It stimulates the limbic part of the brain, which elevates the mind, helping to overcome stress and despair. It is used in European medicine to combat depression.

Jasmine *(Jasminum officinale)* is exhilarating to the mind and emotions, unlocking past blocks. It also alleviates nervous exhaustion, depression, and listlessness.

Juniper *(Juniperus osteosperma and J. scopulorum)* elevates spiritual awareness and creates feelings of love and peace.

Orange *(Citrus sinensis)* is elevating to the mind and body and brings joy and peace. A Brazilian university evaluated the potential anxiolytic effect of *Citrus sinensis* essential oil and found in a placebo-controlled study that the aroma of sweet orange oil was acutely anxiolytic, giving support to its calming use as a tranquilizer by aromatherapists (Goes TC, et al., 2012).

Cedarwood *(Cedrus atlantica)* is high in sesquiterpenes, which can stimulate the limbic part of the brain, the center of emotions and memory. It stimulates the pineal gland, which releases melatonin, thereby improving thoughts, cognition, and memory.

White Lotus *(Nymphaea lotus)* is calming and relaxing. It helps a person move forward, overcoming self-defeating thoughts. It also uplifts and brings deep peace and comfort.

Applications:

- Diffuse, directly inhale, or add 2-4 drops to bath water.
- Apply 1 to 2 drops on edge of ears, over heart, on wrists, neck, or temples.
- Dilute 1:15 with V-6 Vegetable Oil Complex for body massage.
- Put 4-8 drops on cotton balls or tissues and put in or on vents.

Caution: Possible sun/skin sensitivity.

Joy™

This beautiful blend produces a magnetic energy that brings joy to the heart, mind, and soul. It inspires romance and helps overcome deep-seated grief and depression.

Ingredients:

Bergamot *(Citrus bergamia)* (furocoumarin-free) is simultaneously uplifting and calming, with a unique ability to relieve anxiety, stress, and tension.

Ylang Ylang *(Cananga odorata)* promotes relaxation, balances male and female energies, restores confidence and equilibrium, and alleviates insomnia.

Geranium *(Pelargonium graveolens)* assists in balancing hormones. It is antispasmodic, relaxant, anti-inflammatory, antibacterial, antifungal, and stimulates the liver and pancreas.

Lemon *(Citrus limon)* is stimulating and invigorating, promoting a deep sense of well-being. A Brazilian university study found that lemon essential oil had sedative, anxiolytic, and antidepressant effects (LM Lopes C, et al., 2011).

Coriander *(Coriandrum sativum)* has long been revered as a home remedy for relieving feelings of nausea, aiding digestion, and supporting healthy immune function.

Tangerine *(Citrus reticulata)* contains esters and aldehydes that are sedating and calming, combating anxiety and nervousness. It is high in limonene, which prevents DNA damage.

Jasmine *(Jasminum officinale)* exudes an exquisite fragrance that revitalizes spirits and brings feelings of love, support, and joy. It is used to relieve sorrow, depression, and nervous exhaustion.

Roman Chamomile *(Anthemis nobilis)* combats restlessness, tension, and insomnia. It releases mental blocks and purges toxins from the liver, where anger is stored.

Palmarosa *(Cymbopogon martini)* is stimulating and revitalizing, enhancing both the nervous and cardiovascular systems and bringing about a feeling of security.

Rose *(Rosa damascena)* has the highest frequency among essential oils. It creates a sense of balance, harmony, and well-being and elevates the mind. It creates a magnetic energy that attracts pure love and brings joy to the heart.

Applications:

- Dilute 1:15 with V-6 Vegetable Oil Complex for a full-body massage.
- Put 2 drops on a wet cloth and put in clothes dryer.
- Put 4-8 drops on cotton balls or tissues and put in or on vents.
- Diffuse, directly inhale, or add 2-4 drops to bath water.
- Apply over the heart, thymus, temples, and wrists.
- It may also be massaged on the lower back, abdomen, and on the heart and brain Vita Flex points.

JuvaCleanse®

The liver is the body's largest internal organ and major detoxifier. Even the toxins in the air we breathe are filtered by the liver, including chemicals from aerosol cleaners, paint, insect sprays, etc., but eventually those filters need to be cleaned. The essential oils of Ledum, Celery Seed, and Helichrysum have long been known for their liver cleansing properties. JuvaCleanse was clinically tested in 2003 for removing mercury from body tissues.

In 2003 a study conducted by Roger Lewis, MD, at the Young Life Research Clinic in Springville, Utah, evaluated the efficacy of Helichrysum, Ledum, and Celery Seed in treating cases of advanced Hepatitis C.

In one case a 20-year-old male diagnosed with Hepatitis C had a viral count of 13,200. After taking two capsules (approx. 750 mg each) of JuvaCleanse per day for one month with no other intervention, the patient's viral count dropped more than 80 percent to 2,580.

Ingredients:

Helichrysum (*Helichrysum italicum*) regenerates tissue and improves circulation. It stimulates liver cell function and removes plaque from the veins and arteries.

Celery Seed (*Apium graveolens*) is a powerful liver cleanser and expectorant and has been used against hepatitis.

Ledum (*Ledum groenlandicum*) has been shown in clinical studies to protect the liver and increase bile flow. It has been used for detoxifying fat from the liver and for other liver dysfunctions, including hepatitis.

Applications:

- Apply over the liver and on the liver and kidney Vita Flex points on the foot.
- It is very beneficial when used with Raindrop Technique.
- Take 1 capsule 2 times daily as a dietary supplement.

JuvaFlex™

This blend helps with liver and lymphatic detoxification. The emotions of anger and hate create toxins that are stored in the liver that can lead to sickness and disease. JuvaFlex helps break addictions to coffee, alcohol, drugs, and tobacco.

Ingredients:

Sesame seed oil (*Sesamum indicum*) is used as a cosmetic carrier oil and is reputed to penetrate the skin easily. It is an antioxidant rich in vitamin E.

Fennel (*Foeniculum vulgare*) is antiseptic and stimulating to the circulatory system. It increases bile flow and hepatocyte function.

Geranium (*Pelargonium graveolens*) improves bile flow from the liver. It is antispasmodic and improves liver, pancreas, and kidney function.

Rosemary (*Rosmarinus officinalis*) is antiseptic and antimicrobial. It balances the endocrine system. It is liver protecting and helps combat hepatitis and other infectious diseases.

Roman Chamomile (*Chamaemelum nobile*) is anti-inflammatory and expels toxins from the liver. It strengthens liver function.

Blue Tansy (*Tanacetum annuum*) is anti-inflammatory and helps cleanse the liver and lymphatic system.

Helichrysum (*Helichrysum italicum*) regenerates tissue and improves circulation. It stimulates liver cell function and removes plaque from the veins and arteries.

Applications:

- Apply 1-2 drops over liver area and massage 3-4 drops on the Vita Flex points on the foot with Raindrop Technique-style along the spine.
- It also works nicely using a warm compress with 3-4 drops of oils with Ortho Sport or Ortho Ease Massage Oils.

Lady Sclareol™

This oil, rich in phytoestrogens, is designed to be worn with its exquisite fragrance. It enhances the feminine nature by improving mood and raising estrogen levels. It may also provide relief for PMS symptoms.

Ingredients:

Coriander (*Coriandrum sativum*) has long been revered as a home remedy for relieving feelings of nausea, aiding digestion, and supporting healthy immune function.

Geranium (*Pelargonium graveolens*) helps release negative memories, opening and elevating the mind. It has been used for centuries for skin care. It revitalizes tissue and nerves and has relaxant, anti-inflammatory, and anti-infectious effects.

Vetiver *(Vetiveria zizanioides)* is psychologically grounding and stabilizing. It has been shown to help with concentration and coping with stress and insomnia.

Orange *(Citrus sinensis)* is elevating to the mind and body. A Brazilian university evaluated the potential anxiolytic effect of *Citrus sinensis* essential oil and found in a placebo-controlled study that the aroma of sweet orange oil was acutely anxiolytic, giving support to its calming use as a tranquilizer by aromatherapists (Goes TC, et al., 2012).

Clary Sage *(Salvia sclarea)* contains natural sclareol, a phytoestrogen that mimics estrogen function to help balance the hormones. It helps with menstrual cramps, PMS, and circulatory problems.

Bergamot *(Citrus bergamia)* (furocoumarin-free) is simultaneously uplifting and calming, with a unique ability to relieve anxiety, stress, and tension.

Ylang Ylang *(Cananga odorata)* promotes relaxation, balances male and female energies, restores confidence and equilibrium, and alleviates insomnia.

Sandalwood *(Santalum album)* is high in sesquiterpenes, which stimulate the pineal gland and the limbic region of the brain, the center of our emotions. It is used traditionally in yoga and meditation.

Spanish Sage *(Salvia lavandulifolia)* is high in limonene, which prevents DNA damage.

Jasmine *(Jasminum officinale)* is used for muscle spasms, frigidity, depression, and nervous exhaustion. It is stimulating to the mind and improves concentration.

Idaho Tansy *(Tanacetum vulgare)* is antiviral, anti-infectious, antibacterial, and fights colds, flu, and infections. According to E. Joseph Montagna's PDR on herbal

formulas, tansy helps skin problems and strengthens the kidneys, heart, joints, and digestive system.[5]

Applications:
- For topical or aromatic use as a perfume.
- Apply 2-4 drops to Vita Flex points on the ankles or at the clavicle notch.
- It may be applied to the abdomen for relief of premenstrual discomfort.

Live with Passion™

This blend revives the zest for life and improves internal energy with a combination of essential oils formulated specifically to help people attain an optimistic attitude.

Ingredients:

Sandalwood *(Santalum album)* is high in sesquiterpene compounds, which stimulate the pineal gland and the limbic region of the brain, the center of emotions and memory. It is used traditionally in yoga and meditation and may help remove negative programming in the cells.

Clary Sage *(Salvia sclarea)* contains natural sclareol, a phytoestrogen that mimics estrogen function that helps balance the hormones. It also helps with menstrual cramps, PMS, and circulatory problems.

Ginger *(Zingiber officinale)* is energizing and uplifting.

Jasmine *(Jasminum officinale)* stimulates the mind, improves concentration, and helps overcome nervous exhaustion and depression. It is also used for muscle spasms and frigidity.

Patchouli *(Pogostemon cablin)* is very high in sesquiterpenes that stimulate the limbic center of the brain. It re-establishes mental and emotional equilibrium and energizes the mind. It promotes grounding and helps center the emotions, allowing the mind to relax and let go of jealousies, obsessions, and insecurities.

Cedarwood *(Cedrus atlantica)* is high in sesquiterpenes, which stimulate the limbic part of the brain, the center of emotions and memory. It stimulates the pineal gland, which releases melatonin, thereby improving thoughts, cognition, and memory. Cedarwood is very stabilizing and grounding.

Helichrysum *(Helichrysum italicum)* improves circulation and helps release feelings of anger, promoting forgiveness.

Angelica *(Angelica archangelica)* helps to calm emotions, bring memories back to the point of origin before trauma and anger were experienced, and helps release negative feelings.

Melissa *(Melissa officinalis)* brings out gentleness. It is calming and balancing to the emotions, affecting the limbic part of the brain, the emotional center of memories. It was used anciently to treat nervous disorders and many different heart ailments.

Neroli (*Citrus sinensis*) was used by the ancient Egyptians for healing the mind, body, and spirit. It helps stabilize the emotions, promoting peace, confidence, and awareness. It brings thoughts and feelings into focus, alleviating anxiety, depression, and insomnia.

Applications:
- Diffuse and/or apply on wrists, temples, chest, and forehead.
- Mix 2 to 4 drops of oil with 2 tablespoons of Sensation, Relaxation, or Evening Peace Bath & Shower Gel or mix with ½ cup bath salts water and pour into the tub. Soak for 20 to 30 minutes or until water cools.
- Be cautious for possible skin sensitivity.
- If pregnant or under a doctor's care, consult your physician.

- Dilution recommended for both topical and internal use. Dilute before using on sensitive areas such as the face, neck, genital area, etc.
- Children love the smell so you could mix a gentle oil like Lavender or RutaVaLa with the KidScents Bath Gel, so they can enjoy a relaxing time when they have their bath.

Longevity™

This oil contains the highest antioxidant and DNA-protecting essential oils. When taken as a dietary supplement, this blend promotes longevity and prevents premature aging.

Ingredients:

Thyme *(Thymus vulgaris)* has been shown in studies to dramatically boost glutathione levels in the heart, liver, and brain. It also prevents lipid peroxidation or degradation of the fats found in many vital organs. The oxidation of fats in the body is directly linked to accelerated aging.

Orange *(Citrus sinensis)* contains over 90 percent d-limonene, one of the most powerful anticancerous compounds studied in recent years and the subject of over 50 peer-reviewed research papers published in leading medical journals throughout the world.

Clove *(Syzygium aromaticum)* has the highest known antioxidant power as measured by ORAC (Oxygen Radical Absorbance Capacity), a test developed by USDA researchers at Tufts University. It is anticoagulant, one of the most antimicrobial and antiseptic of all essential oils, and prevents cellular DNA damage.

Frankincense *(Boswellia carterii)* stimulates the limbic part of the brain, which elevates the mind, helping to overcome stress and despair. It is also anticancerous.

Applications:
- Dilute 1 part essential oil to 4 parts V-6 Vegetable Oil Complex.

161

- As a dietary supplement, put a few drops of oil diluted with V-6 in a capsule and swallow, or put 2-3 drops in Agave, Yacon Syrup, or maple syrup in a spoon; mix and swallow; or mix in about 4 fl. oz. of NingXia Red, goat milk, or rice milk, etc.

M-Grain™

This blend helps relieve pain from slight headaches to severe migraine headaches. It is anti-inflammatory and antispasmodic.

Ingredients:

Basil *(Ocimum basilicum)* combats muscle spasms and inflammation. It is relaxing to both striated and smooth muscles (involuntary muscles such as the heart and digestive system).

Marjoram *(Origanum majorana)* is anti-inflammatory and is used to treat sore and aching muscles. It relieves muscle spasms and migraine headaches and calms nerves.

Lavender *(Lavandula angustifolia)* is anti-inflammatory and antispasmodic. It is high in aldehydes and esters, and it combats insomnia, stress, and nervous tension. It is extremely relaxing and grounding.

Roman Chamomile *(Anthemis nobilis)* is a strong anti-inflammatory with antispasmodic effects. It helps with insomnia, restlessness, and tension.

Peppermint *(Mentha piperita)* has powerful pain-blocking, anti-inflammatory, and antispasmodic properties. A 2013 study conducted at the South African Tshwane University in Pretoria found that the main constituent of peppermint, menthol, not only is a highly effective skin penetrator but has analgesic effects (Kamatou GP, et al., 2013).

Helichrysum *(Helichrysum italicum)* is a powerful anesthetic and analgesic and reduces pain, inflammation, and muscle spasms.

Applications:

- Dilute 1 part essential oil to 1 part V-6 Vegetable Oil Complex.
- Diffuse, directly inhale, or add 2-4 drops to bath water.
- Apply on brain stem, forehead, crown of head, shoulders, back of neck, temples, and Vita Flex points on the feet.
- Put 4-8 drops on cotton balls or tissues and put in or on vents.

Caution: Possible skin sensitivity.

Magnify Your Purpose™

This blend stimulates the endocrine system for greater energy flow to the right hemisphere of the brain, activating creativity, motivation, and focus. This helps strengthen commitment to purpose, desire, and intentions until you realize your goals.

Ingredients:

Sandalwood *(Santalum album)* is high in sesquiterpene compounds, which stimulate the pineal gland and the limbic region of the brain, the center of emotions and memory. It is used traditionally in yoga and meditation and may help remove negative programming in the cells.

Sage *(Salvia officinalis)* strengthens the vital centers. It has been used for purifying, healing, and dispelling negative emotions.

Coriander *(Coriandrum sativum)* has long been revered as a home remedy for relieving feelings of nausea, aiding digestion, and supporting healthy immune function.

Patchouli *(Pogostemon cablin)* is very high in sesquiterpenes that stimulate the limbic center of the brain. It re-establishes mental and emotional equilibrium and energizes the mind. It promotes grounding and helps center the emotions, allowing the mind to relax and let go of jealousies, obsessions, and insecurities.

Nutmeg (*Myristica fragrans*) supports the adrenal glands for increased energy and is powerfully stimulating and energizing.

Bergamot (*Citrus bergamia*) (furocoumarin-free) is simultaneously uplifting and calming, with a unique ability to relieve anxiety, stress, and tension.

Cinnamon Bark (*Cinnamomum zeylanicum*) is the oil of wealth from the Orient and part of the formula the Lord gave to Moses (Exodus 30:22-27). It has a frequency that attracts wealth and abundance. It has been used traditionally to release malice or spite.

Ginger (*Zingiber officinale*) is energizing and uplifting.

Ylang Ylang (*Cananga odorata*) promotes relaxation, balances male and female energies, restores confidence and equilibrium, and alleviates insomnia.

Geranium (*Pelargonium graveolens*) assists in balancing hormones. It is antispasmodic, relaxant, anti-inflammatory, antibacterial, antifungal, and stimulates the liver and pancreas.

Applications:
- Dilute 1 part essential oil to 1 part V-6 Vegetable Oil Complex.
- Diffuse directly, inhale, or add 2-4 drops to bath water.
- Apply on heart, solar plexus, thymus, temples, ears, or wrists.
- Put 4-8 drops on cotton balls or tissues and put in or on vents.
- Add 2 drops to a wet cloth and put in clothes dryer.

Caution: Possible skin sensitivity.

Melrose™

This is a blend of four essential oils that have strong antiseptic properties to cleanse and disinfect cuts, scrapes, burns, rashes, and bruised tissue. These oils help regenerate damaged tissue and reduce inflammation. It is powerful when diffused to dispel odors, purify the air, and protect against daily radiation bombardment.

Ingredients:
Rosemary (*Rosmarinus officinalis* CT cineol) is antiseptic, antifungal, and antimicrobial.

Melaleuca (*M. alternifolia*), also known as tea tree oil, is antiseptic, antibacterial, antifungal, antiparasitic, and anti-inflammatory.

Clove (*Syzygium aromaticum*) is one of the most antimicrobial and antiseptic of all essential oils. It is antifungal, antiviral, anti-infectious, and antibacterial.

Niaouli (*Melaleuca quinquenervia*) is anti-infectious, antiparasitic, and antibacterial.

Applications:
- Dilute 1 part essential oil to 1 part V-6 Vegetable Oil Complex.
- Diffuse, directly inhale, or add 2-4 drops to bath water.
- Apply to broken skin, cuts, scrapes, burns, rashes, and infection. Follow with Rose Ointment to keep oils sealed in wound.
- Put 1 to 2 drops on a piece of cotton and place in the ear for earaches.

Caution: Possible skin sensitivity.

Mister™

This blend helps to decongest the prostate and promote greater male hormonal balance.

Ingredients:
Sesame seed oil (*Sesamum indicum*) is used as a cosmetic carrier oil and is reputed to penetrate the skin easily. It is an antioxidant rich in vitamin E.

Sage (*Salvia officinalis*) has been used in Europe for hair loss. It strengthens vital centers, relieves depression, and reduces mental fatigue.

Fennel (*Foeniculum vulgare*) has hormone-like activity and is stimulating to the circulatory, cardiovascular, and respiratory systems.

Lavender *(Lavandula angustifolia)* is antispasmodic, hypotensive, anti-inflammatory, anti-infectious, and an anticoagulant. It is very relaxing, grounding, and combats depression.

Myrtle *(Myrtus communis)* helps normalize hormonal imbalances of the thyroid and sex glands. Stimulates and balances functions of the prostate.

Yarrow *(Achillea millefolium)* is a prostate decongestant and hormone balancer and is anti-inflammatory.

Peppermint *(Mentha piperita)* strengthens the liver and glandular function.

Applications:

- Diffuse, directly inhale, or add 2-4 drops to bath water.
- Apply to ankle Vita Flex points, lower pelvis, or areas of concern.
- Use in a hot compress.
- Dilute 1:15 with V-6 Vegetable Oil Complex for body massage.

Motivation™

Motivation stimulates feelings of action and accomplishment, providing positive energy to help overcome feelings of fear and procrastination.

Ingredients:

Roman Chamomile *(Anthemis nobilis)* combats restlessness, tension, and insomnia. It purges toxins from the liver, where anger is stored.

Spruce *(Picea mariana)* helps to open and release emotional blocks, creating a feeling of balance and grounding.

Ylang Ylang *(Cananga odorata)* increases relaxation and balances male and female energies. It also restores confidence and equilibrium.

Lavender *(Lavandula angustifolia)* has been documented to improve concentration and mental acuity.

Japanese researchers at Yamanashi Prefectural University tested lavender aroma for concentration in the late afternoon, when work concentration was at its lowest. Of three groups of young men tested in the 2005 study (control group, jasmine group, and lavender group), the lavender group had significantly higher concentration levels than the other two groups (Sakamoto R, et al., 2005).

A study at Kyushu University in Japan corroborated this finding after tests of lavender outperformed a control group and helped to maintain sustained attention during a long-term vigilance task (Shimizu K, et al., 2008).

Applications:

- Diffuse, directly inhale, or add 2-4 drops to bath water.
- Apply on feet (big toe), chest, nape of the neck, behind ears, wrists, or around navel.
- Put 4-8 drops on cotton balls or tissues and put in or on vents.

Oola®* Balance

Young Living and Oola have partnered together to offer this one-of-a-kind essential oil blend, Oola Balance. This blend is designed to align and balance your center, giving you an increase in concentration with a positive outlook. As mind and body are balanced, the ability to focus on passions, behaviors, and health are amplified for the better.

Ingredients:

Lavender *(Lavandula angustifolia)* has been documented to improve concentration and mental acuity.

Frankincense *(Boswellia carterii)* stimulates the limbic part of the brain, which elevates the mind, helping to overcome stress and despair. It is used in European medicine to combat depression.

Ylang Ylang *(Cananga odorata)* promotes relaxation, balances male and female energies, restores confidence and equilibrium, and alleviates insomnia.

Sacred Frankincense *(Boswellia sacra)* is considered a holy anointing oil in the Middle East and has been used in religious ceremonies for thousands of years. It stimulates the limbic part of the brain, which elevates the mind, helping to overcome stress and despair.

Idaho Balsam Fir *(Abies balsamea)* opens emotional blocks and recharges vital energy.

Jasmine *(Jasminum officinale)* has therapeutic effects, both emotional and physical. It is uplifting, antidepressant, and counteracts indifference, frigidity, and hopelessness.

Sandalwood *(Santalum album)* is high in sesquiterpene compounds, which stimulate the pineal gland and the limbic region of the brain, the center of our emotions and memory. It has been used traditionally in yoga and meditation. It also promotes and enhances deep sleep.

Galbanum *(Ferula galbaniflua)* was used for both medicinal and spiritual purposes. When combined with frankincense and sandalwood, its frequency increases dramatically. ("And the Lord said unto Moses, Take unto thee sweet spices, stacte, and onycha, and galbanum; sweet spices with pure frankincense:" Exodus 30:34).

Orange *(Citrus sinensis)* is elevating to the mind and body, bringing security, joy, and peace.

Angelica *(Angelica archangelica)* helps to calm emotions and bring memories back to the point of origin before trauma or anger was experienced, helping to let go of negative feelings.

Geranium *(Pelargonium graveolens)* helps release negative memories, thereby opening and elevating the mind.

Myrrh *(Commiphora myrrha)* is referenced throughout the Bible, constituting a part of a holy anointing formula given to Moses (Exodus 30:22-27). It has one of the highest levels of sesquiterpenes, a class of compounds that stimulate the hypothalamus, pituitary, and amygdala, the control center for emotions and hormone release in the brain.

Hyssop *(Hyssopus officinalis)* is very balancing for emotions and can be spiritually uplifting.

Ocotea *(Octotea quixos)* has high levels of alpha-humulene to balance the body's response to stress and difficult situations.

Spanish Sage *(Salvia lavandulifolia)* is high in limonene, which prevents DNA damage.

Spruce *(Picea mariana)* opens and releases emotional blocks, fostering a sense of balance and grounding.

Cistus *(Cistus ladaniferus)* enhances immunity and immune cell regeneration. It is anti-infectious, antiviral, and antibacterial.

Spikenard *(Nardostachys jatamansi)* was used by Mary of Bethany to anoint the feet of Jesus. It strengthens immunity and hypothalamus function.

Coriander *(Coriandrum sativum)* has long been revered as a home remedy for relieving feelings of nausea, aiding digestion, and supporting healthy immune function.

Bergamot *(Citrus bergamia)* (furocoumarin-free) is simultaneously uplifting and calming, with a unique ability to relieve anxiety, stress, and tension.

Lemon *(Citrus limon)* has an extremely cleansing smell. This oil helps purify and uplift.

Roman Chamomile *(Anthemis nobilis)* combats restlessness, tension, and insomnia.

It purges toxins from the liver, where anger is stored. It also clears mental blocks.

Palmarosa (*Cymbopogon martini*) is stimulating and revitalizing and enhances both the nervous and cardiovascular system.

Rose (*Rosa damascena*) has the highest frequency among essential oils. It creates a sense of balance, harmony, and well-being and elevates the mind. It creates a magnetic energy that attracts love and brings joy to the heart.

Applications:

- Dilute 1 part essential oil to 1 part V-6 Vegetable Oil Complex.
- Diffuse or directly inhale.
- Apply 1 to 2 drops on edge of ears, wrists, neck, or temples or other areas as desired.

*Registered trademark of OolaMoola, LLC

Oola®* Grow

Young Living and Oola have partnered together to offer this one-of-a-kind essential oil blend, Oola Grow. This blend is designed to help you reach unlimited potential and growth in many aspects of life. Whether it's emotional, spiritual, or mental, Oola Grow gives you courage to focus on the task at hand and helps you move forward toward positive advancements and progression.

Ingredients:

Fractionated (virgin) coconut oil (*Cocos nucifera*) has been processed or "fractioned" to create a strong shelf life. With its antiseptic and disinfectant properties, it gives a strong, stabilizing foundation to the formulation.

Sweet almond oil (*Prunus amygdalus dulcis*) is used in this blend as a carrier oil. In the ancient Ayurveda system of health care native to India, the almond is considered a nutrient for the brain and nervous system.

Roman Chamomile (*Anthemis nobilis*)

combats restlessness, tension, and insomnia. It purges toxins from the liver, where anger is stored. It also clears mental blocks.

Spruce (*Picea mariana*) opens and releases emotional blocks, fostering a sense of balance and grounding.

Blue Cypress (*Callitris intratropica*) improves circulation and increases the flow of oxygen to the brain, stimulating the amygdala, pineal gland, pituitary gland, and hypothalamus.

Coriander (*Coriandrum sativum*) has long been revered as a home remedy for relieving feelings of nausea, aiding digestion, and supporting healthy immune function.

Clary Sage (*Salvia sclarea*) balances the hormones. It contains natural sclareol, a phytoestrogen that mimics estrogen function.

Ylang Ylang (*Cananga odorata*) promotes relaxation, balances male and female energies, restores confidence and equilibrium, and alleviates insomnia.

Geranium (*Pelargonium graveolens*) helps release negative memories, thereby opening and elevating the mind.

Bergamot (*Citrus aurantium bergamia*) is simultaneously uplifting and calming, with a unique ability to relieve anxiety, stress, and tension.

Jasmine (*Jasminum officinale*) has therapeutic effects, both emotional and physical. It is uplifting, antidepressant, and counteracts indifference, frigidity, and hopelessness.

Rosewood (*Aniba rosaeodora*) is high in linalool, which has a relaxing, empowering, and uplifting effect. It is also very grounding and strengthening.

Cedarwood (*Cedrus atlantica*) is high in sesquiterpenes, which can stimulate the limbic part of the brain, the center of emotions and memory. It stimulates the pineal gland, which releases melatonin, thereby improving thoughts, cognition, and memory.

White Fir *(Abies concolor)* is antimicrobial, antiseptic, antiarthritic, and stimulating. It supports the body and reduces the symptoms of arthritis, rheumatism, bronchitis, coughs, and sinusitis. It creates a feeling of grounding, anchoring, and empowering.

Lavender *(Lavandula angustifolia)* has been documented to improve concentration and mental acuity.

Frankincense (*Boswellia carterii*) stimulates the limbic part of the brain, which elevates the mind, helping to overcome stress and despair. It is used in European medicine to combat depression.

Galbanum *(Ferula galbaniflua)* was used for both medicinal and spiritual purposes. When combined with Frankincense and Sandalwood, its frequency increases dramatically. ("And the Lord said unto Moses, Take unto thee sweet spices, stacte, and onycha, and galbanum; sweet spices with pure frankincense:" Exodus 30:34).

Juniper *(Juniperus osteosperma)* elevates spiritual awareness to create feelings of love and peace. Juniper has also been used to cleanse the spirit.

Orange *(Citrus sinensis)* is elevating to the mind and body, bringing security, joy, and peace.

Sandalwood *(Santalum album)* is high in sesquiterpene compounds, which stimulate the pineal gland and the limbic region of the brain, the center of our emotions and memory. It has been used traditionally in yoga and meditation. It also promotes and enhances deep sleep.

Blue Tansy *(Tanacetum annuum)* is anti-inflammatory and combats anger and negative emotions, promoting a feeling of self-control.

Idaho Tansy *(Tanacetum vulgare)* is antiviral, anti-infectious, antibacterial, and fights colds, flu, and infections. According to E. Joseph Montagna's *Herbal Desk Reference*, tansy tones the entire body.

Neroli (*Citrus Aurantium amara*) was used by the ancient Egyptians for healing the mind, body, and spirit. It helps stabilize the emotions, promoting peace, confidence, and awareness. It brings thoughts and feelings into focus, alleviating anxiety, depression, and insomnia.

Cinnamon Bark *(Cinnamomum zeylanicum)* is the oil of wealth from the Orient and part of the formula the Lord gave to Moses (Exodus 30:22-27).

Emperors of China and India measured their wealth partly by the amount of cinnamon they possessed. Traditionally, it was thought to have a frequency that attracted wealth and abundance.

It is highly antiviral, antifungal, and antibacterial. It brings back memories of wassail, home-cooked food, and fond memories of the holidays.

Rose *(Rosa damascena)* has the highest frequency among essential oils. It creates a sense of balance, harmony, and well-being and elevates the mind. It creates a magnetic energy that attracts love and brings joy to the heart.

White Lotus *(Nymphaea lotus)* is calming and relaxing. It helps a person move forward, overcoming self-defeating thoughts. It also uplifts and brings deep peace and comfort.

Applications:

- Dilute 1 part essential oil to 1 part V-6 Vegetable Oil Complex.
- Diffuse or directly inhale.
- Apply 1 to 2 drops on edge of ears, wrists, neck, or temples or other areas as desired.

*Registered trademark of OolaMoola, LLC

PanAway®

This very popular blend reduces pain and inflammation, increases circulation, and accelerates healing. It relieves swelling and discomfort from arthritis, sprains, muscle spasms, cramps, bumps, and bruises.

Ingredients:

Wintergreen *(Gaultheria procumbens)* has strong anti-inflammatory and antispasmodic properties. It is analgesic and reduces all types of pain.

Helichrysum *(Helichrysum italicum)* is a powerful anesthetic and analgesic and reduces pain from inflammation and muscle spasms.

Clove *(Syzygium aromaticum)* is used in the dental industry to numb gum and kill pain. It is one of the most antimicrobial and antiseptic of all essential oils.

Peppermint *(Mentha piperita)* has powerful pain-blocking, anti-inflammatory, and antispasmodic properties. A recent study conducted at the South African Tshwane University in Pretoria found that the main constituent of peppermint, menthol, not only is a highly effective skin penetrator but has analgesic effects (Kamatou GP, et al., 2013).

Applications:

- Dilute 1 part essential oil to 1 part V-6 Vegetable Oil Complex.
- Diffuse, humidify, directly inhale, or add 2-4 drops to bath water.
- Apply 1-2 drops on location or on temples, back of neck, or forehead.
- Use as a compress or for a Raindrop Technique-style massage along spine.
- It relieves deep tissue pain. Additional Helichrysum may be added to enhance the effect of PanAway.
- When the pain is bone related, more Wintergreen may be a good addition.

- All of the oils may be diluted with Ortho Ease or Ortho Sport massage oils.

Caution: Possible skin sensitivity.

Peace & Calming®

This blend promotes relaxation and a deep sense of peace and emotional well-being, helping to dampen tensions and uplift spirits. When massaged on the bottoms of feet, it can be a wonderful prelude to a peaceful night's rest. It may calm overactive and hard-to-manage children. It also reduces depression, anxiety, stress, and insomnia.

Ingredients:

Tangerine *(Citrus reticulata)* contains esters and aldehydes that are sedating and calming, helping to combat anxiety and nervousness.

Orange *(Citrus sinensis)* is elevating to the mind and body and brings joy and peace. A Brazilian university evaluated the potential anxiolytic effect of *Citrus sinensis* essential oil and found in a placebo-controlled study that the aroma of sweet orange oil was acutely anxiolytic, giving support to its calming use as a tranquilizer by aromatherapists (Goes TC, et al., 2012).

Ylang Ylang *(Cananga odorata)* increases relaxation and balances male and female energies, restoring confidence and equilibrium.

Patchouli *(Pogostemon cablin)* is very high in sesquiterpenes that stimulate the limbic center of the brain. It re-establishes mental and emotional equilibrium and energizes the mind. It promotes grounding and helps center the emotions to clarify thoughts, allowing the mind to relax and let go of jealousies, obsessions, and insecurities.

Blue Tansy *(Tanacetum annuum)* helps cleanse the liver and lymphatic system and combats anger and negative emotions.

Applications:

- Diffuse, directly inhale, or add 2-4 drops to bath water.
- Apply to wrists, edge of ears, or foot Vita Flex points.
- Dilute 1:15 with vegetable oil for body massage.
- Put 4-8 drops on cotton balls or tissues and put in or on vents.
- Combine with Lavender for insomnia and German Chamomile for calming.

Caution: Possible sun/skin sensitivity.

Present Time™

This blend is an empowering fragrance that creates a feeling of being in the moment. Disease develops when we live in the past and with regret. Being in the present time is the key to progressing and moving forward.

Ingredients:

Almond oil *(Prunus dulcis)* is a carrier oil in this blend but adds a rich source of vitamin E. In the ancient Ayurveda system of health care native to India, the almond is considered a nutrient for the brain and nervous system.

Neroli *(Citrus sinensis)* was used by the ancient Egyptians for healing the mind, body, and spirit. It is stabilizing and strengthening to the emotions, promoting peace, confidence, and awareness. It brings thoughts and mental awareness to alleviate anxiety, depression, and insomnia.

Spruce *(Picea mariana)* opens and releases emotional blocks, fostering a sense of balance and grounding.

Ylang Ylang *(Cananga odorata)* promotes relaxation, balances male and female energies, restores confidence and equilibrium, and alleviates insomnia.

Applications:

- Diffuse, directly inhale, or add 2-4 drops to bath water.
- Apply to sternum and thymus area, neck, and forehead.

Purification®

This purifying blend cleanses and disinfects the air and neutralizes mildew, cigarette smoke, and disagreeable odors. It disinfects and cleans cuts, scrapes, and bites from spiders, bees, hornets, and wasps.

Ingredients:

Citronella *(Cymbopogon nardus)* is antiseptic, antibacterial, antispasmodic, anti-inflammatory, insecticidal, and insect-repelling.

Lemongrass *(Cymbopogon flexuosus)* has strong antifungal properties and is purifying and antibacterial.

Rosemary *(Rosmarinus officinalis* CT cineol*)* is antiseptic, antifungal, and antimicrobial and may be beneficial for skin conditions and dandruff. It helps fight candida and is anti-infectious.

Melaleuca Alternifolia *(M. alternifolia)*, also known as tea tree, is antibacterial, anti-fungal, antiparasitic, antiseptic, and anti-inflammatory.

Lavandin *(Lavandula* x *hybrida)* is antifungal, antibacterial, a strong antiseptic, and a tissue regenerator.

Myrtle *(Myrtus communis)* is antibacterial and may support immune function in fighting colds, flu, and other infectious disease.

Applications:

- Dilute 1 part essential oil to 1 part V-6 Vegetable Oil Complex.
- Diffuse 15 to 30 minutes every 3 to 4 hours.
- Directly inhale or add 2-4 drops to bath water.
- Apply on location to cuts, sores, bruises, or wounds.
- Put 4-8 drops on cotton balls or tissues and

- put in or on vents.
- Add 2 drops to a wet cloth and put in clothes dryer.

Caution: Possible skin sensitivity.

Raven™

The oils of this blend fight against respiratory disease and infections such as tuberculosis, influenza, and pneumonia. It is highly antiviral and antiseptic.

Ingredients:

Ravintsara *(Cinnamomum camphora)* is referred to by the people of Madagascar as the oil that heals. It is antiseptic, anti-infectious, antiviral, antibacterial, antifungal, and expectorant. It has been used to treat influenza, sinusitis, bronchitis, and herpes.

Lemon *(Citrus limon)* increases microcirculation and promotes immunity.

Wintergreen *(Gaultheria procumbens)* has strong anti-inflammatory and antispasmodic properties. It is analgesic, reduces pain, and helps increase respiratory capacity.

Peppermint *(Mentha piperita)* is a powerful anti-inflammatory and antiseptic for the respiratory system. It is used to treat bronchitis and pneumonia. It is high in menthol and menthone, helps suppress coughs, and clears lung and nasal congestion.

Eucalyptus Radiata *(E. radiata)* may have a profound antiviral effect upon the respiratory system. It may also help reduce inflammation of the nasal mucous membrane.

Applications:

- Dilute 1 part essential oils to 1 part V-6 Vegetable Oil Complex.
- Diffuse, humidify, directly inhale, or add 2-4 drops to bath water.
- Apply to throat and lung area and to foot Vita Flex points.

- Use as a hot compress over lungs or with Raindrop Technique.
- To use in suppository, dilute with V-6 1:10 and retain during the night.

Caution: Possible sun/skin sensitivity.

R.C.™

R.C. gives relief from colds, bronchitis, sore throats, sinusitis, coughs, and respiratory congestion. It decongests sinus passages, combats lung infections, and relieves allergy symptoms.

Ingredients:

Myrtle *(Myrtus communis)* supports the respiratory system and helps treat chronic coughs and tuberculosis. It is suitable to use for coughs and chest complaints with children. It is a sinus decongestant and alleviates throat infections.

Eucalyptus Globulus *(E. globulus)* has shown to be a powerful antimicrobial and germ killer. It is expectorant, mucolytic, antibacterial, antifungal, antiviral, and antiseptic. It reduces infections in the throat and lungs, such as rhinopharyngitis, laryngitis, flu, sinusitis, bronchitis, and pneumonia.

Marjoram *(Origanum majorana)* supports the respiratory system and reduces spasms. It is anti-infectious, antibacterial, and antiseptic.

Pine *(Pinus sylvestris)* opens and disinfects the respiratory system, particularly the bronchial tract. It has been used since the time of Hippocrates to support respiratory function and fight infection. According to Daniel Pénoël, MD, pine is one of the best oils for bronchitis and pneumonia.

Eucalyptus Citriodora *(E. citriodora)* decongests and disinfects the sinuses and lungs. It is anti-inflammatory, anti-infectious, and antispasmodic.

Lavender *(Lavandula angustifolia)* is antispasmodic, hypotensive, anti-inflammatory, and antiseptic. It is relaxing and grounding.

Cypress (*Cupressus sempervirens*) promotes blood circulation and lymph flow. It is anti-infectious, antibacterial, antimicrobial, mucolytic, antiseptic, refreshing, and relaxing.

Eucalyptus Radiata (*E. radiata*) is anti-infectious, antibacterial, antiviral, an expectorant, and anti-inflammatory. It has strong action against bronchitis and sinusitis.

Spruce (*Picea mariana*) helps the respiratory and nervous systems. It is anti-infectious, antiseptic, and anti-inflammatory.

Peppermint (*Mentha piperita*) is a powerful nasal and lung decongestant with antiseptic properties. It opens nasal passages, reduces cough, improves airflow to the lungs, and kills airborne bacteria, fungi, and viruses. A study conducted at the South African Tshwane University in Pretoria found that the main constituent of peppermint, menthol, not only is a highly effective skin penetrator but has analgesic effects (Kamatou GP, et al., 2013).

Applications:

- Dilute 1 part essential oil to 1 part V-6 Vegetable Oil Complex.
- Diffuse, humidify, directly inhale, apply on chest, neck, throat, or over sinus area.
- Use as a hot compress or with Raindrop Technique.
- Dilute 1:15 with V-6 Vegetable Oil Complex for body massage.
- Put 4-8 drops on cotton balls and put in or on vents.
- To combat sinus and lung congestion, add R.C., Raven, Dorado Azul, or Eucalyptus Blue to a bowl of steaming hot water. Place a towel over your head and inhale the steam from the mixture. Combine with Raven and

Thieves (alternating morning and night) to enhance effects.

Caution: Possible skin sensitivity.

Release™

This is a helpful blend to release anger and memory trauma from the liver in order to create emotional well-being. It helps open the subconscious mind through pineal stimulation to release deep-seated trauma. It is one of the most powerful of the emotionally supporting essential oil blends.

Ingredients:

Ylang Ylang (*Cananga odorata*) increases relaxation, balances male and female energies, and restores confidence and equilibrium.

Olive oil (*Olea europea*) is an ancient beauty secret discovered over 5,000 years ago. It promotes a smooth complexion with youthful elasticity; conditions dry, brittle nails; and makes the hair shine with vibrancy.

The Egyptians, Greeks, and Romans were all enamored with this prized oil as they enjoyed its radiant, youthful benefits. Olive oil preserves the taste, aroma, vitamins, and properties of the olive fruit. In ancient times it was considered a magical source for the fountain of youth, wealth, and power. It mixes well with the essential oils, offering nutrients with greater skin penetration.

Lavandin (*Lavandula* x *hybrida*) is antifungal, antibacterial, a strong antiseptic, and a tissue regenerator.

Geranium (*Pelargonium graveolens*) stimulates nerves and assists in balancing hormones. Its aromatic influence helps release negative memories, thereby opening and elevating the mind.

Sandalwood (*Santalum album*) is high in sesquiterpene compounds, which stimulate the pineal gland and the limbic region of the brain, the center of emotions and memory. It was used traditionally in yoga and meditation and may help remove negative programming in the cells.

Blue Tansy (*Tanacetum annuum*) helps cleanse the liver and lymphatic system. Emotionally, it combats anger and negative emotions and promotes a feeling of self-control.

Applications:

- Diffuse, directly inhale, or add 2-4 drops to bath water.
- Apply over liver, anywhere trauma has occurred, or as a compress.
- Massage on bottoms of feet and behind ears.
- Dilute 1:15 with V-6 Vegetable Oil Complex for body massage.
- Put 4-8 drops on cotton balls or tissues and put in or on vents.

Relieve It™

This blend is high in anti-inflammatory compounds that relieve deep tissue pain and muscle soreness.

Ingredients:

Spruce (*Picea mariana*) is anti-infectious, antiseptic, and anti-inflammatory.

Black Pepper (*Piper nigrum*) is anti-inflammatory and combats deep tissue pain. It has been traditionally used to treat arthritis.

Hyssop (*Hyssopus officinalis*) is anti-inflammatory and anti-infectious.

Peppermint (*Mentha piperita*) has powerful, pain-blocking, anti-inflammatory, and antispasmodic properties. A study conducted at the South African Tshwane University in Pretoria found that the main constituent of peppermint, menthol, not only is a highly

effective skin penetrator but has analgesic effects (Kamatou GP, et al., 2013).

Applications:

- Dilute 1 part essential oil to 1 part V-6 Vegetable Oil Complex.
- Apply on location to relieve pain.
- Use as a cold or hot compress.
  Caution: Possible skin sensitivity.

RutaVaLa™

RutaVaLa is a proprietary blend of *Ruta graveolens* (Ruta), Lavender, and Valerian essential oils that promotes relaxation of the body and mind, soothes stressed nerves, and induces sleep. Ruta has long been used in South America to promote the relaxation of body and mind, relieve and soothe stressed nerves, and revitalize passion.

Ingredients:

Lavender (*Lavandula angustifolia*) has been shown in endless research to calm and relax physical and mental tension. Its unique sedative properties add even more relaxation power to the RutaVaLa blend. A German university study suggested clinical use of lavender oil in patients suffering from anxiety (Schuwald AM, et al., 2013).

Valerian (*Valeriana officinalis*) is well known for its sedative and relaxation properties and is used both as an herb and as an essential oil to promote mental balance and as a sleep aid.

Ruta (*Ruta graveolens*) is harvested and distilled in Ecuador. It is sometimes referred to as "rue." Its use dates back to biblical times as an herb to be tithed. It is antiseptic and was one of the oils used in the original Vinegar of Four Thieves during the Black Plague.

Applications:

- Diffuse or inhale every hour or as needed.

RutaVaLa™ Roll-On

RutaVaLa Roll-On is a proprietary blend of *Ruta graveolens* (Ruta), Lavender, and Valerian essential oils that promotes relaxation of the body and mind, soothes stressed nerves, and induces sleep. Ruta has long been used in South America to promote the relaxation of body and mind, relieve and sooth stressed nerves, and revitalize passion.

Ingredients:

Fractionated (virgin) coconut oil *(Cocos nucifera)* has been processed or "fractioned" to create a strong shelf life. With its antiseptic and disinfectant properties, it gives a strong, stabilizing foundation to the delicate roll-on formulation.

Lavender *(Lavandula angustifolia)* has been shown in endless research to calm and relax physical and mental tension. Its unique sedative properties add even more relaxation power to the RutaVaLa blend.
A German university study suggested clinical use of lavender oil in patients suffering from anxiety (Schuwald AM, et al., 2013).

Valerian *(Valeriana officinalis)*, well known for its sedative and relaxation properties, is used both as an herb and as an essential oil to promote mental balance and aid sleep.

Ruta *(Ruta graveolens)* is harvested and distilled in Ecuador. It is sometimes referred to as "rue." Its use dates back to biblical times as an herb to be tithed. It is antiseptic and was one of the oils used in the original Vinegar of Four Thieves during the Black Plague.

Applications:

- Apply several drops to wrists, temples, neck, or any desired area as needed.
- It works very well on the bottoms of feet, and children love it.

Cautions: Possible skin/sun sensitivity. If you are pregnant or have a medical condition, consult with a health professional prior to use. Do a skin test before using by putting one drop on the sensitive skin area under the arm. Keep away from eyes and mucus membranes.

Sacred Mountain™

Mountain aromas instill strength, empowerment, grounding, and protection with the spiritual feeling of being in a sacred environment.

Ingredients:

Spruce *(Picea mariana)* opens and releases emotional blocks, fostering a sense of balance and grounding. Traditionally, it was believed to possess the frequency of prosperity.

Ylang Ylang *(Cananga odorata)* increases relaxation, balances male and female energies, and restores confidence and equilibrium.

Idaho Balsam Fir *(Abies balsamea)* has been researched for its ability to kill airborne germs and bacteria. As a conifer oil, it creates a feeling of grounding, anchoring, and empowering.

Cedarwood *(Cedrus atlantica)* is high in sesquiterpenes, which stimulate the limbic part of the brain, the center of emotions and memory. It stimulates the pineal gland, which releases melatonin, thereby improving thoughts, cognition, and memory. Cedarwood is very stabilizing and grounding.

Applications:

- Dilute 1 part essential oil to 1 part V-6 Vegetable Oil Complex.
- Diffuse, directly inhale, or add 2-4 drops to bath water.
- Apply to crown of head, back of neck, behind ears, and on thymus and wrists.
- Dilute 1:15 with vegetable oil for body massage.

- Put 4-8 drops on cotton balls or tissues and put in or on vents.
- Add 2 drops to a wet cloth and put in clothes dryer.

Caution: Possible skin sensitivity.

SARA™

This very specific blend enables one to relax into a mental state to facilitate the release of trauma from sexual and/or ritual abuse. SARA also helps unlock other traumatic experiences such as physical and emotional abuse.

Ingredients:

Almond oil *(Prunus dulcis)* is a carrier oil in this blend but adds a rich source of vitamin E.

In the ancient Ayurveda system of health care native to India, the almond is considered a nutrient for the brain and nervous system.

Ylang Ylang *(Cananga odorata)* increases relaxation, balances male and female energies, and restores confidence and equilibrium.

Geranium *(Pelargonium graveolens)* helps release negative memories, thereby opening and elevating the mind.

Lavender *(Lavandula angustifolia)* is relaxing and grounding.

A German university study suggested clinical use of lavender oil in patients suffering from anxiety (Schuwald AM, et al., 2013). Japanese researchers at Yamanashi Prefectural University tested lavender aroma for concentration in the late afternoon, when work concentration was at its lowest. Of three groups of young men tested in the study (control group, jasmine group, and lavender group), the lavender group had significantly higher concentration levels than the other two groups (Sakamoto R, et al., 2005).

Orange *(Citrus sinensis)* is elevating to the mind and body and brings joy and peace. A Brazilian university evaluated the potential anxiolytic effect of *Citrus sinensis* essential oil and found in a placebo-controlled study that the aroma of sweet orange oil was acutely anxiolytic, giving support to its calming use as a tranquilizer by aromatherapists (Goes TC, et al., 2012).

Blue Tansy *(Tanacetum annuum)* helps cleanse the liver and calm the lymphatic system, helping one to overcome anger and negative emotions, promoting a feeling of self-control. Its primary constituents are limonene and sesquiterpenes.

Cedarwood *(Cedrus atlantica)* is high in sesquiterpenes, which stimulate the limbic part of the brain, the center of emotions and memory.

It stimulates the pineal gland, which releases melatonin, thereby improving thoughts, cognition, and memory. Cedarwood is very stabilizing and grounding.

White Lotus *(Nymphaea lotus)* helps overcome self-defeating thoughts. It may also help release negative trauma and bring one a sense of comfort and ease.

Rose *(Rosa damascena)* possesses the highest frequency of all essential oils, creating balance, harmony, and well-being as it elevates the mind and brings joy to the heart.

Applications:

- Apply over energy centers and areas of abuse, on navel, lower abdomen, temples, nose, and Vita Flex points on the feet.

Caution: Possible sun sensitivity.

SclarEssence™

This blend balances hormones naturally using essential oil phytoestrogens. It helps to increase estrogen levels by supporting the body's own production of hormones. It combines the soothing effects of Peppermint with the balancing power of Fennel and Clary Sage and the calming action of Spanish Sage for an extraordinary dietary supplement.

Ingredients:

Clary Sage *(Salvia sclarea)* contains natural sclareol, a phytoestrogen that mimics estrogen function to help balance hormones. It helps with menstrual cramps, PMS, and circulatory problems.

Spanish Sage *(Salvia lavandulifolia)* is high in limonene, which prevents DNA damage.

Peppermint *(Mentha piperita)* strengthens the liver and glandular function.

Fennel *(Foeniculum vulgare)* is antiseptic and stimulating to the gastrointestinal system. It is antispasmodic so it may provide relief from cramps. It also has estrogen-like properties and helps balance hormones.

Applications:

- Put 1-10 drops in a 00 capsule mixed with V-6 Vegetable Oil Complex.
- Ingest 1 capsule daily as needed.

Caution: Do not use in conjunction with any other hormone products.

Sensation™

This beautiful smell is profoundly romantic, refreshing, and arousing. It amplifies the excitement of experiencing new heights of self-expression and awareness.

Sensation is also nourishing and hydrating for the skin and is beneficial for many skin problems.

Ingredients:

Coriander *(Coriandrum sativum)* has long been revered as a home remedy for relieving feelings of nausea, aiding digestion, and supporting healthy immune function.

Ylang Ylang *(Cananga odorata)* promotes relaxation, balances male and female energies, restores confidence and equilibrium, and alleviates insomnia.

Bergamot *(Citrus bergamia)* (furocoumarin-free) is simultaneously uplifting and calming, with a unique ability to relieve anxiety, stress, and tension.

Jasmine *(Jasminum officinale)* is beneficial for dry, oily, irritated, or sensitive skin. It combats muscle spasms, frigidity, depression, listlessness, and brings joy and harmony to the heart.

Geranium *(Pelargonium graveolens)* assists in balancing hormones. It is antispasmodic, relaxant, anti-inflammatory, antibacterial, antifungal, and stimulates the liver and pancreas.

Applications:

- Diffuse or add 2-4 drops to bath water.
- Apply on location, neck, or wrists.
- Use as a compress over abdomen.
- Dilute 1:15 with V-6 Vegetable Oil Complex for body massage.
- Put 4-8 drops on cotton balls or tissues and put in or on vents.
- Add 2 drops to a wet cloth and put in clothes dryer.

Caution: Possible skin sensitivity.

Slique™ Essence

Slique Essence combines powerful essential oils and stevia extract to support healthy weight-management goals. It suppresses food cravings, especially when used in conjunction with Slique™ Tea or any of the Slique™ products. The oils in this blend add a flavorful and uplifting element to any day, with the added support of Spearmint to aid proper digestion. Ocotea essential oil was chosen for its irresistible cinnamon-esque aroma, which can help trigger feelings of fullness and reduce the number of unexpected cravings. Slique Essence is antibacterial, antifungal, a lipid regulator, and a glucose regulator.

Stevia is added as an all-natural sweetener that

provides a pleasant, sweet taste with no added calories.

Ingredients:

Grapefruit *(Citrus paradisi)* is decongesting and fat dissolving. It is high in limonene, which prevents DNA damage, and has anticoagulant properties. Its aroma can be very calming and can bring a sense of wholeness.

Tangerine *(Citrus reticulata)* contains esters and aldehydes that are sedating and calming, combating anxiety and nervousness. It is high in limonene, which prevents DNA damage.

Spearmint *(Mentha spicata)* has been used orally for digestive disorders, flatulence, nausea, sore throat, diarrhea, colds, headaches, toothaches, and cramps.

Lemon *(Citrus limon)* has an extremely cleansing aroma. This oil helps purify and uplift.

Ocotea *(Ocotea quixos)* has high levels of alpha-humulene to balance the body's response to stress and difficult situations.

Stevia *(Stevia rebaudioside A)* is a super-sweet, low-calorie dietary supplement that helps regulate blood sugar and supports the pancreas. It supports weight loss and weight management because it contains no calories.

Applications:

- Add 2-4 drops to 4-6 oz. of Slique Tea or water.
- Take internally as a dietary supplement.
- Apply topically; dilute with V-6 Vegetable Oil Complex.
- Inhale directly.
- Use as needed throughout the day.

Note: The Stevia extract in this formula may impede diffuser performance.

Stress Away™ and Stress Away™ Roll-On

This is a gentle, fragrant blend that brings a feeling of peace and tranquility to both children and adults and helps to relieve daily stress and nervous tension. It helps with normal, everyday stress, improves mental response, restores equilibrium, promotes relaxation, and lowers hypertension.

Ingredients:

Copaiba *(Copaifera reticulata/langsdorfii)* is an oleoresin like Frankincense and is exuded from the trunk of the copaiba tree in South America. Historically it is used for anti-inflammatory and antitumoral healing in folk medicines.

In modern pharmacology it is used in products that soothe and protect the skin. Its hypnotic-like properties work as a sedative to the nervous system and can induce sleep. It is stimulating to the nervous or sympathetic nervous system.

Lime *(Citrus lime/aurantifolia)* is well known in folklore for its ability to cleanse, purify, and renew the spirit and is said to be effective in cleansing the aura. It can stimulate and refresh a tired mind and can help with depression. It has also been used for acne, asthma, colds, flu, and varicose veins.

Cedarwood *(Cedrus atlantica)* is high in sesquiterpenes, which stimulate the limbic part of the brain, the center of emotions and memory. It stimulates the pineal gland, which releases melatonin, thereby improving thoughts, cognition, and memory. Cedarwood is very stabilizing and grounding.

Vanilla *(Vanilla planifolia)* is a species of vanilla orchid that is native to Mexico and is one of the primary sources for vanilla flavoring, due to its high vanillin content.

Ocotea *(Ocotea quixos)* has a complex aroma that induces feelings of fullness or completeness, creating an environment of peace and tranquility.

Lavender *(Lavandula officinalis)* has been documented to improve concentration and mental acuity.

Japanese researchers at Yamanashi Prefectural University tested lavender aroma for concentration in the late afternoon, when work concentration was at its lowest. Of three groups of young men tested in the 2005 study (control group, jasmine group, and lavender group), the lavender group had significantly higher concentration levels than the other two groups (Sakamoto R, et al., 2005).

A study at Kyushu University in Japan corroborated this finding after tests of lavender outperformed a control group and helped to maintain sustained attention during a long-term vigilance task (Shimizu K, et al., 2008).

Applications:
- Apply liberally to temples, neck, or wrists as needed.

Surrender™

This inviting oil helps one surrender aggression and a controlling attitude. Stress and tension are released quickly when we surrender willfulness.

Ingredients:

Lavender *(Lavandula angustifolia)* has sedative and calming properties. It helps overcome nervous tension, depression, and chaotic energy.

Lemon *(Citrus limon)* is stimulating and invigorating, promoting a deep sense of well-being. It is very calming and reassuring to many individuals. A Brazilian university study found that lemon essential oil had sedative, anxiolytic, and antidepressant effects (LM Lopes C, et al., 2011).

Roman Chamomile *(Anthemis nobilis)* combats restlessness, tension, and insomnia. It purges toxins from the liver, where anger is stored. It also opens mental blocks.

Spruce *(Picea mariana)* opens and releases emotional blocks, creating a feeling of balance and grounding. Traditionally, it was believed to possess the frequency of prosperity.

Angelica *(Angelica archangelica)* helps to calm emotions and bring memories back to the point of origin before trauma or anger was experienced, helping us to let go of negative feelings.

German Chamomile *(Matricaria recutita)* has an electrical frequency that promotes peace and harmony, creating a feeling of security.

Mountain Savory *(Satureja montana)* is stimulating and energizing.

Applications:
- Diffuse, directly inhale, or add 2-4 drops to bath water.
- Apply on location, forehead, solar plexus, along ear rim, chest, and nape of neck.
- Dilute 1:15 with V-6 Vegetable Oil Complex for body massage.
- Put 4-8 drops on cotton balls or tissues and put in or on vents.

Caution: Possible sun/skin sensitivity.

The Gift™

The Gift is the very "essence of Arabia," blending the oils of antiquity into a most unique and exotic fragrance. It combines seven ancient therapeutic oils to capture the spirit of Arabia. This oil blend represents Mary's gift to Gary in honor of Shutran's noble journey through the book *The One Gift*, a historical novel depicting the wit, intrigue, sorrow, and romance of the ancient frankincense and myrrh caravans.

Out of the writings and legends of antiquity, the mysteries unfold as we discover their powerful uses for healing the injuries of war, accidents, scorpion stings, and snakebites and in sacred rituals for attaining greater spiritual attunement for healing and protecting the body.

Present-day science is now documenting the properties of these oils that augment the immune system, stimulate healing, and overcome depression. Myrrh and Frankincense are being touted for their anticancer, anti-infectious, antibacterial and antiviral abilities, as well as being a topical anesthesia and having the ability to regenerate bone and cartilage. They are the oldest known substances for their immune stimulating and healing powers to ever come out of the ancient world.

Ingredients:

Sacred Frankincense *(Boswellia sacra)* is considered a holy anointing oil in the Middle East and has been used in religious ceremonies for thousands of years. It stimulates the limbic part of the brain, which elevates the mind, helping to overcome stress and despair.

Idaho Balsam Fir *(Abies balsamea)* opens emotional blocks and recharges vital energy. It gives a feeling of strength and inner peace. As a conifer oil, it creates a feeling of grounding, anchoring, and empowering.

Jasmine *(Jasminum officinale)* stimulates the mind and improves concentration.

Galbanum *(Ferula galbaniflua)* has been a prized oil for healing since biblical times ("And the Lord said unto Moses, Take unto thee sweet spices, stacte, and onycha, and galbanum; sweet spices with pure frankincense:" Exodus 30:34).

Myrrh *(Commiphora myrrha)* possesses the frequency of wealth, according to legends, and is referenced throughout the Old and New Testaments, "A bundle of myrrh is my well-beloved unto me. . . ." Song of Solomon 1:13. It was also part of a formula the Lord gave to Moses (Exodus 30:22-27). It was used traditionally in the royal palaces by the queens during pregnancy and birthing and confers a sense of dignity and stateliness; myrrh is a kingly oil.

Cistus *(Cistus ladanifer)* enhances immunity and immune cell regeneration. It is anti-infectious, antiviral, and antibacterial, and in ancient times it was known as rockrose.

Spikenard *(Nardostachys jatamansi)* was used by Mary of Bethany to anoint the feet of Jesus. It strengthens immunity and hypo-thalamus function. It uplifts and gives spiritual strength and resoluteness for action.

Applications:

• It can be worn as a perfume, diffused, or massaged on the bottoms of feet.

Thieves®

This is a most amazing blend of highly anti-viral, antiseptic, antibacterial, and anti-infectious essential oils.

It was created from research based on legends about a group of 15th-century thieves who rubbed oils on themselves to avoid contracting the plague while they robbed the bodies of the dead and dying. When apprehended, the thieves were forced to tell what their secret was and disclosed the formula of the herbs, spices, and oils they used to protect themselves in exchange for more lenient punishment.

Studies conducted at Weber State University (Ogden, UT) during 1997 demonstrated the killing power of these amazing oils against air-borne microorganisms. The analysis showed that after 10 minutes of Thieves diffusion in the air, there was an 82% reduction in the gram positive

Micrococcus luteus organism bioaerosol, a 96% reduction in gram negative *Pseudomonas aeruginosa* organism bioaerosol, and a 44% reduction in *S. aureus* bioaerosol (Chao SC, et al., 1998).

Ingredients:

Clove *(Syzygium aromaticum)* is one of the most antimicrobial, antiseptic, antifungal, antiviral, and anti-infectious of all essential oils.

Lemon *(Citrus limon)* has antiseptic-like properties and contains compounds that amplify immunity. It promotes circulation, leukocyte formation, and lymphatic function.

Cinnamon Bark *(Cinnamomum zeylanicum)* is one of the most powerful antiseptics known and is strongly antibacterial, antiviral, and antifungal.

Eucalyptus Radiata *(E. radiata)* is anti-infectious, antibacterial, antiviral, and anti-inflammatory.

Rosemary *(Rosmarinus officinalis* CT cineol*)* is antiseptic and antimicrobial. It is high in cineole—a key ingredient in antiseptic drugs.

Applications:

- Dilute 1 part essential oil to 4 parts V-6 Vegetable Oil Complex.
- Diffuse for 15 minutes every 3 to 4 hours.
- Apply neat to bottoms of feet.
- Dilute 1:15 in vegetable oil and massage over thymus.
- For headaches, put 1 drop on tongue and push against roof of mouth.
- Dilute 1:15 with V-6 Vegetable Oil Complex for body massage.
- Put 4-8 drops on cotton balls or tissues and put in or on vents.
- Add 2 drops to a wet cloth and put in clothes dryer.

Caution: Possible sun/skin sensitivity.

Three (3) Wise Men™

This blend of 3 Wise Men promotes feelings of reverence and spiritual awareness combined with the power of therapeutic-grade essential oils that open the subconscious. It is considered a gift by many and enhances emotional equilibrium as it soothes and uplifts the heart.

Ingredients:

Almond oil *(Prunus dulcis)* is a rich source of vitamin E.

In the ancient Ayurveda system of health care native to India, the almond is considered a nutrient for the brain and nervous system, inducing intellectual acuity and longevity.

Sandalwood *(Santalum album)* is very high in sesquiterpene compounds that stimulate the pineal gland and the limbic region of the brain, the center of emotions and memory. It is used traditionally in yoga and meditation.

Juniper *(Juniperus osteosperma* and *J. scopulorum)* elevates spiritual awareness, creating feelings of love and peace.

Frankincense *(Boswellia carterii)* is considered a holy anointing oil in the Middle East and has been used in religious ceremonies for thousands of years. It stimulates the limbic part of the brain, which elevates the mind.

Spruce *(Picea mariana)* opens and releases emotional blocks, creating a feeling of balance and grounding. Traditionally, it was believed to possess the frequency of prosperity.

Myrrh *(Commiphora myrrha)* is referenced throughout the Bible, constituting a part of a holy anointing formula given to Moses (Exodus 30:22-27). It has one of the highest levels of sesquiterpenes, a class of compounds that stimulate the hypothalamus, pituitary, and amygdala, the control center for emotions and hormone release in the brain.

Applications:

- Diffuse, directly inhale, or add 2-4 drops to bath water.
- Add 2 drops on crown of head, behind ears, over eyebrows, on chest, over thymus, and at back of neck.
- Dilute 1:15 with V-6 Vegetable Oil Complex for body massage.
- Put 4-8 drops on cotton balls or tissues and put in or on vents.
- Add 2 drops to a wet cloth and put in clothes dryer.

Tranquil™ Roll-On

This proprietary blend of Lavender, Cedarwood, and Roman Chamomile essential oils, packaged in a roll-on applicator, provides convenient and portable relaxation and stress relief. All three of these oils have been well documented as being effective in reducing restlessness, decreasing anxiety, and inducing a calming feeling to mind and body. Their combined effect is uplifting as well as relaxing and can be useful in promoting sleep as well as reducing stress.

Ingredients:

Lavender *(Lavandula angustifolia)* is used in the traditional medicine of many cultures as a calmative. One of the most versatile of the essential oils, Lavender can be applied topically or used for aromatherapy to contribute to overall relaxation.

Cedarwood *(Cedrus atlantica)* has a very high level of sesquiterpenes, which can act directly on the limbic system in the brain to induce relaxation and calmness. Like conifer oils, Cedarwood provides a feeling of "grounding" that contributes to relaxation. It can also be applied topically, diffused, or inhaled directly.

Fractionated (virgin) coconut oil *(Cocos nucifera)* has been processed or "fractioned" to create a strong shelf life. With its antiseptic and disinfectant properties, it gives a strong stabilizing foundation to the delicate roll-on formulation.

Roman Chamomile *(Anthemis nobilis)* has traditionally been used to calm and soothe small children. It combats restlessness, tension, and insomnia.

Applications:

- Apply liberally to temples, neck, or wrists as needed.

Transformation™

Repressed trauma and tragedy from the past may be out of sight, but they are definitely not out of mind. Memories are imprinted in our cells for better or worse. Stored negative emotions need to be replaced with joy, hope, and courage.

Transformation blend radiates with the purifying oils of Lemon and Peppermint, along with the revitalizing power of sesquiterpenes from Sandalwood and Frankincense. Idaho Blue Spruce anchors new mental programming.

Reaching into the deepest recesses of memory, Transformation empowers and upholds the changes you want to make in your belief system. Positive, uplifting beliefs are foundational for the transformation of behavior.

Ingredients:

Lemon *(Citrus limon)* has antiseptic-like properties and contains compounds that amplify immunity. A Brazilian university study found that lemon essential oil had sedative, anxiolytic, and antidepressant effects (LM Lopes C, et al., 2011).

Peppermint *(Mentha piperita)* is stimulating, energizing, and empowering. The Human Cognitive Neuroscience Unit at the University of Northumbria in the UK documented the ability of peppermint to enhance memory and increase alertness (Moss M, et al., 2008).

Clary Sage *(Salvia sclarea)* balances the hormones. It contains natural sclareol, a phytoestrogen that mimics estrogen function.

Sandalwood *(Santalum album)* is very high in sesquiterpenes, which stimulate the pineal gland and the limbic region of the brain, the center of our emotions. It is used traditionally in yoga and meditation and may help remove negative programming in the cells.

Idaho Blue Spruce *(Picea pungens)* has an aroma that is grounding, stimulating to the mind, and relaxing to the body.

Sacred Frankincense *(Boswellia sacra)* is considered a holy anointing oil in the Middle East and has been used in religious ceremonies for thousands of years. It stimulates the limbic part of the brain, which elevates the mind, helping to overcome stress and despair.

Cardamom *(Elettaria cardamomum)* is uplifting, refreshing, and invigorating. It may be beneficial for clearing confusion.

Palo Santo *(Bursera graveolens)*, harvested in Ecuador, is similar to Frankincense and has traditionally been used to purify and cleanse the spirit from negative energies.

Ocotea *(Ocotea quixos)* has high levels of alpha-humulene to balance the body's response to stress and difficult situations.

Applications:
- Diffuse for most effective use.
- It may also be applied topically on appropriate Vita Flex points.

Trauma Life™

The emotional trauma from accidents, death of loved ones, assault, abuse, etc., can implant its devastation deep within the hidden recesses of the mind, causing life-long problems that seem endless.

Being able to release such burdens can bring about a new "lease on life" with a return to motivation and vitality.

This blend combats stress and uproots trauma that cause insomnia, anger, restlessness, and a weakened immune response.

Ingredients:

Sandalwood *(Santalum album)* is high in sesquiterpene compounds, which stimulate the pineal gland and the limbic region of the brain, the center of emotions and memory. It is used traditionally in yoga and meditation. It may help remove negative programming in the cells.

Frankincense *(Boswellia carterii)* elevates the mind and helps overcome stress and despair. It stimulates the limbic region of the brain, the center of emotions. In ancient times, Frankincense was known for its anointing and healing powers.

Valerian *(Valeriana officinalis)*, well known for its sedative and relaxation properties, is used both as an herb and as an essential oil to promote mental balance and aid sleep. It is calming, relaxing, grounding, and emotionally balancing. It also helps minimize shock, anxiety, and the stress that accompanies traumatic situations.

Spruce *(Picea mariana)* opens and releases emotional blocks, fostering a sense of balance and grounding.

Davana *(Artemisia pallens)* is high in sesquiterpenes, which help overcome anxiety.

Lavender *(Lavandula angustifolia)* is a relaxant and helps overcome insomnia and anxiety. It combats nervous anxiety, depression, and chaotic energy.

Geranium *(Pelargonium graveolens)* stimulates the nerves and helps release negative memories.

Helichrysum *(Helichrysum italicum)* improves circulation and helps release feelings of anger, promoting forgiveness.

Citrus Hystrix *(Citrus hystrix)* has aldehydes and esters that are calming and sedating.

Rose *(Rosa damascena)* has the highest frequency among essential oils. It creates a sense of balance, harmony, and well-being and elevates the mind. It creates a magnetic energy that attracts love and brings joy to the heart.

Applications:

- Diffuse, directly inhale, or add 2-4 drops to bath water.
- Apply to bottoms of feet, chest, forehead, nape of neck, behind ears, and along spine Raindrop Technique-style.
- Dilute 1:15 with V-6 Vegetable Oil Complex for body massage.
- Put 4-8 drops on cotton balls or tissues and put in or on vents.

Caution: Possible sun/skin sensitivity.

Valor®

This blend was formulated to balance energies and instill courage, confidence, and self-esteem. It helps the body self-correct its balance and alignment.

Ingredients:

Fractionated (virgin) coconut oil *(Cocos nucifera)* has been processed or "fractioned" to create a strong shelf life. With its antiseptic and disinfectant properties, it gives a strong, stabilizing foundation to the formulation.

Spruce *(Picea mariana)* opens and releases emotional blocks, fostering a sense of balance and grounding. Traditionally, it was believed to possess the frequency of prosperity.

Rosewood *(Aniba rosaeodora)* is anti-infectious, antibacterial, antifungal, antispasmodic, and is very grounding and strengthening.

Blue Tansy *(Tanacetum annuum)* helps cleanse the liver and lymphatic system, helping one to overcome anger and negative emotions, promoting a feeling of self-control.

Frankincense *(Boswellia carterii)* is considered a holy anointing oil in the Middle East and has been used in religious ceremonies for thousands of years.

It stimulates the limbic part of the brain, elevating the mind and helping to overcome stress and despair. It is used in European medicine to combat depression.

Applications:

- Diffuse, directly inhale, or add 2-4 drops to bath water.
- Apply 4 to 6 drops to wrists, chest, and base of neck, bottoms of feet, or along spine in Raindrop Technique.
- When using a series of oils, apply Valor first and wait 5 to 10 minutes before applying other oils.
- Dilute 1:15 with V-6 Vegetable Oil Complex for body massage.

Valor® Roll-On

Valor Essential Oil Roll-On is an empowering combination of therapeutic-grade essential oils that works with both the physical and spiritual aspects of the body to increase feelings of strength, courage, and self-esteem in the face of adversity. Renowned for its strengthening qualities, Valor enhances an individual's internal resources. It has also been found to help energy alignment in the body.

This has become a very popular blend, now offered in a portable, convenient, roll-on application.

Ingredients:

Fractionated (virgin) coconut oil *(Cocos nucifera)* has been processed or "fractioned" to create a strong shelf life. With its antiseptic and disinfectant properties, it gives a strong, stabilizing foundation to the delicate roll-on formulation.

Spruce *(Picea mariana)* helps open and release emotional blocks, bringing about a feeling of balance and grounding.

Rosewood *(Aniba rosaeodora)* is high in linalool, which has a relaxing, empowering, and uplifting effect. It is also very grounding and strengthening.

Frankincense *(Boswellia carterii)* is high in sesquiterpenes, which have a stimulating effect on the limbic system, elevating the mind and helping to replace feelings of sadness and despair with courage and determination.

Blue Tansy *(Tanacetum annuum)* cleanses and calms the lymphatic system and the liver, helping to overcome anger and negative emotions and promoting a feeling of self-control.

Applications:
- Apply generously to feet, wrists, or back of the neck.
- It can be worn as a fragrance.

White Angelica™

Increases and strengthens the aura around the body to bring a renewed sense of strength and protection, creating a feeling of wholeness in the realm of one's own spirituality. Its frequency neutralizes negative energy and gives a feeling of security.

Ingredients:

Fractionated (virgin) coconut oil *(Cocos nucifera)* has been processed or "fractioned" to create a strong shelf life. With its antiseptic and disinfectant properties, it gives a strong, stabilizing foundation to the formulation.

Myrrh *(Commiphora myrrha)* is referenced throughout the Old and New Testaments, constituting a part of a holy anointing

formula given to Moses (Exodus 30:22-27). It contains sesquiterpenes, a class of compounds that stimulate the hypothalamus, pituitary, and amygdala, the control center for emotions and hormone release in the brain.

Bergamot *(Citrus bergamia)* (furocoumarin-free) is simultaneously uplifting and calming, with a unique ability to relieve anxiety, stress, and tension.

Sandalwood *(Santalum album)* is high in sesquiterpene compounds, which stimulate the pineal gland and the limbic region of the brain, the center of emotions and memory. It is used traditionally in yoga and meditation.

Geranium *(Pelargonium graveolens)* stimulates the nerves and helps release negative memories, thereby opening and elevating the mind.

Ylang Ylang *(Cananga odorata)* increases relaxation, balances male and female energies, and restores confidence and equilibrium.

Spruce *(Picea mariana)* opens and releases emotional blocks, fostering a sense of balance and grounding. Traditionally, it was believed to possess the frequency of prosperity.

Rosewood *(Aniba rosaeodora)* is high in linalool, which has a relaxing, empowering, and uplifting effect. It is also very grounding and strengthening.

Coriander *(Coriandrum sativum)* has long been revered as a home remedy for relieving feelings of nausea, aiding digestion, and supporting healthy immune function.

Hyssop *(Hyssopus officinalis)* is strongly balancing for emotions. Helps stimulate creativity and meditation.

Melissa *(Melissa officinalis)* brings out gentleness. It is calming and balancing to the emotions, affecting the limbic part of the brain, the emotional center of memories. It was used anciently to treat nervous disorders and many different ailments of the heart.

Rose *(Rosa damascena)* has the highest frequency among essential oils. It creates a sense of balance, harmony, and well-being and elevates the mind. It creates a magnetic energy that attracts love and brings joy to the heart.

Angelica *(Angelica archangelica)* helps to calm emotions and to bring memories back to the point of origin before trauma or anger was experienced, helping to let go of negative feelings.

Applications:
- Diffuse, directly inhale, or add 2-4 drops to bath water.
- Apply to shoulders, along spine, on crown of head, on wrists, behind ears, on base of neck, or on foot Vita Flex points.

- Dilute 1:15 with V-6 Vegetable Oil Complex for body massage.
- Put 4-8 drops on cotton balls or tissues and put in or on vents.
- Add 2 drops to a wet cloth and put in clothes dryer.

ENDNOTES:
1. Göbel H, et al. Effect of peppermint and eucalyptus oil preparations on neurophysiological and experimental algesimetric headache parameters. *Cephalalgia*. 1994; 14(3):228-234.
2. Diego MA, et al. Aromatherapy positively affects mood, EEG patterns of alertness and math computations. *Int J Neurosci*. 1998 Dec;96(3-4):217-224.
3. Motomura N, et al. Reduction of mental stress with lavender odorant. *Percept Mot Skills*. 2001 Dec;93(3):713-718.
4. Komori T, et al. Effects of citrus fragrance on immune function and depressive states. *Neuroimmunomodulation*. 1995 May;2(3):174-180.
5. Montagna FJ. *Herbal Desk Reference*. Dubuque: Kendall/Hunt Publishing Company, 1990.
6. Chao SC, et al. Effect of a diffused essential oil blend on bacterial bioaerosols. *J Essent Oil Res*. 1998 Sep;10(5):517-523.

Chapter 6
Techniques for Essential Oil Application

The Use of Different Techniques

There are many creative ways to use essential oils for healing and supporting the human body that open a world of great discovery and untapped potential. It does not seem to matter how the essential oils are used, as long as their energy penetrates the body through direct application, inhalation, or ingestion.

The possibilities become very exciting as the essential oils are used by individuals new and/or inexperienced, and they begin to discover unexpected and fascinating benefits. However, as with any natural substance, essential oils should be used carefully, intelligently, and most importantly, with common sense. Keeping this in mind, common sense will enable you to enjoy the benefits and immense pleasure in using the essential oils as you learn to apply them through these techniques that have brought Peace & Calming, Joy, Harmony, and Abundance to thousands of people throughout the world.

The five specific techniques explained in this chapter have been studied and used in research as the development of their application has been refined and documented. Numerous doctors and health professionals are now acknowledging the benefits of these natural techniques, and thousands of individuals throughout the world have had tremendous benefits.

This knowledge is available to those who are interested in learning about essential oils, God's gift that Mother Nature eagerly provides, and how to use these brilliant but simple techniques in order to help themselves, their families, friends, and those in their world of influence.

Neuro Auricular Technique

D. Gary Young developed the Neuro Auricular Technique, NAT, which integrates the use of pure, therapeutic-grade essential oils with acupressure by using a small, pen-shaped instrument with a rounded end to apply the oils to the acupressure meridians or Vita Flex points on the ears.

He discovered that using essential oils in conjunction with acupressure was extremely beneficial. Interestingly, he found that acupressure stimulation on specific neurological points with the essential oils evoked a quicker response to specific conditions. The combination of acupressure with essential oils seemed to substantially increase benefits in targeted areas.

The Neuro Auricular Technique has shown remarkable benefits in both the emotional and physical realm. When working on a physical need, an emotional release is often experienced that can bring about a positive attitude of hope and renewed vitality.

In relationship to the spine and dealing with neurological problems that exist because of spinal cord injury, the Neuro Auricular Technique has been extremely beneficial in delivering the oils to the exact location of the neurological damage.

The Neuro Auricular Technique is a program that Gary continues to research, develop, and teach worldwide to doctors and other health practitioners. It has proven to have tremendous results and has the potential to be a well-known modality in the future.

Emotional Ear Chart

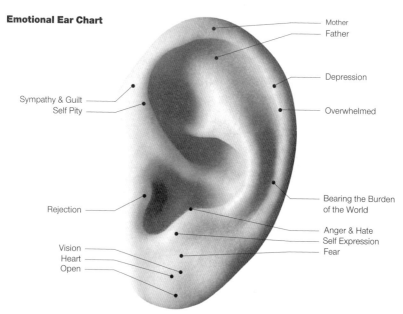

Mother
Father
Depression
Overwhelmed
Sympathy & Guilt
Self Pity
Bearing the Burden of the World
Rejection
Anger & Hate
Self Expression
Fear
Vision
Heart
Open

Physical Ear Chart

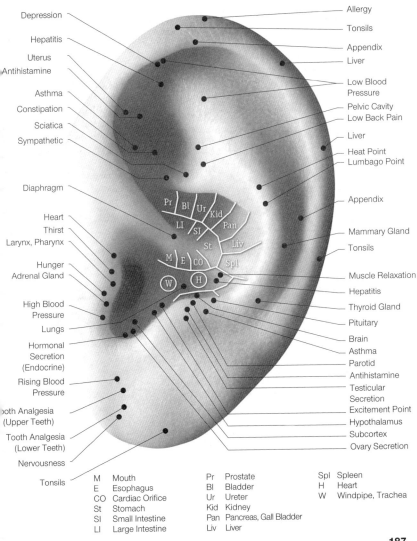

Depression
Hepatitis
Uterus
Antihistamine
Asthma
Constipation
Sciatica
Sympathetic
Diaphragm
Heart
Thirst
Larynx, Pharynx
Hunger
Adrenal Gland
High Blood Pressure
Lungs
Hormonal Secretion (Endocrine)
Rising Blood Pressure
Tooth Analgesia (Upper Teeth)
Tooth Analgesia (Lower Teeth)
Nervousness
Tonsils

Allergy
Tonsils
Appendix
Liver
Low Blood Pressure
Pelvic Cavity
Low Back Pain
Liver
Heat Point
Lumbago Point
Appendix
Mammary Gland
Tonsils
Muscle Relaxation
Hepatitis
Thyroid Gland
Pituitary
Brain
Asthma
Parotid
Antihistamine
Testicular Secretion
Excitement Point
Hypothalamus
Subcortex
Ovary Secretion

M	Mouth	Pr	Prostate	Spl	Spleen
E	Esophagus	Bl	Bladder	H	Heart
CO	Cardiac Orifice	Ur	Ureter	W	Windpipe, Trachea
St	Stomach	Kid	Kidney		
SI	Small Intestine	Pan	Pancreas, Gall Bladder		
LI	Large Intestine	Liv	Liver		

187

Lymphatic Pump

Maintaining lymph circulation is one of the keys to keeping the immune system adequately functioning. This technique is designed to promote lymph circulation. It is an excellent tool for those who are sedentary or bedridden.

1. With the recipient lying on his or her back, hold one leg with one hand just above the ankle with your palm on the underside of the leg (covering the Achilles tendon).

2. Place the other hand on the bottom of the recipient's foot with your palm over the ball of the foot and your fingers curled around the toes.

3. Push the top of the foot away from you (See Figure A).

4. Then pull the foot toward you by the toes until the ball of the foot is as close to the table as possible (See Figure B).

5. Check with the recipient during the pump to verify that the muscles in the foot are not being overextended. This should be an active process, but not a painful one.

6. Pull and push the foot using this "pumping motion" at least 10 times on each leg for maximum benefit. Note that the recipient's entire body should move during each step of the Lymphatic Pump.

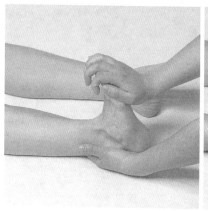

Figure A — Pushing the foot

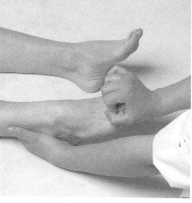

Figure B — Pulling the foot

Vita Flex Technique

Vita Flex means "vitality through the reflexes" and is an easy way to apply essential oils through the bottoms of the feet. It is a very important technique that can facilitate the relief of pain and suffering quickly as well as improving physical and emotional well-being.

It helps identify different structural and health needs of the body and together with the Raindrop Technique increases the opportunity for healing and rejuvenation. Vita Flex is a specialized form of hand and foot massage that is exceptionally effective in delivering the benefits of essential oils throughout the body.

It is said to have originated in Tibet thousands of years ago and was perfected in the 1960s by Stanley Burroughs long before acupuncture was popular in Western medicine.

It is based on a complete network of reflex points that stimulate all the internal body systems. When the fingertips connect to specific reflex points with essential oils using the special Vita Flex application, an electrical charge is released that sends energy through the neuroelectrical pathways.

This electrical charge follows the pathways of the nervous system to where there is a break in the electrical circuit, usually related to an energy block caused by toxins, damaged tissues, or loss of oxygen.

There are more than 1,500 Vita Flex points throughout the body in comparison to only 365 acupuncture points used in reflexology. Vita Flex is similar to but different from reflexology. As it is used today, reflexology has a tendency to ground out the electrical charge from constant compression and rotation pressure that causes cell separation and loss of oxygen to subdermal tissues, causing further injury.

In contrast to the steady stimulation of reflexology, Vita Flex uses a rolling and releasing motion that involves placing the fingers flat on the skin, rolling up onto the fingertips, and continuing over onto the fingernails, using medium pressure, and then sliding the hand forward about ½ inch, continually repeating this rolling and releasing technique until the specific Vita Flex area is covered. This rolling motion is repeated over the area three times.

Vita Flex corrects weakened or injured areas through the electrical reflex points, preventing further injury and less stress and allowing for quicker, more efficient healing. Combining the electrical frequency of the oils and that of the person receiving the application creates rapid and phenomenal results.

This ancient technique has brought healing of a greater dimension to our modern world with its complete, scientific, workable system of controls that releases the unlimited healing power within the human body.

The diagram of the nervous system shows the points on the spine and their electrical connection to specific areas throughout the entire body.

Vita Flex on the Hands

The hands also have specific reflex points that correspond to different organs and systems of the body. Although the hands are smaller and perhaps not as comfortable to work on, if you are in a hurry or are unable to get to the feet, there are still definite benefits in using the Vita Flex technique on the hands.

Vita Flex Foot Chart

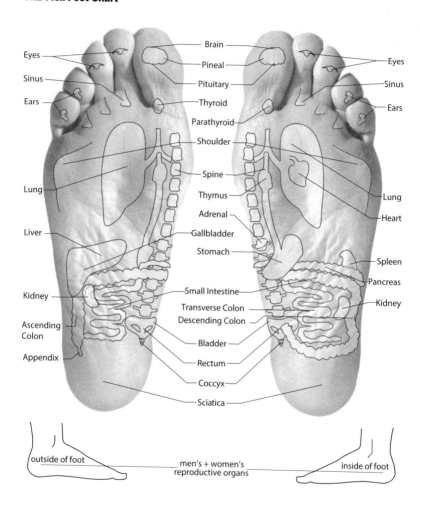

Brain
Pineal
Pituitary

Eyes
Sinus
Ears

Eyes
Sinus
Ears

Thyroid
Parathyroid
Shoulder
Spine
Thymus
Adrenal
Gallbladder
Stomach

Lung

Lung
Heart

Liver

Spleen
Pancreas

Kidney

Small Intestine
Transverse Colon
Descending Colon

Kidney

Ascending
Colon

Appendix

Bladder
Rectum
Coccyx
Sciatica

outside of foot

men's + women's
reproductive organs

inside of foot

Nervous System Connection Points

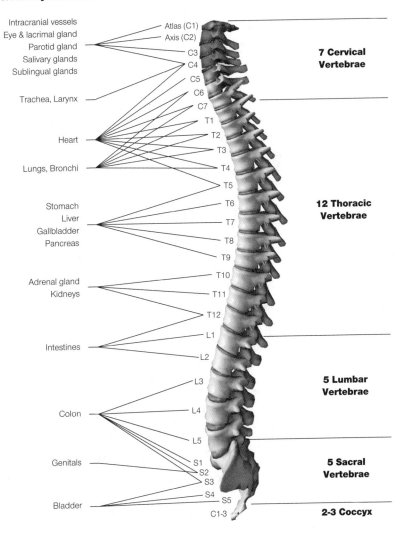

Intracranial vessels
Eye & lacrimal gland
Parotid gland
Salivary glands
Sublingual glands

Trachea, Larynx

Heart

Lungs, Bronchi

Stomach
Liver
Gallbladder
Pancreas

Adrenal gland
Kidneys

Intestines

Colon

Genitals

Bladder

Atlas (C1)
Axis (C2)
C3
C4
C5
C6
C7
T1
T2
T3
T4
T5
T6
T7
T8
T9
T10
T11
T12
L1
L2
L3
L4
L5
S1
S2
S3
S4
S5
C1-3

7 Cervical Vertebrae

12 Thoracic Vertebrae

5 Lumbar Vertebrae

5 Sacral Vertebrae

2-3 Coccyx

Palm of Left Hand

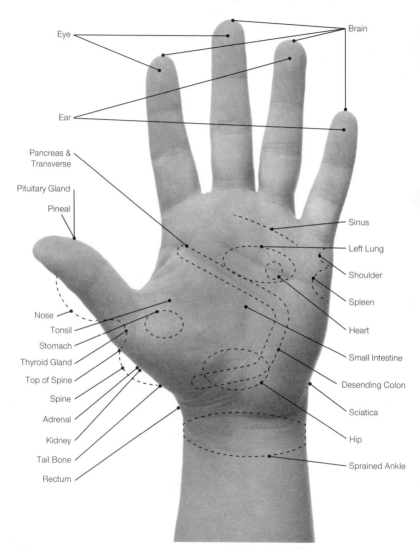

Eye

Brain

Ear

Pancreas & Transverse

Pituitary Gland

Pineal

Sinus

Left Lung

Shoulder

Spleen

Nose

Tonsil

Stomach

Thyroid Gland

Top of Spine

Spine

Adrenal

Kidney

Tail Bone

Rectum

Heart

Small Intestine

Desending Colon

Sciatica

Hip

Sprained Ankle

Palm of Right Hand

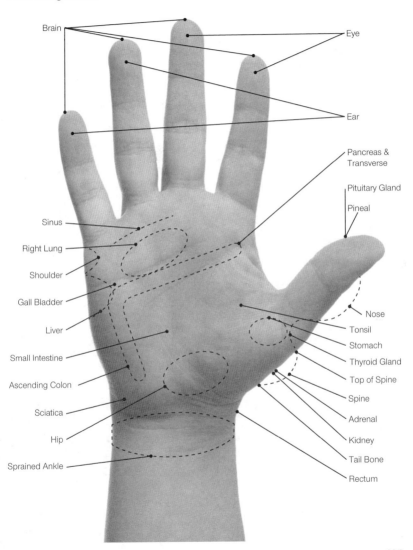

Brain

Eye

Ear

Pancreas & Transverse

Pituitary Gland

Pineal

Sinus

Right Lung

Shoulder

Gall Bladder

Liver

Small Intestine

Ascending Colon

Sciatica

Hip

Sprained Ankle

Nose

Tonsil

Stomach

Thyroid Gland

Top of Spine

Spine

Adrenal

Kidney

Tail Bone

Rectum

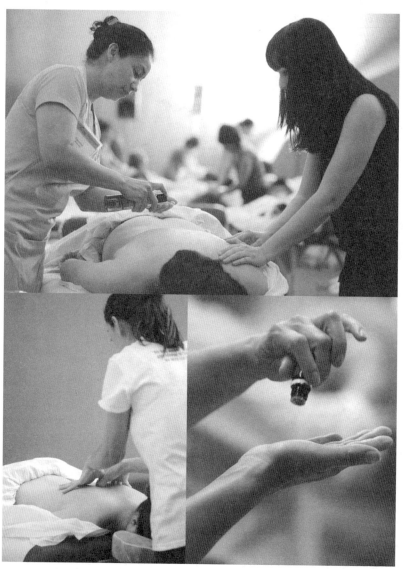

Raindrop Technique™

Most people would agree that massage is soothing, relaxing, and pleasurable. But Raindrop Technique is unquestionably far superior as it combines essential oils with special massage techniques to add greater therapeutic benefits to a pleasurable massage.

Anyone who has experienced Raindrop Technique is very quick to get on the massage table again to enjoy and discover new benefits of this most remarkable application of essential oils.

Raindrop Technique is one of the safest, noninvasive regimens available for spinal health. It is also an invaluable method to promote healing from within using topically applied essential oils.

The Development of the Raindrop Technique

D. Gary Young developed the Raindrop Technique based on his research of essential oils and their antimicrobial properties, his knowledge of the Vita Flex technique and its reflex points on the feet, and fascinating information on the light stroking called effleurage and its effect on the muscles and the nervous system.

Lakota Indians

While visiting with the Lakota people, Gary learned that for several generations before the U.S./Canadian border was established, the Lakota Indians migrated across the Canadian border into the northern regions of Saskatchewan and Manitoba. There, they often witnessed the Northern Lights, or Aurora Borealis.

Those who were ill or had complicated health problems would stand facing the Aurora Borealis, hold their hands toward the lights, and inhale deeply.

The Lakota believed that when the Aurora Borealis was visible, the air was charged with healing energy. They would mentally "inhale" this energy, allowing it to pass through their spine and on to other afflicted areas of the body through neurological pathways. Many experienced dramatic healing effects through this practice.

Eventually, after the border divided the U.S. from Canada, making migrations to the north impossible, the Lakota began practicing this energy process mentally, coupled with light stroking to facilitate the spreading of energy through the body.

Effleurage

Gary has said that he does not know if this is where the effleurage he teaches (feathered finger-stroking) first originated, but it has become associated with this healing technique. It is believed that the Lakota people continued their practice of mentally processing energy, coupled with effleurage, to distribute healing energy throughout the body.

Gary found that when this practice of effleurage was coupled with the therapeutic power of essential oils and the stimulation of Vita Flex, its effects were greatly heightened. Since this therapeutic practice was adopted in 1989, Raindrop Technique has been embraced by massage therapists, chiropractors, and other medical professionals around the world for its help with relaxation, correcting spinal misalignments, and antiviral effects.

Statistical Validation

In 2001, David Stewart, PhD, circulated a questionnaire to over 2,000 health practitioners, massage therapists, aromatherapists, and their clients to gain insight on the results that were accruing from Raindrop Technique.

He received 422 responses summarizing the experiences of some 14,000 Raindrop sessions.

His findings are summarized in his booklet *A Statistical Validation of Raindrop Technique* (available through Life Science Publishing; order online at lifesciencepublishers.com or by calling toll-free 800-336-6308).

Overall, the 416 respondents who had received a Raindrop Technique rated it positive (97 percent), pleasant (98 percent), resulted in improved health (89 percent), resulted in an improved emotional state (86 percent), and would choose to receive Raindrop Technique again (99.9 percent).

Consistent with the French Model

The use of undiluted essential oils in Raindrop Technique is consistent with the French model for aromatherapy—which is the most extensively practiced and studied model in the world. With over 40 years of experience using essential oils clinically, the French have consistently recommended neat (undiluted) use of essential oils.

An illustrious roster of 20th century French physicians provides convincing evidence that undiluted essential oils have a valuable place in the therapeutic arsenal of clinical professionals. René Gattefossé, PhD; Jean Valnet, MD; Jean-Claude Lapraz, MD; Daniel Pénoël, MD; and many others have long attested to the safe and effective use of undiluted essential oils and the dramatic and powerful benefits they can impart.

Skin Warming or Reddening

In the case of Raindrop Technique, the use of certain undiluted essential oils typically causes minor reddening and "heat" in the tissues. Normally, this is perfectly safe and not something to be overly concerned about. Individuals who have fair skin such as blondes and redheads or those persons whose systems are toxic are more susceptible to this temporary reddening.

Should the reddening or heat become excessive, it can be remedied within a minute or two by immediately applying several drops of V-6 Vegetable Oil Complex or a pure, high quality vegetable oil like jojoba, almond, or coconut oil on the affected area. This effectively dilutes the oils and the warming effect.

Temporary, mild warming is normal for Raindrop Technique. Typically, it is even milder than that of many capsicum creams or sports ointments. Indeed, rather than being a cause of concern, this warming indicates that positive benefits are being received.

In cases where the warmth or heat exceeds the comfort zone of the recipient, as mentioned before, the facilitator can apply any pure vegetable oil to the area until the comfort level is regained and reddening dissipates (usually within 2-5 minutes).

Note: If a rash should appear, it is an indication of a chemical reaction between the oils and synthetic compounds in the skin cells and the interstitial fluid of the body (usually from conventional personal care products).

Some misconstrue this as an allergic reaction, when in fact the problem is not caused by an allergy but rather by foreign chemicals already imbedded in the tissues. Essential oils are known to digest toxic waste, chemicals, and other unwanted toxins in the body, and sometimes that process starts to work very quickly.

Medical Professionals

A number of medical professionals throughout the United States have adopted Raindrop Technique in their clinical practice and have found it to be an outstanding method to relieve the problems associated with sciatica, scoliosis, kyphosis, and chronic back pain.

Ken Krieger, DC, a chiropractor practicing in Scottsdale, Arizona, states, "As a chiropractor, I believe that the dramatic results of Raindrop

Technique are enough for me to rewrite the books on scoliosis."

Similarly, Terry Friedmann, MD, of Westminster, Colorado, stated that " . . . these essential oils truly represent a new frontier of medicine; they have resolved cases that many professionals had regarded as hopeless."

Microorganisms May Cause Scoliosis and Sciatica

A growing amount of scientific research shows that certain microorganisms lodge near the spinal cord and contribute to deformities. These pathogens create inflammation, which, in turn, contorts and disfigures the spinal column.

Raindrop Technique uses a sequence of highly antimicrobial essential oils dropped on the back as a noninvasive therapy for fighting against pathogens lying dormant against the spine, which alleviates symptoms of scoliosis, kyphosis, and other back ailments while strengthening the immune system.

Studies at Western General Hospital in Edinburgh, Scotland, linked virus-like particles to idiopathic scoliosis.[1,2]

Researchers at the University of Bonn have also found that the varicella zoster virus can lodge in the spinal ganglia throughout life.[3]

Research in 2001 further corroborated the existence of infectious microorganisms as a cause of spine pain and inflammation. Alistair Stirling and his colleagues at the Royal Orthopedic Hospital in Birmingham, England, found that 53 percent of patients with severe sciatica tested positive for chronic, low-grade infection by gram-negative bacteria (particularly *Propionibacterium acnes*), which triggered inflammation near the spine. Stirling suggested that the reason these bacteria had not been identified earlier was because of the extended time required to incubate disc material (7 days).[4]

The tuberculosis mycobacterium has also been shown to contribute to spinal disease and possibly deformations. Research at the Pasteur Institute in France, published in *The New England Journal of Medicine*, documented increasing numbers of patients showing evidence of spinal disease (Pott's disease) caused by tuberculosis.[5, 6, 7, 8]

In addition, vaccines made from live viruses have been linked to spinal problems. A 1982 study by Pincott and Taff found a connection between oral poliomyelitis vaccines and scoliosis.[9]

Raindrop Technique is a powerful, noninvasive technique utilizing the antiviral, antibacterial, and anti-inflammatory action of several key essential oils to assist the body in maintaining or retraining the spinal column's natural curvature.

During the past 18 years, this technique has helped alleviate or resolve many cases of scoliosis, kyphosis, and chronic back pain and has eliminated the need for back surgery for hundreds of people.

Powerful Antibacterial Agents

Essential oils are some of the most powerful inhibitors of microbes known and as such are an important, new weapon in combating many types of tissue infections. A 1999 study by Marilena Marino and colleagues found that thyme oil exhibited strong action against stubborn gram-negative bacteria.[10]

Similarly, basil essential oil also demonstrated strong bactericidal action against microorganisms *Aeromonas hydrophila* and *Pseudomonas fluorescens*.[11]

A study at the Central Food Technological Institute in Mysore, India, found that a large number of essential oil components had tremendous germ-killing effects, inhibiting the growth of Staphylococcus, Micrococcus, Bacillus, and Enterobacter strains of bacteria.

These compounds included menthol (found in Peppermint), eucalyptol (found in Rosemary,

Eucalyptus Radiata, and Geranium), linalool (found in Marjoram), and citral (found in Lemongrass).[12]

A 2001 study conducted by D. Gary Young, Diane Horne, Sue Chao, and colleagues at Weber State University in Ogden, Utah, found that Oregano, Thyme, Peppermint, and Basil exhibited very strong antimicrobial effects against pathogens such as *Streptococcus pneumoniae*, a major cause of illness in young children and death in elderly and immune-weakened patients.[13] Many other studies confirm these findings.[14]

The ability of essential oils to penetrate the skin quickly and pass into body tissues to produce therapeutic effects has also been studied. Hoshi University researchers in Japan found that cyclic monoterpenes (including menthol, which is found in Peppermint) are so effective in penetrating the skin that they can actually enhance the absorption of water-soluble drugs.[15] North Dakota State University researchers have similarly found that cyclic monoterpenes such as limonene and other terpenoids such as menthone and eugenol easily pass through the dermis, magnifying the penetration of pharmaceutical drugs such as tamoxifen.[16]

Ingesting Essential Oils

It is interesting to note that many essential oils used in Raindrop Technique—in addition to being highly antimicrobial—are also among those classified as GRAS (Generally Regarded As Safe) for internal use by the U.S. Food and Drug Administration. These include Basil, Marjoram, Peppermint, Oregano, and Thyme. These and many other essential oils on the GRAS list have had a long history for decades as foods or flavorings with virtually no adverse reactions. It is interesting how the people of the world were ingesting essential oils long before the FDA determined they were safe.

In sum, Raindrop Technique is a safe, noninvasive way to achieve spinal health. It is

an invaluable method to promote healing from within using topically applied essential oils.

The Raindrop Technique Experience

Most people would agree that massage is soothing, relaxing, and pleasurable. But Raindrop Technique is unquestionably far superior as it combines essential oils with special massage techniques to add greater therapeutic benefits to a pleasurable massage.

Anyone who has experienced Raindrop Technique is very quick to get on the massage table again to enjoy and discover new benefits of this most remarkable application of essential oils.

Physical Relief and Emotional Release

When D. Gary Young developed Raindrop Technique in 1991, he first chose nine pure, therapeutic-grade essential oils that would synergistically combine to kill viral and bacterial pathogens, reduce inflammation, support the immune system, ease respiratory discomfort, relax stressed muscles, and relieve the body of bone and joint discomfort.

He felt this combination of oils would also balance the energy, lift the spirit by reducing stress, and calm a troubled and confused mind. This began a new realm of healing that emerged from within the confines of emotional bondage.

In the cerebral cortex is a structure called the amygdala that is affected only by scent. It is here that the emotions and memories of life are stored. Since essential oils have the ability to cross the blood barrier and stimulate the amygdala, buried feelings of past trauma, emotional upset, and unhappy memories are often released to the cognizant mind, bringing those feelings and consequences to the surface of awareness.

Many physical and emotional problems become dim or completely disappear as the foundation of the emotion is discovered and released. Raindrop Technique has vast benefits only to be realized by the individual receiving the application. It is different for each individual, unlike anyone else, and is very personal and specific to each person's needs.

Children tend to respond even faster than adults because they do not have any preconceived ideas about what they want to have happen or experience. They just love it and often fall asleep while the essential oils and the touch of massage fill them with peace and contentment as body systems harmonize together.

Raindrop Technique is an experience for everyone at any age for whatever the need or desire may be, and perhaps it is just a time of quiet relaxation and enjoyment.

Raindrop Technique and Essential Oils

Raindrop Technique is one of the safest, most noninvasive regimens available for spinal health. It is also an invaluable method to promote healing from within using topically applied essential oils.

Single oils

- **Oregano** (*Origanum vulgare*) may also use **Plectranthus Oregano** (Plectranthus amboinicus): Awakens receptors, kills pathogens, and helps digest toxic substances on the receptor sites
- **Thyme** (*Thymus vulgaris*): Kills pathogens and digests waste and toxic substances on the receptor sites
- **Basil** (*Ocimum basilicum*): Releases muscle tension
- **Cypress** (*Cupressus sempervirens*): Improves circulation and is oil for the pituitary gland
- **Wintergreen** (*Gaultheria procumbens*): Reduces pain
- **Marjoram** (*Origanum majorana*): Strengthens muscles
- **Peppermint** (*Mentha piperita):* Promotes greater oil penetration

Essential oil blends

- **Valor:** Structural balancing and alignment
- **Aroma Siez:** Muscle relaxation and pain reduction
- **White Angelica:** Protection for adversarial energies

Simple Explanation

The oils are dispensed like drops of rain from a height of about 6 inches above the back. Starting from the low back, the oils are feathered with the back of the fingers up along the vertebrae, out over the back muscles, and over the shoulders to the neck. Although the entire technique takes from 30-45 minutes to complete, the oils continue to work for several days as the healing and realignment process takes place.

Many recipients feel the benefits of the oils for several days afterwards, as they recognize that the pain has decreased or is completely gone, there is no fever, they have more mobility, and they have an overall feeling of peace and a renewed zest for life.

Experiencing the wonderful results of a first-time Raindrop application does not mean that all the desired benefits will be realized. One Raindrop session might be just a time to balance and relax the body. Some individuals may feel they want to have Raindrop once a week, once a month, or every three or four months. Other individuals working on structural realignment or needing emotional support may choose to have Raindrop done on a weekly basis to continue with their progress.

It is important to recognize that a healthy body is not attained by doing just one thing. It is a result of a well-rounded program of exercise, proper diet, and sufficient sleep. Health is everything we do, say, see, eat, and think, along with drinking plenty of water and getting enough sleep.

Overview of Application

The "facilitator(s)" is the person giving the Raindrop Technique, and the "receiver" refers to the person receiving it.

Preparation

To properly perform the Raindrop Technique, it is necessary to obtain the following:

1. A massage table or comfortable, flat surface. The surface should be high enough that the facilitator can perform the technique without back strain. Use sheets or towels as a barrier, being sensitive to the fact that essential oils may damage or stain vinyl and other fabrics.

2. It is important to respect the receiver's modesty at all times. The use of a blanket or sheet provides the best protection. Make sure the environment and your actions promote a sense of security and protection for the receiver.

3. Raindrop Technique Kit:
   - Valor
   - Oregano
   - Thyme
   - Basil
   - Cypress
   - Wintergreen
   - Marjoram
   - Aroma Siez
   - Peppermint
   - White Angelica*
   - V-6 Vegetable Oil Complex
   - Ortho Ease Massage Oil

   * White Angelica is needed but is not included in the kit.

Step 1: Balance energy. Apply **Valor** on the soles of the feet. If a second person is assisting, then that person can put the oils on the shoulders.

Step 2: Vita Flex Technique. Work the same Raindrop Technique oils into the spinal reflex areas of the feet.
Vita Flex facilitates quick absorption of the oils through the bottoms of the feet and prepares the body for Raindrop on the back. It is also highly relaxing.

Step 3: The 5-step Feathering Technique. Use with each of the oils as they are applied on the back, starting at the base of the spine and working upwards to stimulate the cell receptors and activate energy centers along the spine, as well as to distribute the oil drops over the back for rapid penetration.

Step 4: Feather 3-5 drops of **Oregano (or Plectranthus Oregano)**—from the spine outwards.

Step 5: Feather 3-5 drops of **Thyme**—from the spine outwards.

Step 6: Stretch and release. Feather 4-6 drops of **Basil** along both sides of the spine and feather out and upwards. Then take hold of the feet and gently pull to stretch the spine, releasing tension from the vertebra, back muscles, and tissue.

Step 7: Finger Straddle Massage. Apply 5-8 drops of **Cypress** on the spine and feather; then perform the Spinal Finger Straddle.

Step 8: Vita Flex Thumb Roll. Apply 5-8 drops of **Wintergreen** on the spine and feather; then perform the Vita Flex Thumb Roll.

Step 9: Circular Hand Massage. Apply 8-10 drops of **Marjoram** on the back and feather; then perform the Circular Hand Massage.

Step 10: Palm Slide. Apply 8-10 drops of **Aroma Siez** over the entire back and feather; then perform the Palm Slide.

Step 11: Feathering Technique. Apply 3-5 drops of **Peppermint** on the spine and feather.

Step 12: Feathering Technique. Apply 8-10 drops of Valor over the back and feather.

Be sure to remember the following

1. The Raindrop Technique should be performed only if the facilitator is feeling balanced and focused. Time should be spent developing clarity and energy for transfer to the receiver during the technique.

2. Both facilitator and receiver should be relaxed and comfortable. Appropriate clothing should be worn.

3. An environment should be created that is warm, quiet, relaxing, and comfortable. Soft music and lighting generally prove to be beneficial to the receiver.

4. Both the facilitator and the receiver should remove all jewelry. This includes watches, pendants, chains, rings, bracelets, belts, earrings, etc. These items produce an electrical energy that may interfere with the technique. Metal eyeglasses are acceptable.

5. Facilitators should make sure their fingernails are clipped and filed to prevent scratching the receiver's skin, particularly when performing Vita Flex. Nails should also be free of polish. (Essential oils can remove polishes and lacquers.)

6. Inquire as to whether the receiver has been exposed to chemicals or has worked in a toxic environment.

7. Ask the receiver if he or she needs to use the restroom prior to beginning.

8. Request permission to begin the Raindrop Technique.

9. It is necessary to access the receiver's back for application of the oils. The use of clothing that fully exposes the spine works best. If modesty can be preserved, remove all clothing from the waist up for easier application.

10. To begin, the receiver should lie as straight as possible on his or her back, face up, on the massage table. Arms should rest alongside the body with the palms touching the sides of the thighs. This will help direct the flow of energy and keep it connected to the receiver.

11. Once contact is made with the receiver, the facilitator should maintain a constant physical connection. This promotes feelings of calmness and security while developing a sense of trust with the facilitator.

12. While applying the Raindrop Technique, use caution when working near the spine or applying direct pressure.

13. Offer assistance to the receiver when dismounting the table.

14. Have plenty of water available for the receiver after the Raindrop Technique is complete.

15. Provide detailed instructions to the receiver for post-Raindrop Technique care.

Application of Raindrop and Vita Flex Techniques

1. BALANCING BODY ENERGY

Application of Valor

Valor serves as the foundation for all work performed during the Raindrop Technique. This essential oil blend helps regulate the electromagnetic energy that flows through the body and balances the receiver's emotional, spiritual, and physical energy. By balancing these energies, the receiver's connections are dramatically improved.

It is only necessary for one facilitator to perform this process by using the foot application. If two facilitators are present, work in unison: one at the shoulders and one at the feet. Both will apply Valor and remain in contact until the energy is balanced.

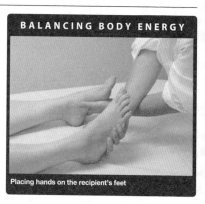

BALANCING BODY ENERGY

Placing hands on the recipient's feet

Shoulder Application

1. The facilitator should put White Angelica essential oil blend on his or her shoulders, back of the neck, and thymus area before starting the Raindrop Technique.
2. The facilitator places 3 drops of Valor in each hand.
3. With both palms up, cup under the receiver's right shoulder with the right hand and cup under the left shoulder with the left hand.
4. Hold this position until the facilitator at the feet completes the same technique.
5. Continue with the foot application as described.

Foot Application

1. Facing the receiver, place 6 drops of Valor in each hand.
2. Make contact with the receiver's feet, with the palm of the right hand to the right foot and the palm of the left hand to the left foot. The feet should be held snug with the palms of the hands against the soles of the feet. The facilitator should have firm, but comfortable, contact with the receiver.

2. VITA FLEX

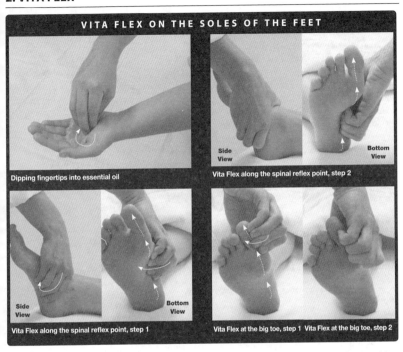

VITA FLEX ON THE SOLES OF THE FEET

Dipping fingertips into essential oil

Side View — Bottom View
Vita Flex along the spinal reflex point, step 2

Side View — Bottom View
Vita Flex along the spinal reflex point, step 1

Vita Flex at the big toe, step 1   Vita Flex at the big toe, step 2

To use this technique, nine essential oils are applied to the spinal Vita Flex area on the soles of the feet. These nine oils, in application sequence, are:

1. Oregano
2. Thyme
3. Basil
4. Cypress
5. Wintergreen
6. Marjoram
7. Peppermint
8. Aroma Siez
9. White Angelica

Things to Remember

1. Always begin with the right foot for consistency purposes.
2. Use firm, but not painful, pressure; roll and press to the first knuckle.
3. Move slowly and evenly, one finger width at a time.
4. Repeat everything in three's.

Procedure

The following procedure is to be repeated for each of the seven oils, using the appropriate sequence (see the *10 Steps for Vita Flex* worksheet for more detailed instructions).

1. Place 2–3 drops of essential oil (1–2 drops for smaller feet) in the palm of the left hand. Dip the fingertips of the right hand in the oil and stir clockwise three times to energize the oil. Apply along the spine Vita Flex

points (bottom inside edge of the foot from heel to the tip of the big toe).

2. Cup the hand so that the fingertips rest on the Vita Flex points at the heel while the thumb rests on the top of the foot.

3. Rock the hand forward so the nail ends up flat against the bottom of the foot (about half a finger length). Then rock backward to the original position.

4. Continue this technique all the way up the foot to the tip of the big toe. End with several Vita Flexes on the neck and center pad of the big toe. Repeat two times before moving to the other foot.

5. Continue this process with the remaining oils.

Remember: Right hand to right foot and left hand to left foot. Do both right and left feet before moving to the next oil in the sequence.

3. SPINAL APPLICATION OF ESSENTIAL OILS

After Vita Flex is complete, have the receiver turn over and lie on his or her stomach. Be sure that the receiver is comfortable and that modesty is respected. The receiver should place his or her arms comfortably along the sides of the body. The entire back needs to be exposed for application of the Raindrop oils. The oils will be applied from the sacrum to the atlas.

Feather strokes are used in addition to stretching, Vita Flex, and rubbing techniques. For both Vita Flex and other procedures within the Raindrop, specific steps are performed three complete times.

The oils used here mirror those that were used in the Vita Flex application and should be used in the same sequential order.

A. Oregano (or Plectranthus Oregano)

1. Hold the bottle 6 inches above the skin and evenly place 2–4 drops of Oregano along the spine, extending from the sacrum to the atlas.

Feather

2. Use 6-inch brush strokes to "feather" up the spine. To feather, gently brush the back of the fingertips up the spine while alternating hands.

3. Use 12-inch brush strokes to feather up the length of the spine.

4. Feather the entire length of the spine using three long brush strokes.

5. Repeat this process two or three more times.

Fan

6. Use 6-inch fanning strokes to fan up the spine and to the sides of the receiver. To fan, gently brush the back of the fingertips up and away from the spine.

7. Fan the entire length of the spine using three long fanning strokes.

Note: Do not repeat this process.

B. Thyme

1. Hold the bottle 6 inches above the skin and evenly place 2–4 drops of Thyme along the spine, extending from the sacrum to the atlas.

2. Immediately feather up the spine according to the technique previously described.

C. Basil

1. Apply 3–4 drops of Basil evenly along both sides of the spine.

2. Immediately feather up the spine according to the technique previously described.

FEATHER STROKES

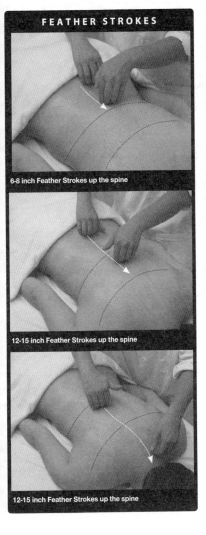

6-8 inch Feather Strokes up the spine

12-15 inch Feather Strokes up the spine

12-15 inch Feather Strokes up the spine

FAN STROKES

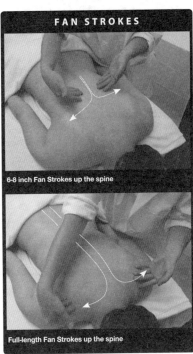

6-8 inch Fan Strokes up the spine

Full-length Fan Strokes up the spine

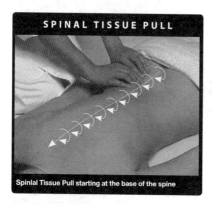

SPINAL TISSUE PULL

Spinal Tissue Pull starting at the base of the spine

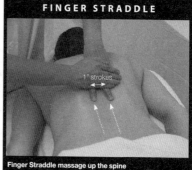

FINGER STRADDLE

1" strokes

Finger Straddle massage up the spine

Spinal Tissue Pull

3. Alongside the spine, place hands side by side with fingers curved and the heels of the hands resting on the back. Complete three rotations using the pads of the fingertips to create small, circular, clockwise motions to gently pull the muscle tissue away from the spine.

4. After finishing one side of the spine, move to the other side of the receiver and repeat the procedure on the opposite side. Do not apply direct pressure to the spinal vertebrae.

5. Repeat this step two more times.

D. Cypress

1. Hold the bottle 6 inches above the skin and evenly place 4–6 drops of Cypress along both sides of the spine, extending from the sacrum to the atlas.

2. Immediately feather up the spine according to the technique previously described.

Finger Straddle

3. Stand on the receiver's left side, near the shoulder area, facing the receiver's feet.

4. With the index and middle fingers of the left hand, straddle the spine at the sacrum. Place the bottom edge of the right hand ulna or pinky-side down, just below the middle joints of the two straddling fingers.

5. Apply moderate, downward pressure with the straddling fingers while pulling them slowly to the atlas of the spine. At the same time, saw with the right hand using short, rapid, back-and-forth motions.

6. Once at the atlas, use the straddled fingers to gently pull toward the head three times.

7. Repeat this process two more times.

E. Wintergreen

1. Hold the bottle 6 inches above the skin and evenly space 6–10 drops of Wintergreen along both sides of the spine, extending from the sacrum to the atlas.

2. Immediately feather up the spine according to the technique previously described.

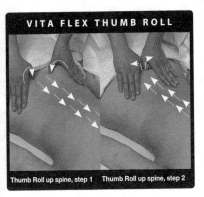

VITA FLEX THUMB ROLL

Thumb Roll up spine, step 1   Thumb Roll up spine, step 2

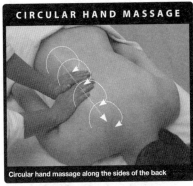

CIRCULAR HAND MASSAGE

Circular hand massage along the sides of the back

Vita Flex Thumb Roll

3. At the sacrum, place both thumbs 1 inch apart on either side of the spine with the tip of the thumbs down, one slightly higher on the back than the other.

4. Begin rolling thumbs from the tip to the nail, back and forth, working up the spine in small increments from the sacrum to the atlas, applying mild pressure the entire time.

5. Continue to roll your thumbs lightly over onto the knuckles and then back to their stand-up position. When doing this process, the knuckles should make contact with the spine. Work up the spine 1 inch at a time.

6. Repeat this step two more times. For clients who have neurological conditions, it is important to work down from the atlas to the sacrum instead of working up the spine.

F. Marjoram

1. Hold the bottle 6 inches above the skin and evenly space 10–15 drops of Marjoram over the entire back, extending from the sacrum to the atlas.

2. Immediately feather as needed to evenly distribute the oil.

Circular Hand Massage

3. Place your hands palms down on the lower right side of the back. Rotate hands in a firm, clockwise motion up the right side of the spine.

4. Walk to the left side of the receiver and place your hands palms down on the lower left side of the back. Rotate hands in a firm, clockwise motion up the left side of the spine. Walk back to the right side of the receiver.

5. Repeat steps 3 and 4 two more times.

G. Aroma Siez

1. Hold the bottle 6 inches above the skin and evenly place 10 drops of Aroma Siez all over the back, extending from the sacrum to the atlas.

2. Immediately feather as needed to evenly distribute the oil.

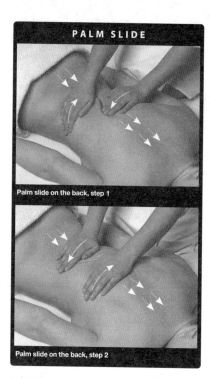

Palm slide on the back, step 1

Palm slide on the back, step 2

Palm Slide

3. Place both hands palms down on the receiver's back on each side of the spine near the sacrum. One hand should be slightly higher than the other.

4. Slide palms, with mild downward pressure, in opposite directions, working slowly up the spine using a back and forth motion up to the nape of the neck.

5. Slide back to the base using the same movements.

6. Repeat this process two more times.

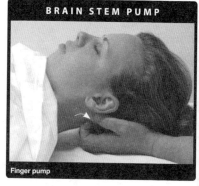

Finger pump

H. Peppermint

1. Hold the bottle 6 inches above the skin and evenly space 3–5 drops of Peppermint along the spine, extending from the sacrum to the atlas.

2. Immediately feather up the spine according to the technique previously described.

I. Valor

1. Hold the bottle 6 inches above the skin and evenly space 10–12 drops of Valor along the spine, extending from the sacrum to the atlas.

2. Immediately feather up the spine according to the technique previously described.

4. LYMPHATIC PUMP
(Brain Stem Pump Technique)

1. Have the receiver lie facing up.

2. Place both hands under the back of the head with fingertips resting at the base of the skull.

3. Gently pull the head toward you in a soft, rocking motion so the entire body moves. Sustain motion for one minute, then rest for one minute.

4. Repeat this process one more time. This movement provides an excellent lymphatic pump effect.

5. STRETCH AND RELAX PULL

1. Sit so that your shoulders are parallel to the receiver's shoulders.
2. Hold the receiver's head, using the cranial hold, with your less dominant hand under the base of the receiver's head and the dominant hand cradling the chin.
3. Next, place together your pointer finger and your middle finger and place them under the receiver's chin, just above the Adam's apple, keeping your ring and pinky fingers from touching the receiver's throat.
4. Pull straight back, gently toward you, with the hand under the base of the skull and gently pull with the fingers on the chin. Hold for three to five seconds and gently release.
5. Repeat this movement two more times.

Note: If there is another facilitator to assist with this process, he or she should stand at the feet of the receiver and hold the ankles. When the gentle pull is being done at the head, the facilitator at the feet holds the ankles and gently pulls and then releases at the same time as the facilitator at the head.

FINAL NOTES

- Finish by having the receiver place White Angelica on his or her shoulders, back of the neck, and thymus.
- It is possible that the receiver may have some emotions surface during the application of the Raindrop Technique. Be sure to have the emotional oils ready to assist him or her through the process of releasing those emotions.
- It is important that BOTH the receiver and facilitator drink plenty of water when giving and receiving the Raindrop Technique.

Customizing Raindrop Technique

Raindrop Technique may be customized to address different health issues that are not directly related to back problems. Lung infections, digestive complaints, hormonal problems, liver insufficiencies, and other problems can all be dealt with by substituting standard Raindrop Technique essential oils with other oils that are specifically targeted for that body system.

As a rule, when customizing, start with Valor, Oregano (or Plectranthus Oregano), and Thyme. For extra antiviral effect, add Mountain Savory. The other essential oils such as Basil, Wintergreen, Marjoram, Thyme, or Cypress can be omitted or replaced by essential oils specific for the condition being targeted.

For example, if targeting a lung infection, replace Basil and Wintergreen with Ravintsara. Cypress is replaced with Eucalyptus Radiata, and Marjoram is replaced with R.C.

Use "The Personal Usage Guide" to see other essential oils that would be applicable for what the individual needs are.

The basic Raindrop Technique has several variations, but these variations are not easy to explain and require class instruction and demonstration.

It would be informative to attend a Raindrop Technique Training with D. Gary Young or one of his trainers and learn the Raindrop Technique from someone who has the knowledge of essential oils and their application.

Raindrop Technique has assisted both professionals and lay people to achieve true balance in the body. Out of the thousands of Raindrop Technique sessions that have been performed, there have been hundreds of instances where the results were amazingly profound and immediate. Here are just a few examples:

A young man from Denver, Colorado, who suffered from chronic scoliosis, was able—for the first time in eight years—to fully bend over after the application of Raindrop Technique. With an overhead camera televising an image of his spine as he bent over, an audience of over 400 watched the vertebrae in his spine literally move into place. When he stood up, he was measured and had gained an inch in height.

Another instance involved a professional model, in her early 40s, who had developed early adult-onset scoliosis. She had to alter clothing so that it would fit properly for modeling sessions. She was not able to sit still for any length of time. After a Raindrop session, her spine straightened to such a degree that she, too, had gained an inch in height. She followed up with more sessions, and in the next few months reported that all discomfort was gone. She now dances and rides horses, pain free.

It is quite common for individuals with scoliosis who receive Raindrop Technique to gain 1/2 inch or more in stature from a single application.

Many others have reported pain relief, congestion relief, and cold and flu relief as a result of Raindrop Technique, which is why it has captured so much interest among those involved in the healing arts.

ENDNOTES

1. Green RJ, Webb JN, Maxwell MH. The nature of virus-like particles in the paraxial muscles of idiopathic scoliosis. *J Pathol.* 1979 Sep;129(1):9-12.

2. Webb JN, Gillespie WJ. Virus-like particles in paraspinal muscle in scoliosis. *Br Med J.* 1976 Oct 16;2(6041):912-3.

3. Wolff MH, Buchel F, Gullotta F, Helpap B, Schneweiss KE. Investigations to demonstrate latent viral infection of varicella-Zoster virus in human spine ganglia. *Verh Dtsch Ges Pathol.* 1981;65:203-7.

4. Stirling A, et al. Association between sciatica and *Propionibacterium acnes. Lancet* 2001 Jun 23:357(9273):2024-5.

5. Nagrath SP, Hazra DK, Pant PC, Seth HC. Tuberculosis spine—a diagnostic conundrum. Case report. *J Assoc Physicians India.* 1974 May;22(5):405-7.

6. Jenks PJ, Stewart B. Images in clinical medicine. Vertebral tuberculosis. *N Engl J Med.* 1998 June 4;338(23):1677.

7. Monaghan D, Gupta A, Barrington NA. Case report: Tuberculosis of the spine—an unusual presentation. *Clin Radiol.* 1991 May;43(5):360-2.

8. Petersen CK, Craw M, Radiological differentiation of tuberculosis and pyogenic osteomyelitis: a case report. *J Manipulative Physiol Ther.* 1986 Mar;9(1):39-42.

9. Pinott JR, Taffs LF. Experimental scoliosis in primates: a neurological cause. *J Bone Joint Surg Br.* 1982;64(4):503-7.

10. Marino M, Bersani C, Comi G. Antimicrobial activity of the essential oils of Thymus vulgaris L. measured using a bioimpedometric method. *Journal of Food Protection,* Vol. 62, No. 9, 1999:1017-1023.

11. Wan J, Wilcock A, Coventry MJ. The effect of essential oils of basil on the growth of Aeromonas fluorescens. *Journal of Applied Microbiology,* 1998, 84: 152-158.

12. Beuchat LR. Antimicrobial properties of spices and their essential oils. Center for Food Safety and Quality Enhancement, Department of Food Science and Technology, University of Georgia, Griffin, Georgia.

13. Horne D, et al. Antimicrobial effects of essential oils on Streptococcus pneumoniae. *Journal of Essential Oil Research,* (September/October 2001), 13: 387-392.

14. Moleyar V, Narasimham P. Antibacterial activity of essential oil components. *International Journal of Food Microbiology,* Vol. 16 (1992): 337-32.

15. Obata Y, et al. Effect of pretreatment of skin with cyclic monoterpenes on permeation of diclofenac in hairless rat. *Biol Pharm Bull.* 1993 Mar;16(3):312-4.

16. Zhao K, Singh J. Mechanisms of percutaneous absorption of tamoxifen by terpenes: eugenol, d-limonene and menthone. *Control Release.* 1998 Nov 13;55(2-3):253-60.

Chapter 7
Personal Usage

Taking Charge of Your Health

Many people think that by taking supplements, they can solve their health challenges. They do not consider the negative impact of the environment and what they could do to change it.

Today's diet is immensely deficient, which greatly affects our health and well-being and is certainly something to be evaluated and perhaps changed. Exercise should be a routine part of weekly activities, but most of us simply do not make the time. It takes discipline and commitment and would definitely have a positive effect on our health.

Emotional and spiritual feelings and attitudes that negatively affect one's life are perhaps the most difficult to recognize. An unhealthy state of being, disease, and even death can be brought on by negative thoughts and emotions.

Many people, including social workers and health practitioners, believe that negative emotions are the precursor to both mental and physical dysfunction of the body, resulting in mental illness and disease. Surely, that is not true in all cases, but it is definitely something to consider.

We must look at all of these things in an effort to bring balance to our lives, overcome body dysfunction and disease, and find happiness and fulfillment.

1. What causes poor nutrition?

Poor diet, especially eating fast food. Over 40,000 chemicals are found in our food today, which includes prepared and processed foods.

Contaminated water and water treated with chemicals like chlorine and fluoride inhibit proper thyroid function and slow down metabolism, circulation, and immune function.

Poor digestion and assimilation caused by nutritionally deficient foods lacking in the necessary enzymes and minerals critical for digestion cause many problems, with constipation as the number one complaint.

2. What is environmental pollution?
- Air pollution
- Chemicals in the home and work environment
- Changes in ozone
- Electromagnetic and radiation pollution from computers, cell phones, televisions, electrical appliances, etc.
-

3. Why do we have poor physical fitness?
- No exercise
- Obesity from bad diet
- No or low self-discipline
- Premature aging
- Fragile bones and weak muscles

4. What causes a negative attitude?

- Depression
- Low energy
- Low self-esteem
- Few or no goals
- Little or no motivation
-

5. Why are we spiritually depressed?

- No specific belief system
- Fear
- Sense of being lost
- Poor relationship with self, spouse, children, extended family, friends, and most importantly: Our Creator, or God

---

Helpful Conversions

1 drop	=	approximately 60 mg
1 ml	=	1/5 teaspoon
1 ml	=	approximately 16 drops
1 ml	=	fills one capsule
5 ml	=	1 teaspoon
5 ml	=	approximately 80 drops
15 ml	=	1 tablespoon
15 ml	=	1/2 fluid ounce
240 ml	=	1 cup (depends on product)
30 ml	=	1 fluid ounce
28 grams	=	1 ounce

We have control over many things—more than those over which we have no control. We can change our diet, change our attitude, start working out to improve our fitness, change what we can in our own personal environment, and start turning to that great universal power for understanding and direction.

We have wonderful nutritional supplements available to us, and we have God's beautiful essential oils to uplift, energize, motivate, and help propel us onto a greater path of success in every walk of life. What we do and how we do it is our choice.

Essential oils are God's medicine today and for the future and can be used in many different ways. Their use and application have become very vast and creative, depending on the oil.

Although their topical use is perhaps the most common, dietary use of essential oils may be one of the most effective ways of unlocking their health benefits. Many essential oils are used for food flavoring and are classified as "GRAS" by the U.S. Food and Drug Administration, meaning they are "generally regarded as safe" for human consumption.

Essential oils have been used for centuries for religious ceremonies, in cosmetics for beautification of the body, and medicinally for many maladies, endowing them with a long history of safe use.

Research indicates that certain essential oils act as potent antioxidants that can actually raise antioxidant levels in the body and prevent premature aging.

According to researcher Jean Valnet, MD, an essential oil applied directly on the skin can pass into the bloodstream and diffuse throughout the tissues in 20 minutes or less.

Inhalation can have a direct influence on both the body and mind due to its ability to stimulate the brain's limbic system, a group of subcortical structures including the hypothalamus, the hippocampus, and the amygdala. This can produce powerful effects that can affect everything from emotional balance and energy levels to appetite control and heart and immune functions.

Some researchers believe that inhalation also enhances the body's immune system. Disease and trauma foster emotional negativity that essential oils often dissipate. Oils with immune-stimulating properties can increase the body's resistance, whether used topically or taken orally, helping to build a healthy environment that prevents the onset of disease.

Getting Started

Methods of Application

Essential oils are very concentrated, natural substances—easily 100 times more concentrated than the natural herbs and plants from which they are distilled. For this reason it is important to dilute certain essential oils before using them therapeutically.

Other essential oils are so mild that dilution is simply not necessary, even for use on infants.

The five standard methods of application are topical, inhalation, ingestion, oral, and retention.

Mixing Single Oils and Blends

The essential oil singles and blends listed for a specific condition may be used either separately or together. Combining two single oils, or one single oil with a blend, may often produce a stronger effect than when using them individually.

Usually 1-3 drops of either a single oil or a blend is sufficient, mixing up to 3 or 4 oils in any given combination at a time.

Using an Essential Oil

The essential oils recommended for specific conditions are not the only oils you can use; these oils are merely a starting point. Other oils not listed can also be just as effective. You have to use the oils to determine what works best for you.

However, the essential oils are listed in a preferred order. Start with the first single oil, blend, or supplement in the list. If results are not apparent after waiting a little while, try another single oil, blend, supplement, or combination on the next application. Sometimes you have to keep experimenting until you find what works for you. This is because one particular oil may be more compatible with one person's body chemistry than with another person's chemistry (see further explanation at the beginning of the Usage Guide).

Essential oils can be used topically for massage, acupuncture, Raindrop Technique, and Vita Flex on the bottoms of the feet. In most cases, 3-4 drops are sufficient to produce significant effects, unless using a specific protocol.

Most single oils and blends should be diluted 50/50 when putting them on the skin. Oils that definitely should be diluted are oils such as Cistus, Clove, Cypress, Lemongrass, Mountain Savory, Oregano, Rosemary, Thyme, etc. For some people, an oil like Basil might be too "hot" if put neat on the skin; for others, Basil will not be "hot" at all. That is why it is best to always do a skin test before applying any oil. When in doubt, dilute.

When diluting the oils, use the V-6 Vegetable Oil Complex for either topical or internal application, particularly if you have not used essential oils previously. Use no more than 10 to 20 drops during one topical application.

Precautions

When using topically, first do a skin test by putting 1 drop of the desired essential oil on the inside of the upper arm. If cosmetics and personal care products made with synthetic chemicals or soaps and cleansers containing synthetic or petroleum-based chemicals have been used on the skin, then the skin may be uncomfortably sensitive.

If any redness or irritation results, the skin should be thoroughly cleansed; then the oil may be reapplied. If skin irritation persists, try using a different oil or oil blend.

You may want to consider starting an internal cleansing program for 30 days before using essential oils. Use ICP, ComforTone, JuvaPower, Essentialzyme, Detoxzyme, and other cleansing supplements.

Internal Use

Many essential oils are taken internally as dietary supplements. Some people put 1-3 drops in water to drink, but others use cold NingXia Red or another juice of their choice.

If you prefer to swallow a capsule, you can fill a "00" capsule with oil using an eyedropper. Fill with the number of drops desired and the rest of the capsule with V-6 Vegetable Oil Complex or any other organic vegetable oil. If you are uncertain, consult with someone who is experienced in taking oils internally.

Always drink more water when using essential oils because they can accelerate the detoxification process in the body. If you are not taking in adequate fluids, the toxins could recirculate, causing nausea, headaches, etc.

Developing Your Program

It is usually best to use one or two application methods at a time. If you were to use all 10 applications for a sore throat at once, it would take more time and probably be inconvenient, costly, and unnecessary.

First, you must decide which oils and supplements you want to use for your program. Choose up to three or four oils, be certain how many drops you are going to use, undiluted or diluted, and if diluted, what the dilution ratio is that you want to try.

Consult Your Health Care Professional

Consult your health care professional about any serious disease or injury. Do not attempt to self-diagnose or prescribe any natural substances such as essential oils for health conditions that require professional attention.

For example: If you have sore shoulder muscles, you could decide to use the following:

Your Oils:

- PanAway: dilution 50/50
- Aroma Siez: dilution 50/50
- Helichrysum: neat
- V-6 Vegetable Oil Complex
- Ortho Sport Massage Oil
- Deep Relief Roll-On to carry with you

Your Supplements: Mineral Essence: 2 droppers in 2 oz. of NingXia Red in water in the morning

- ICP: 2 tablespoons in water in the morning
- Essentialzyme: 2 each morning, 1 in the evening
- BLM: 1 teaspoon in water and drink 2 x daily
- Power Meal: 2 scoops in water or juice 2 x daily
- Detoxzyme: 4-6 in the evening before or after dinner
- MegaCal: 1 teaspoon in water and drink at night
- ImmuPro: 2 before going to bed

Make sure you understand the proper essential oil dilution level. Have your V-6 Vegetable Oil Complex that you are going to use for the dilution and your Ortho Ease Massage Oil or Ortho Sport Massage Oil together with all of the essential oils.

Write down your program so that it is easy to follow each day, and make sure you have enough so that you do not run out and then have to stop your program while you wait for your next order to arrive.

Developing Your Program

Addressing the overall health of the body is important when considering a specific solution. Although essential oils have powerful, therapeutic effects, they are not, by themselves, a total solution. They must be accompanied by a program of internal cleansing, proper diet, and supplementation. This may also include lifestyle changes such as exercise, meditation or yoga, and stress-free situations.

Cleanse

Cleansing the colon and liver is the first and most important step to take when dealing with any disease. Many imbalances may be corrected by cleansing alone. Products that cleanse the body include the Cleansing Trio (Comfor-Tone, Essentialzyme, and ICP), JuvaTone, JuvaFlex, Detoxzyme, Digest & Cleanse, DiGize, and ParaFree.

Note: It would be difficult, if not impossible, for infants or children under age 8 to try a colon and liver cleanse. Instead, use 3 drops of DiGize in a teaspoon of V-6 Vegetable Oil Complex, rub around the navel, and place moderately warm packs on the stomach. Apply 2-3 drops of DiGize, Fennel, or Peppermint on the bottoms of the feet.

Put 1 drop of any of the same oils in a glass of water or juice for a child over the age of 4 to drink. Those same drops could also be mixed in a teaspoon of yogurt or kefir that any child can easily swallow.

Balance and Build

After the body has been cleansed, it is easier to balance and nourish the systems of the body. This includes rebuilding and nourishing beneficial intestinal flora and re-mineralizing the blood and tissues. Products that build the body include Mineral Essence, Esssentialzyme, Essentialzymes-4, MultiGreens, Power Meal, MegaCal, Master Formula HIS or HERS, NingXia Red, Life 5, Balance Complete, OmegaGize^3, Sulfurzyme, Super B, Super C, Super C Chewables, MightyVites, Mightyzyme, and MightyMist.

Nourish and Support

Supporting the endocrine and immune systems comprises the third phase. Products include Exodus II, Thieves, ImmuPro, Mineral Essence, Essentialzyme, Essentialzymes-4, MightyVites, Mightyzyme, MightyMist, Super B, Super C, Master Formula HIS or HERS, Thyromin, EndoGize, Prostrate Health, Progessence Plus, and Power Meal.

Note: For children or adults who have difficulty swallowing capsules and tablets, Essentialzymes-4, may be emptied into other food products such as yogurt, oatmeal, NingXia Red, etc., and ingested.

Be Consistent with Your Regimen

Therapeutic-grade essential oils are powerful, natural, healing substances that work extremely well with the body's own defenses to solve problems. However, they are not drugs, and they may not always work in seconds, or even minutes. Essential oils will enhance and speed up the benefits of dietary supplements, but it is still a "natural" process. Sometimes it can take hours or even days to see the improvement.

Application
Topical

- Apply neat or undiluted to specific area.
- Dilute 50/50: Add 1 part essential oil to 1 part V-6 Vegetable Oil Complex.
- Dilute 20/80: Add 1 part essential oil to 4 parts V-6 Vegetable Oil Complex.
- Vita Flex: Apply 1-3 drops neat to the Vita Flex points on the feet as directed (see Vita Flex chart in Application section).
- Compress: After applying oils to the skin, soak a hand towel in warm water, wring it out, and lay it over the targeted skin area. Then cover the wet towel with a dry towel to hold the heat in for 10-15 minutes or until the wet towel is no longer warm.

If the individual becomes uncomfortable or has a hot sensation, remove towel and apply V-6 Vegetable Oil Complex.

A cool towel instead of a warm towel can be used to create a cold compress.

Bath Salts

Put 10-15 drops of essential oil into ½ cup of Epsom salts or baking soda. Add warm water, mix, and pour into warm bathwater. Soak in the tub for 20 to 30 minutes before using soap or shampoo.

Special showerheads are available that are designed to hold salt mixtures for a revitalizing shower.

Body Massage

You can use any dilution of essential oils desired with the V-6 Vegetable Oil Complex. It depends on the oil or oils being used. Usually a few drops of oil are sufficient with the massage oil.

You can also apply oils directly to the skin and then apply a massage oil such as Relaxation, Sensation, Cel-Lite Magic, Dragon Time, Ortho Easel, or Ortho Sport for a full-body massage.

Ortho Ease and Ortho Sport massage oils have a stronger therapeutic action and help immensely with sore and aching muscles and joints.

Oil blends such as Valor, White Angelica, or RutaVaLa do not need to be diluted. Oil blends such as PanAway, Raven, and Relieve It should always be diluted.

Read the instructions or ask for advice if you are just beginning to use the oils in massage.

Vita Flex / Auricular / Lymphatic Pump

See the Application section for more information.

Raindrop Technique

Have a Raindrop Technique 1-2 times weekly. See Application section for more information.

Inhalation

- **Diffuse:** Diffuse undiluted oils in a cold-air diffuser. Cold air diffusers are not designed to handle vegetable oils because they are thicker and may clog the diffuser mechanism.
- **Direct:** Put 2-3 drops of oil in the palm of one hand, rub palms together, cup hands over your nose and mouth, and inhale.

You may even want to put a dab of oil under your nose.

If you touch the skin near your eyes, they may water or sting, but it will dissipate in a few minutes.

- **Steam**: Run hot, steaming water into a sink or large bowl. Water should be at least 2 inches deep to retain heat for a few minutes.

Add 3-6 drops of oil to the hot water; then drape a towel over your head, covering the hot water so that you enclose your face over the steam.

Inhale vapors deeply through the nose as they rise with the steam. Add more hot water to continue vaporizing, if desired.

Ingestion

- **Capsule**: Use a clean medicine dropper to fill the larger half of an empty "00" gelatin capsule half-way with oil. Then fill the remainder with V-6 Vegetable Oil Complex or a high quality, cold-pressed, vegetable oil; put the other half of the gel cap on; and swallow.

If your hand is steady, you can simply hold the bottle and let the oil drip from the bottle into the capsule.

Take the capsule (s) immediately, as it will become soft quickly, making it hard to pick up.

- **Dosages**: There are two sizes of capsules: (1) a "00" size capsule holds 400 mg, and (2) a "0" size capsule holds 200 mg.

The "00" size capsule is easier to use because it is bigger, there is less chance of spilling, and you can fill it with whatever amount you want.

If the "00" is not available, then use the "0" size. You just have to be more careful when filling, and you have to swallow more capsules.

Retention

- **Rectal**: Mix a 40/60 ratio (4 parts essential oil to 6 parts V-6 Vegetable Oil Complex), insert 1-2 tablespoons in the rectum with a bulb syringe, and retain up to 8 hours or overnight.
- **Vaginal**: Tampon: Mix a 40/60 ratio (4 parts essential oil to 6 parts V-6 Vegetable Oil Complex), put 1-2 tablespoons on a tampon, and insert into the vagina for internal infection. Put oil on a sanitary pad for external lesions. Retain up to 8 hours or overnight. Use only tampons or sanitary pads made with non-perfumed, non-scented, organic cotton.

Quick Usage Guide

Body Defense: Antiviral, Antibacterial, Anti-inflammatory, and Disease

Singles: Cinnamon Bark, Idaho Balsam Fir, Idaho Blue Spruce, Cistus, Clove, Dorado Azul, Lemon, Oregano, Ocotea, Palo Santo, Spearmint, Spikenard, Tangerine, Thyme, Eucalyptus Blue, Hinoki, Yuzu

Blends: Breathe Again Roll-On, Melrose, Purification, R.C., Raven, Sacred Mountain, The Gift, Thieves

Nutritionals: ImmuPro, Inner Defense, NingXia Red, ParaFree

Oral Care, Sprays: Thieves Toothpastes, Thieves Fresh Essence Plus Mouthwash, Thieves Spray, Thieves Hard Lozenges

Bones, Joints, and Muscles

Singles: Basil, Black Pepper, Copaiba, Idaho Balsam Fir, Idaho Blue Spruce, Lemongrass, Marjoram, Roman Chamomile, Spruce, Wintergreen

Blends: Aroma Siez, Deep Relief Roll-On, M-Grain, PanAway, Relieve It

Nutritionals: BLM, Balance Complete, Master Formula HIS or HERS, MegaCal, Mineral Essence, Power Meal, Sulfurzyme

Massage Oils: Ortho Ease Massage Oil, Ortho Sport Massage Oil

Digestive Dysfunction, Constipation, Bloating, Gas, and Cleansing

Singles: Coriander, Eucalyptus Radiata, Fennel, Ginger, Grapefruit, Juniper, Ledum, Melaleuca Alternifolia, Peppermint, Idaho Blue Spruce, Tarragon, Hinoki

Blends: DiGize, EndoFlex, Exodus II, GLF, JuvaCleanse, JuvaFlex, Longevity

Nutritionals: AlkaLime, ComforTone, Digest & Cleanse, ICP, JuvaPower, JuvaSpice (for salads and cooking), JuvaTone, Life 5; all enzymes: Allerzyme, Detoxzyme, Essentialzyme, Essentialzymes-4, Mightyzyme (Children)

Massage Oil: Cel-Lite Magic Massage Oil

Emotional and Spiritual

Singles: Bergamot, Clary Sage, Frankincense, Galbanum, Lavender, Lemon, Orange, Patchouli, Pine, Sacred Frankincense, Tsuga, Ylang Ylang, Idaho Blue Spruce, Hinoki

Blends: Abundance, Acceptance, Australian Blue, Believe, Chivalry, Egyptian Gold, Forgiveness, Gathering, Gentle Baby, Gratitude, Grounding, Harmony, Hope, Humility, Inner Child, Inspiration, Into the Future, Joy, Lady Sclareol, Live With Passion, Motivation, Present Time, RutaVaLa, SARA, SclarEssence, Sensation, Surrender, The Gift, 3 Wise Men, Transformation, Trauma Life, Valor, White Angelica

Nutritionals: CortiStop Women's, EndoGize, FemiGen, PD 80/20

Creams, Massage Oil, Serum: Dragon Time Massage Oil, Prenolone Plus Body Cream, Progessence Plus, Regenolone Moisturizing Cream

Fortifying and Maintaining the Body— Antioxidants

Singles: Idaho Blue Spruce, Juniper, Lemon, Nutmeg, Peppermint, Rosemary

Blends: En-R-Gee, Hope, ImmuPower, Joy, Motivation

Nutritionals: Balance Complete, Blue Agave, EndoGize, Essentialzyme, Essentialzymes-4, Inner Defense, JuvaTone, Master Formula HIS or HERS, MegaCal, MightyMist (Children), MightyVites (Children), Mightyzyme (Children), Mineral Essence, MultiGreens, NingXia Red, OmegaGize³, Power Meal,

Prostate Health, Pure Protein, Super B, Super C, Super C Chewable, Thyromin, JuvaSpice (for salads and cooking)

Memory, Confusion, Lack of Mental Clarity, Brain Fog

Singles: Frankincense, Lavender, Peppermint, Rosemary, Sacred Frankincense

Blends: Awaken, Brain Power, Citrus Fresh, Clarity, Common Sense, Dream Catcher, Envision, Gathering, Into the Future, Joy

Nutritionals: Essentialzyme, Essentialzymes-4, Detoxzyme, Master Formula HIS or HERS, MegaCal, NingXia Red, Thyromin, Ultra Young Plus

Overweight, Metabolism

Singles: Fennel, Grapefruit, Lemon, Nutmeg, Patchouli, Spearmint

Blends: DiGize, EndoFlex, GLF, Joy, JuvaFlex, Motivation, SclarEssence

Nutritionals: Allerzyme, ComforTone, Detoxzyme, Digest & Cleanse, EndoGize, Essentialzyme, Essentialzymes-4, ICP, JuvaPower, JuvaTone, NingXia Red, PD 80/20, Power Meal, Thyromin, JuvaSpice (for salads and cooking), Ultra Young Plus

Protection—Antioxidants

Singles: Cinnamon Bark, Copaiba, Dorado Azul, Eucalyptus Blue, Frankincense, Sacred Frankincense, Idaho Blue Spruce, Helichrysum, Melaleuca Alternifolia, Melissa, Mountain Savory, Ocotea, Oregano, Palo Santo, Ravintsara, Roman Chamomile, Thyme

Blends: Aroma Life, DiGize, Exodus II, Melrose, PanAway, Purification, R.C., Raven, The Gift, Thieves

Nutritionals: Longevity Softgels, Master Formula HIS or HERS, Super C, Super C Chewable

Sprays, Body Oils: LavaDerm Cooling Mist, Protec

Skin Care

Note: After applying essential oils on the skin, use a skin cream to sooth the natural drying effect of some oils: A·R·T (Age Refining Technology) Day Activator, A·R·T Night Reconstructor, A·R·T Gentle Foaming Cleanser, A·R·T Purifying Toner, Boswellia Wrinkle Cream, Genesis Hand & Body Lotion, Lavender Hand & Body Lotion, Sandalwood Moisture Cream, Sensation Hand & Body Lotion

Singles: Frankincense, Sacred Frankincense, Idaho Blue Spruce, Galbanum, German Chamomile, Helichrysum, Idaho Tansy, Jasmine, Lavender, Melaleuca Ericifolia, Myrrh, Myrtle, Roman Chamomile, Rose, Sandalwood, Vetiver, Western Red Cedar, Ylang Ylang

Blends: Gentle Baby, Highest Potential, Sensation, 3 Wise Men, Valor

Lotions, Serums, Sprays, Nutritionals: Sulfurzyme, ClaraDerm, Progessence Plus, Regenolone Moisturizing Cream, Prenolone Plus Body Cream, Rose Ointment, Essential Beauty Serum

Stress

Singles: Dill, Lavender, Lemon, Orange, Yuzu, Rosemary, Valerian, Vetiver, Hinoki

Blends: Harmony, Joy, Peace & Calming, RutaVaLa, RutaVaLa Roll-On, Sacred Mountain, Stress Away Roll-On, Tranquil Roll-On, Trauma Life, Valor, White Angelica

Nutritionals: Master Formula HIS or HERS, MegaCal, Mineral Essence, Sleep Essence, Super B, Thyromin

Massage Oils: Relaxation Massage Oil, Sensation Massage Oil

Personal Usage

In "Recommendations," products are listed in order beginning with the first, or preferred, recommendation. In other words, **the first one or two oils listed would be the first ones that you would try**. However, any single oil or blend listed would have application.

Whenever you are working with natural products, you never know which product will work the best for you until you try it. Your body will tell you. Different oils work for different people. You have to experiment until you make that determination based on your body's chemistry and need.

Supplements vary considerably in their usage. You may want to try the first three or four products recommended to see how your body responds. You may find that your body responds to one product over another.

In the case of enzymes, it is simply your choice. However, it is important to read the chapter on enzymes and minerals, the chapter on nutritionals, and consult the Enzyme Quick Reference Guide, located in both chapters. Enzymes may be combined in the way you determine you need them.

As always, just follow the guidelines and use common sense. Trust your body, focus on your intuitive feelings and what you have learned, and you will make the right choice.

No matter what you take, your body will benefit as long as you do not "go overboard." You are the best one to decide what is best for your body. Just start slowly and enjoy your new rejuvenation and vitality.

ABUSE, MENTAL AND PHYSICAL

The trauma from mental and physical abuse can result in self-defeating behavior that can undermine success later in life. Through their powerful effect on the limbic system of the brain (the center of stored memories and emotions), essential oils can help release pent-up trauma, emotions, or memories. All memories alter the RNA and DNA and create a blueprint in the DNA. This is why trauma imprinting can be passed from generation to generation. Always start with Frankincense.

Recommendations

Singles: Sacred Frankincense, Frankincense, Idaho Balsam Fir, Sandalwood, Melissa, Ylang Ylang, Amazonian Ylang Ylang

Blends: Trauma Life, SARA, Release, Acceptance, Forgiveness, Surrender, Humility, White Angelica, Inner Child, Harmony, Hope, Tranquil Roll-On, Valor, Valor Roll-On, Peace & Calming, The Gift, Oola Grow, Common Sense

Nutritionals: OmegaGize³, NingXia Red, EndoGize, Mineral Essence, Master Formula HIS or HERS

Application and Usage

Inhalation

- Diffuse your choice of oils for 1 hour every 2 hours or as desired.
- Put 2-3 drops of your chosen oil in your hands and rub them together, cup your hands over your nose, and inhale throughout the day as needed.
- Put 8-10 drops of oil on a cotton ball or tissue and put it in an air vent in your house, vehicle, hotel room, etc.
- If diffusing while sleeping, set your timer for

the desired length of time for automatic shut off.

Topical

You may apply single oils or blends neat or diluted, depending on the oil or oils being used. Please see the instructions at the beginning of this chapter for more information on applying oils to the skin.

Specific Types of Abuse

Physical Abuse: Apply 2-3 drops of SARA and Forgiveness over the abuse area and around the navel. Follow with 1-2 drops of Release over the Vita Flex points on the feet, especially the liver point of the right foot, under the nose, and directly over the liver. Then apply Trauma Life.

Parental, Sexual, or Ritual Abuse: Apply 1-3 drops of SARA over the area where abuse took place; then Forgiveness, Trauma Life, Release, Joy, Present Time.

Spousal Abuse: Apply SARA, Forgiveness, Trauma Life, Release, Valor, Joy, Envision, Hope.

Feelings of Revenge: Apply 1-2 drops of Surrender on the sternum over the heart, 2-3 drops of Present Time on the thymus, and 2-3 drops of Forgiveness over the navel.

Suicidal: Apply 2 drops of Hope on the rim of the ears. Melissa, Brain Power, Surrender, RutaVaLa, Common Sense, or Present Time may also be beneficial.

Protection and Balance: Apply 1-2 drops of White Angelica on each shoulder and 1-2 drops of Harmony on energy points or chakras. Finish with Valor followed by Sacred Frankincense or Frankincense to set the DNA blueprint.

ACIDOSIS
(See also HEARTBURN, FUNGUS)

Acidosis is a condition where the pH of the blood serum becomes excessively acidic. This condition should not be confused with an acid stomach. Acidic blood can stress the liver and eventually lead to many forms of chronic and degenerative diseases. Dietary changes will help in raising the serum pH (making it more alkaline). Cleansing is an essential dietary step in balancing pH.

Recommendations

Singles: Peppermint, Fennel, Tarragon, Lemon
Blends: DiGize, EndoFlex, BLF, JuvaCleanse
Nutritionals: AlkaLime, Essentialzyme, MultiGreens, JuvaPower, MegaCal, Essentialzymes-4, Mineral Essence

Application and Usage
Ingestion

The amount of oil ingested varies with different oils. Whether putting the oils in a capsule or drinking them in a liquid, please refer to the instructions at the beginning of this chapter.

- Take 1 capsule with desired oil 2 times daily.
- Put 2-3 drops of oil in a spoonful of Blue Agave, Yacon Syrup, Stevia, maple syrup, or milk. Honey and yogurt are too acidic.
- Put the desired amount of oils in a glass of rice milk, almond milk, goat milk, carrot juice, NingXia Red, or even water and then drink it.
- Take an Essentialzymes-4 yellow capsule with Peppermint until acid level is balanced; then add Essentialzyme.
- To reduce acid indigestion and prevent fermentation that can contribute to bad dreams and interrupted sleep, take 1 teaspoon of AlkaLime in water before bedtime.
- To raise pH, take 2-6 capsules of MultiGreens 3 times daily and take 1 teaspoon of AlkaLime in water 1 hour before or 2 hours after meals each day. For maintenance, take 1 teaspoon of AlkaLime once per week at bedtime.

- To stimulate enzymatic action in the digestive tract, mix together raw carrot juice, NingXia Red, alfalfa juice, and papaya juice with 1 dropper of Mineral Essence and 1 drop of DiGize.

Topical

You may apply single oils or blends neat or diluted, depending on the oil or oils being used. Please see the instructions at the beginning of this chapter for more information on applying oils to the skin.

ADDICTIONS

Many foods and plants—such as tobacco, caffeine, drugs, alcohol, breads, sugar, and other sweeteners—create chemical dependencies.

Cleansing and detoxifying the liver is a crucial first step toward breaking free of these addictions. Alkaline calcium can help bind bile acids and prevent fatty liver. A colon and tissue cleanse is also important.

A body lacking in sufficient enzymes, vitamins, minerals, and other nutrients may also play a part in some addictions. Blue Agave, Yacon Syrup, Stevia, maple syrup, honey, molasses, and other natural sweeteners are good substitutes for sugar, which should be restricted in a diet.

The Thieves oil blend has been very helpful in curbing an addiction. One or two drops on the tongue are very sufficient to stop the onset of a craving. JuvaTone, JuvaPower, and Juva-Cleanse may be used long term to help detoxify the liver. They suppress the addiction and eventually change the addiction blueprint in the cells of the body.

Recommendations

Singles: Orange, Ledum, Fennel, Tarragon
Blends: GLF, Thieves, Harmony, Peace & Calming, JuvaCleanse, JuvaFlex
Nutritionals: Detoxzyme, ComforTone, Digest & Cleanse, JuvaPower, ICP, JuvaTone, Power

Meal, MegaCal, Essentialzyme, Balance Complete, Blue Agave, Yacon Syrup, Omega-Gize³, Slique Tea, Slique Bars

Application and Usage
Inhalation
- Diffuse your choice of oils for 1 hour every 2 hours or as desired.
- Put 2-3 drops of your chosen oil in your hands and rub them together, cup your hands over your nose, and inhale throughout the day as needed.
- Put 8-10 drops of oil on a cotton ball or tissue and put it in an air vent in your house, vehicle, hotel room, etc.
- If diffusing while sleeping, set your timer for the desired length of time for automatic shut off.

Topical
You may apply single oils or blends neat or diluted, depending on the oil or oils being used. Please see the instructions at the beginning of this chapter for more information on applying oils to the skin.
- Apply 1-2 drops neat (undiluted) on temples and back of neck 4 times daily or as desired.
- Place a warm compress with 1-2 drops of chosen oil over the liver.

Ingestion
The amount of oil ingested varies with different oils. Whether putting the oils in a capsule or drinking them in a liquid, please refer to the instructions at the beginning of this chapter.
- Take 1 capsule with desired oil 2 times daily.
- Put 2-3 drops of oil in a spoonful of Blue Agave, Yacon Syrup, Stevia, maple syrup, coconut oil, or milk. Honey and yogurt are too acidic.
- Put the desired amount of oils in a glass of rice milk, almond milk, goat milk, carrot juice, NingXia Red, or even water and then drink it.

ADRENAL GLAND DISORDERS

The adrenal glands consist of two sections: An inner part called the medulla, which produces stress hormone, and an outer part called the cortex, which secretes critical hormones called glucocorticoids and aldosterone. Because of these hormones, the cortex has a far greater impact on overall health than the medulla.

Aldosterone and glucocorticoids are very important because they directly affect blood pressure and minerals that help regulate the conversion of carbohydrates into energy.

In cases like Addison's disease, adrenal cortex hormones fail to produce sufficient amounts or none of the critical hormones, which can lead to life-threatening fluid and mineral loss, unless these hormones are replaced.

On the other hand, Cushing's disease, or syndrome, occurs when the body has too much of the hormone cortisol or other steroid hormones.

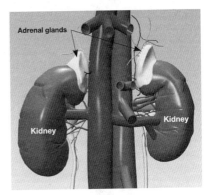

Adrenal Glands

....

Addison's Disease

Addison's disease is an autoimmune disease in which the body's own immune cells begin to destroy the adrenal glands. Sulfurzyme, an important source of organic sulfur, is known to have positive effects in fighting many types of autoimmune diseases, including lupus, arthritis, and fibromyalgia.

Symptoms associated with Addison's disease

- Severe fatigue
- Lightheadedness when standing
- Nausea
- Depression/ irritability
- Craving salty foods
- Loss of appetite
- Muscle spasms
- Dark, tan-colored skin

Some essential oils have chemical components or structures that have adrenal-like action, enabling them to give support to the body's own system, which may help correct those deficiencies by strengthening adrenal cortex function. The EndoFlex oil blend promotes adrenal-like activity that raises energy levels.

Recommendations

Singles: Nutmeg, Fennel, German Chamomile, Clove, Sacred Frankincense, Frankincense, Spikenard

Blends: EndoFlex, En-R-Gee, Brain Power, Common Sense, Clarity

Nutritionals: Thyromin, Sulfurzyme, EndoGize, MultiGreens, Balance Complete, MegaCal, Mineral Essence, Super B, Life 5

Support the Adrenal Glands

Add the following amounts of essential oils to ¼ teaspoon of massage oil and apply as a warm compress over the adrenal glands (located on top of the kidneys):

- 3 drops Clove
- 3 drops Nutmeg
- 7 drops Rosemary

Application and Usage
Inhalation
- Diffuse your choice of oils for ½ hour every 4-6 hours or as desired.
- Put 2-3 drops of your chosen oil in your hands and rub them together, cup your hands over your nose, and inhale throughout the day as needed.
- Put 8-10 drops of oil on a cotton ball or tissue and put it in an air vent in your house, vehicle, hotel room, etc.
- If diffusing while sleeping, set your timer for the desired length of time for automatic shut off.

Topical
You may apply single oils or blends neat or diluted, depending on the oil or oils being used. Please see the instructions at the beginning of this chapter for more information on applying oils to the skin.

Ingestion and Oral
The amount of oil ingested varies with different oils. Whether putting the oils in a capsule or drinking them in a liquid, please refer to the instructions at the beginning of this chapter.
- Take 1 capsule with desired oil 2 times daily.

....

Cushing's Syndrome (Disease)
Adrenal gland imbalance is characterized by the overproduction of adrenal cortex hormones such as cortisol. While these hormones are crucial to sound health in normal amounts, their unchecked overproduction can cause as much harm as their underproduction. This results in the following symptoms:

- Slow wound healing
- Obesity
- Low resistance
- Acne
- Infection
- Moon-shaped face
- Easily bruised skin
- Osteoporosis
- Weak or wasted muscles

Although Cushing's disease can be caused by a malfunction in the pituitary, it is usually triggered by excessive use of immune-suppressing corticosteroid medications, such as those used for asthma and arthritis. Once these are stopped, the disease often abates.

The key to reducing excess cortisol is often reducing stress.

Recommendations
Singles: Canadian Fleabane (Conyza), Spearmint, Dorado Azul, Sacred Frankincense, Frankincense, Idaho Balsam Fir

Blends: EndoFlex, Exodus II, Peace & Calming, Acceptance, Grounding, Harmony, DiGize

Nutritionals: Ultra Young Plus, ImmuPro, PD 80/20, Mineral Essence, CortiStop Women's, Digest & Cleanse, JuvaPower, OmegaGize[3]

Application and Usage
Inhalation
- Diffuse your choice of oils for ½ hour every 4-6 hours or as desired.
- Put 2-3 drops of your chosen oil in your hands and rub them together, cup your hands over your nose, and inhale throughout the day as needed.
- Put 8-10 drops of oil on a cotton ball or tissue and put it in an air vent in your house, vehicle, hotel room, etc.
- If diffusing while sleeping, set your timer for the desired length of time for automatic shut off.

Topical
You may apply single oils or blends neat or diluted, depending on the oil or oils being used. Please see the instructions at the beginning of this chapter for more information on applying oils to the skin.
- Apply warm compress over adrenal area (on back, over kidneys) with 1-2 drops of recommended oil.

Ingestion and Oral

The amount of oil ingested varies with different oils. Whether putting the oils in a capsule or drinking them in a liquid, please refer to the instructions at the beginning of this chapter.

- Take 2 capsules with Exodus II or other desired oil 2 times daily.
- Put 2-3 drops of oil in a spoonful of Blue Agave, Yacon Syrup, maple syrup, etc.
- Put the desired amount of oils in a glass of rice milk, almond milk, goat milk, carrot juice, NingXia Red, or even water and then drink it.

AGITATION

Agitation is caused by a weakened nervous system, lack of sleep, frustration, and is often a result of a congested liver or over stimulation of the sympathetic system.

Recommendations

Singles: Lavender, Roman Chamomile, Vetiver, Ocotea, Valerian, Idaho Balsam Fir, Myrrh, Sacred Frankincense, Frankincense, Frereana Frankincense, Melissa, Helichrysum, Marjoram

Blends: RutaVaLa, RutaVaLa Roll-On, Tranquil Roll-On, Stress Away Roll-On, Forgiveness, Peace & Calming, Surrender, Humility, White Angelica

Nutritionals: ImmuPro, Super B, JuvaTone, MegaCal, EndoGize

Application and Usage

Inhalation

- Diffuse recommended oils for 1 hour every 2 hours as needed.
- Put 2-3 drops of recommended oil in your hands and rub them together, cup your hands over your nose, and inhale 2-3 times per day or as needed.
- Put 2-3 drops of recommended oil on a cotton ball or tissue and put it in an air vent in your house, vehicle, hotel room, etc.
- If diffusing while sleeping, set your timer for the desired length of time for automatic shut off.

Topical

You may apply single oils or blends neat or diluted, depending on the oil or oils being used. Please see the instructions at the beginning of this chapter for more information on applying oils to the skin.

- Apply 1-2 drops neat or undiluted on temples and back of neck as desired.
- You may also apply 1-2 drops on the Vita Flex brain and heart points.
- Applying a single drop under the nose is helpful and refreshing.
- Place a warm compress with 3-4 drops of chosen oil over the back.

AIDS (ACQUIRED IMMUNE DEFICIENCY SYNDROME)

The AIDS virus attacks and infects immune cells that are essential for life. Frankincense and Myrrh have immune-building properties. Other oils like Cumin *(Cuminum cyminum)* have an inhibitory effect on viral replication.

In May 1994, Dr. Radwan Farag of Cairo University demonstrated that cumin seed oil had an 88 to 92 percent inhibition effect in vitro against HIV, the virus responsible for AIDS. Other antiviral essential oils include Oregano, Sandalwood, Ocotea, and Melaleuca Alternifolia.

Recommendations

Singles: Ocotea, Cumin, Cypress, Oregano, Plectranthus Oregano, Sandalwood, Melaleuca Alternifolia, Myrrh, Sacred Frankincense, Frankincense, Peppermint, Cistus, Cumin

Blends: Exodus II, Thieves, Inner Defense, Release, Acceptance

Nutritionals: NingXia Red, Power Meal, Im-muPro, Longevity, Essentialzyme, Essential-zymes-4, EndoGize, Pure Protein

Body Care: Raindrop Technique application

Application and Usage
Inhalation

- Diffuse your choice of oils for 1 hour every 2-4 hours or as desired.
- Put 2-3 drops of your chosen oil in your hands and rub them together, cup your hands over your nose, and inhale throughout the day as needed.
- Put 10 drops of oil on a cotton ball or tissue and put it in an air vent in your house, ve-hicle, hotel room, etc.
- If diffusing while sleeping, set your timer for the desired length of time for automatic shut off.

Topical

You may apply single oils or blends neat on feet and spine or diluted, depending on the oil or oils being used. Please see the instructions at the beginning of this chapter for more informa-tion on applying oils to the skin.

Ingestion and Oral

The amount of oil ingested varies with dif-ferent oils. Whether putting the oils in a cap-sule or drinking them in a liquid, please refer to instructions at the beginning of this chapter.

- Take 2 capsules with 50:50 Cistus and Cy-press 2 times daily.
- Put 2-3 drops of oil in a spoonful of Blue Agave, Yacon Syrup, maple syrup, etc.
- Put the desired amount of oils in a glass of rice milk, almond milk, goat milk, carrot juice, NingXia Red, or even water and then drink it.

ALCOHOLISM
(See Also ADDICTIONS)

Alcoholism, also known as alcohol depen-dence, includes alcohol craving and continued drinking. It includes four symptoms:

1. Craving: A strong compulsion, or need, to drink alcohol
2. Impaired control: The inability to limit drinking
3. Physical dependence: Inability to stop drink-ing without experiencing withdrawal symp-toms such as nausea, shakiness, sweating, and anxiety
4. Tolerance: The need for increasing amounts of alcohol

Recommendations

Singles: Sacred Frankincense, Frankincense, Lavender, Roman Chamomile, Ledum, He-lichrysum, Orange

Blends: JuvaCleanse, GLF, Forgiveness, Re-lease, Acceptance, Valor, Valor Roll-On, Motivation, White Angelica, The Gift, Com-mon Sense

Nutritionals: JuvaTone, ICP, ComforTone, Super B, Power Meal, Detoxzyme, Master Formula HIS or HERS, Mineral Essence

Application and Usage
Inhalation

- Diffuse your choice of oils for 1 hour every 2 hours or as desired.
- Put 2-3 drops of your chosen oil in your hands and rub them together, cup your hands over your nose, and inhale throughout the day as needed.
- Put 8-10 drops of oil on a cotton ball or tis-sue and put it in an air vent in your house, vehicle, hotel room, etc.
- If diffusing while sleeping, set your timer for the desired length of time for automatic shut off.

Topical

You may apply single oils or blends neat or diluted, depending on the oil or oils being used. Please see the instructions at the beginning of this chapter for more information on applying oils to the skin.

- Apply 1-2 drops neat on temples and back of neck several times daily.
- Place a warm compress with 6-8 drops of chosen oil over the liver.

Ingestion and Oral

The amount of oil ingested varies with different oils. Whether putting the oils in a capsule or drinking them in a liquid, please refer to the instructions at the beginning of this chapter.

- Take 1 capsule with desired oil 2 times daily.
- Put 2-3 drops of oil in a spoonful of Blue Agave, Yacon Syrup, maple syrup, etc.
- Put the desired amount of oils in a glass of rice milk, almond milk, goat milk, carrot juice, NingXia Red, or even water and then drink it.

ALKALOSIS

Alkalosis is a condition where the pH of the intestinal tract and the blood become excessively alkaline. While moderate alkalinity is essential for good health, excessive alkalinity can cause problems and result in fatigue, depression, irritability, and sickness.

The best way to lower the internal pH of the body is to eat a high protein diet (meat, eggs, dairy, seeds, nuts, legumes, etc.).

Recommendations

Singles: Peppermint, Lemon, Orange, Tarragon, Fennel, Ginger, Patchouli, Lemongrass

Blends: DiGize, GLF, EndoFlex

Nutritionals: Essentialzyme, ICP, Allerzyme, ComforTone, Digest & Cleanse, Pure Protein, Power Meal, Life 5

Application and Usage

Inhalation

Diffuse your choice of oils for ½ hour every 4-6 hours or as desired.

- Put 2-3 drops of your chosen oil in your hands and rub them together, cup your hands over your nose, and inhale throughout the day as needed.
- Put 8-10 drops of oil on a cotton ball or tissue and put it in an air vent in your house, vehicle, hotel room, etc.
- If diffusing while sleeping, set your timer for the desired length of time for automatic shut off.

Topical

You may apply single oils or blends neat or diluted, depending on the oil or oils being used. Please see the instructions at the beginning of this chapter for more information on applying oils to the skin.

Ingestion

The amount of oil ingested varies with different oils. Whether putting the oils in a capsule or drinking them in a liquid, please refer to the instructions at the beginning of this chapter.

- Take 1 capsule with desired oil 2 times daily.
- Put 2-3 drops of oil in a spoonful of Blue Agave, Yacon Syrup, maple syrup, etc.
- Put the desired amount of oils in a glass of rice milk, almond milk, goat milk, carrot juice, NingXia Red, or even water and then drink it.

ALLERGIES

Allergies are a result of the response to many different situations. They can be triggered by food, pollen, environmental chemicals, dander, dust, insect bites, to name just a few, and can affect the following:

- Respiration—wheezing, labored breathing
- Mouth—swelling of the lips or tongue,

itching lips

- Digestive tract—diarrhea, vomiting, cramps
- Skin—rashes, dermatitis
- Nose—sneezing, congestion, bloody nose

Food Allergies

Food allergies are different from food intolerances. Food allergies involve an immune system reaction, whereas food intolerances involve gastrointestinal reactions and are far more common.

For example, peanuts often produce a lifelong allergy due to peanut proteins being targeted by immune system antibodies as foreign invaders. In contrast, intolerance of pasteurized cow's milk that causes cramping and diarrhea is due to the inability to digest lactose (milk sugar) because of a lack of the enzyme lactase.

Food allergies are often associated with the consumption of peanuts, shellfish, nuts, wheat, cow's milk, eggs, and soy. Infants and children are far more prone to have food allergies than adults, due to the immaturity of their immune and digestive systems.

A thorough intestinal cleansing is one of the best ways to combat most allergies. Start with ICP, ComforTone, Essentialzyme, Essentialzymes-4, JuvaTone, and Life 5.

Hay Fever (Allergic Rhinitis)

Hay fever is an allergic reaction triggered by airborne allergens (pollen, animal hair, feathers, dust mites, etc.) that cause the release of histamines and subsequent inflammation of nasal passages and sinus-related areas. A more serious form of respiratory allergy is asthma, which manifests in the chest and lungs.

Symptoms: Inflammation of the nasal passages, sinuses, and eyelids that cause sneezing, runny nose, wheezing, and watery and red itchy eyes.

Recommendations

Singles: Fennel, Eucalyptus Blue, Lavender, Ocotea, Roman Chamomile, Peppermint, German Chamomile, Marjoram, Sacred Frankincense, Frankincense

Blends: DiGize, Harmony, JuvaCleanse, Valor, Valor Roll-On, R.C., Raven

Nutritionals: Allerzyme, Mineral Essence, ComforTone, Detoxzyme, Essentialzyme, JuvaPower, JuvaTone, MultiGreens, Sulfurzyme, Essentialzymes-4 yellow capsule, AlkaLime

Application and Usage
Inhalation

- Diffuse your choice of oils for 1 hour every 2 hours or as desired.
- Put 2-3 drops of your chosen oil in your hands and rub them together, cup your hands over your nose, and inhale throughout the day as needed.
- Put 8-10 drops of oil on a cotton ball or tissue and put it in an air vent in your house, vehicle, hotel room, etc.
- If diffusing while sleeping, set your timer for the desired length of time for automatic shut off.

Topical

You may apply single oils or blends neat or diluted, depending on the oil or oils being used. Please see the instructions at the beginning of this chapter for more information on applying oils to the skin.

Ingestion and Oral

The amount of oil ingested varies with different oils. Whether putting the oils in a capsule or drinking them in a liquid, please refer to the instructions at the beginning of this chapter.

- Take 1 capsule with DiGize or other desired oil 2 times daily.
- Put 2-3 drops of oil in a spoonful of Blue

Agave, Yacon Syrup, maple syrup, coconut oil, milk, etc.

- Put the desired amount of oils in a glass of rice milk, almond milk, goat milk, carrot juice, NingXia Red, or even water and then drink it.

ANALGESIC

An analgesic is defined as a compound that binds with a number of closely related, specific receptors in the central nervous system to block the perception of pain or affect the emotional response to pain. A number of essential oils have analgesic properties.

Recommendations

Singles: Clove, Helichrysum, Dorado Azul, Palo Santo, Elemi, Wintergreen, Copaiba

Blends: PanAway, Aroma Siez, Deep Relief Roll-On, Thieves, Inner Defense, Brain Power, Relieve It

Pain Relief Blend: Equal parts Wintergreen, Spruce, and Black Pepper

Application and Usage

Inhalation

- Diffuse your choice of oils for ½ hour every 4-6 hours or as desired.
- Applying a single drop under the nose is helpful and refreshing.
- Put 2-3 drops of your chosen oil in your hands and rub them together, cup your hands over your nose, and inhale throughout the day as needed.
- Put 8-10 drops of oil on a cotton ball or tissue and put it in an air vent in your house, vehicle, hotel room, etc.
- If diffusing while sleeping, set your timer for the desired length of time for automatic shut off.

Topical

You may apply single oils or blends neat or diluted, depending on the oil or oils being used.

Please see the instructions at the beginning of this chapter for more information on applying oils to the skin.

- Mix equal parts of Wintergreen, Spruce, and Black Pepper and massage with V-6 Vegetable Oil Complex.
- You may also apply 2-3 drops on the Vita Flex liver point of the right foot.

ANTHRAX

The anthrax bacterium *(Bacillus anthracis)* is one of the oldest and deadliest diseases known. There are three predominant types:

- External, acquired from contact with infected animal carcasses
- Internal, obtained from breathing airborne anthrax spores
- Battlefield, developed for biological warfare that is a far more lethal variety

When the airborne variety of anthrax invades the lungs, it is 90 percent fatal unless antibiotics are administered at the very beginning of the infection, but anthrax often goes undiagnosed until it is too late for antibiotics.

External varieties of anthrax may be contracted by exposure to animal hides and wool. While vaccinations and antibiotics have stemmed anthrax infection in recent years, new strains have developed that are resistant to all countermeasures.

According to Jean Valnet, MD, Thyme oil may be effective for killing the anthrax bacillus.[1] Two highly antimicrobial phenols in Thyme, carvacrol and thymol, are responsible for this action.

Recommendations

Singles: Ravintsara, Thyme, Oregano, Plectranthus Oregano, Clove, Cinnamon, Citronella, Lemongrass

Blends: Raven, Exodus II, Thieves, The Gift, ImmuPower, Melrose, Longevity

Nutritionals: Life 5, Inner Defense, ImmuPro, NingXia Red, Super C, Super C Chewable

Household Cleaners and Disinfectants: Thieves Household Cleaner, Thieves Spray, Thieves Waterless Hand Purifier, Thieves Foaming Hand Soap, Thieves Wipes

Application and Usage
Inhalation

- Diffuse your choice of oils for ½ hour every 4-6 hours or as desired to purify the air.
- Put 2-3 drops of your chosen oil in your hands and rub them together, cup your hands over your nose, and inhale throughout the day as needed.
- Put 8-10 drops of oil on a cotton ball or tissue and put it in an air vent in your house, vehicle, hotel room, etc.
- If diffusing while sleeping, set your timer for the desired length of time for automatic shut off.

Topical

You may apply single oils or blends neat or diluted, depending on the oil or oils being used. Please see the instructions at the beginning of this chapter for more information on applying oils to the skin.

- Use oils neat or dilute 50:50 for hands and other exposed skin areas.

Ingestion and Oral

The amount of oil ingested varies with different oils. Whether putting the oils in a capsule or drinking them in a liquid, please refer to the instructions at the beginning of this chapter.

- Take 1 capsule with desired oil 2 times daily.
- Put 2-3 drops of oil in a spoonful of Blue Agave, Yacon Syrup, maple syrup, coconut oil, milk, etc.
- Put the desired amount of oils in a glass of rice milk, almond milk, goat milk, carrot juice, NingXia Red, or even water and then drink it.
- Take 1 capsule 4 times daily, alternating oils.

ANTIBIOTIC REACTIONS

Synthetic antibiotic drugs indiscriminately kill both beneficial and harmful bacteria. This can result in yeast infections, including candida, diarrhea, poor nutrient assimilation, fatigue, sulfur toxicity, degenerative diseases, and many other conditions.

The average adult has 3-4 pounds of beneficial bacteria or flora constantly in the intestinal tract that support the body in healthy digestion and immune function and promote the following body functions:

- Constitutes the first line of defense against bacterial and viral infection
- Produces B vitamins
- Maintains pH balance
- Combats yeast and fungus overgrowth
- Aids in the digestive process

Recommendations

Singles: Peppermint, Spearmint, Lemon
Blends: JuvaCleanse, DiGize, Purification, Thieves, GLF, EndoFlex
Nutritionals: Life 5, Essentialzyme, Detoxzyme, Balance Complete, Power Meal, Mineral Essence, Inner Defense, Digest & Cleanse

Application and Usage
Inhalation

- Diffuse your choice of oils for ½ hour every 4-6 hours or as desired.
- Put 2-3 drops of your chosen oil in your hands and rub them together, cup your hands over your nose, and inhale throughout the day as needed.
- Put 8-10 drops of oil on a cotton ball or tissue and put it in an air vent in your house, vehicle, hotel room, etc.
- If diffusing while sleeping, set your timer for the desired length of time for automatic shut off.

Topical

You may apply single oils or blends neat or diluted, depending on the oil or oils being used. Please see the instructions at the beginning of this chapter for more information on applying oils to the skin.

Ingestion

The amount of oil ingested varies with different oils. Whether putting the oils in a capsule or drinking them in a liquid, please refer to the instructions at the beginning of this chapter.

- Take 1 capsule with desired oil 2 times daily.
- Put 2-3 drops of oil in a spoonful of Blue Agave, Yacon Syrup, maple syrup, coconut oil, etc.
- Put the desired amount of oils in a glass of rice milk, almond milk, goat milk, carrot juice, NingXia Red, or even water and then drink it.
- Life 5: Take 2-3 capsules on an empty stomach before meals during antibiotic treatment.
- After completing antibiotic treatment, continue using Life 5 for 10-15 days.

ANTISEPTICS AND DISINFECTANTS

Antiseptics prevent the growth of pathogenic microorganisms. Many essential oils have powerful, antiseptic properties. Clove and Thyme essential oils have been documented to kill over 50 types of bacteria and 10 types of fungi.

Other potent antiseptic essential oils include Cinnamon, Cassia, Melaleuca Alternifolia, Oregano, Plectranthus Oregano, Mountain Savory, Dorado Azul, and Ocotea.

Recommendations

Singles: Thyme, Clove, Oregano, Plectranthus Oregano, Rosemary, Mountain Savory, Eucalyptus Radiata, Eucalyptus Globulus, Eucalyptus Dives, Eucalyptus Polybractea, Lavandin, Cinnamon, Cassia, Ravintsara, Melaleuca Alternifolia, Ocotea

Blends: Raven, Purification, Melrose, R.C., Breathe Again Roll-On, Thieves

Nutritionals: Inner Defense, Exodus, Thieves Lozenges (Hard/Soft), Thieves Fresh Essence Plus Mouthwash

Household Cleaners and Disinfectants: Thieves Foaming Hand Cleanser, Thieves Waterless Hand Purifier, Thieves Household Cleaner, Thieves Cleansing Bar Soap

Application and Usage
Inhalation

- Diffuse your choice of oils for ½ hour every 4-6 hours or as desired.
- Put 2-3 drops of your chosen oil in your hands and rub them together, cup your hands over your nose, and inhale throughout the day as needed.
- Put 8-10 drops of oil on a cotton ball or tissue and put it in an air vent in your house, vehicle, hotel room, etc.
- If diffusing while sleeping, set your timer for the desired length of time for automatic shut off.

Topical

You may apply single oils or blends neat or diluted, depending on the oil or oils being used. Please see the instructions at the beginning of this chapter for more information on applying oils to the skin.

- Apply 1-2 drops diluted 50:50 and gently rub over affected areas.

APNEA

Apnea is a temporary cessation of breathing during sleep. It can lessen the quality of sleep, resulting in chronic fatigue, lowered immune function, and lack of energy.

Recommendations

Singles: Spruce, Idaho Balsam Fir, Cedarwood, Juniper, Ylang Ylang, Amazonian Ylang Ylang, Lavender, Sacred Frankincense,

Frankincense, Sandalwood

Blends: Clarity, Valor, Valor Roll-On, Common Sense, Stress Away Roll-On, RutaVaLa, RutaVaLa Roll-On, White Angelica, Sacred Mountain, Present Time

Nutritionals: Thyromin, MultiGreens, Super B, Inner Defense, Ultra Young Plus, SleepEssence

Application and Usage
Inhalation

- Diffuse your choice of oils for ½ hour every 4-6 hours or as desired.
- Put 2-3 drops of your chosen oil in your hands and rub them together, cup your hands over your nose, and inhale throughout the day as needed.
- Put 8-10 drops of oil on a cotton ball or tissue and put it in an air vent in your house, vehicle, hotel room, etc.
- If diffusing while sleeping, set your timer for the desired length of time for automatic shut off.

Topical

You may apply single oils or blends neat or diluted, depending on the oil or oils being used. Please see the instructions at the beginning of this chapter for more information on applying oils to the skin.

- Massage 2-4 drops of oil neat on the soles of the feet just before bedtime.

ARTHRITIS

More than 100 different kinds of arthritis have been identified. Two of the most common kinds are osteoarthritis and rheumatoid arthritis.

....

Osteoarthritis

Osteoarthritis involves the breakdown of the cartilage that forms a cushion between two joints. As this cartilage is eaten away, the two bones of the joint start rubbing together and wearing down.

In contrast, rheumatoid arthritis is caused from a swelling and inflammation of the synovial membrane, the lining of the joint.

Natural anti-inflammatories such as German Chamomile and Wintergreen when combined with cartilage builders (glucosamine/chondroitin) are powerful, natural cures for arthritis.

The best natural anti-inflammatories include fats rich in omega-3s and essential oils such as Nutmeg, Wintergreen, German Chamomile, and Idaho Balsam Fir. The best cartilage builders include Type II collagen and glucosamine contained in BLM powder.

Nutmeg, a source of myristicin, has been researched for its anti-inflammatory effects in several studies. It works by inhibiting pro-inflammatory prostaglandins when taken internally or applied topically. Clove exhibits similar action.

Chamazulene, the blue sesquiterpene in German Chamomile, also shows strong anti-inflammatory activity when used both topically and orally.

Methyl salicylate is a major compound in Wintergreen, similar to the active agent in aspirin that is found naturally in PanAway. It has strong anti-inflammatory and analgesic properties.

Glucosamine and chondroitin are the two most powerful natural compounds for rebuilding cartilage and are the key ingredients in the supplement BLM.

Recommendations

Singles: Wintergreen, Peppermint, Vetiver, Valerian, Palo Santo, Idaho Balsam Fir, Eucalyptus Globulus, Sacred Frankincense, Frankincense, Frereana Frankincense, Idaho Ponderosa Pine, German Chamomile, Helichrysum, Dorado Azul, Spruce, Pine

Blends: PanAway, Relieve It, Aroma Siez, Deep

Relief Roll-On

Nutritionals: Essentialzyme, Essentialzymes-4, BLM, Sulfurzyme, ImmuPro, ICP, JuvaPower, JuvaTone, Detoxzyme, MegaCal, Longevity Softgels, Rehemogen, OmegaGize^3, Estro, EndoGize

Body Care Massage Oils and Creams: Ortho Sport Massage Oil, Ortho Ease Massage Oil

Application and Usage
Inhalation
- Diffuse your choice of oils for ½ hour every 4-6 hours or as desired.
- Put 2-3 drops of your chosen oil in your hands and rub them together, cup your hands over your nose, and inhale throughout the day as needed.
- Put 8-10 drops of oil on a cotton ball or tissue and put it in an air vent in your house, vehicle, hotel room, etc.
- If diffusing while sleeping, set your timer for the desired length of time for automatic shut off.

Topical
You may apply single oils or blends neat or diluted, depending on the oil or oils being used. Please see the instructions at the beginning of this chapter for more information on applying oils to the skin.
- Dilute 5-10 drops of oil in 1 teaspoon V-6 Vegetable Oil Complex and apply on location. Essential oils can also be applied neat and then followed by application of V-6 Vegetable Oil Complex.
- Applying a single drop of oil under the nose is helpful and refreshing.
- Body Massage: Ortho Sport Massage Oil or Ortho Ease Massage Oil offer tremendous relief.

Ingestion
The amount of oil ingested varies with different oils. Whether putting the oils in a capsule or drinking them in a liquid, please refer to the instructions at the beginning of this chapter.
- Take 1 capsule with desired oil 2 times daily.
- Put 2-3 drops of oil in a spoonful of Blue Agave, Yacon Syrup, maple syrup, coconut oil, milk, etc.
- Put the desired amount of oils in a glass of rice milk, almond milk, goat milk, carrot juice, NingXia Red, or even water and then drink it.
- Detoxification of the body and strengthening the joints is important. Cleanse the colon and liver.

BLM: Take 2-4 capsules 2 times daily.

MegaCal: Mix 1 teaspoon in water before going to bed.

ImmuPro: Take 2-3 tablets 3 times daily.

ComforTone: Take 3 capsules 2 times daily; increase if needed.

ICP: Take 2 scoops in water or juice in the morning.

JuvaPower: Take 2 scoops in water or juice before going to bed.

Rehemogen: Cleans and purifies the blood, which may have toxins blocking nutrient and oxygen absorption into cells (See Circulation).

OmegaGize^3: Take 1-3 capsules daily.

···

Rheumatoid Arthritis
Rheumatoid arthritis is a painful, inflammatory condition of the joints marked by swelling, thickening, and inflammation of the synovial membrane lining the joint. In contrast, osteoarthritis is characterized by a breakdown of the joint cartilage, without any swelling or inflammation.

Rheumatoid arthritis is classified as an autoimmune disease because it is caused by the body's own immune system attacking the joints.

Inflammation from rheumatoid arthritis has been ameliorated by the boswellic acids found in most frankincense species.[2]

Other factors can aggravate arthritis such as:

- Deficiencies of minerals and other nutrients
- Microbes and toxins
- Lack of water intake
- Eating bread

Essential oils are effective in helping to combat pain and infection. In cases where arthritis is caused by infectious organisms, such as Lyme disease (*Borrelia burgdorferi*), chlamydia, and salmonella, essential oils may counteract and prevent infection.

Highly antimicrobial essential oils include Mountain Savory, Rosemary, Melaleuca Alternifolia, and Oregano. Essential oils easily pass into the bloodstream when applied topically.

MSM, the main ingredient in the supplement Sulfurzyme, has been documented to be one of the most effective, natural supplements for reducing the pain associated with rheumatism and arthritis.

MSM has been a subject of a number of clinical studies and was used extensively by Ronald Lawrence, MD, in his clinical practice to successfully treat rheumatism and arthritis.

Glucosamine and chondroitin are also powerful, natural compounds for reducing inflammation, halting the progression of arthritis, and rebuilding cartilage. These are the key ingredients in the supplement BLM.

Recommendations

Singles: Wintergreen, Peppermint, Sacred Frankincense, Frankincense, Frereana Frankincense, Palo Santo, Vetiver, Nutmeg, Clove, Mountain Savory, Rosemary, Melaleuca Alternifolia, Helichrysum, Idaho Balsam Fir, Idaho Ponderosa Pine, Pine, Eucalyptus Globulus, Copaiba, Myrrh, Valerian, Dorado Azul, Spruce

Blends: PanAway, Relieve It, Aroma Siez, Deep Relief Roll-On

Nutritionals: BLM, Detoxzyme, Sulfurzyme, MegaCal, Master Formula HIS or HERS, Mineral Essence, Essentialzyme, Longevity Softgels, ImmuPro, Rehemogen, EndoGize

Body Care Massage Oils and Creams: Ortho Ease Massage Oil, Ortho Sport Massage Oil

Application and Usage

Inhalation

- Diffuse your choice of oils for ½ hour every 4-6 hours or as desired.
- Put 2-3 drops of your chosen oil in your hands and rub them together, cup your hands over your nose, and inhale throughout the day as needed.
- Put 8-10 drops of oil on a cotton ball or tissue and put it in an air vent in your house, vehicle, hotel room, etc.
- If diffusing while sleeping, set your timer for the desired length of time for automatic shut off.

Topical

You may apply single oils or blends neat or diluted, depending on the oil or oils being used. Please see the instructions at the beginning of this chapter for more information on applying oils to the skin.

- Dilute 5-10 drops of essential oils in 1 teaspoon of V-6 Vegetable Oil Complex and apply on location. Essential oils can also be applied neat and then followed by V-6 Vegetable Oil Complex.
- Massage 2-4 drops of oil neat on the soles of the feet just before bedtime.
- Place a warm compress once daily with oils of your choice on the back.
- Massage with oils of your choice mixed with V-6 Vegetable Oil Complex, Relaxation Massage Oil, Sensation Massage Oil, Ortho Ease Massage Oil, or Ortho Sport Massage Oil.

Ingestion and Oral

The amount of oil ingested varies with different oils. Whether putting the oils in a capsule or drinking them in a liquid, please refer to the instructions at the beginning of this chapter.

- Take 1 capsule with desired oil 2 times daily.
- Put 2-3 drops of oil in a spoonful of Blue Agave, Yacon Syrup, maple syrup, coconut oil, milk, etc.
- Put the desired amount of oils in a glass of rice milk, almond milk, goat milk, carrot juice, NingXia Red, or even water and then drink it.

ATTENTION DEFICIT DISORDER (ADD AND ADHD)

Terry Friedmann, MD, in 2001 completed pioneering studies using essential oils to combat ADD and ADHD. Using twice-a-day inhalation of essential oils, including Vetiver, Cedarwood, and Lavender, Dr. Friedmann was able to achieve clinically significant results in 60 days.

Researchers postulate that essential oils mitigate ADD and ADHD through their stimulation of the limbic system of the brain.

Because attention deficit disorder may be caused by mineral deficiencies in the diet, increasing nutrient intake and absorption of magnesium, potassium, and other trace minerals can also have a significant, beneficial effect in resolving ADD.

Recommendations

Singles: Vetiver, Lavender, Cedarwood, Sandalwood, Cardamom, Peppermint, Sacred Frankincense, Frankincense

Blends: Brain Power, Peace & Calming, Clarity

Nutritionals: OmegaGize[3], Mineral Essence, NingXia Red, Power Meal, Balance Complete, Essentialzyme, Detoxzyme, Multi-Greens, Master Formula HIS or HERS

Application and Usage

Inhalation

- Diffuse your choice of oils for 1 hour 4-8 times daily as desired.
- Put 2-3 drops of the desired oil in your hands and rub them together, cup your hands over your nose, and inhale throughout the day as needed.
- Put 8-10 drops of oil on a cotton ball or tissue and put it in an air vent in your house, vehicle, hotel room, etc.
- If diffusing while sleeping, set your timer for the desired length of time for automatic shut off.

Topical

You may apply single oils or blends neat or diluted, depending on the oil or oils being used. Please see the instructions at the beginning of this chapter for more information on applying oils to the skin.

- Apply 1-2 drops of the oil of your choice neat or diluted 4-8 times daily on the neck, brain stem, and even on the head.
- Applying a single drop under the nose is helpful and refreshing.
- Massage 2-4 drops of oil neat on the soles of the feet just before bedtime. Children love it.

Ingestion and Oral

The amount of oil ingested varies with different oils. Whether putting the oils in a capsule or drinking them in a liquid, please refer to the instructions at the beginning of this chapter.

- Take 1 capsule with desired oil 2 times daily.
- Put 2-3 drops of oil in a spoonful of Blue Agave, Yacon Syrup, maple syrup, coconut oil, milk, etc.
- Put the desired amount of oils in a glass of rice milk, almond milk, goat milk, carrot juice, NingXia Red, or even water and then drink it.
- Drink 3-6 oz. of NingXia Red daily.

AUTISM

Improving diet can be the key to reducing the problems associated with autism. Eliminating refined and synthetic sugars and replacing them with natural sweeteners such as Blue Agave, natural fruit sweeteners, maple syrup, etc., has produced outstanding results in numerous cases of autism.

Autism is a neurologically based developmental disorder that is four times more common in boys than girls. It is characterized by the following:

- Social ineptness (loner)
- Nonverbal and verbal communication difficulties
- Repetitive behavior (rocking, hair twirling)
- Self-injurious behavior (head banging)
- Very limited or peculiar interests
- Reduced or abnormal responses to pain, noises, or other outside stimuli

Autism is being increasingly linked to certain vaccinations; and MMR, the one-shot combination for measles, mumps, and rubella, is most often cited by researchers. British researcher Andrew Wakefield, MD, suggests using single shots for children for measles, mumps, and rubella (instead of the combined MMR shot) until further research is done.

Dr. Wakefield's suggestions may be acceptable to people who know little about vaccinations, but the research that has been done on vaccines sends a very loud warning. Vaccinations given in combination or singularly are damaging to anyone of any age. Unfortunately, children are usually the innocent victims who suffer the most.

Until very recently, children were receiving large doses of thimerosal, a vaccine preservative that contains 49.6 percent mercury, which is well above the limit recommended by the EPA through vaccination. Some success in reversing autism has resulted through mercury detoxifi-cation along with nutritional supplementation.

Some researchers believe that gastrointestinal disorders may be linked to the brain dysfunctions that cause autism in children (Horvath, et al., 1998). In fact, there have been several cases of successful treatment of autism using pancreatic enzymes.

Stimulation of the limbic region of the brain may also help treat autism. The aromas from essential oils have a powerful ability to stimulate this part of the brain, since the sense of smell (olfaction) is tied directly to the emotional centers. As a result, the aroma of an essential oil has the potential to exert a powerful influence on disorders such as ADD and autism.

Recommendations

Singles: Vetiver, Patchouli, Lavender, Eucalyptus Globulus, Melissa, Cedarwood, Sandalwood, Frankincense

Blends: Brain Power, GLF, Valor, Valor Roll-On, Clarity, Peace & Calming, Common Sense, The Gift

Nutritionals: Essentialzyme, Essentialzymes-4, NingXia Red, ½ Super B for children, Sulfurzyme, Detoxzyme, Power Meal, Balance Complete, AlkaLime

Application and Usage
Inhalation

- Diffuse your choice of oils for 1 hour 4-6 times daily or as desired.
- Put 2-3 drops of your chosen oil in your hands and rub them together, cup your hands over your nose, and inhale throughout the day as needed.
- Put 8-10 drops of oil on a cotton ball or tissue and put it in an air vent in your house, vehicle, hotel room, etc.
- If diffusing while sleeping, set your timer for the desired length of time for automatic shut off.

Topical

You may apply single oils or blends neat or diluted, depending on the oil or oils being used. Please see the instructions at the beginning of this chapter for more information on applying oils to the skin.

- Apply 1-2 drops neat (undiluted) on temples and back of neck, as desired.
- Applying a single drop under the nose is helpful and refreshing.
- Massage 2-4 drops of oil neat on the soles of the feet just before bedtime. Children love it.

Ingestion and Oral

The amount of oil ingested varies with different oils. Whether putting the oils in a capsule or drinking them in a liquid, please refer to the instructions at the beginning of this chapter.

- Take 1 capsule with desired oil 2 times daily.
- Put 2-3 drops of oil in a spoonful of Blue Agave, Yacon Syrup, maple syrup, coconut oil, milk, etc.
- Put the desired amount of oils in a glass of rice milk, almond milk, goat milk, carrot juice, NingXia Red, or even water and then drink it.

Autism Blend

- 15 drops Sacred Frankincense or Frankincense
- 12 drops Myrrh
- 10 drops Idaho Balsam Fir
- 10 drops Canadian Fleabane (Conyza)
- 4 drops Peppermint

Take 3 capsules daily: morning, noon, and night.

Use this blend for Raindrop Technique 2 times daily: morning and night.

Using this regimen, a 7-year-old boy with cerebral palsy and autism, after one month, was able to walk flat footed without his walker, test scores in school improved by 28 percent, and his attention span increased 30 percent, his mother reported.

BED BUGS

Having bed bugs is a very miserable experience. Some bed bugs are so small they just look like specks of dirt that you brush off the sheets. You cannot tell they are alive unless you look at them with a microscope. They thrive in a moist, warm environment, and when you wake up in the morning, you are astounded at all the bites you have in the most unexpected places.

The itching is horrible and lasts for about one week. It is amazing that a tiny, almost microscopic bug can give such an intense bite. Essential oils are the answer to treating without dreaded chemicals. Some of the oils have a powerful ability to kill on contact. The thought of sleeping with those little, hungry critters is not a pleasant thought, and to some, it's repulsive; but knowing the bugs are dead is a positive feeling.

If you suspect bed bugs, wash all of your bedding in hot water and add 10 to 15 drops of Thieves, Palo Santo, Oregano, Plectranthus Oregano, Thyme, Citrus Fresh, Melrose, etc., and see what works best for you. After you make the bed, spray with a single oil or with one of the blends morning and night to ensure that they do not return.

If you live in a warm or hot, humid environment, then you will probably have to spray at least once every day or perhaps twice. If you see any little specks, make sure they are not biting bugs that have come to visit.

Recommendations

These blends work for most bugs but have been tried and tested with bed bugs.

Bed Bug Killer Blend No. 1

- 20 drops Palo Santo
- 20 drops Idaho Tansy

Mix together and spray. Dilute with water as much as you think you can and still have results. You will have to experiment to determine that. Spray sheets and clothing to kill any insects that might be imbedded in the cloth or anywhere else that you might suspect their presence.

Insect Bite Blend No. 2
- 20 drops Palo Santo
- 20 drops Idaho Tansy
- 10 drops Eucalyptus Blue

Apply on bites as needed.

Bed Bug Killer Blend No. 3
- Mix 20 drops Thieves with 2-3 cups water, shake well, and spray sheets and pillows.

BLADDER / URINARY TRACT INFECTION (CYSTITIS)

Bladder infections and inflammation known as cystitis are caused by bacteria that travel up the urethra. This disorder is more common in women than men because of the woman's shorter urethra. If the infection travels up the ureters and reaches the kidneys, kidney infection can result.

Symptoms of infection
- Frequent urge to urinate with only a small amount of urine passing
- Strong smelling urine
- Blood in urine
- Burning or stinging during urination
- Tenderness or chronic pain in bladder and pelvic area
- Pain intensity fluctuates as bladder fills or empties
- Symptoms worsen during menstruation

Recommendations
Singles: Myrrh, Spikenard, Melaleuca Alternifolia, Juniper, Oregano, Plectranthus Oregano, Lemon, Melissa, Mountain Savory, Thyme, Cistus, Rosemary, Clove

Blends: Inspiration, Melrose, Thieves, DiGize, EndoFlex, R.C., Purification

Nutritionals: K&B, ImmuPro, AlkaLime

Application and Usage
Topical

You may apply single oils or blends neat or diluted, depending on the oil or oils being used. Please see the instructions at the beginning of this chapter for more information on applying oils to the skin.

- Dilute 50:50 and apply a few drops on location 3-6 times daily.
- Dilute 2-4 drops of Melrose, Purification, or other oil and use in a warm compress over bladder 1-2 times daily.
- Receive a Raindrop Technique 3 times weekly.
- First Week: Use Myrrh, Thyme, Mountain Savory, Palo Santo, and Inspiration and follow with a hot compress.

Ingestion

The amount of oil ingested varies with different oils. Whether putting the oils in a capsule or drinking them in a liquid, please refer to the instructions at the beginning of this chapter.

- Take 1 capsule with desired oil 2 times daily.
- Put 2-3 drops of oil in a spoonful of Blue Agave, Yacon Syrup, maple syrup, coconut oil, milk, etc.
- Put the desired amount of oils in a glass of rice milk, almond milk, goat milk, carrot juice, NingXia Red, or even water and then drink it.
- Use K&B tincture (2-3 droppers in distilled water) 3-6 times daily. K&B helps strengthen and tone weak bladder, kidneys, and urinary tract.
- Take ½ teaspoon of AlkaLime daily, in water only, 1 hour before or after meal.
- Drink unsweetened cranberry juice and sweeten with honey, Yacon Syrup, Blue Agave, or maple syrup.
- Drink 4 liters of purified water daily.

BLOATING/SWELLING
(See also MENSTRUAL AND FEMALE HORMONE CONDITIONS)

Bloating is caused by many imbalances in the body. Bloating during menstrual cycle or swelling in the lower extremities is caused by pH imbalance and low estrogen. Bloating can also be caused by enzyme deficiencies, resulting in poor digestion and allergies. Swelling in the legs can be from low potassium and poor circulation, which will cause fluid retention.

It is important to determine whether it is bloating or fluid retention; there is a very significant difference.

Recommendations
Singles: Juniper, Tangerine, Clary Sage, Cypress, Peppermint, Fennel, Tarragon, Nutmeg

Blends: DiGize, GLF, Citrus Fresh

Nutritionals: Essentialzyme, Essentialzymes-4, Mineral Essence, AlkaLime, Detoxzyme, Allerzyme, ICP, ComforTone, JuvaPower, Super B

 Serum: Progessence Plus

Application and Usage
Inhalation
- Diffuse your choice of oils for ½ hour every 4-6 hours or as desired.
- Put 2-3 drops of your chosen oil in your hands and rub them together, cup your hands over your nose, and inhale throughout the day as needed.
- Put 8-10 drops of oil on a cotton ball or tissue and put it in an air vent in your house, vehicle, hotel room, etc.
- If diffusing while sleeping, set your timer for the desired length of time for automatic shut off.

Topical
You may apply single oils or blends neat or diluted, depending on the oil or oils being used.

Please see the instructions at the beginning of this chapter for more information on applying oils to the skin.

Ingestion and Oral
The amount of oil ingested varies with different oils. Whether putting the oils in a capsule or drinking them in a liquid, please refer to the instructions at the beginning of this chapter.
- Take 1 capsule with desired oil 2 times daily.
- Put 2-3 drops of oil in a spoonful of Blue Agave, Yacon Syrup, maple syrup, coconut oil, milk, etc.
- Put the desired amount of oils in a glass of rice milk, almond milk, goat milk, carrot juice, NingXia Red, or even water and then drink it.
- Take 2 capsules of DiGize 3 times daily.
- Take 1 capsule of peppermint 3 times daily.

BONE PROBLEMS
Symptoms of bone problems include pain, brittleness, and lumps. Treatment depends on the nature and cause of the problems; unexplained symptoms can be serious and should always receive medical attention.

....

Broken Bones
A health professional should always be involved in the diagnosis and setting of a broken bone or a suspected broken bone.

Recommendations
Singles: Thyme, Helichrysum, Wintergreen, Peppermint, Spruce, Idaho Balsam Fir, Pine, Copaiba, Palo Santo, Myrrh, Lemongrass, Ginger, Vetiver

Blends: Aroma Siez, PanAway, Relieve It, Deep Relief Roll-On

Nutritionals: MegaCal, BLM, PD 80/20, SuperCal, Mineral Essence, OmegaGize[3]

 Massage Oils and Creams: Ortho Ease Massage Oil, Ortho Sport Massage Oil,

Regenolone, Progessence Plus

The following blends can also help relieve pain and speed the bone mending process:

Broken Bone Blend No. 1

- 8 drops Idaho Balsam Fir
- 6 drops Helichrysum
- 1 drop Myrrh, Sacred Frankincense, or Frankincense
- 1 drop Wintergreen

Broken Bone Blend No. 2

- 10 drops Wintergreen
- 4 drops Palo Santo
- 4 drops Vetiver
- 3 drops Pine
- 3 drops Helichrysum
- 2 drops Lemongrass

Application and Usage
Topical

You may apply single oils or blends neat or diluted, depending on the oil or oils being used. Please see the instructions at the beginning of this chapter for more information on applying oils to the skin.

- Dilute 50:50 and apply a few drops on location 3-6 times daily.
- Prior to casting a broken bone, mix one of the above blends and very gently apply 5-10 drops (depending on size) neat to break area. If there are any signs of skin sensitivity or irritation, apply a small amount of V-6 Vegetable Oil Complex.

Note: Apply extremely gently if bone break is suspected.

Bone Pain

Bone pain can be caused from injuries, arthritis, or other more serious reasons. See your health-care professional for the correct diagnosis and proper treatment.

Recommendations

Singles: Wintergreen, Spruce, Copaiba, Pine, Idaho Balsam Fir, Helichrysum

Blends: PanAway, Relieve It, Deep Relief Roll-On

Nutritionals: MegaCal, BLM, Master Formula HIS or HERS, Essentialzyme, Essentialzymes-4

Application and Usage
Topical

You may apply single oils or blends neat or diluted, depending on the oil or oils being used. Please see the instructions at the beginning of this chapter for more information on applying oils to the skin.

- Dilute 50:50 and apply a few drops on location 3-6 times daily as needed.
- Poor bone and muscle development can indicate HGH, potassium, and/or mineral deficiency.

Osteoporosis (Bone Density Loss)

Osteoporosis is primarily caused by six main factors:

- Progesterone deficiency
- Estradiol deficiency
- Testosterone deficiency
- Lack of magnesium and boron in diet
- Lack of vitamin D in diet
- Lack of dietary calcium

Natural progesterone is the single most effective way to increase bone density in women over age 40. Clinical studies by John Lee, MD, showed dramatic increases in bone density using just 20 mg of daily, topically applied progesterone.

Calcium, magnesium, and boron are a few of the most important minerals for bone health and are usually lacking or deficient in most modern diets. Magnesium is especially important for bone strength, but most Americans consume only a fraction of the 400 mg daily value needed for bone health.

Calcium and magnesium may not be adequately metabolized when consumed because of poor intestinal flora and excess phytates in the diet (a problem with vegetarians). Phytates occur in many nuts, grains, and seeds, including rice. Enzymes like phytase are essential for increasing calcium absorption by liberating calcium from insoluble phytate complexes.

Lack of vitamin D (cholecalciferol) has become epidemic among older people and has contributed to a lack of absorption of calcium in the diet.

MegaCal, AlkaLime, and Mineral Essence are all excellent sources of calcium and magnesium, which are essential for strong bones. Mineral Essence is an excellent source of magnesium and other trace minerals.

Avoid drinking anything that is carbonated because it can leach calcium from the bones due to its phosphoric acid content.

Studies show that the majority of women who do resistance training 3-4 times a week do not develop osteoporosis.

Recommendations

Singles: Wintergreen, Idaho Balsam Fir, Palo Santo, Sacred Frankincense, Frankincense, Thyme, Cypress, Peppermint, Marjoram, Rosemary, Basil, Elemi, Spruce, Pine

Blends: SclarEssence, PanAway, Aroma Siez, Purification, Melrose, Sacred Mountain, Relieve It

Nutritionals: Estro, FemiGen, EndoGize, BLM, MegaCal, Essentialzyme, Detoxzyme, AlkaLime, Mineral Essence, Essentialzymes-4, SuperCal, Sulfurzyme, Thyromin

  Creams and Serums: Prenolone Plus Body Cream, Progessence Plus

Application and Usage
Topical

You may apply single oils or blends neat or diluted, depending on the oil or oils being used. Please see the instructions at the beginning of this chapter for more information on applying oils to the skin.

- Massage 6-10 drops diluted 50:50 on spine (or area affected) 2-3 times daily.

BRAIN DISORDERS AND PROBLEMS

As the control center of the body, the brain controls speech, movement, thoughts, and memory and regulates the function of many organs. When problems occur, the results can be devastating.

Absentmindedness

Clinical studies on Ningxia wolfberry *(Lycium barbarum)* have shown that it has an anti-senility effect.[3] Clinical studies at Tufts University and the Department of Veterans Affairs Medical Center, Denver, Colorado, and Boston, Massachusetts, found that high antioxidant foods such as spinach found in JuvaPower and blueberry found in NingXia Red dramatically improved learning and cognition.[4, 5]

Recommendations

Singles: Peppermint, Sacred Frankincense, Frankincense, Rosemary, Cardamom, Canadian Fleabane (Conyza)

Blends: Clarity, M-Grain, Brain Power, Common Sense, Oola Balance, Oola Grow

Nutritionals: NingXia Red, PD 80/20, OmegaGize[3], NingXia Nitro, Master Formula HIS or HERS, Essentialzyme

Application and Usage
Inhalation

- Diffuse your choice of oils for 1 hour every 2 hours or as desired.
- Put 2-3 drops of your chosen oil in your hands and rub them together, cup your hands over your nose, and inhale throughout the day as needed.

- Put 8-10 drops of oil on a cotton ball or tissue and put it in an air vent in your house, vehicle, hotel room, etc.
- If diffusing while sleeping, set your timer for the desired length of time for automatic shut off.

Topical

You may apply single oils or blends neat or diluted, depending on the oil or oils being used. Please see the instructions at the beginning of this chapter for more information on applying oils to the skin.

- Apply 1-2 drops neat (undiluted) on temples and back of neck, as desired.

....

Alzheimer's

Over 4 million Americans suffer from Alzheimer's. Alzheimer's was found to nearly double in subjects with high levels of homocysteine in the Framingham Study. The Center for Disease Control and Prevention has concluded that the primary cause of Alzheimer's disease is probably not aluminum, although it could be a contributing factor in patients who were already at risk of developing the disease. In spite of this fact, people are still being urged to get yearly flu shots, which contain aluminum as an adjuvant. Pepper, Grapefruit, and Fennel oils have been found to stimulate brain activity.[6] Peppermint oil has been helpful in protecting against stresses and toxins in brain cells.[7]

Dr. Richard Restick, a leading neurologist in Washington, D.C., stated that maintaining normal synaptic firing would forestall many types of neurological deterioration in the body.

Essential oils high in sesquiterpenes, such as Vetiver, Cedarwood, Patchouli, German Chamomile, Myrrh, Melissa, and Sandalwood, are known to cross the blood-brain barrier. Frankincense is a general cerebral stimulant.

Recommendations

Singles: Melissa, Sandalwood, Helichrysum, Ginger, Nutmeg, German Chamomile, Spikenard, Eucalyptus Globulus, Sacred Frankincense, Frankincense, Patchouli, Cedarwood, Myrrh

Helichrysum supports neurotransmitter activity and has shown the possibility of chelating aluminum. Nutmeg is a general cerebral stimulant and has adrenal cortex-like activity.

Blends: Brain Power, Common Sense, Valor, Valor Roll-On, Clarity, Oola Balance, Oola Grow, Harmony, RutaVaLa, RutaVaLa Roll-On

Nutritionals: MultiGreens, Power Meal, Sulfurzyme, Essentialzyme, Mineral Essence, NingXia Red, NingXia Nitro, Master HIS or HERS, Super C, Super C Chewable, MegaCal, OmegaGize[3]

Application and Usage

Inhalation

- Diffuse your choice of oils for ½ hour every 4-6 hours or as desired.
- Put 2-3 drops of your chosen oil in your hands and rub them together, cup your hands over your nose, and inhale throughout the day as needed.
- Put 8-10 drops of oil on a cotton ball or tissue and put it in an air vent in your house, vehicle, hotel room, etc.
- If diffusing while sleeping, set your timer for the desired length of time for automatic shut off.

Topical

You may apply single oils or blends neat or diluted, depending on the oil or oils being used. Please see the instructions at the beginning of this chapter for more information on applying oils to the skin.

- Apply 1-2 drops directly onto the brain reflex centers. These points include the forehead, temples, and mastoids (the bones just behind the ears). Apply oils and mild, direct pressure to the brainstem area (center top of neck at base of skull) and work down the spine.

- Apply 1-2 drops neat to Vita Flex brain points on feet 1-2 times daily.
- Receive a Raindrop Technique once every 2 weeks.

Ingestion and Oral

The amount of oil ingested varies with different oils. Whether putting the oils in a capsule or drinking them in a liquid, please refer to the instructions at the beginning of this chapter.

- Take 1 capsule with desired oil 2 times daily.
- Put 2-3 drops of oil in a spoonful of Blue Agave, Yacon Syrup, maple syrup, coconut oil, milk, etc.
- Put the desired amount of oils in a glass of rice milk, almond milk, goat milk, carrot juice, NingXia Red, or even water and then drink it.

....

Concentration, Impaired

Impaired concentration is very common and may not always lead to a debilitating condition. Some common reasons why people can't concentrate are lack of sleep, lack of exercise, improper diet, and too much technology. A study in *Research in Higher Education* showed that students who texted the professor during a lecture scored 42.81 on a test following the lecture while non-texting students had a higher score of 58.67.[8]

Recommendations

Singles: Peppermint, Basil, Lemon, Bergamot, Rosemary, Sacred Frankincense, Frankincense, Dorado Azul

Blends: Brain Power, Clarity, RutaVaLa, RutaVaLa Roll-On, Harmony, Valor, Valor Roll-On, Oola Balance, Oola Grow, Common Sense, 3 Wise Men

Nutritionals: MegaCal, Super B, OmegaGize[3], Digest & Cleanse, Mineral Essence, NingXia Nitro

Application and Usage

Inhalation

- Diffuse your choice of oils for ½ hour every 4-6 hours or as desired.
- Put 2-3 drops of your chosen oil in your hands and rub them together, cup your hands over your nose, and inhale throughout the day as needed.
- Put 8-10 drops of oil on a cotton ball or tissue and put it in an air vent in your house, vehicle, hotel room, etc.
- If diffusing while sleeping, set your timer for the desired length of time for automatic shut off.

Topical

You may apply single oils or blends neat or diluted, depending on the oil or oils being used. Please see the instructions at the beginning of this chapter for more information on applying oils to the skin.

- Apply 1-2 drops neat directly onto the brain reflex centers 2-4 times daily, as needed. These points include the forehead, temples, and mastoids (the bones just behind the ears). Apply oils and mild, direct pressure to the brainstem area (center top of neck at base of skull) and work down the spine.
- Apply 1-2 drops neat to Vita Flex brain points on feet 1-2 times daily.
- Receive a Raindrop Technique once every 2 weeks.

Ingestion and Oral

The amount of oil ingested varies with different oils. Whether putting the oils in a capsule or drinking them in a liquid, please refer to the instructions at the beginning of this chapter.

- Put 2-3 drops of oil in a spoonful of Blue Agave, Yacon Syrup, maple syrup, coconut oil, milk, etc.
- Take 1 capsule with desired oil 2 times daily.
- Put the desired amount of oils in a glass of

rice milk, almond milk, goat milk, carrot juice, NingXia Red, or even water and then drink it.

....

Confusion

Confusion is when a person is not able to think with his or her usual level of clarity. Decision-making ability is reduced, and feeling disoriented is common. Confusion may develop gradually or arise suddenly and has multiple causes, including medical conditions, medications, injuries, environmental factors, substance abuse, stress, low hormones, and low thyroid.

Recommendations

Singles: Peppermint, Lemon, Rosemary, Basil, Sacred Frankincense, Frankincense, Cardamom

Blends: M-Grain, Gathering, Brain Power, Clarity, Oola Balance, Oola Grow, Common Sense, Harmony

Nutritionals: MegaCal, Super B, OmegaGize³, Digest & Cleanse, Mineral Essence, Thyromin, NingXia Red, EndoGize

Application and Usage
Inhalation

- Diffuse your choice of oils for ½ hour every 4-6 hours or as desired.
- Put 2-3 drops of your chosen oil in your hands and rub them together, cup your hands over your nose, and inhale throughout the day as needed.
- Put 8-10 drops of oil on a cotton ball or tissue and put it in an air vent in your house, vehicle, hotel room, etc.
- If diffusing while sleeping, set your timer for the desired length of time for automatic shut off.

Topical

You may apply single oils or blends neat or diluted, depending on the oil or oils being used. Please see the instructions at the beginning of

this chapter for more information on applying oils to the skin.

- Applying a single drop under the nose is helpful and refreshing.
- Dilute 50:50 and apply on location 3-6 times daily.
- Massage 2-4 drops of oil neat on the soles of the feet just before bedtime.

....

Convulsions

Convulsions, also called seizures, are involuntary contractions of the voluntary muscles. Monitor diet and discontinue sugar, dairy products, and fried and processed foods.

Recommendations

Singles: Sacred Frankincense, Frankincense, Palo Santo, Eucalyptus Blue, Copaiba, Western Red Cedar, Wintergreen

Blends: Brain Power, Valor, Valor Roll-On, RutaVaLa, RutaVaLa Roll-On, Tranquil Roll-On, Clarity, Common Sense

Nutritionals: Detoxzyme, AlkaLime, Inner Defense, Mineral Essence

Application and Usage
Inhalation

- Diffuse your choice of oils for ½ hour every 4-6 hours or as desired.
- Put 2-3 drops of your chosen oil in your hands and rub them together, cup your hands over your nose, and inhale throughout the day as needed.
- Put 8-10 drops of oil on a cotton ball or tissue and put it in an air vent in your house, vehicle, hotel room, etc.
- If diffusing while sleeping, set your timer for the desired length of time for automatic shut off.

Topical

You may apply single oils or blends neat or diluted, depending on the oil or oils being used. Please see the instructions at the beginning of

this chapter for more information on applying oils to the skin.

- Apply 2-4 drops neat at base of skull, across the neck, top of spine (C1-C6 vertebrae), and bottom of feet.
- Apply 1-2 drops neat on temples and back of neck as desired.
- Place a warm compress with 1-2 drops of chosen oil on the back.

....

Memory, Impaired

Many areas of the brain help create and retrieve memories. Malfunction of or damage to any of these areas can lead to memory loss.

Recommendations

Singles: Rosemary, Peppermint, Cardamom, Basil, Vetiver, Rose, Lemon, Lemongrass, Helichrysum, Lavender, Rosewood, Tangerine, Spearmint, Idaho Tansy, Palo Santo

Note: Peppermint improves mental concentration and memory. Dr. Dember conducted a study at the University of Cincinnati in 1994 showing that inhaling Peppermint increased mental accuracy by 28 percent. [9]

The fragrances of diffused oils such as Lemon have also been reported to increase memory retention and recall.

Blends: Brain Power, Clarity, M-Grain, En-R-Gee, Oola Balance, Oola Grow

Nutritionals: Longevity Softgels, MultiGreens, Mineral Essence, Thyromin, NingXia Red

Memory Blend No. 1

- 5 drops Basil
- 10 drops Rosemary
- 4 drops Helichrysum
- 2 drops Peppermint
- 2 drops Cardamom

Memory Blend No. 2

- 4 drops Lavender
- 3 drops Geranium
- 3 drops Rosewood

- 3 drops Rosemary
- 2 drops Tangerine
- 1 drop Spearmint

Application and Usage

Inhalation

- Diffuse your choice of oils for ½ hour every 4-6 hours or as desired.
- Put 2-3 drops of your chosen oil in your hands and rub them together, cup your hands over your nose, and inhale throughout the day as needed.
- Put 8-10 drops of oil on a cotton ball or tissue and put it in an air vent in your house, vehicle, hotel room, etc.
- If diffusing while sleeping, set your timer for the desired length of time for automatic shut off.

Topical

You may apply single oils or blends neat or diluted, depending on the oil or oils being used. Please see the instructions at the beginning of this chapter for more information on applying oils to the skin.

- Applying a single drop under the nose is helpful and refreshing.
- Dilute 50:50 and apply 2-3 drops on temples, forehead, mastoids (bone behind ears), and/or brainstem (back of neck) as needed 3-6 times daily.
- Massage 2-4 drops of oil neat on the soles of the feet just before bedtime.

Ingestion and Oral

The amount of oil ingested varies with different oils. Whether putting the oils in a capsule or drinking them in a liquid, please refer to the instructions at the beginning of this chapter.

- Take 1 capsule with desired oil 3 times daily.
- Put 2-3 drops of oil in a spoonful of Blue Agave, Yacon Syrup, maple syrup, coconut oil, milk, etc.

- Put the desired amount of oils in a glass of rice milk, almond milk, goat milk, carrot juice, NingXia Red, or even water and then drink it.

Cleansing
Vascular cleansing may improve mental function by supporting improved blood flow, boosting distribution of oxygen and nutrients (see Vascular Cleansing).

Mental Fatigue
Some of the causes of mental fatigue are being overworked, having poor sleep patterns, lacking exercise, and having a poor diet.

Recommendations
Singles: Sacred Frankincense, Frankincense, Frereana Frankincense, Rosemary, Vetiver, Cedarwood, Peppermint

Blends: Brain Power, Clarity, Valor, Valor Roll-On, RutaVaLa, RutaVaLa Roll-On, Tranquil Roll-On, Oola Balance, Oola Grow

Nutritionals: Thyromin, Super B, EndoGize, MultiGreens, NingXia Red, NingXia Nitro, Master Formula HIS and HERS

Application and Usage
Inhalation
- Diffuse your choice of oils for ½ hour every 4-6 hours or as desired.
- Put 2-3 drops of your chosen oil in your hands and rub them together, cup your hands over your nose, and inhale throughout the day as needed.
- Put 8-10 drops of oil on a cotton ball or tissue and put it in an air vent in your house, vehicle, hotel room, etc.
- If diffusing while sleeping, set your timer for the desired length of time for automatic shut off.

Topical
You may apply single oils or blends neat or diluted, depending on the oil or oils being used.

Please see the instructions at the beginning of this chapter for more information on applying oils to the skin.

- Applying a single drop under the nose is helpful and refreshing.
- Dilute 50:50 and apply 2-3 drops on temples, forehead, mastoids (bone behind ears), and/or brainstem (back of neck) as needed 3-6 times daily.
- Massage 2-4 drops of oil neat on the soles of the feet just before bedtime.

Ingestion and Oral
The amount of oil ingested varies with different oils. Whether putting the oils in a capsule or drinking them in a liquid, please refer to the instructions at the beginning of this chapter.

- Take 1 capsule with desired oil 3 times daily.
- Put 2-3 drops of oil in a spoonful of Blue Agave, Yacon Syrup, maple syrup, coconut oil, milk, etc.
- Put the desired amount of oils in a glass of rice milk, almond milk, goat milk, carrot juice, NingXia Red, or even water and then drink it.

Cleansing
Vascular cleansing may improve mental function by supporting improved blood flow, boosting distribution of oxygen and nutrients (see Vascular Cleansing).

BREASTFEEDING
The most common causes of sore or cracked nipples are poor breastfeeding technique, dehydration, or infection.

Dry, Cracked Nipples

Recommendations
Singles: Myrrh, Vetiver, Sandalwood
Blends: Valor, Valor Roll-on, Harmony, The Gift
Nutritionals: MultiGreens, Master Formula

HIS and HERS, NingXia Red

Creams, Serums, and Oils: Rose Ointment, KidScents Tender Tush, Essential Beauty Serum for Dry Skin, virgin coconut oil

Application and Usage
Topical

You may apply single oils or blends neat or diluted, depending on the oil or oils being used. Please see the instructions at the beginning of this chapter for more information on applying oils to the skin.

- Dilute 50:50 and massage over breast and on Vita Flex points of the feet.

....

Mastitis (Infected Breast)

Mastitis is an infection of the breast tissue that results in pain, swelling, redness, and warmth of the breast. It most commonly affects women who are breastfeeding.

Recommendations

Singles: Myrrh, Melissa, Melaleuca Alternifolia, Thyme, Patchouli, Roman Chamomile, Rosemary, Lavender

Blends: ImmuPower

Nutritionals: Longevity

Massage either of these blends on the breasts and under armpits 2 times daily.

Breast Blend No. 1
- 3 drops Thyme
- 7 drops PanAway
- 1 teaspoon V-6 Vegetable Oil Complex

Breast Blend No. 2
- 3 drops Lemon
- 4 drops Thyme
- 2 drops Melissa
- 1 teaspoon V-6 Vegetable Oil Complex

Breast Blend No. 3
- 3 drops Myrrh
- 3 drops Vetiver
- 2 drops Copaiba
- 1 drop Blue Spruce

- ½ teaspoon V-6 Vegetable Oil Complex

Breast Blend No. 4
- 4 drops Melissa
- 10 drops Myrrh
- 1 drop Thyme
- 1 drop Mountain Savory

Application and Usage
Topical

You may apply single oils or blends neat or diluted, depending on the oil or oils being used. Please see the instructions at the beginning of this chapter for more information on applying oils to the skin.

- Dilute 20:80 and massage over breast and on Vita Flex points of the feet.

BURSITIS

Bursitis is an inflammation of the bursa, which are small, fluid-filled sacs located near the joints. Bursa act as shock absorbers when muscles or tendons come into contact with bone. As the bursa become swollen, they result in pain, particularly when the affected joint is used.

Bursitis can be caused by injury, infection, or arthritis, and usually involves the joints of the knees, elbows, shoulders, and Achilles tendon. Occasionally bursitis can occur in the base of the big toe. Bursitis may signal the beginning of arthritis.

Recommendations

Singles: Wintergreen, Idaho Blue Spruce, Peppermint, Copaiba, Dorado Azul, Palo Santo, Sacred Frankincense, Frankincense, Idaho Balsam Fir, Basil, Lavender, Black Pepper, Idaho Tansy, Elemi, Oregano, Plectranthus Oregano, Marjoram

Blends: PanAway, Relieve It, Sacred Mountain, Deep Relief Roll-On

Nutritionals: Sulfurzyme, MegaCal, BLM

Massage Oil: Ortho Ease Massage Oil, Ortho Sport Massage Oil

Application and Usage
Inhalation
- Diffuse your choice of oils for ½ hour every 4-6 hours or as desired.
- Put 2-3 drops of your chosen oil in your hands and rub them together, cup your hands over your nose, and inhale throughout the day as needed.
- Put 8-10 drops of oil on a cotton ball or tissue and put it in an air vent in your house, vehicle, hotel room, etc.
- If diffusing while sleeping, set your timer for the desired length of time for automatic shut off.

Topical
You may apply single oils or blends neat or diluted, depending on the oil or oils being used. Please see the instructions at the beginning of this chapter for more information on applying oils to the skin.
- Apply 2-4 drops neat or diluted 50:50 on affected area or joint 3-5 times daily or as needed to soothe pain
- Apply a cold compress around affected joint 1-3 times daily.

Ingestion
The amount of oil ingested varies with different oils. Whether putting the oils in a capsule or drinking them in a liquid, please refer to the instructions at the beginning of this chapter.
- Take 1 capsule with desired oil 2 times daily.
- Put 2-3 drops of oil in a spoonful of Blue Agave, Yacon Syrup, maple syrup, coconut oil, milk, etc.
- Put the desired amount of oils in a glass of rice milk, almond milk, goat milk, carrot juice, NingXia Red, or even water and then drink it.

CANCER
Cancer is among the most complex and difficult of any human disease to treat. A patient diagnosed with cancer should always defer to his or her physician for primary care. Keeping this in mind, a number of individuals have achieved successful remission by following a natural protocol and some of the principles outlined in this section.

It is important to note that many natural therapies—especially those using essential oils—work best in the early stages of cancer. In fact, all clinical trials are showing that Frankincense is the number one inhibitor of many cancers. Citrus oils, high in d-limonene, including Orange, Grapefruit, and Tangerine, work better as cancer preventatives than cancer treatments, although they have been tested to have powerful, anticancer properties in all stages of cancer.

A study at Charing Cross Hospital in London, England, published in 1998 achieved close to a 15 percent remission rate in patients with advanced colon and breast cancer using doses from 1 to 15 grams of d-limonene from Orange oil as their only treatment. In patients with only weeks or months to live, limonene treatment extended patients' lives by up to 18 months in some cases.[10]

The Foundation of Natural Cancer Treatment
Natural treatment of cancer or any illness is a highly debated topic, but when you are faced with cancer, finding solutions becomes important.

Emotions and Cancer
Cancer should always be treated first by discovering the underlying emotions that contributed to the onset of the disease. In many cases, negative emotions and trauma not only trigger the beginning of cancer but can further its me-

tastasis. Any kind of negative emotion—anger, fear, rage, helplessness, abandonment—can cause the cancer to spread faster.

When essential oils are used as the basis of an emotional care program, they can have powerfully positive effects in improving the attitude and emotional well-being and potential outcome of the disease. Essential oil blends such as White Angelica, Release, Grounding, Inner Child, Trauma Life, Forgiveness, Joy, Common Sense, Hope, Believe, Peace & Calming, Valor, and SARA can form the center of any emotional care regimen.

Cleansing and Removing Toxins

Industrial pollutants such as benzene and lead, along with lifestyle toxins such as cigarette smoke, chemicals, heterocyclic amines from overcooked meat, and many others contribute to a vast majority of cancers. Even daily radiation from computers, cell phones, and a vast number of electrical appliances may contribute to a toxic overload within the body.

Today's fast-food industry is a major culprit in selling so much nutritionally deficient food that we eat. Processed food is fast and convenient, but is it worth the threat to our health? Cosmetics, hair sprays, dyes, soaps, paints, and household cleaners add to an endless list of pollutants in our environment and toxicity to which we are subjected.

To help lower the risk of cancer, it is important to reduce the exposure to these chemicals and change our diet and the products that we use in our environment. The chemicals should be avoided at all cost, as they can damage DNA, decrease immunity, promote oncogenes (genes that can turn normal cells into cancer cells), and accelerate cancer development.

Cleansing and Chelation

The foundation of any cancer program should begin with a period of cleansing. Cleansing and chelation can help remove some of the toxin- and petrochemical-buildup that may have triggered the cancer initially.

Fasting can be one of the single, most powerful, anticancer tools available, particularly in the early stages. Anyone who is in advanced stages of cancer must cleanse very slowly to see how the body responds. Going without food and drinking only juices immediately could be detrimental to a sick body. Common sense needs to be used in all situations.

Essential oils that improve liver function and promote glutathione can form the center of any detoxification program. Lemon and Orange oils, in studies at Johns Hopkins University, have shown to substantially increase glutathione levels in the liver and colon, which have beneficial effects in detoxification.

Chelation can be particularly important in removing carcinogenic metals from the body. Studies in Germany have shown that transition metals such as iron, mercury, lead, zinc, nickel, and cadmium can accumulate to high levels in tumors, particularly in breast cancer tissue. A series of chelations to eliminate these metals can produce tremendous benefits in the earliest stage of cancer.[11]

Rice bran is a good chelator of metals and contains anticancer phytonutrients such as gamma oryzanol and other compounds. It is also rich in immune stimulating arabinoxylans that increase cancer cell death.[12]

The Ningxia wolfberry is rich in polysaccharides that similarly amplify immunity. A number of clinical research trials have shown that wolfberry compounds can dramatically improve cancer remission, particularly when combined with immune-stimulating therapies.[13]

Cleansing Products Suitable for Most Cancers

Many products support the body in its cleansing process. You will not be able to take all the cleansing products, so decide which ones you want to take and how much you want to take of each product. Write down your program so you can follow it consistently. Start slowly so your body can adjust and begin to cleanse.

Cleansing: Essentialzyme, Detoxzyme, Essentialzymes-4, JuvaPower, JuvaTone, ComforTone, DiGize, GLF, JuvaCleanse, JuvaFlex, NingXia Red

Emotional Support: Sacred Frankincense, Frankincense, Lavender, Palo Santo, Rose, Ylang Ylang, Amazonian Ylang Ylang, Acceptance, Believe, Brain Power, Common Sense, Dream Catcher, Gathering, Envision, Forgiveness, Gratitude, Harmony, Hope, Joy, Live with Passion, Motivation, Present Time, Peace & Calming, RutaVaLa, RutaVaLa Roll-On, The Gift, Transformation, Valor, White Angelica

Enzymes Ramping Protocol

Essentialzyme was formulated in 1984 with this protocol for someone suffering from a degenerative disease.

Phase 1: Take 3 tablets 3 times daily. Increase by 1 tablet every day until you become nauseous and then discontinue Essentialzyme for 24 to 36 hours.

Phase 2: Take 4 tablets 3 times daily. Increase daily by 1 tablet until you become nauseous. Rest (discontinue) again for 24-36 hours.

Phase 3: Take 5 tablets 3 times daily. Increase daily by 1 tablet until you become nauseous. Rest for 24-36 hours.

Phase 4: Start again with the amount that you were taking before the nausea occurred the third time. For example: If you were taking 18 tablets, you would have been taking 6 tablets 3 times daily when you became nauseous. Therefore, start Phase 4 again with 6 tablets 3 times daily and continue with this amount for 6 weeks.

Phase 5: In the 7th week, start the enzyme-ramping program all over again. This means to begin phase 1 again and increase the amount by 1 each day until nausea or vomiting starts again. Repeat and continue for 6 weeks as previously described.

If your doctor determines that you are in remission, you can maintain with 5-10 tablets daily for one year, 6 days a week.

Maintenance: Take 5-10 Essentialzyme tablets 3 times daily.

Caution: This is a very rigorous program, so you should consult with your doctor or health-care professional before starting and have that person monitor your progress during the program.

Why Fasting Works

New research has uncovered that insulin receptors make cancer cells different from normal cells. Cancer cells have over 10 times the number of receptors for insulin as a normal cell. Excess insulin can stimulate cancer cells disproportionately compared to well-differentiated cells. Similarly, because cancer cells are fast-growing, they require far more glucose (blood sugar) than normal cells.

The most effective way of lowering both insulin and blood glucose levels is with a fast. Bernard Jensen, ND, used a 180-day fast, made initially of only barley grass juice, to fight and eliminate metastatic prostate cancer. Even a partial fast in which refined carbohydrates are eliminated and caloric intake is reduced to 500-1,000 calories can be potentially very therapeutic.

Determining Hormone Sensitivity

Women dealing with breast, ovarian, uterine, and cervical cancer in most cases can be estrogen receptor sensitive, yet doctors will continue to give and recommend HRT (hormone replacement therapy) made from xenoestrogens that come from petrochemicals, compounds that are known to promote and cause cancer, before determining if a patient has cancer in the early stages of development.

However, we must understand the mechanism of what happens. First cholesterol cascades down to pregnenolone to progestogens and then to androgens that divide and go to the ovaries and testes.

In the ovaries, the androgens, called androstenedione, cross the basal membrane, where they are converted to the estradiol sex hormones such as estradiol, estrone, and estriol. The ovaries produce primarily estradiol. Most free circulating estrone stems from a conversion of estradiol in the liver, even though the ovaries produce small amounts of estrone.

The liver plays a major role as the chemistry laboratory of the body. Because the liver is the body's largest fat-storing organ, it will hold petrochemicals known as xenoestrogens that are cancer-causing agents. Xenoestrogens disrupt the conversion of estradiol and cause a division of the estrone.

This division will be either negative or positive. If estradiol converts to 16-alpha-hydroxyestrone, a cancer-causing agent, this estrone will then bind to the estrogen receptors in female and male reproductive organs. If estradiol converts to 2-hydroxyestrone, a cancer-*preventing* steroid hormone, it will bind or stick to the receptors, protecting them from the harmful estrone. This has caused a lot of controversy among the natural health and allopathic practitioners for years.

Natural hormones produced in the body are referred to as steroid hormones. Synthetic hormones are called nonsteroid hormones. Most people do not understand that plant hormones are neither steroid nor nonsteroid hormones. They are natural phytohormones that encourage the production of 2-hydroxyestrone, the cancer preventive hormone that does not bind or stick to the receptor sites contrary to the nonsteroid hormones that cause inflammation and cysts on the ovaries.

There is no evidence that phytohormones will stimulate estrogen-sensitive cancer. Phytohormones are the same as the hormone-supporting chemical compounds found in the essential oils of Fennel, Clary Sage, Melissa, Lemongrass, Sage, etc.

There is also no reason to be concerned about food unless it is a GMO food like soy. Herbs like black cohosh do not stimulate estrogen-sensitive cancer. Quite simply they are neither steroid- nor nonsteroid-stimulating hormones.

Another concern is to understand that metabolic enzymes are required to help facilitate steroid hormone conversion. When the body and liver are toxic, this becomes a serious problem, creating a metabolic enzyme deficiency. In the absence of metabolic enzymes and a toxic liver, estradiol is converted to 16-alpha-hydroxyestrone, the cancer-causing hormone.

The hormones that naturally occur in milk require metabolic hormones to ensure they are converted to 2-hydroxyestrone. When the milk goes through the pasteurization process, it kills the enzymes necessary for the 2-hydroxyestrone conversion and converts to the cancer-causing 16-alpha-hydroxyestrone.

Essentialzyme is the metabolic enzyme, which makes it so important for daily prevention and good health.

Pasteurized milk is also a concern because milk contains steroid hormones fed to cows.

When milk products are pasteurized and homogenized, whether it is milk, cheese, butter, cottage cheese, or any other product containing steroid hormones, the pasteurization destroys the natural enzymes, thus preventing the production of 2-hydroxyestrone, the cancer-prevention steroid, and instead converts it to 16-alpha-hydroxyestrone, the cancer-causing hormone.

This is where the controversy begins and the misunderstanding of estrogen-sensitive cancers becomes a problem. It is easy to see how processed and non-processed foods affect the outcome of our health.

This does not apply only to women but applies to men as well. Men have estrogen also and will respond the same way to both phytoestrogens and mycoestrogens (estrogens produced by fungi found in stored grain) that stimulate the production of 16-alpha-hydroxyestrone. If there were more focus on eating unprocessed foods; cleansing the liver of toxins, petrochemicals, and undigested pollutants; and improving and building a reserve of metabolic enzymes, there would be much less cancer.

Cancer and Antioxidants

It is recommended to seek the advice from a health-care professional before embarking on any antioxidant program. Some studies have reported that certain antioxidants can reduce the effectiveness of some types of chemotherapy such as cisplatin.

A large number of other studies have found the opposite, showing that antioxidants can improve patient remissions and prognosis. In the case of radiation treatments, a number of well-controlled studies have similarly found that antioxidants can improve patient outcomes dramatically and counter the injury and immune suppression caused by these therapies.

In fact, a 2010 human study by A. Pace [1] that vitamin E had a neuroprotective effect against the serious, adverse effects of cisplatin.[14]

Similar to DNA-protective essential oils, antioxidants produce their best results as cancer preventatives and in the earliest stages of cancer. As cancer progresses, the likelihood of meaningful remissions using only antioxidants declines rapidly.

Research conducted at Brigham Young University in Provo, Utah, and the UNLV Cancer Research Institute identified some of the most inhibitory essential oils against a variety of cancer cell lines. The oils were also tested for their lack of toxicity to normal cells.

Inflammation and Cancer

The link between cancer and inflammation has become stronger in recent years. It is well known that the salicylates in aspirin have high anti-inflammatory effects and reduce the risk of colon cancer dramatically.

The natural salicylates found in the essential oil of Wintergreen are very close in structure to the acetyl salicylic acid found in aspirin. According to Erica Leibert of Harvard University, Wintergreen oil is 40 percent stronger than an aspirin equivalent with very similar anti-inflammatory properties.

Clove has been researched as a potential chemopreventive agent for lung cancer because of its powerful anti-inflammatory effects.[15] The biochemical alpha-humulene in the oil, also found in Idaho Balsam Fir and Copaiba, has been shown to have significant cancer prevention properties through its anti-inflammatory action.[16]

Frankincense and conifer oils like Idaho Balsam Fir containing l-limonene are coming to the forefront of attention in cancer research in various cancer-treatment study programs at Oklahoma State University, Wake Forest University, and Virginia-Maryland Regional College of Veterinary Medicine.

The l-limonene found in Frankincense, Idaho Blue Spruce, and Idaho Balsam Fir shows a remarkable ability to suppress tumor growth, particularly in melanoma. Boswellic acids found in frankincense gum resin have also been shown to have powerful, anti-inflammatory effects. Myrrh gum has been studied for its ability to combat various cancers, including breast cancer.

Anti-inflammatory Essential Oils Suitable for Most Cancers: Frankincense, Clove, Idaho Balsam Fir, Palo Santo, Ledum, Myrrh, Wintergreen

Immunity and Cancer

Enhancing immune function is a vital component of both traditional and complementary approaches to cancer. Typically, chemotherapy and radiation can drastically break down populations of T-cells and NK (natural killer) cells that are responsible for fighting tumor growth. Certain natural compounds can restore levels of these critical immune components.

Singles: Sacred Frankincense, Frankincense, Idaho Blue Spruce, Idaho Balsam Fir, Sandalwood, Palo Santo, Hyssop, Thyme, Clove, Melaleuca Alternifolia

Blends: Citrus Fresh, Thieves, Exodus II, Melrose, GLF, ImmuPower, 3 Wise Men, DiGize

Immune-Enhancing Supplements Suitable for Most Cancers: ImmuPro, Super C, Super C Chewable, Master Formulas HIS or HERS, Essentialzyme, Detoxzyme, Essentialzymes-4, MultiGreens, NingXia Red

Breast Cancer

Recommendations

Singles: Sacred Frankincense, Frankincense, Sandalwood, Myrtle, Tsuga

Nutritionals: NingXia Red, Super C, Essentialzyme, AlkaLime

Cervical Cancer

Recommendations

Singles: Patchouli, Sandalwood, Galbanum, Valerian, Sacred Frankincense, Frankincense, Tsuga, Douglas Fir, Hyssop, Nutmeg, Tarragon

Nutritionals: NingXia Red, Super C, Essentialzyme, AlkaLime

Leukemia

Recommendations

Singles: Clove, Hyssop, Idaho Blue Spruce, Sacred Frankincense

Nutritionals: NingXia Red, Super C, Essentialzyme, AlkaLime

Lung Cancer

Recommendations

Singles: Sacred Frankincense, Frankincense, Idaho Blue Spruce, Palo Santo, Sandalwood, Clove, Thyme, Hyssop

Nutritionals: NingXia Red, Super C, Essentialzyme, AlkaLime

Prostate Cancer

Recommendations

Singles: Sacred Frankincense, Frankincense, Sage, Western Red Cedar, Thyme, Sandalwood, Myrtle, Dill, Idaho Blue Spruce

Nutritionals: Protec, NingXia Red, Super C, Essentialzyme, AlkaLime

Skin Cancer (Melanoma)

Recommendations

Singles: Sacred Frankincense, Frankincense, Thyme, Sandalwood, Grapefruit, Hyssop, Tarragon

Nutritionals: NingXia Red, Super C, Essentialzyme, AlkaLime

Tumors

Recommendations

Singles: Sacred Frankincense, Frankincense, Western Red Cedar, Sage, Sandalwood, Grapefruit, Hyssop, Myrtle, Idaho Blue Spruce

Nutritionals: NingXia Red, Super C, Essentialzyme, AlkaLime

Uterine Cancer

Recommendations

Singles: Sacred Frankincense, Frankincense, Sage, Western Red Cedar, Thyme, Sandalwood, Myrtle, Dill, Idaho Blue Spruce

Nutritionals: Protec

CARDIOVASCULAR CONDITIONS AND PROBLEMS

Cardiovascular conditions are those that affect the heart and other circulatory organs.

Anemia

Anemia is a condition caused from insufficient red blood cells. There can be many different causes of anemia, which would suggest that you should see your physician for proper diagnosis. Nutritional deficiencies of iron or vitamin B12 can contribute to this disorder as well as to improper liver function. A liver cleanse and nutritional support will certainly help in rebuilding red blood cell counts.

Recommendations

Singles: German Chamomile, Thyme, Sacred Frankincense, Frankincense, Helichrysum, Lemon, Mountain Savory, Rosemary

Blends: JuvaCleanse, DiGize, EndoFlex, JuvaFlex

Nutritionals: JuvaPower, MultiGreens, Super B, Rehemogen, NingXia Red, JuvaSpice (for salads and cooking), Master HIS or HERS, Mineral Essence

Application and Usage

Inhalation

- Diffuse your choice of oils for ½ hour every 4-6 hours or as desired.
- Put 2-3 drops of your chosen oil in your hands and rub them together, cup your hands over your nose, and inhale throughout the day as needed.
- Put 8-10 drops of oil on a cotton ball or tissue and put it in an air vent in your house, vehicle, hotel room, etc.
- If diffusing while sleeping, set your timer for the desired length of time for automatic shut off.

Topical

•You may apply single oils or blends neat or diluted, depending on the oil or oils being used. Please see the instructions at the beginning of this chapter for more information on applying oils to the skin.

Ingestion and Oral

The amount of oil ingested varies with different oils. Whether putting the oils in a capsule or drinking them in a liquid, please refer to the directions at the beginning of this chapter.

- Take 2 capsules 2 times daily filled with half Helichrysum and half Cistus.
- Put 2-3 drops of oil in a spoonful of Blue Agave, Yacon Syrup, maple syrup, coconut oil, milk, etc.
- Put the desired amount of oils in a glass of rice milk, almond milk, goat milk, carrot juice, NingXia Red, or even water and then drink it.

Aneurysm

Aneurysms are weak spots on the blood vessel walls that balloon out and may eventually rupture. In cases of brain aneurysms, a bursting blood vessel can cause a stroke, which can result in death or paralysis. (The fatality rate is over 50 percent in the U.S.) See your physician immediately.

Some essential oils and nutritional supplements support the cardiovascular system and help with blood regulation. Cypress strengthens capillary and vascular walls. Helichrysum helps dissolve blood clots.

Recommendations

Singles: Cistus, Helichrysum, Cypress, Lemon
Blends: Aroma Life, JuvaCleanse, Purification
Nutritionals: NingXia Red, BLM, Essentialzyme, Pure Protein, Ningxia Wolfberries (Dried), Digest & Cleanse, Detoxzyme

Aneurysm Blend

- 5 drops Cistus
- 1 drop Helichrysum
- 1 drop Cypress

Inhalation

- Diffuse your choice of oils for 1 hour every 4-6 hours or as desired.
- Put 2-3 drops of your chosen oil in your hands and rub them together, cup your hands over your nose, and inhale throughout the day as needed.
- Put 8-10 drops of oil on a cotton ball or tissue and put it in an air vent in your house, vehicle, hotel room, etc.
- If diffusing while sleeping, set your timer for the desired length of time for automatic shut off.

Topical

You may apply single oils or blends neat or diluted, depending on the oil or oils being used. Please see the instructions at the beginning of this chapter for more information on applying oils to the skin.

- Dilute essential oils with V-6 Vegetable Oil Complex 50:50 and massage on back of neck and head 3-5 times daily.

Ingestion and Oral

The amount of oil ingested varies with different oils. Whether putting the oils in a capsule or drinking them in a liquid, please refer to the instructions at the beginning of this chapter.

- Take 1 capsule with cistus or cypress or other desired oil 2 times daily.
- Take 2 capsules 2 times daily 50:50 with Cistus and Cypress.
- Put 2-3 drops of oil in a spoonful of Blue Agave, Yacon Syrup, maple syrup, coconut oil, milk, etc.
- Put the desired amount of oils in a glass of rice milk, almond milk, goat milk, carrot juice, NingXia Red, or even water and then drink it.

....

Angina

Angina is a severe and crushing chest pain caused from an inadequate supply of oxygen to the heart muscle.

Recommendations

Singles: Clove, Marjoram, Helichrysum, Goldenrod, Orange, Lemon, Wintergreen
Blends: DiGize, Aroma Life, Peace & Calming, Stress Away Roll-On, Valor, Valor Roll-On, RutaVaLa, RutaVaLa Roll-On, Longevity
Nutritionals: NingXia Red, Ningxia Wolfberries (Dried), OmegaGize[3], MegaCal, Longevity Softgels, Essentialzyme, Detoxzyme

Application and Usage

Inhalation

- Diffuse your choice of oils for ½ hour every 4-6 hours or as desired.
- Put 2-3 drops of your chosen oil in your hands and rub them together, cup your hands over your nose, and inhale throughout the day as needed.
- Put 8-10 drops of oil on a cotton ball or tissue and put it in an air vent in your house, vehicle, hotel room, etc.
- If diffusing while sleeping, set your timer for the desired length of time for automatic shut off.

Topical

You may apply single oils or blends neat or diluted, depending on the oil or oils being used. Please see the instructions at the beginning of this chapter for more information on applying oils to the skin.

- Massage 1-3 drops neat over the heart area 1-3 times daily.
- Apply on left side of chest, left shoulder, and back of neck.
- Massage 1 drop each of 2 or 3 of the recommended oils on the heart Vita Flex points on foot, hand, and arm, as needed.

Ingestion and Oral

The amount of oil ingested varies with different oils. Whether putting the oils in a capsule or drinking them in a liquid, please refer to the instructions at the beginning of this chapter.

- Take 1-2 capsules with desired oil 2 times daily.
- Put 2-3 drops of oil in a spoonful of Blue Agave, Yacon Syrup, maple syrup, coconut oil, milk, etc.
- Put the desired amount of oils in a glass of rice milk, almond milk, goat milk, carrot juice, NingXia Red, or even water and then drink it.

....

Arteriosclerosis (Hardening of the Arteries)

This condition is defined as any one of a group of diseases that causes a thickening and a loss of elasticity of arterial walls. It can be caused by inflammation and is frequently an underlying cause of a heart attack or stroke.

Recommendations

Singles: Clove, Helichrysum, Geranium, Lavender, German Chamomile, Cumin, Dorado Azul

Blends: Longevity, Aroma Life

Nutritionals: Longevity Softgels, OmegaGize³, MegaCal, Ningxia Wolfberries (Dried), NingXia Red, Master Formula HIS or HERS

Application and Usage

Inhalation

- Diffuse your choice of oils for ½ hour every 4-6 hours or as desired.
- Put 2-3 drops of your chosen oil in your hands and rub them together, cup your hands over your nose, and inhale throughout the day as needed.
- Put 8-10 drops of oil on a cotton ball or tissue and put it in an air vent in your house, vehicle, hotel room, etc.
- If diffusing while sleeping, set your timer for the desired length of time for automatic shut off.

Topical

You may apply single oils or blends neat or diluted, depending on the oil or oils being used. Please see the instructions at the beginning of this chapter for more information on applying oils to the skin.

- Massage 1-3 drops neat over the heart area 2-3 times weekly.
- Apply on left side of chest, left shoulder, and back of neck.
- Massage 1 drop each of 2 or 3 of the recommended oils on the heart Vita Flex points on foot, hand, and arm, as needed.

Ingestion and Oral

The amount of oil ingested varies with different oils. Whether putting the oils in a capsule or drinking them in a liquid, please refer to the instructions at the beginning of this chapter.

- Take 1 capsule with desired oil 2 times daily.
- Put 2-3 drops of oil in a spoonful of Blue Agave, Yacon Syrup, maple syrup, coconut oil, milk, etc.
- Put the desired amount of oils in a glass of rice milk, almond milk, goat milk, carrot juice, NingXia Red, or even water and then drink it.

Bleeding (Hemorrhaging)

Some essential oils, when topically applied or used on pressure bandages, are excellent for slowing bleeding and initiating healing.

Recommendations

Singles: Helichrysum, Geranium, Cistus, Cypress, Lavender, Myrrh

Blends: Purification, Trauma Life, Deep Relief Roll-On

Nutritionals: JuvaPower, Master Formula HIS or HERS

Application and Usage
Topical

You may apply single oils or blends neat or diluted, depending on the oil or oils being used. Please see the instructions at the beginning of this chapter for more information on applying oils to the skin.

- Apply 1-2 drops neat (undiluted) on the location of small wounds.
- You may also apply 2-3 drops on the Vita Flex points of the feet.
- Place a cold compress diluted with 1-2 drops of Helichrysum, Myrrh, etc.

Blood Circulation, Poor

Essential oils, when used regularly, can improve circulation as much as 20 percent.

Recommendations

Singles: Helichrysum, Cypress, Clove, Idaho Balsam Fir, Cistus, Idaho Blue Spruce

Blends: Aroma Life, EndoFlex, En-R-Gee, Longevity, Valor, Valor Roll-On

Nutritionals: NingXia Red, Longevity Softgels, Ningxia Wolfberries (Dried), Mineral Essence

Application and Usage
Topical

You may apply single oils or blends neat or diluted, depending on the oil or oils being used.

Please see the instructions at the beginning of this chapter for more information on applying oils to the skin.

- Apply neat 2-3 drops on Vita Flex points of feet or on inside of wrists 2-3 times daily.

Ingestion and Oral

The amount of oil ingested varies with different oils. Whether putting the oils in a capsule or drinking them in a liquid, please refer to the instructions at the beginning of this chapter.

- Take 1 capsule with Helichrysum, Cypress, or other desired oil 2 times daily.
- Put 2-3 drops of oil in a spoonful of Blue Agave, Yacon Syrup, maple syrup, coconut oil, milk, etc.
- Put the desired amount of oils in a glass of rice milk, almond milk, goat milk, carrot juice, NingXia Red, or even water and then drink it.

Blood Clots (Embolism, Hematoma, Thrombus)

A blood clot, or hematoma, is a tumor-like mass of coagulated blood, caused by a break in the blood vessel or capillary wall.

Essential oils such as Helichrysum, Geranium, and Cistus are excellent for balancing blood viscosity and dissolving clots. Clove oil and citrus rind oils, such as Lemon and Grapefruit, exert a blood-thinning effect that can help speed the dissolution of the clot.

These oils are also some of the most powerful antioxidants known and can slow the formation of oxidized cholesterol in cells, which contributes to atherosclerosis. Helichrysum is effective in preventing blood clot formation and promoting the dissolution of clots.

As people age, the viscosity or thickness of the blood increases and so does the tendency of the blood to clot excessively.

If blood clots, known as embolisms, occur

in the brain, they can cause strokes; if they obstruct a coronary artery, they can cause ischemic heart attacks.

People with diabetes or high blood pressure are far more likely to die from blood clots.

Foods rich in vitamin E, vitamin A, and omega-3 fats are vital for proper blood viscosity.

Recommendations

Singles: Helichrysum, Cistus, Clove, Geranium, Lemon, Grapefruit, Nutmeg, Cypress, Wintergreen

Blends: Aroma Life, PanAway, Relieve It, Longevity, DiGize

Nutritionals: OmegaGize^3, Super C, Super C Chewable, Mineral Essence, Longevity Softgels, Thieves, Inner Defense, NingXia Red

> **Oral Care:** Thieves Dentarome toothpastes contain Clove, which has natural blood-thinning properties.

Application and Usage

Inhalation

- Diffuse your choice of oils for ½ hour every 4-6 hours or as desired.
- Put 2-3 drops of your chosen oil in your hands and rub them together, cup your hands over your nose, and inhale throughout the day as needed.
- Put 8-10 drops of oil on a cotton ball or tissue and put it in an air vent in your house, vehicle, hotel room, etc.
- If diffusing while sleeping, set your timer for the desired length of time for automatic shut off.

Topical

You may apply single oils or blends neat or diluted, depending on the oil or oils being used. Please see the instructions at the beginning of this chapter for more information on applying oils to the skin.

- Massage equal parts Lemon, Lavender, and Helichrysum on location with or without hot packs.
- Massage equal parts Cistus, Lavender, and Helichrysum on location.
- Place a warm compress with 1-2 drops of chosen oil on the back for 15 minutes 2 times daily.

Ingestion and Oral

The amount of oil ingested varies with different oils. Whether putting the oils in a capsule or drinking them in a liquid, please refer to the instructions at the beginning of this chapter.

- Take 1 capsule with desired oil 2 times daily.
- Take 2 capsules diluted 50:50 with Helichrysum and Cistus 2 times daily between meals.
- Put 2-3 drops of oil in a spoonful of Blue Agave, Yacon Syrup, maple syrup, coconut oil, milk, etc.
- Put the desired amount of oils in a glass of rice milk, almond milk, goat milk, carrot juice, NingXia Red, or even water and then drink it.

....

Blood Detoxification

When there are fewer toxins in the blood, it is easier for the blood to function properly and to continually carry the needed nutrients throughout the body and the digested waste and toxins out of the body, which is the key for staying healthy and being able to fight disease and expel chemicals and other pollutants.

Recommendations

Singles: Helichrysum, Goldenrod, Geranium, German Chamomile, Clove, Idaho Balsam Fir, Mountain Savory

Blends: DiGize, GLF

Nutritionals: JuvaCleanse, MultiGreens, Rehemogen, ICP, JuvaPower, JuvaSpice (for salads and cooking), Sulfurzyme, Balance Complete, Slique Tea

> MSM (found in Sulfurzyme) purifies the body and blood.

Application and Usage
Topical
You may apply single oils or blends neat or diluted, depending on the oil or oils being used. Please see the instructions at the beginning of this chapter for more information on applying oils to the skin.

- Massage 2-3 drops neat (undiluted) on the Vita Flex points of the feet and on the inside of the wrists 2-3 times daily.

Ingestion and Oral
Look up the specific action of these oils and decide what best targets your desired results.

The amount of oil ingested varies with different oils. Whether putting the oils in a capsule or drinking them in a liquid, please refer to the instructions at the beginning of this chapter.

- Take 1 capsule of GLF or JuvaCleanse, plus rosemary or other desired oil, 2 times daily.
- Put 2-3 drops of oil in a spoonful of Blue Agave, Yacon Syrup, maple syrup, coconut oil, milk, etc.
- Put the desired amount of oils in a glass of rice milk, almond milk, goat milk, carrot juice, NingXia Red, or even water and then drink it.

....

Blood Platelets (Low)
Blood platelets (thrombocytes) are necessary for fighting infections and for blood clotting. To avoid a drastic drop in the platelet level, consume leafy vegetables, fruits like bananas and oranges, and dairy products.

Recommendations
Singles: Lemon, Thyme, Melaleuca Alternifolia, Geranium, Cypress

Blends: Aroma Life

Nutritionals: JuvaTone, Rehemogen, JuvaPower, JuvaSpice

To enhance the effects of Rehemogen, use it with JuvaTone, JuvaPower, or JuvaSpice (for salads and cooking).

....

Blood Pressure, High (Hypertension)
One way to help normalize blood pressure is to cleanse the liver and colon for better circulation. Cleansing the colon will help rid the body of wastes and toxins that could be clogging the normal process of digestion. Cleansing and digestion are critical to normal body function.

Recommendations
Singles: Ocotea, Rosemary, Clove, Lavender, Marjoram, Ylang Ylang, Amazonian Ylang Ylang, Cypress, Cinnamon

Blends: Aroma Life, Peace & Calming, Citrus Fresh, Humility, Slique Essence

Nutritionals: Essentialzyme, Detoxzyme, OmegaGize^3, ImmuPro, Super B, Mineral Essence, Balance Complete, MegaCal, Ningxia Wolfberries (Dried), Slique Tea

Application and Usage
Inhalation
- Diffuse your choice of oils for ½ hour 3 times daily.
- Inhalation of Jasmine reduces anxiety in some people and thereby lowers blood pressure.
- Put 2-3 drops of your chosen oil in your hands and rub them together, cup your hands over your nose, and inhale throughout the day as needed.
- Put 8-10 drops of oil on a cotton ball or tissue and put it in an air vent in your house, vehicle, hotel room, etc.
- If diffusing while sleeping, set your timer for the desired length of time for automatic shut off.

Topical
You may apply single oils or blends neat or diluted, depending on the oil or oils being used. Please see the instructions at the beginning of this chapter for more information on applying oils to the skin.

- Apply 1-3 drops oil diluted 20:80 for a full

body massage daily.
- Rub 1-2 drops of oil on the temples and back of neck several times daily.
- Place a warm compress with 1-2 drops of chosen oil on the back.
- For 3 minutes, massage 1-2 drops each of Aroma Life and Ylang Ylang (or Amazonian Ylang Ylang) on the heart Vita Flex point and over the heart and carotid arteries along the neck.
- Notice how the blood pressure will begin to drop within 5-20 minutes. Monitor the pressure and reapply as desired.

Ingestion

The amount of oil ingested varies with different oils. Whether putting the oils in a capsule or drinking them in a liquid, please refer to the instructions at the beginning of this chapter.
- Take 1 capsule with desired oil 2 times daily.
- Put 2-3 drops of oil in a spoonful of Blue Agave, Yacon Syrup, maple syrup, coconut oil, milk, etc.
- Put the desired amount of oils in a glass of rice milk, almond milk, goat milk, carrot juice, NingXia Red, or even water and then drink it.
- Increase the intake of magnesium, which acts as a smooth-muscle relaxant and as a natural calcium channel blocker for the heart, lowering blood pressure and dilating the heart blood vessels.
- Take 1 teaspoon of MegaCal before going to bed.
- Take 1-2 droppers of Mineral Essence 2 times daily.
- Take 1 Super B daily with your meal. Vitamin B3 (niacin) 20 mg daily is an excellent vasodilator found in Super B.

Bruising
(See also Bruised Muscles)

Some people bruise easily because the capillary walls are weak and break easily, particularly in the skin. Those who bruise easily may be deficient in vitamin C.

Essential oils can help speed the healing of bruises and reduce the risk of blood clot formation. Oils like Cypress help to strengthen capillary walls, while oils like Helichrysum help speed the reabsorption of the blood that has collected in the tissue.

Recommendations

Singles: Helichrysum, Cistus, Geranium, Lavender, Spikenard, Cypress, Roman Chamomile, Idaho Blue Spruce, Dorado Azul

Blends: Deep Relief Roll-On

Nutritionals: MultiGreens, JuvaTone, JuvaPower, JuvaSpice, Super C, Super C Chewable, NingXia Red, Slique Tea

Bruise Blend No. 1
- 5 drops Helichrysum
- 4 drops Lavender
- 3 drops Cypress
- 3 drops Cistus
- 3 drops Geranium

Bruise Blend No. 2
- 6 drops Clove
- 4 drops Black Pepper
- 3 drops Peppermint
- 2 drops Marjoram
- 2 drops Geranium
- 2 drops Cypress

Application and Usage
Topical

You may apply single oils or blends neat or diluted, depending on the oil or oils being used. Please see the instructions at the beginning of this chapter for more information on applying oils to the skin.

- Apply 2-3 drops neat 2-3 times daily, depending on which oil you choose. Helichrysum is especially beneficial in healing bruises when applied neat on location.
- Dilute the oil you choose 50:50 with V-6 Vegetable Oil Complex and apply 1-3 drops on bruised area 2-5 times daily.
- Apply a cold compress on location 2-4 times daily or as needed.

Ingestion and Oral

The amount of oil ingested varies with different oils. Whether putting the oils in a capsule or drinking them in a liquid, please refer to the instructions at the beginning of this chapter.

- Take 1 capsule with desired oil 2 times daily.
- Put 2-3 drops of oil in a spoonful of Blue Agave, Yacon Syrup, maple syrup, coconut oil, milk, etc.
- Put the desired amount of oils in a glass of rice milk, almond milk, goat milk, carrot juice, NingXia Red, or even water and then drink it.
- Take 1-4 tablets of Super C Chewable daily.
- Take 2-3 capsules of MultiGreens 3 times daily.

....

Cholesterol, High

When fatty cholesterol deposits accumulate in the arteries, physical symptoms like chest pains and heart attacks may take place.

Recommendations

Singles: Lemongrass, Rosemary, Clove, German Chamomile, Roman Chamomile, Spikenard

Blends: Aroma Life, Longevity, Slique Essence

Nutritionals: OmegaGize³, Essentialzyme, Detoxzyme, Mineral Essence, MegaCal, JuvaPower, JuvaSpice, MultiGreens, Super C, Super C Chewable, SuperCal, Longevity Softgels, ICP, Essentialzymes-4, Balance Complete, Slique Tea, Slique Bars

Cholesterol Reducing Blend
- 5 drops Roman Chamomile
- 5 drops Lemongrass
- 4 drops Rosemary
- 3 drops Helichrysum

Application and Usage
Topical

You may apply single oils or blends neat or diluted, depending on the oil or oils being used. Please see the instructions at the beginning of this chapter for more information on applying oils to the skin.

- Apply neat or dilute 50:50, if needed, 2-4 drops at pulse points, where arteries are close to the surface (wrists, inside elbows, base of throat), 2-3 times daily.
- Also rub 6-10 drops along spine 3 times daily.
- Have a body massage 2 times weekly.

Ingestion and Oral

The amount of oil ingested varies with different oils. Whether putting the oils in a capsule or drinking them in a liquid, please refer to the instructions at the beginning of this chapter.

- Take 1 capsule with desired oil 2 times daily.
- Put 2-3 drops of oil in a spoonful of Blue Agave, Yacon Syrup, maple syrup, coconut oil, milk, etc.
- Put the desired amount of oils in a glass of rice milk, almond milk, goat milk, carrot juice, NingXia Red, or even water and then drink it.

Supplementation regimens

1. Do a colon and liver cleanse using ICP, ComforTone, Essentialzyme, JuvaTone, JuvaPower or JuvaSpice, JuvaFlex, and Juva-Cleanse. JuvaTone is particularly useful for high cholesterol.
2. Magnesium acts as a smooth muscle relaxant and supports the cardiovascular system. It acts as a natural calcium channel blocker

for the heart, lowering blood pressure and dilating the heart blood vessels (Dr. T. Friedmann). Mineral Essence and MegaCal are good sources of magnesium.

....

Congestive Heart Failure
(See also Heart Attack)

Congestive heart failure is the inability of the heart to supply enough blood to meet the demands of the body. The most common cause is coronary artery disease, a narrowing of the small blood vessels that supply oxygen and blood to the heart.

Symptoms include shortness of breath, loss of appetite, cough, fatigue, weakness, swollen abdomen, need to urinate at night, weight gain, and swollen feet and ankles.

Coenzyme Q10 is one of the most effective supplements for supporting the heart muscle.

Recommendations

Singles: Helichrysum, Goldenrod, Clove, Marjoram, Cypress

Blends: Aroma Life, Longevity

Nutritionals: MegaCal, Mineral Essence, Coenzyme Q10

Application and Usage
Topical

You may apply single oils or blends neat or diluted, depending on the oil or oils being used. Please see the instructions at the beginning of this chapter for more information on applying oils to the skin.

- Apply 1-2 drops neat to heart Vita Flex points on foot, hand, and arm, as described under the "Heart Vita Flex" section under the topic Heart Health.
- Apply neat or dilute 50:50, if needed, 2-4 drops at pulse points, where arteries are close to the surface (wrists, inside elbows, base of throat), 2-3 times daily.
- Also rub 6-10 drops along spine 3 times daily.

- Have a body massage 2 times weekly.

Ingestion and Oral

The amount of oil ingested varies with different oils. Whether putting the oils in a capsule or drinking them in a liquid, please refer to the instructions at the beginning of this chapter.

- Take 1 capsule with desired oil 2 times daily.
- Put 2-3 drops of oil in a spoonful of Blue Agave, Yacon Syrup, maple syrup, coconut oil, milk, etc.
- Put the desired amount of oils in a glass of rice milk, almond milk, goat milk, carrot juice, NingXia Red, or even water and then drink it.

....

Fibrillation

This is a specific form of heart arrhythmia that occurs when the upper heart chambers contract at a rate of over 300 pulsations per minute. The lower chambers cannot keep this pace, so efficiency is reduced and not enough blood is pumped. Palpitations, a feeling that the heart is beating irregularly, more strongly, or more rapidly than normal, is the most common symptom.

Recommendations

Singles: Ylang Ylang, Amazonian Ylang Ylang, Valerian, Goldenrod, Marjoram, Lavender, Rosemary, Idaho Tansy

Blends: Aroma Life, Peace & Calming

Nutritionals: OmegaGize[3], Mineral Essence, MegaCal, Sulfurzyme, Ningxia Wolfberries (Dried), Master Formula HIS or HERS

Application and Usage
Inhalation

- Diffuse your choice of oils for ½ hour every 4-6 hours or as desired.
- Put 2-3 drops of your chosen oil in your hands and rub them together, cup your hands over your nose, and inhale throughout the

day as needed.

- Put 8-10 drops of oil on a cotton ball or tissue and put it in an air vent in your house, vehicle, hotel room, etc.
- If diffusing while sleeping, set your timer for the desired length of time for automatic shut off.

Topical

You may apply single oils or blends neat or diluted, depending on the oil or oils being used. Please see the instructions at the beginning of this chapter for more information on applying oils to the skin.

- Apply 1-3 drops neat 1-3 times daily of 2-3 of the recommended oils on the heart Vita Flex points on foot, hand, and arm as described in the "Heart Vita Flex" section under the topic Heart Health.
- Apply neat or dilute 50:50, if needed, 2-4 drops at pulse points, where arteries are close to the surface (wrists, inside elbows, base of throat), 2-3 times daily.
- Also apply to left chest, left shoulder, and back of neck.
- Also rub 6-10 drops along spine 3 times daily.
- Have a body massage 2 times weekly.

Ingestion and Oral

The amount of oil ingested varies with different oils. Whether putting the oils in a capsule or drinking them in a liquid, please refer to the instructions at the beginning of this chapter.

- Take 1 capsule with desired oil 2 times daily.
- Put 2-3 drops of oil in a spoonful of Blue Agave, Yacon Syrup, maple syrup, coconut oil, milk, etc.
- Put the desired amount of oils in a glass of rice milk, almond milk, goat milk, carrot juice, NingXia Red, or even water and then drink it.

Heart Attack (Myocardial Infarction)

A heart attack is a circulation blockage resulting in an interruption of blood supply to an area of the heart. Depending on the size of the area affected, it can be mild or severe.

Note: Contact your physician immediately if you suspect a heart attack.

Many people do not understand how someone who is relatively healthy, with low cholesterol levels, suffers a heart attack with no explanation. The explanation is actually inflammation, the fundamental cause of heart disease.

Inflammation of the heart is caused when blood vessels leading to the heart are clogged and damaged. This releases a protein into the bloodstream called C-reactive protein. The level of this protein indicates the degree of inflammation in the linings of the arteries. Certain essential oils have been documented to be excellent for reducing inflammation. German Chamomile contains azulene, a blue compound with highly anti-inflammatory properties. Peppermint is also highly anti-inflammatory. Other oils also have anti-inflammatory properties such as Helichrysum, Spruce, Wintergreen, and Valerian. Clove, Nutmeg, and Wintergreen are natural blood thinners and help reduce blood clotting.

Magnesium, the most important mineral for the heart, acts as a smooth muscle relaxant and supports the cardiovascular system. Magnesium will act as a natural calcium channel blocker for the heart, lowering blood pressure and dilating the heart blood vessels (according to Terry Friedmann, MD).

Recommendations

Singles: Wintergreen, Lavender, Roman Chamomile, Helichrysum, Dorado Azul, Ocotea, Idaho Tansy, Clove, Nutmeg, Copaiba, Palo Santo

Blends: PanAway, Longevity, Aroma Life, Peace & Calming, Relieve It, Valor, Valor Roll-On

Nutritionals: MegaCal, Longevity Softgels, Mineral Essence, OmegaGize³, Sulfurzyme, Rehemogen, NingXia Red

Application and Usage
Inhalation

- Diffuse your choice of oils for ½ hour 3 times daily or as often as needed to bring calm.
- Put 2-3 drops of your chosen oil in your hands and rub them together, cup your hands over your nose, and inhale throughout the day as needed.
- Put 8-10 drops of oil on a cotton ball or tissue and put it in an air vent in your house, vehicle, hotel room, etc.
- If diffusing while sleeping, set your timer for the desired length of time for automatic shut off.

Topical

You may apply single oils or blends neat or diluted, depending on the oil or oils being used. Please see the instructions at the beginning of this chapter for more information on applying oils to the skin.

- If there is not enough time to remove shoes to get at the feet, apply the "pumping" action to left hand and arm points. Using 1-2 drops of Aroma Life on each point will increase effectiveness and may even revive an individual having a heart attack while waiting for medical attention.
- Apply 1-3 drops neat 1-3 times daily of 2-3 of the recommended oils on the heart Vita Flex points on foot, hand, and arm as described in the "Heart Vita Flex" section under the topic Heart Health.
- Apply neat or dilute 50:50, if needed, 2-4 drops at pulse points, where arteries are close to the surface (wrists, inside elbows, base of throat), 2-3 times daily.
- Also apply to left chest, left shoulder, and back of neck.
- Also rub 6-10 drops along spine 3 times

daily.
- Have a body massage 2 times weekly.

Ingestion and Oral

The amount of oil ingested varies with different oils. Whether putting the oils in a capsule or drinking them in a liquid, please refer to the instructions at the beginning of this chapter.

- Take 1 capsule with desired oil 2 times daily.
- Put 2-3 drops of oil in a spoonful of Blue Agave, Yacon Syrup, maple syrup, coconut oil, milk, etc.
- Put the desired amount of oils in a glass of rice milk, almond milk, goat milk, carrot juice, NingXia Red, or even water and then drink it.

....

Heart Health

Heart disease is the leading cause of death in the United States. Keys to prevention include quitting smoking, controlling high blood pressure, lowering cholesterol, exercising, and maintaining a healthy weight.

....

Heart Vita Flex

The foot Vita Flex point related to the heart is on the sole of the left foot, below the ring toe (fourth toe) and approximately 1 inch below the base of the toe. Massaging this point is as effective as massaging the hand and arm points together (see charts in Application).

The hand Vita Flex point related to the heart is in the palm of the left hand, 1 inch below the ring finger joint at the lifeline. A secondary heart point is on the inside of the lower end of the upper left arm, approximately 2 inches up the arm from the elbow, not on the muscle but up under the muscle. Have another person use his or her thumbs to firmly press these two points alternately for 3 minutes in a kind of pumping action. Work all three points when possible. Start with the foot first; then go to the hand and arm.

Heart Stimulant

The effects of heart stimulants include increased heart rate and blood pressure.

Recommendations

Singles: Rosemary, Peppermint, Ylang Ylang, Amazonian Ylang Ylang, Goldenrod, Anise Seed, Mandarin, Thyme, Marjoram

Blends: Aroma Life, Peace & Calming, Release, Joy, Sacred Mountain, RutaVaLa, RutaVaLa Roll-On, Valor, Valor Roll-On, Stress Away Roll-On

Nutritionals: Master HIS or HERS

Application and Usage
Inhalation

- Diffuse your choice of oils for ½ hour every 4-6 hours or as desired.
- Put 2-3 drops of your chosen oil in your hands and rub them together, cup your hands over your nose, and inhale throughout the day as needed to calm.
- Put 8-10 drops of oil on a cotton ball or tissue and put it in an air vent in your house, vehicle, hotel room, etc.
- If diffusing while sleeping, set your timer for the desired length of time for automatic shut off.

Topical

You may apply single oils or blends neat or diluted, depending on the oil or oils being used. Please see the instructions at the beginning of this chapter for more information on applying oils to the skin.

- Apply 1-3 drops neat over the heart area 1-3 times daily.
- Massage the Vita Flex points with one drop each of the 2-3 recommended oils on the heart Vita Flex points along the foot, hand, and arm as needed.

Phlebitis (Inflammation of Veins) (See also EDEMA)

Phlebitis refers to inflammation of a blood vein, usually due to a thrombus or blood clot. Symptoms include pain and tenderness along the course of the vein, discoloration of the skin, inflammatory swelling, joint pain, and acute edema below the inflamed site.

Natural progesterone is an effective anti-inflammatory.

Recommendations

Singles: Juniper, Helichrysum, Cistus, Cypress, Wintergreen, Tangerine, Copaiba, German Chamomile, Geranium, Lavender, Clove, Nutmeg, Lemon

Blends: Aroma Life, Longevity

Nutritionals: Longevity Softgels

Serums and Creams: Progessence Plus, Prenolone Plus Body Cream

Phlebitis Blend

- 10 drops Tangerine
- 7 drops Lemon
- 5 drops Cypress
- 4 drops Juniper

Application and Usage
Topical

- You may apply single oils or blends neat or diluted, depending on the oil or oils being used. Please see the instructions at the beginning of this chapter for more information on applying oils to the skin.
- The essential oil of Cypress may help strengthen vascular walls.
- You may apply single oils or blends neat or diluted, depending on the oils that are used.
- Massage 2-4 drops of oil neat on the soles of the feet just before bedtime.
- Apply 2-4 drops neat on location 2-4 times daily.
- Apply a cold compress on location 2-4 times daily.

Plaque

Plaque is a cholesterol build up along the walls of the arteries, which causes the arteries to narrow. This is often when the physical symptoms of high cholesterol are noticed.

Singles: Rosemary, Helichrysum, Dorado Azul
Blends: Aroma Life, DiGize
Nutritionals: Detoxzyme, Digest & Cleanse, JuvaPower, Life 5

Application and Usage
Inhalation

- Diffuse your choice of oils for ½ hour every 4-6 hours or as desired.
- Put 2-3 drops of your chosen oil in your hands and rub them together, cup your hands over your nose, and inhale throughout the day as needed.
- Put 8-10 drops of oil on a cotton ball or tissue and put it in an air vent in your house, vehicle, hotel room, etc.
- If diffusing while sleeping, set your timer for the desired length of time for automatic shut off.

Topical

You may apply single oils or blends neat or diluted, depending on the oil or oils being used. Please see the instructions at the beginning of this chapter for more information on applying oils to the skin.

- Apply 1-3 drops, diluted 50:50, on temples, forehead, mastoids, back of neck, and at base of throat just above clavicle notch.
- Applying a single drop under the nose is helpful and refreshing.
- Massage 2-4 drops of oil neat on Vita Flex brain points on the soles of the feet just before bedtime.

Ingestion and Oral

The amount of oil ingested varies with different oils. Whether putting the oils in a capsule or drinking them in a liquid, please refer to the instructions at the beginning of this chapter.

- Take 1 capsule with Helichrysum or other desired oil 2 times daily.
- Take 1-2 capsules 50:50 with Helichrysum and Cistus 2 times daily.
- Put 2-3 drops of oil in a spoonful of Blue Agave, Yacon Syrup, maple syrup, coconut oil, milk, etc.
- Put the desired amount of oils in a glass of rice milk, almond milk, goat milk, carrot juice, NingXia Red, or even water and then drink it.

Strokes

Two principal kinds of strokes can damage the brain: hemorrhagic strokes and thrombotic strokes.

Some essential oils can be used topically to help strengthen the integrity of capillary walls. In particular, the essential oils of Helichrysum, Cistus, and Nutmeg are known to have anti-clotting properties and can be used as a preventative measure to reduce the risk of thrombotic stroke.

Hemorrhagic Strokes

A hemorrhagic stroke is caused by an aneurysm or a weakness in the blood vessel wall that balloons out and ruptures, spilling blood into the surrounding brain tissue. Strokes are very serious events, and if you suspect that you may be susceptible, immediately see a physician.

Recommendations
Singles: Cypress, Cistus, Helichrysum, Sandalwood
Blends: Brain Power, Common Sense, Clarity, Longevity, Stress Away Roll-On, Peace & Calming
Nutritionals: Sulfurzyme, MegaCal, Mineral Essence, Essentialzyme, Rehemogen, Master Formula HIS or HERS, NingXia Red

Application and Usage
Inhalation
- Diffuse your choice of oils for ½ hour every 4-6 hours or as desired.
- Put 2-3 drops of your chosen oil in your hands and rub them together, cup your hands over your nose, and inhale throughout the day as needed.
- Put 8-10 drops of oil on a cotton ball or tissue and put it in an air vent in your house, vehicle, hotel room, etc.
- If diffusing while sleeping, set your timer for the desired length of time for automatic shut off.

Topical
You may apply single oils or blends neat or diluted, depending on the oil or oils being used. Please see the instructions at the beginning of this chapter for more information on applying oils to the skin.
- Apply 1-3 drops, diluted 50:50, on temples, forehead, mastoids, back of neck, and at base of throat just above clavicle notch.
- Applying a single drop under the nose is helpful and refreshing.
- Massage 2-4 drops of oil neat on Vita Flex brain points on the soles of the feet just before bedtime.

Ingestion and Oral
The amount of oil ingested varies with different oils. Whether putting the oils in a capsule or drinking them in a liquid, please refer to the instructions at the beginning of this chapter.
- Take 1 capsule with Helichrysum or other desired oil 2 times daily.
- Take 1-2 capsules 50:50 with Helichrysum and Cistus 2 times daily.
- Put 2-3 drops of oil in a spoonful of Blue Agave, Yacon Syrup, maple syrup, coconut oil, milk, etc.

- Put the desired amount of oils in a glass of rice milk, almond milk, goat milk, carrot juice, NingXia Red, or even water and then drink it.

Thrombotic Strokes
Thrombotic strokes are caused by a blood clot lodging in a cerebral blood vessel and cutting blood supply to a part of the brain.

Recommendations
Singles: Helichrysum, Cistus, Nutmeg, Cypress, Sandalwood, Juniper, Grapefruit, Orange, Clove

Blends: Longevity, Aroma Life, JuvaCleanse

Nutritionals: Sulfurzyme, MegaCal, Omega-Gize[3], Essentialzyme, Pure Protein, Master Formula HIS or HERS, Power Meal, NingXia Red

These supplements are rich in essential minerals, fatty acids, and nutrients necessary for regenerating and rebuilding damaged nerve tissues.

Application and Usage
Inhalation
- Diffuse your choice of oils for ½ hour every 4-6 hours or as desired.
- Put 2-3 drops of your chosen oil in your hands and rub them together, cup your hands over your nose, and inhale throughout the day as needed.
- Put 8-10 drops of oil on a cotton ball or tissue and put it in an air vent in your house, vehicle, hotel room, etc.
- If diffusing while sleeping, set your timer for the desired length of time for automatic shut off.

Topical
You may apply single oils or blends neat or diluted, depending on the oil or oils being used. Please see the instructions at the beginning of this chapter for more information on applying

oils to the skin.

- Applying the essential oil of Cypress may help strengthen vascular walls.
- You may apply single oils or blends neat or diluted, depending on the oils that are used.
- Apply 1-2 drops neat on temples and back of neck as desired.
- Applying a single drop under the nose is helpful and refreshing.
- Massage 2-4 drops of oil neat on the soles of the feet just before bedtime.

....

Tachycardia

Tachycardia is another form of heart arrhythmia in which the heart rate suddenly increases to 160 beats per minute or faster.

Recommendations

Singles: Ylang Ylang, Amazonian Ylang Ylang, Rosemary, Sandalwood, Wintergreen, Marjoram, German Chamomile, Lavender, Goldenrod, Idaho Tansy

Blends: Peace & Calming, Aroma Life, Acceptance

Nutritionals: Sulfurzyme, NingXia Red, Coenzyme Q10

Application and Usage
Inhalation

- Diffuse your choice of oils for ½ hour every 4-6 hours or as desired.
- Put 2-3 drops of your chosen oil in your hands and rub them together, cup your hands over your nose, and inhale throughout the day as needed.
- Put 8-10 drops of oil on a cotton ball or tissue and put it in an air vent in your house, vehicle, hotel room, etc.
- If diffusing while sleeping, set your timer for the desired length of time for automatic shut off.

Topical

You may apply single oils or blends neat or diluted, depending on the oil or oils being used. Please see the instructions at the beginning of this chapter for more information on applying oils to the skin.

- Massage 1-3 drops over heart area 1-3 times daily. Also apply to left chest, left shoulder, and back of neck.
- Massage 1 drop each of 2 or 3 of the recommended oils on heart Vita Flex points on foot, hand, and arm as needed.

Ingestion and Oral

The amount of oil ingested varies with different oils. Whether putting the oils in a capsule or drinking them in a liquid, please refer to the instructions at the beginning of this chapter.

- Take 1 capsule with desired oil 3 times daily.
- Put 2-3 drops of oil in a spoonful of Blue Agave, Yacon Syrup, maple syrup, coconut oil, milk, etc.
- Put the desired amount of oils in a glass of rice milk, almond milk, goat milk, carrot juice, NingXia Red, or even water and then drink it.

....

Varicose Veins (Spider Veins)

The blue color of varicose veins is coagulated blood in the surrounding tissue from hemorrhaging of capillaries around the veins. This blood has to be dissolved and re-absorbed.

Recommendations

Singles: Helichrysum, Cypress, Cistus, Elemi, Geranium, Clove, Peppermint, Lemon, Lavender

Helichrysum helps dissolve the coagulated blood in the surrounding tissue.

Blends: Aroma Life, Citrus Fresh, Aroma Siez

Nutritionals: MultiGreens, Super B, Longevity Softgels

Other Topical Products: Ortho Ease Massage Oil, Essential Beauty Serum (Acne-Prone Skin), Thieves Spray

Application and Usage
Topical

You may apply single oils or blends neat or diluted, depending on the oil or oils being used. Please see the instructions at the beginning of this chapter for more information on applying oils to the skin.

Varicose Vein Blend

- 3-4 drops Geranium
- 1 drop Cistus
- 1 drop Cypress
- 1 drop Helichrysum

Apply 2-4 drops on location, massaging toward the heart, 3-6 times daily.

Nightly Varicose Vein Regimen (Legs)

1. Apply 1-3 drops varicose vein blend, neat, on location. Rub very gently towards heart with smooth strokes along the vein, then up and over the vein until the oil is absorbed.
2. Apply 6 drops Tangerine and 6 drops Cypress to the area. Gently massage until absorbed.
3. Do the lymphatic pump procedure described in Application.
4. Follow with a soft massage of the whole leg using 10-15 drops of Aroma Life diluted 50:50.
5. Wrap and elevate the leg. It is best to do this at night before retiring and to gradually elevate the foot off the bed, an inch more each night, until it is 4 inches higher than the head.
6. Wear support hose during the daytime. It may take up to a year to achieve desired results.

....

Vascular Cleansing

Keeping your blood clean will help you stay healthy.

1. Drink plenty of water.
2. Cleanse the blood by taking blood-cleansing herbs and essential oils.
3. Cleanse the kidneys.

4. Consider fasting for one to three days.
5. Take enzymes.

Singles: Helichrysum, Idaho Blue Spruce, Sacred Frankincense, Frankincense, Dorado Azul

Blends: GLF, DiGize, JuvaCleanse

Nutritionals: JuvaPower, NingXia Red

Application and Usage
Inhalation

- Diffuse your choice of oils for ½ hour every 4-6 hours or as desired.
- Put 2-3 drops of your chosen oil in your hands and rub them together, cup your hands over your nose, and inhale throughout the day as needed.
- Put 8-10 drops of oil on a cotton ball or tissue and put it in an air vent in your house, vehicle, hotel room, etc.
- If diffusing while sleeping, set your timer for the desired length of time for automatic shut off.

Topical

You may apply single oils or blends neat or diluted, depending on the oil or oils being used. Please see the instructions at the beginning of this chapter for more information on applying oils to the skin.

- Apply 1-3 drops, diluted 50:50, on temples, forehead, mastoids, back of neck, and at base of throat just above the clavicle notch.
- Applying a single drop under the nose is helpful and refreshing.
- Massage 2-4 drops of oil neat on Vita Flex brain points on the soles of the feet just before bedtime.

Ingestion and Oral

The amount of oil ingested varies with different oils. Whether putting the oils in a capsule or drinking them in a liquid, please refer to the instructions at the beginning of this chapter.

- Take 1 capsule with Helichrysum or other desired oil 2 times daily.

- Take 1-2 capsules 2 times daily 50:50 with Helichrysum and Cistus.
- Put 2-3 drops of oil in a spoonful of Blue Agave, Yacon Syrup, maple syrup, coconut oil, milk, etc.
- Put the desired amount of oils in a glass of rice milk, almond milk, goat milk, carrot juice, NingXia Red, or even water and then drink it.

CANKER SORES
(See also MOUTH ULCERS)

These are technically known as aphthous ulcers, are not regarded as an infectious disease, and are not caused by the herpes virus.

Canker sores tend to occur because of stress, illness, weakened immune system, and injury caused by such things as hot food, rough brushing of teeth, or dentures. They appear under the tongue more commonly than cold sores.

Recommendations

Singles: Melissa, Clove, Lavender, Sandalwood, Cypress, Thyme

Blends: Thieves, Melrose

Nutritionals: Inner Defense, ImmuPro, AlkaLime

Oral Care: Thieves Spray, Thieves Fresh Essence Mouthwash

Application and Usage
Topical

You may apply single oils or blends neat or diluted, depending on the oil or oils being used. Please see the instructions at the beginning of this chapter for more information on applying oils to the skin.

- Gently apply 1 drop neat with fingertip to canker sore 4-8 times daily.

Ingestion and Oral

- Gargle with Thieves mouthwash 2-4 times daily.
- Take maple syrup 2-4 times daily.

CELLULITE

Cellulite is one of the harder types of fats to dissolve in the body. Cellulite is an accumulation of old fat cell clusters that solidify and harden as the surrounding tissue loses its elasticity.

Excess fat is undesirable for two reasons:

1. The extra weight puts an extra load on all body systems, particularly the heart and cardiovascular system, as well as the joints (knees, hips, spine, etc.).

2. Toxins and petrochemicals (pesticides, herbicides, and metals) tend to accumulate in fatty tissue. This can contribute to hormone imbalance, neurological problems, and a higher risk of cancer.

Essential oils such as Ledum, Tangerine, and Grapefruit may help reduce fat cells. Cypress enhances circulation to support the elimination of fatty deposits. The essential oils of Lemongrass and Spearmint also may help fat metabolism. Cel-Lite Magic Massage Oil contains many of these oils and may help reduce cellulite deposits.

Cellulite is slow to dissolve, so target areas should be worked for a month or more in conjunction with weight training, a weight-loss program, and drinking purified water—one-and-a-half times the body weight in ounces each day. Be patient. You should begin to see results in 4-6 weeks when using the oils in combination with a muscle-building and weight-loss regimen.

Recommendations

Singles: Grapefruit, Spearmint, Rosemary, Lemon, Tangerine, Cypress, Fennel, Juniper, Lemongrass

Blends: EndoFlex, Digest & Cleanse

Nutritionals: Thyromin, Power Meal, Omega-Gize³, Essentialzymes-4, Balance Complete Thyromin balances and boosts metabolism.

Topical Treatments: Cel-Lite Magic Massage Oil

Application and Usage
Topical
You may apply single oils or blends neat or diluted, depending on the oil or oils being used. Please see the instructions at the beginning of this chapter for more information on applying oils to the skin.

- Dilute 50:50 and massage 3-6 drops vigorously on cellulite locations at least 3 times daily, especially before exercising.

Cellulite Blend No. 1
- 10 drops Grapefruit
- 5 drops Lavender
- 3 drops Helichrysum
- 3 drops Patchouli
- 4 drops Cypress
  Use as bath salt 2-4 times weekly.

Cellulite Blend No. 2 (Bath)
- 5 drops Juniper
- 3 drops Orange
- 3 drops Cypress
- 3 drops Rosemary
  Mix the above blend together with 2 tablespoons Epsom salts or Bath Gel Base and dissolve in warm bath water. Massage with Cel-Lite Magic after bath.
- Apply 3-5 drops of Grapefruit neat 1-2 times daily to increase fat-reducing action in areas of fat rolls, puckers, and dimples.

CEREBRAL PALSY
The effects of cerebral palsy vary greatly, causing impaired movement associated with exaggerated reflexes or rigidity of the limbs and trunk, abnormal posture, involuntary movements, unsteadiness of walking, or a combination of these.

It is caused most often by abnormal development in the brain before birth or injury during delivery. Individuals stricken with cerebral palsy often have other conditions related to developmental brain abnormalities such as intellectual disabilities, vision and hearing problems, or seizures.

Signs and symptoms
- Stiff muscles and exaggerated reflexes (spasticity)
- Stiff muscles with normal reflexes (rigidity)
- Lack of muscle coordination, tremors, or involuntary movements
- Slow development of motor skills such as pushing with arms, sitting up, or crawling
- Reaching with only one hand or dragging a leg while crawling
- Difficulty eating and swallowing, excessive drooling
- Slow speech development or difficulty speaking
- Difficulty in picking up toys, spoons, etc.

Medical researchers have not found an answer but offer different therapies and medication in an effort to help. Natural medicine offers help with the same desire of seeing improvement. Because essential oils cross the blood brain barrier, they can stimulate brain activity in a nontoxic way, and one can hope and wait to see what possible benefits will appear.

Different people have tried different things that have resulted in the information below. By investigating further with supplements and natural remedies, many new things will be discovered. The risk is minimal and the gain could be slight to immense.

Recommendations
Singles: Sacred Frankincense, Frankincense, Myrrh, Idaho Balsam Fir, Peppermint, Canadian Fleabane (Conyza)

Blends: PanAway, Aroma Siez, Relieve It, Deep Relief Roll-On

Nutritionals: BLM, Sulfurzyme, Essentialzymes-4, Power Meal, Pure Protein, MultiGreens, Mineral Essence, Essentialzyme, Super B, NingXia Red

Body Care Massage Oils: Ortho Ease Massage Oil, Ortho Sport Massage Oil

Application and Usage
Inhalation
- Diffuse your choice of oils for ½ hour every 4-6 hours or as desired.
- Put 2-3 drops of your chosen oil in your hands and rub them together, cup your hands over your nose, and inhale throughout the day as needed.
- Put 8-10 drops of oil on a cotton ball or tissue and put it in an air vent in your house, vehicle, hotel room, etc.
- If diffusing while sleeping, set your timer for the desired length of time for automatic shut off.

Topical
You may apply single oils or blends neat or diluted, depending on the oil or oils being used. Please see the instructions at the beginning of this chapter for more information on applying oils to the skin.
- Use blend for Raindrop Technique 2 times daily: morning and night.

Ingestion and Oral
The amount of oil ingested varies with different oils. Whether putting the oils in a capsule or drinking them in a liquid, please refer to the instructions at the beginning of this chapter.
- Take 1 capsule with desired oil 2 times daily.
- Put 2-3 drops of oil in a spoonful of Blue Agave, Yacon Syrup, maple syrup, coconut oil, milk, etc.
- Put the desired amount of oils in a glass of rice milk, almond milk, goat milk, carrot juice, NingXia Red, or even water and then drink it.

Cerebral Palsy Blend
- 15 drops Sacred Frankincense or Frankincense
- 12 drops Myrrh
- 10 drops Idaho Balsam Fir
- 10 drops Canadian Fleabane (Conyza)
- 4 drops Peppermint
- Take 3 capsules daily: morning, noon, and night.

Using this regimen, a 7-year-old boy with cerebral palsy and autism, after one month, was able to walk flat footed without his walker, test scores in school improved by 28 percent, and his attention span increased 30 percent, his mother reported.

CHEMICAL SENSITIVITY REACTION
Environmental poisoning and chemical sensitivity are becoming a major cause of discomfort and disease. Strong chemical compounds, such as insecticides, herbicides, and formaldehyde found in paints, glues, cosmetics, and finger nail polish, enter the body easily. Symptoms include indigestion, upper and lower gas, poor assimilation, poor electrolyte balance, rashes, hypoglycemia, allergic reaction to foods and other substances, along with emotional mood swings, fatigue, irritability, lack of motivation, lack of discipline and creativity.

Recommendations
Singles: Wintergreen, Sacred Frankincense, Frankincense, Lemon, Sandalwood, Copaiba, Eucalyptus Globulus

Blends: PanAway, Citrus Fresh, Inner Child, Christmas Spirit

Resins: Frankincense Gum Resin, Myrrh Gum Resin

Nutritionals: Detoxzyme, JuvaPower, JuvaSpice, JuvaTone, Balance Complete, ICP, ComforTone, Essentialzyme, Life 5, Allerzyme

Application and Usage
Inhalation
- Diffuse your choice of oils for ½ hour every 4-6 hours or as desired.

- Put 2-3 drops of your chosen oil in your hands and rub them together, cup your hands over your nose, and inhale throughout the day as needed.
- Put 8-10 drops of oil on a cotton ball or tissue and put it in an air vent in your house, vehicle, hotel room, etc.
- If diffusing while sleeping, set your timer for the desired length of time for automatic shut off.

Topical

You may apply single oils or blends neat or diluted, depending on the oil or oils being used. Please see the instructions at the beginning of this chapter for more information on applying oils to the skin.

- Dilute oil 50:50 and apply on affected areas 2-4 times daily.

Ingestion and Oral

The amount of oil ingested varies with different oils. Whether putting the oils in a capsule or drinking them in a liquid, please refer to the instructions at the beginning of this chapter.

- Take 1 capsule with desired oil 2 times daily.
- Put 2-3 drops of oil in a spoonful of Blue Agave, Yacon Syrup, maple syrup, coconut oil, milk, etc.
- Put the desired amount of oils in a glass of rice milk, almond milk, goat milk, carrot juice, NingXia Red, or even water and then drink it.

  For headache relief, take the following:
- 4 Essentialzyme
- 1/8 teaspoon M-Grain diluted 50:50 in vegetable oil

  Drink 2-3 large glasses of water immediately after taking these products.

CHICKEN POX (HERPES ZOSTER) (See also COLD SORES, BLISTERS)

Chicken pox (also known as shingles, *Varicella zoster*, or *Herpes zoster*) is caused by a virus that is closely related to the herpes simplex virus. This virus is prone to hiding along nerves under the skin and may cause recurring infection through life.

When *Herpes zoster* infection occurs in children, it is known as chicken pox; when infection occurs or recurs in adults, it is known as shingles.

A childhood bout with chicken pox may leave the virus dormant in sensory (skin) nerves. If the immune system is taxed by severe emotional stress, illness, or long-term use of cortico-steroids, the dormant viruses may become active and start to infect the pathway of the skin nerves.

Recommendations

Singles: Lemongrass, Lavender, Melaleuca Alternifolia, Sandalwood, Melissa, Clove, Cypress, Geranium, Wintergreen

Blends: Thieves, Australian Blue, Melrose

Nutritionals: Inner Defense, ImmuPro, Balance Complete, Power Meal, SuperCal, PD 80/20

Body Care: Thieves Spray, Ortho Ease Massage Oil, LavaDerm Cooling Mist

Application and Usage
Inhalation

- Diffuse your choice of oils for ½ hour every 4-6 hours or as desired.
- Put 2-3 drops of your chosen oil in your hands and rub them together, cup your hands over your nose, and inhale throughout the day as needed.
- Put 8-10 drops of oil on a cotton ball or tissue and put it in an air vent in your house, vehicle, hotel room, etc.
- If diffusing while sleeping, set your timer for

the desired length of time for automatic shut off.

Topical

You may apply single oils or blends neat or diluted, depending on the oil or oils being used. Please see the instructions at the beginning of this chapter for more information on applying oils to the skin.

- Add 20 drops of essential oils (using any of the above oils) to 1 tablespoon of calamine lotion or V-6 Vegetable Oil Complex and lightly dab on spots (lesions).

Ingestion and Oral

The amount of oil ingested varies with different oils. Whether putting the oils in a capsule or drinking them in a liquid, please refer to the instructions at the beginning of this chapter.

- Take 1 capsule with desired oil 2 times daily.
- Put 2-3 drops of oil in a spoonful of Blue Agave, Yacon Syrup, maple syrup, coconut oil, milk, etc.
- Put the desired amount of oils in a glass of rice milk, almond milk, goat milk, carrot juice, NingXia Red, or even water and then drink it.

CHOLERA

Cholera is an acute diarrheal disease caused by an interotoxin produced by a gram negative bacterium called *Vibrio cholerae*. Severe cases are marked by vomiting, muscle cramps, and constant watery diarrhea, which can result in serious fluid loss, saline depletion, acidosis, and shock. The disease is typically found in India and Southeast Asia and is spread by feces-contaminated water and food. If you suspect cholera, you should immediately seek professional medical advice.

A recent study shows that lemon—freshly squeezed juice, peel, and essential oil—act as a biocide against *Vibrio cholerae* with no harmful side effects.[17]

Recommendations

Singles: Lemon, Clove, Thyme, Rosemary, Oregano

Blends: DiGize

Nutritionals: Digest & Cleanse

Application and Usage

Inhalation

- Diffuse your choice of oils for ½ hour every 4-6 hours or as desired.
- Put 2-3 drops of your chosen oil in your hands and rub them together, cup your hands over your nose, and inhale throughout the day as needed.
- Put 8-10 drops of oil on a cotton ball or tissue and put it in an air vent in your house, vehicle, hotel room, etc.
- If diffusing while sleeping, set your timer for the desired length of time for automatic shut off.

Topical

You may apply single oils or blends neat or diluted, depending on the oil or oils being used. Please see the instructions at the beginning of this chapter for more information on applying oils to the skin.

Ingestion and Oral

The amount of oil ingested varies with different oils. Whether putting the oils in a capsule or drinking them in a liquid, please refer to the instructions at the beginning of this chapter.

- Take 1 capsule with desired oil 2 times daily.
- Put 2-3 drops of oil in a spoonful of Blue Agave, Yacon Syrup, maple syrup, coconut oil, milk, etc.
- Put the desired amount of oils in a glass of rice milk, almond milk, goat milk, carrot juice, NingXia Red, or even water and then drink it.

CHRONIC FATIGUE SYNDROME

The cause of chronic fatigue syndrome is somewhat of a mystery, but scientists believe it may be caused by a combination of factors, including immune system problems, hormone imbalances, genetic factors, psychiatric or emotional conditions, brain abnormalities, and viruses, including Epstein-Barr virus, human herpes virus 6, and mouse leukemia viruses. However, no primary cause has been found.

Recommendations

Singles: Peppermint, Lemon, Orange
Blends: Awaken, DiGize, Joy
Nutritionals: Detoxzyme, EndoGize, PD80/20, Super B, Thyromin, Ultra Young Plus, NingXia Red, NingXia Nitro
Serum: Progessence Plus

Application and Usage
Inhalation

- Diffuse your choice of oils for ½ hour every 4-6 hours or as desired.
- Put 2-3 drops of your chosen oil in your hands and rub them together, cup your hands over your nose, and inhale throughout the day as needed.
- Put 8-10 drops of oil on a cotton ball or tissue and put it in an air vent in your house, vehicle, hotel room, etc.
- If diffusing while sleeping, set your timer for the desired length of time for automatic shut off.

Topical

You may apply single oils or blends neat or diluted, depending on the oil or oils being used. Please see the instructions at the beginning of this chapter for more information on applying oils to the skin.

Ingestion and Oral

The amount of oil ingested varies with different oils. Whether putting the oils in a capsule or drinking them in a liquid, please refer to the instructions at the beginning of this chapter.

- Take 1 capsule with desired oil 2 times daily.
- Put 2-3 drops of oil in a spoonful of Blue Agave, Yacon Syrup, maple syrup, coconut oil, milk, etc.
- Put the desired amount of oils in a glass of rice milk, almond milk, goat milk, carrot juice, NingXia Red, or even water and then drink it.

COLD SORES
(HERPES SIMPLEX TYPE 1)

Cold sores are also known as *Herpes labialis*. Diets high in the amino acid lysine can reduce the incidence of herpes. Conversely, the amino acid arginine can worsen herpes outbreaks.

Studies have shown neat applications of Melissa to be effective against herpes simplex type 1 and type II. The healing period was shortened, the spread of infection was prevented, and symptoms such as itching, tingling, and burning were lessened.

Peppermint and Melaleuca Alternifolia oils have also been studied for positive effects on the pain of herpes.

Recommendations

Singles: Peppermint, Ravintsara, Melissa, Melaleuca Alternifolia, Lavender, Sandalwood, Mountain Savory, Oregano, Plectranthus Oregano, Thyme, Clove
Blends: Thieves, Melrose, Purification
Nutritionals: Inner Defense, ImmuPro, Super C, Super C Chewable, MultiGreens, ICP, ComforTone, Essentialzyme, JuvaTone, JuvaPower
Sprays and Ointments: Thieves Spray, Rose Ointment

Application and Usage
Topical

You may apply single oils or blends neat or

diluted, depending on the oil or oils being used. Please see the instructions at the beginning of this chapter for more information on applying oils to the skin.

- Apply single oils or blends neat or diluted, depending on the oils being used.
- Apply 1 drop neat as soon as the cold sore appears. Repeat 5-10 times daily.
- If needed, dilute 50:50 with V-6 Vegetable Oil Complex or Rose Ointment to reduce discomfort of drying skin after applying essential oils to an open sore.

COLDS
(See also LUNG INFECTIONS, SINUS INFECTIONS, THROAT INFECTIONS)

The best treatment for a cold or flu is prevention. Because many essential oils have strong antimicrobial properties, they can be diffused to prevent the spread of airborne bacteria and viruses. Antiviral essential oils, blends, and supplements are very effective as preventative aids in avoiding colds as well as in helping the body's defenses fight colds once an infection has started. ImmuPro is a powerful immune stimulant that can also increase infection resistance.

Recommendations
Singles: Ravintsara, Cypress, Peppermint, Thyme, Laurus Nobilis, Hyssop, Oregano, Plectranthus Oregano, Eucalyptus Blue, Eucalyptus Radiata, Melaleuca Alternifolia, Rosemary, Clove, Mountain Savory

Blends: Raven, Thieves, Melrose, Australian Blue, Purification, ImmuPower, Sacred Mountain, R.C., Exodus II, Breathe Again Roll-On

Nutritionals: Inner Defense, ImmuPro, Thieves Lozenges (Hard/Soft), Super C, Super C Chewable, Longevity Softgels, Master Formula HIS or HERS, Detoxzyme, AlkaLime

Oral Treatment: Thieves Spray
Cold Blend No. 1
- 5 drops Rosemary
- 4 drops Eucalyptus Radiata
- 4 drops Peppermint
- 3 drops Cypress
- 2 drops Lemon

Cold Blend No. 2
- 5 drops Rosemary
- 4 drops R.C.
- 4 drops Sacred Frankincense or Frankincense
- 2 drops Peppermint
- 1 drop Oregano

Application and Usage
Inhalation
- Diffuse your choice of oils for ½ hour every 4-6 hours or as desired.
- Put 2-3 drops of your chosen oil in your hands and rub them together, cup your hands over your nose, and inhale throughout the day as needed.
- Put 8-10 drops of oil on a cotton ball or tissue and put it in an air vent in your house, vehicle, hotel room, etc.
- If diffusing while sleeping, set your timer for the desired length of time for automatic shut off.

Topical
You may apply single oils or blends neat or diluted, depending on the oil or oils being used. Please see the instructions at the beginning of this chapter for more information on applying oils to the skin.

- Dilute 50:50 and massage 1-3 drops on each of the following areas: forehead, nose, cheeks, lower throat, chest, and upper back 1-3 times daily.
- Massage 1-3 drops on Vita Flex points on the feet 1-2 times daily.
- Receive a Raindrop Technique 1-2 times weekly.
- Bath salts (see below)

Bath Blend for Relief of Cold Symptoms

- 15 drops Ravintsara
- 8 drops Wintergreen
- 6 drops Spruce
- 6 drops Sacred Frankincense or Frankincense
- 3 drops Laurus Nobilis
- 2 drops Eucalyptus Radiata

Stir essential oils into ½ cup Epsom salt or baking soda and then add the mixture to hot bath water while tub is filling. Soak in hot bath until water cools.

Ingestion and Oral

The amount of oil ingested varies with different oils. Whether putting the oils in a capsule or drinking them in a liquid, please refer to the instructions at the beginning of this chapter.

- Take 1 capsule with desired oil 2 times daily.
- Put 2-3 drops of oil in a spoonful of Blue Agave, Yacon Syrup, maple syrup, coconut oil, milk, etc.
- Put the desired amount of oils in a glass of rice milk, almond milk, goat milk, carrot juice, NingXia Red, or even water and then drink it.
- Take syrup 3-6 times daily.
- Gargle 3-6 times daily.

COLITIS
(See also CROHN'S, DIVERTICULOSIS/ DIVERTICULITIS)

Also known as ileitis or proctitis, ulcerative colitis is marked by the inflammation of the top layers of the lining of the colon, the large intestine. It is different from both irritable bowel syndrome, which has no inflammation, and Crohn's disease, which usually occurs deeper in the colon wall.

The inflammation and ulcerous sores that are characteristic of ulcerative colitis occur most frequently in the lower colon and rectum and occasionally throughout the entire colon.

Symptoms include fatigue, nausea, weight loss, loss of appetite, bloody diarrhea, loss of body fluids and nutrients, frequent fevers, abdominal cramps, arthritis, liver disease, and skin rash.

Take Essentialzymes-4 along with Comfor-Tone and wait about 2 weeks or more before adding JuvaPower. Start with a small amount and increase slowly. If any discomfort is experienced, reduce the amount taken.

....

Ulcerative Colitis

Recommendations

Singles: Spearmint, Wintergreen, Peppermint, Tarragon, Anise Seed, Fennel

Blends: DiGize, GLF, JuvaCleanse

Nutritionals: Digest & Cleanse, AlkaLime, Life 5, JuvaPower, Detoxzyme, ICP, Essentialzyme, Essentialzymes-4, MegaCal

Application and Usage
Inhalation

- Diffuse your choice of oils for ½ hour every 4-6 hours or as desired.
- Put 2-3 drops of your chosen oil in your hands and rub them together, cup your hands over your nose, and inhale throughout the day as needed.
- Put 8-10 drops of oil on a cotton ball or tissue and put it in an air vent in your house, vehicle, hotel room, etc.
- If diffusing while sleeping, set your timer for the desired length of time for automatic shut off.

Topical

You may apply single oils or blends neat or diluted, depending on the oil or oils being used. Please see the instructions at the beginning of this chapter for more information on applying oils to the skin.

- Apply 4-6 drops of your choice of oil, diluted 50:50, on lower abdomen 3-6 times daily.

- Massage 2-4 drops of oil neat on the soles of the feet just before bedtime.

Ingestion and Oral

The amount of oil ingested varies with different oils. Whether putting the oils in a capsule or drinking them in a liquid, please refer to the instructions at the beginning of this chapter.

- Take 1 capsule with desired 2 or 3 oils 2 times daily.
- Take 2 capsules with any 2 of the oils above 2-3 times daily.
- Put 2-3 drops of oil in a spoonful of Blue Agave, Yacon Syrup, maple syrup, coconut oil, milk, etc.
- Put the desired amount of oils in a glass of rice milk, almond milk, goat milk, carrot juice, NingXia Red, or even water and then drink it.

....

Viral Colitis

Use the remedies below for colitis that may be caused by virus rather than bacteria.

Recommendations

Singles: Melissa, Lemongrass, Clove, Blue Cypress, Oregano, Plectranthus Oregano, Cumin, Melaleuca Alternifolia, Tarragon, Thyme, Roman Chamomile, German Chamomile, Rosemary, Peppermint, Cinnamon Bark

Blends: Melrose, Thieves, Purification, DiGize

Nutritionals: Digest & Cleanse, Inner Defense, Longevity Softgels, Essentialzymes-4, Essentialzyme, Life 5

Application and Usage
Topical

You may apply single oils or blends neat or diluted, depending on the oil or oils being used. Please see the instructions at the beginning of this chapter for more information on applying oils to the skin.

- Apply several drops diluted 50:50 over colon area 4-6 times daily.
- You may also apply 2-3 drops on the Vita Flex colon points.
- Have Raindrop Technique 1-2 times weekly.
- Place a warm compress diluted 20:80 using equal parts Helichrysum and DiGize over the colon area.
- Use the blend below in a rectal implant 3 times weekly.

Colitis-Colon Blend

- 3 drops Melaleuca Quinquenervia (Niaouli)
- 2 drops Oregano
- 2 drops Thyme
- 2 drops German Chamomile
- 2 drops Melissa
- 2 drops Peppermint
  Mix above oils with 1 tablespoon V-6 Vegetable Oil Complex.

Ingestion and Oral

The amount of oil ingested varies with different oils. Whether putting the oils in a capsule or drinking them in a liquid, please refer to the instructions at the beginning of this chapter.

- Take 1 capsule with desired oil 2 times daily.
- Put 2-3 drops of oil in a spoonful of Blue Agave, Yacon Syrup, maple syrup, coconut oil, milk, etc.
- Put the desired amount of oils in a glass of rice milk, almond milk, goat milk, carrot juice, NingXia Red, or even water and then drink it.

COMA

Patients in a coma will likely be in a hospital or care center. Discuss with the patient's physician about rubbing essential oils on the bottoms of the patient's feet and diffusing the oils. After the patient returns home, the oils listed below could be helpful.

Recommendations

Singles: Valerian, Vetiver, Sandalwood, Blue Cypress, Black Pepper, Peppermint, Idaho Balsam Fir, Copaiba, Sacred Frankincense, Frankincense

Blends: Hope, Valor, Valor Roll-On, Surrender, The Gift, Inspiration, Brain Power, Trauma Life, R.C.

Serums, Creams, and Massage Oils: Progessence Plus, Regenolone Moisturizing Cream, Sensation Massage Oil

Application and Usage
Inhalation

- Diffuse your choice of oils for 15 minutes 4-7 times daily.

Topical

You may apply single oils or blends neat or diluted, depending on the oil or oils being used. Please see the instructions at the beginning of this chapter for more information on applying oils to the skin.

- Apply 3-5 drops diluted 50:50 on temples, neck, and shoulders.
- Receive a Raindrop Technique with the above mentioned oils.

CONNECTIVE TISSUE DAMAGE (CARTILAGE, LIGAMENTS, TENDONS)

Tendonitis, often called tennis elbow and golfer's elbow, is a torn or inflamed tendon. Repetitive use or infection may be the cause.

MegaCal and BLM provide critical nutrients for connective tissue repair. Sulfurzyme, an outstanding source of organic sulfur, equalizes water pressure inside the cells and reduces pain.

PanAway reduces pain and lemongrass promotes the repair of connective tissue. Lavender with Lemongrass and Marjoram with Lemongrass work well together for inflamed tendons. Deep Relief Roll-On is a convenient way to apply a blend of oils that is both pain relieving and anti-inflammatory.

When selecting oils for injuries, think through the cause and type of injury and select appropriate oils. For instance, tendonitis could encompass muscle damage, nerve damage, ligament strain/tear, inflammation, infection, and possibly an emotion. Therefore, select an oil or oils for each potential cause and apply in rotation or prepare a blend to address multiple causes. The oils in Ortho Sport and Ortho Ease massage oils reduce pain and promote healing.

Recommendations

Singles: Sacred Frankincense, Frankincense, Lemongrass, Lavender, Marjoram, Eucalyptus Blue, Dorado Azul

Blends: PanAway, Deep Relief Roll-On, Aroma Siez, Melrose

Nutritionals: MegaCal, Super B, Super C, Super C Chewable, MultiGreens, Mineral Essence, Sulfurzyme, BLM, PD 80/20

Body Care Massage Oils and Creams: Ortho Ease Massage Oil, Ortho Sport Massage Oil, Regenolone Moisturizing Cream

Application and Usage
Topical

You may apply single oils or blends neat or diluted, depending on the oil or oils being used. Please see the instructions at the beginning of this chapter for more information on applying oils to the skin.

- Apply oils neat or diluted 50:50 on location 3-6 times daily.
- Massage 4-6 drops of oil on affected area. For swelling, elevate and apply ice packs.
- Place a cold compress with 1-2 drops of chosen oil on area 2-4 times daily.

....

Cartilage Injury on Knee, Elbow, Etc.

People with cartilage damage often experience decreased range of motion, stiffness, joint pain, and/or swelling in the affected area.

Recommendations

Singles: Wintergreen, Copaiba, Lemongrass, Palo Santo, Peppermint, Idaho Balsam Fir, Marjoram, Eucalyptus Blue, Dorado Azul, Idaho Blue Spruce

Blends: PanAway, Relieve It, Aroma Siez, Deep Relief Roll-On

Nutritionals: MegaCal, Super B, Super C, Super C Chewable, MultiGreens, Mineral Essence, BLM, Master Formula HIS or HERS, Sulfurzyme

Body Care Massage Oils and Creams: Ortho Ease Massage Oil, Ortho Sport Massage Oil, Regenolone Moisturizing Cream

Cartilage Blend

- 12 drops Wintergreen
- 10 drops Marjoram
- 9 drops Lemongrass

Application and Usage

Topical

You may apply single oils or blends neat or diluted, depending on the oil or oils being used. Please see the instructions at the beginning of this chapter for more information on applying oils to the skin.

- Apply neat or diluted 50:50 on location 3-6 times daily.
- Massage 4-6 drops of oil on affected area. For swelling, elevate and apply ice packs.
- Place a cold compress with 1-2 drops of chosen oil in Ortho Ease or Ortho Sport Massage Oil on area 2-4 times daily.

....

Ligament Sprain or Tear

Note: For sprains, use cold packs. For any serious sprain or constant skeletal pain, always consult a health-care professional. Anytime there is tissue damage, there is always inflammation. Reduce this first.

Recommendations

Singles: Lemongrass, Helichrysum, Lavender, Elemi, Basil, Marjoram, Peppermint, Palo Santo

Blends: PanAway, Relieve It, Aroma Siez, Deep Relief Roll-On

Nutritionals: BLM, MegaCal, Super B, Super C, MultiGreens, Essentialzyme, Mineral Essence, Sulfurzyme

Body Care Massage Oils and Creams: Ortho Ease Massage Oil, Ortho Sport Massage Oil, Regenolone Moisturizing Cream

Sprain Blend

- 15 drops Aroma Siez
- 5 drops Lemongrass

Application and Usage

Topical

You may apply single oils or blends neat or diluted, depending on the oil or oils being used. Please see the instructions at the beginning of this chapter for more information on applying oils to the skin.

- Apply oils neat or diluted 50:50 on location 3-6 times daily.
- Massage 4-6 drops of oil on affected area. For swelling, elevate and apply ice packs.
- Place a cold compress with 1-2 drops of chosen oil on area 2-4 times daily.

....

Tendonitis

Tendons are cords of tough, fibrous connective tissue that attach muscles to bones and are found throughout the entire human body. Tendonitis is the irritation and inflammation of those tendons.

Recommendations

Singles: Lemongrass, Marjoram, Copaiba, Basil, Elemi

Blends: Deep Relief Roll-On, Aroma Siez, PanAway, Relieve It

Nutritionals: MegaCal, Super B, Super C, Super C Chewable, MultiGreens, Mineral Essence, Sulfurzyme, BLM

Body Care Massage Oils and Creams: Regenolone Moisturizing Cream, Ortho Sport Massage Oil, Ortho Ease Massage Oil

Tendonitis Blend No. 1
- 8 drops Wintergreen
- 4 drops Vetiver
- 4 drops Valerian

Tendonitis Relief Blend No. 2 (for Pain Relief)
- 10 drops Rosemary
- 10 drops Eucalyptus Radiata
- 10 drops Peppermint
- 5 drops Palo Santo

Application and Usage
Topical

You may apply single oils or blends neat or diluted, depending on the oil or oils being used. Please see the instructions at the beginning of this chapter for more information on applying oils to the skin.

- Apply oils neat or diluted 50:50 on location 3-6 times daily.
- Massage 4-6 drops of oil on affected area. For swelling, elevate and apply ice packs.
- Place a cold compress with 1-2 drops of chosen oil on area 2-4 times daily.

....

Scleroderma

Also known as systemic sclerosis, scleroderma is a noninfectious, chronic, autoimmune disease of the connective tissue. Caused by an overproduction of collagen, the disease can involve either the skin or internal organs and can be life threatening.

Scleroderma is far more common among women than men.

Recommendations
Singles: Myrrh, Wintergreen, German Chamomile, Sacred Frankincense, Frankincense, Copaiba, Lavender, Patchouli, Sandalwood
Blends: Melrose, Aroma Siez, Thieves, Purification, SclarEssence
Nutritionals: PD 80/20, ICP, ComforTone, Essentialzyme, JuvaTone, JuvaPower, JuvaSpice (for salads and cooking), Thyromin, Mineral Essence, Power Meal, Sulfurzyme, Detoxzyme, Longevity Softgels
Body Care Products: Prenolone Plus Body Cream, LavaDerm Cooling Mist

Scleroderma Blend No. 1
- 2 drops German Chamomile
- 2 drops Myrrh
- 1 drop Lavender
- 1 drop Patchouli

Scleroderma Blend No. 2
- 3 drops Myrrh
- 2 drops Sandalwood

Application and Usage
Topical

You may apply single oils or blends neat or diluted, depending on the oil or oils being used. Please see the instructions at the beginning of this chapter for more information on applying oils to the skin.

- Apply 4-6 drops diluted 50:50 on location 3 times daily. Alternate between using Blend No. 1 and Bend No. 2 each day.

CROHN'S DISEASE (See also COLITIS, DIVERTICULOSIS / DIVERTICULITIS)

Crohn's disease creates inflammation, sores, and ulcers on the intestinal wall. These sores occur deeper than ulcerative colitis. Unlike other forms of colitis, Crohn's disease can affect the entire digestive tract from the mouth all the way to the rectum.

Symptoms
- Abdominal cramping
- Lower-right abdominal pain
- Diarrhea
- A general sense of feeling ill

Attacks may occur once or twice a day for

life. If the disease continues for years, it can cause deterioration of bowel function, leaky gut syndrome, poor absorption of nutrients, loss of appetite and weight, intestinal obstruction, severe bleeding, and increased susceptibility to intestinal cancer.

Most researchers believe that Crohn's disease is caused by an overreacting immune system and is actually an autoimmune disease where the immune system mistakenly attacks the body's own tissues. MSM has been extensively researched for its ability to treat many autoimmune diseases and is the subject of research by University of Oregon researcher Stanley Jacobs. MSM is a key ingredient in Sulfurzyme.

Recommendations

Singles: Ginger, Nutmeg, Wintergreen, German Chamomile, Peppermint, Copaiba, Fennel, Patchouli

Blends: DiGize, PanAway

Nutritionals: OmegaGize[3], Life 5, Detoxzyme, Sulfurzyme, Essentialzymes-4, AlkaLime, ICP, ComforTone, MultiGreens, Digest & Cleanse, NingXia Red, Balance Complete

Application and Usage

Inhalation

- Diffuse your choice of oils for ½ hour every 4-6 hours or as desired.
- Put 2-3 drops of your chosen oil in your hands and rub them together, cup your hands over your nose, and inhale throughout the day as needed.
- Put 8-10 drops of oil on a cotton ball or tissue and put it in an air vent in your house, vehicle, hotel room, etc.
- If diffusing while sleeping, set your timer for the desired length of time for automatic shut off.

Topical

You may apply single oils or blends neat or diluted, depending on the oil or oils being used.

Please see the instructions at the beginning of this chapter for more information on applying oils to the skin.

- Receive a Raindrop Technique 1-2 times weekly incorporating ImmuPower.
- Place a warm compress with 1-2 drops of chosen oil on the back.

Ingestion and Oral

The amount of oil ingested varies with different oils. Whether putting the oils in a capsule or drinking them in a liquid, please refer to the instructions at the beginning of this chapter.

- Take 1 capsule with desired oil 2 times daily.
- Put 2-3 drops of oil in a spoonful of Blue Agave, Yacon Syrup, maple syrup, coconut oil, milk, etc.
- Put the desired amount of oils in a glass of rice milk, almond milk, goat milk, carrot juice, NingXia Red, or even water and then drink it.

Regimen for Crohn's disease

Each phase lasts 3 days and should be added to the previous phases.

- **Phase I:** Essentialzymes-4: Take 1-2 capsules 3 times daily.
- **Phase II:** Take the Essentialzymes-4 in yogurt or liquid acidophilus and charcoal tablets. Do not use ICP, ComforTone, or Essentialzyme yet.
- **Phase III:** Drink 6 oz. raw juice (cherry, prune, celery, carrot, or NingXia Red) 2 times daily.
- **Phase IV:** Take 2 scoops Balance Complete in water or juice 2 times daily.
- **Phase V:** (Start only if there is no sign of bleeding.)
- **ComforTone:** Take 1 capsule morning and night until stools loosen.
- **ICP:** Start with 1 level teaspoon 2 times daily and gradually increase.
- **Essentialzyme:** Start with 1 tablet 3 times daily. If irritation occurs, discontinue for a few days and start again.

CYSTS

Cysts are closed, saclike structures that contain fluid, gas, or semisolid material that is not a normal part of the tissue where it is located. There are hundreds of types, are common, vary in size, and can occur anywhere in the body in people of all ages. Two of the most common types of cysts are ganglion and ovarian.

....

Ganglion Cysts

Ganglion cysts develop in the tissues near joints and tendons, often in the ankles, in the wrists, and behind the knees. They cause painful swelling and are often filled with a thick fluid.

Recommendations

Singles: Oregano, Plectranthus Oregano, Thyme,
Myrrh, Mountain Savory
Blends: Purification, Thieves
Nutritionals: Super C, Mineral Essence, Detoxzyme
Body Care: LavaDerm Cooling Mist, Thieves Spray

Application and Usage
Topical

You may apply single oils or blends neat or diluted, depending on the oil or oils being used. Please see the instructions at the beginning of this chapter for more information on applying oils to the skin.

• Apply 2 drops of chosen oil neat the first day.
• Apply 2 drops of Thyme the second day.
• Apply on location as often as needed.

....

Ovarian and Uterine Cysts
(See also MENSTRUAL AND FEMALE HORMONE CONDITIONS)

Ovarian cysts can be painless or painful if they grow large and affect the ovary. They may be caused by an egg sac that doesn't properly break open or dissolve as part of the menstrual cycle.

Recommendations

Singles: Myrrh, Geranium, Sacred Frankincense, Frankincense, Melaleuca Alternifolia
Blends: Dragon Time, SclarEssence
Nutritionals: PD 80/20, EndoGize, Estro, FemiGen, Mineral Essence, Essentialzyme
Body Creams and Serums: Protec, Prenolone Plus Body Cream, Progessence Plus, Estro, FemiGen

Female Cyst Blend No. 1
• 9 drops Sacred Frankincense or Frankincense
• 5 drops Clary Sage
• 5 drops Myrrh
• 2 drops Thyme
• 2 drops Rosemary

Female Cyst Blend No. 2
• 4 drops Sacred Frankincense or Frankincense
• 4 drops Geranium
• 2 drops Oregano

Application and Usage
Topical

You may apply single oils or blends neat or diluted, depending on the oil or oils being used. Please see the instructions at the beginning of this chapter for more information on applying oils to the skin.

• Apply 1-3 drops on the reproductive Vita Flex points, located around the anklebone on either side of the foot. Work from the ankle bone down to the arch of the foot.
• Place a warm compress with 1-2 oils of your choice on location as needed.
• Retention: Apply 1-2 drops diluted 50:50 on a tampon and insert nightly for 4 nights.
Note: If irritation occurs, discontinue use for 3 days before resuming.

DEPRESSION
(See also INSOMNIA)

Diffusing or directly inhaling essential oils can have an immediate, positive impact on mood. Olfaction (smell) is the only sense that can have direct effects on the limbic region of the brain. Studies at the University of Vienna have shown that some essential oils and their primary constituents (cineole) can stimulate blood flow and activity in the emotional regions of the brain.[18]

Clinical studies at the Department of Psychiatry at the Mie University of Medicine showed that Lemon not only reduced depression, but it also reduced stress when inhaled.[19]

Recommendations

Singles: Lavender, Roman Chamomile, Melissa, Jasmine, Sacred Frankincense, Frankincense, Peppermint, Ylang Ylang, Amazonian Ylang Ylang, Frereana Frankincense, Rosemary, Lemon, Cedarwood

Blends: Valor, Valor Roll-On, Live with Passion, Hope, Joy, Common Sense, The Gift, Oola Balance, Oola Grow, RutaVaLa, RutaVaLa Roll-On

Nutritionals: MultiGreens, Life 5, Super B, Mineral Essence, Balance Complete, Thyromin, EndoGize, SclarEssence, Chocolessence, Einkorn Nuggets

Application and Usage
Inhalation

- Diffuse recommended oils for 20 minutes 3 times daily.
- Put 2-3 drops of your chosen oil in your hands and rub them together, cup your hands over your nose, and inhale 4-6 times daily.
- Put 8-10 drops of oil on a cotton ball or tissue and put it in an air vent in your house, vehicle, hotel room, etc.
- If diffusing while sleeping, set your timer for the desired length of time for automatic shut off.

Topical

You may apply single oils or blends neat or diluted, depending on the oils being used. Please see the instructions at the beginning of this chapter for more information on applying oils to the skin.

- Apply 1-2 drops of recommended oil neat on temples and back of neck as desired.

....

Postpartum Depression

"Baby blues" are normal for a few days after childbirth. Postpartum depression can follow and feel like more of the same or feel worse than before. It can also happen months after childbirth or pregnancy loss.

Recommendations

Singles: Lemon, Melissa, Clary Sage, Cedarwood, Sandalwood, Sacred Frankincense, Frankincense, Frereana Frankincense, Ocotea

Blends: Joy, Trauma Life, Peace & Calming, Hope, RutaVaLa, RutaVaLa Roll-On, Transformation, Dragon Time, Oola Balance, Oola Grow

Nutritionals: Super B, EndoGize, Estro, FemiGen, Chocolessence, Einkorn Nuggets
  Body Serums and Creams: Progessence Plus, Prenolone Plus Body Cream

Application and Usage
Inhalation

- Diffuse recommended oils for 20 minutes 3 times daily.
- Put 2-3 drops of recommended oil in your hands and rub them together, cup your hands over your nose, and inhale 4-6 times daily.
- Put 8-10 drops of oil on a cotton ball or tissue and put it in an air vent in your house, vehicle, hotel room, etc.
- If diffusing while sleeping, set your timer for the desired length of time for automatic shut off.

Topical

You may apply single oils or blends neat or diluted, depending on the oil or oils being used. Please see the instructions at the beginning of this chapter for more information on applying oils to the skin.

- Apply 2-4 drops neat on temples and back of neck 2-4 times daily or as needed.
- Applying a single drop under the nose is helpful and refreshing.
- Place a warm compress with 1-2 drops of chosen oil on the back.

Ingestion and Oral

The amount of oil ingested varies with different oils. Whether putting the oils in a capsule or drinking them in a liquid, please refer to the instructions at the beginning of this chapter.

- Take 1 capsule with desired oil 2 times daily.
- Put 2-3 drops of oil in a spoonful of Blue Agave, Yacon Syrup, maple syrup, coconut oil, milk, etc.
- Put the desired amount of oils in a glass of rice milk, almond milk, goat milk, carrot juice, NingXia Red, or even water and then drink it.

DIABETES

Diabetes is the leading cause of cardiovascular disease and premature death in Westernized countries today. Diabetes causes low energy and persistently high blood glucose.

Type I diabetes usually manifests by age 30 and is often considered to be genetic. Type II diabetes generally manifests later in life and may have a nutritional origin.

Chromium has been shown to help the body metabolize sugars properly.

Wolfberry balances the pancreas and is a detoxifier and cleanser. Diabetes is not common in certain regions of China where wolfberry is consumed regularly.

Stevia leaf extract is one of the most health-restoring plants known. It is a natural sweetener, has no calories, and does not have the harmful side effects of processed sugar or sugar substitutes. Substituting stevia for sugar helps rebuild glucose tolerance and normalize blood sugar fluctuations.

An East Indian herbal formula was shown in a *Journal of the National Medical Association* study to possess hypoglycemic activity. The herbs are: *Cinnamomum tamale, Pterocarpus marsupium, Momordica charantia, Azadirachta indica, Tinospora cordifolia, Aegle marmelos, Gymnema sylvestre, Syzygium cumini, Trigonella foenum-graecum,* and *Ficus racemosa.*

Recommendations

Singles: Ocotea, Clove, Coriander, Fennel, Dill, Cinnamon, Lemongrass

Blends: EndoFlex, DiGize, Thieves, Slique Essence

Nutritionals: MultiGreens, Stevia, MegaCal, Balance Complete, Essentialzyme, Essentialzymes-4, Master Formula HIS or HERS, Ningxia Wolfberries (Dried), Pure Protein, Slique Tea

Application and Usage

Inhalation

- Diffuse your choice of oils for ½ hour every 4-6 hours or as desired.
- Put 2-3 drops of your chosen oil in your hands and rub them together, cup your hands over your nose, and inhale throughout the day as needed.
- Put 8-10 drops of oil on a cotton ball or tissue and put it in an air vent in your house, vehicle, hotel room, etc.
- If diffusing while sleeping, set your timer for the desired length of time for automatic shut off.

Topical

You may apply single oils or blends neat or

diluted, depending on the oil or oils being used. Please see the instructions at the beginning of this chapter for more information on applying oils to the skin.

Ingestion and Oral

The amount of oil ingested varies with different oils. Whether putting the oils in a capsule or drinking them in a liquid, please refer to the instructions at the beginning of this chapter.

- Take 2 capsules 50:50 Ocotea and Coriander 2 times daily.
- Put 2-3 drops of oil in a spoonful of Blue Agave, Yacon Syrup, maple syrup, coconut oil, milk, etc.
- Put the desired amount of oils in a glass of rice milk, almond milk, goat milk, carrot juice, NingXia Red, or even water and then drink it.

DIGESTIVE PROBLEMS

Digestive problems often result in symptoms such as stomach pain, constipation, gas, cramps, bloating, and diarrhea.

....

Constipation (Impacted Bowel)

The principle causes of constipation are inadequate fluid intake and low fiber consumption. Constipation can eventually lead to diverticulosis and diverticulitis, conditions common among older people.

Certain essential oils have demonstrated their ability to improve colon health through supporting intestinal flora, stimulating intestinal motility and peristalsis, fighting infections, and eliminating parasites.

Recommendations

Singles: Ginger, Fennel, Tarragon, Anise Seed, Peppermint

Blends: DiGize, JuvaCleanse

Nutritionals: Digest & Cleanse, ICP, Comfor-Tone, Detoxzyme, Life 5, MegaCal, Mineral Essence, Balance Complete, Essentialzyme, Essentialzymes-4, OmegaGize³, JuvaPower

Application and Usage

Inhalation

- Diffuse your choice of oils for ½ hour every 4-6 hours or as desired.
- Put 2-3 drops of your chosen oil in your hands and rub them together, cup your hands over your nose, and inhale throughout the day as needed.
- Put 8-10 drops of oil on a cotton ball or tissue and put it in an air vent in your house, vehicle, hotel room, etc.
- If diffusing while sleeping, set your timer for the desired length of time for automatic shut off.

Topical

You may apply single oils or blends neat or diluted, depending on the oil or oils being used. Please see the instructions at the beginning of this chapter for more information on applying oils to the skin.

- Apply 6-10 drops neat or diluted 50:50 on stomach area as desired.
- Applying a single drop under the nose is helpful and refreshing.
- Place a warm compress with 1-3 drops of recommended oil over the stomach area and Vita Flex points of the feet.

Ingestion and Oral

The amount of oil ingested varies with different oils. Whether putting the oils in a capsule or drinking them in a liquid, please refer to the instructions at the beginning of this chapter.

- Take 1 capsule with desired oil 2 times daily.
- Put 2-3 drops of oil in a spoonful of Blue Agave, Yacon Syrup, maple syrup, coconut oil, milk, etc.
- Put the desired amount of oils in a glass of rice milk, almond milk, goat milk, carrot juice, NingXia Red, or even water and then drink it.

Regimen

- **Essentialzyme:** Take 3-6 tablets 3 times daily.
- **ComforTone:** Start with 1 capsule and increase the next day to 2 capsules. Continue to increase 1 capsule each day until bowels start moving.
- **ICP:** 1 week after ComforTone, start with 1 tablespoon ICP 2 times daily and then increase to 3 times daily up to 2 tablespoons 3 times daily.
- **Balance Complete:** 3 scoops daily or as needed.
- **Drink** at least ½ cup unsweetened cherry juice, prune juice, pineapple juice, or other raw fruit and vegetable juices each morning.
- **Drink** 8 glasses of pure water daily.

....

Cramps, Stomach

Stomach cramps may be caused by constipation, diarrhea, anxiety, gas, bloating, and PMS. Although stomach cramps are fairly common, paying attention to them is important.

Recommendations

Singles: Ginger, Peppermint, Rosemary, Lavender

Blends: DiGize

Nutritionals: AlkaLime, Digest & Cleanse, Life 5, Essentialzymes-4

Application and Usage

Topical

You may apply single oils or blends neat or diluted, depending on the oil or oils being used. Please see the instructions at the beginning of this chapter for more information on applying oils to the skin.

- Dilute 50:50 and apply 6-10 drops over stomach area 2 times daily.
- Apply a warm compress 1-2 times daily.
- Apply 1-3 drops on stomach Vita Flex points of feet.

Constipation Causes Body Dysfunction

The reason constipation creates diverticulosis is because the muscles of the colon must strain to move an overly hard stool, which puts excess pressure on the colon. Eventually, weak spots in the colon walls form, creating abnormal pockets called diverticula.

These pockets can also be created by parasites that burrow and embed in the lining of the colon wall, lay eggs there, and leave waste matter that hardens on the colon walls, kinking and twisting the colon unnaturally. It is always wise to consider the possibility of parasites and their treatment when diverticula are present.

Enzymes such as Detoxzyme, Essentialzyme, Essentialzymes-4, Allerzyme, and Mightyzyme (for children) are critical to help in the digestion and softening of waste material. ICP and JuvaPower add fiber that help scrub the colon wall, absorb toxins, and help with the elimination process. ParaFree is always a good cleanse at least once a year and certainly when parasites are suspected.

Ingestion and Oral

The amount of oil ingested varies with different oils. Whether putting the oils in a capsule or drinking them in a liquid, please refer to the instructions at the beginning of this chapter.

- Take 1 capsule with desired oil 2 times daily.
- Put 2-3 drops of oil in a spoonful of Blue Agave, Yacon Syrup, maple syrup, coconut oil, milk, etc.
- Put the desired amount of oils in a glass of rice milk, almond milk, goat milk, carrot juice, NingXia Red, or even water and then drink it.

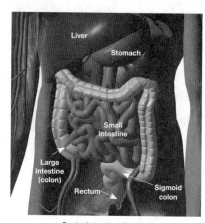

Gastrointestinal System

....

Diarrhea

Diarrhea is the second most commonly reported illness in the U.S. and happens to nearly everyone. It may be caused by bacteria, viruses, food, medication, stress, or chronic medical conditions.

Recommendations

Singles: Ginger, Oregano, Plectranthus Oregano, Mountain Savory, Clove, Lemon, Peppermint, Nutmeg

Blends: DiGize, JuvaFlex, Thieves

Nutritionals: Life 5, ComforTone, Essentialzyme, Detoxzyme, MegaCal, SuperCal, Inner Defense, ICP

Diarrhea Blend

- 4 drops Lemon
- 3 drops Mountain Savory
- 2 drops Wintergreen

Application and Usage

Topical

You may apply single oils or blends neat or diluted, depending on the oil or oils being used. Please see the instructions at the beginning of

this chapter for more information on applying oils to the skin.

- Apply 6-10 drops neat on stomach area as desired.
- Applying a single drop under the nose is helpful and refreshing.
- Dilute 50:50 and apply on location 3-6 times daily.
- Place a warm compress with 1-2 drops of chosen oil on the back.

Ingestion and Oral

The amount of oil ingested varies with different oils. Whether putting the oils in a capsule or drinking them in a liquid, please refer to the instructions at the beginning of this chapter.

- Take 1 capsule with desired oil 2 times daily.
- Put 2-3 drops of oil in a spoonful of Blue Agave, Yacon Syrup, maple syrup, coconut oil, milk, etc.
- Put the desired amount of oils in a glass of rice milk, almond milk, goat milk, carrot juice, NingXia Red, or even water and then drink it.
- A maintenance dosage of ComforTone has helped to protect travelers going to other countries from diarrhea and other digestive discomforts.
- Nutmeg has been shown to have powerful action against diarrhea in a number of medical studies.[18,19]

....

Diverticulosis/Diverticulitis
(See also COLITIS, CROHN'S DISEASE)

Diverticulosis is one of the most common conditions in the U.S. and is caused by a lack of fiber in the diet. Diverticulosis is characterized by small, abnormal pockets (diverticula) that bulge out through weak spots in the wall of the intestine. It is estimated that half of all Americans from age 60 to 80 have diverticulosis.

Symptoms

- Cramping
- Bloating
- Constipation
- Fever and chills
- Cramping tenderness on lower left side of abdomen

One of the easiest ways to resolve this condition is by increasing fiber intake to 20-30 grams daily. Peppermint oil can also stimulate contractions in the colon.

While diverticulosis involves the condition of merely having colon abnormalities, diverticulitis occurs when these abnormalities or diverticula become infected or inflamed. Diverticulitis is present in 10-25 percent of people with diverticulosis.

Many of these symptoms are similar to those of irritable bowel syndrome.

Recommendations

Singles: Oregano, Plectranthus Oregano, Patchouli, Anise, Tarragon, Rosemary, Fennel, Peppermint, Thyme, Nutmeg, Clove, Ocotea, Tangerine, Sacred Frankincense, Frankincense, Cedarwood

Blends: DiGize, Melrose, Thieves, Exodus II, ImmuPower

Nutritionals: AlkaLime, Detoxzyme, Inner Defense, Digest & Cleanse, ICP, ComforTone, Essentialzyme, Balance Complete, JuvaPower

Diverticulitis Blend

- 15 drops DiGize
- 5 drops Melrose

Application and Usage

Inhalation

- Diffuse your choice of oils for ½ hour every 4-6 hours or as desired.
- Put 2-3 drops of your chosen oil in your hands and rub them together, cup your hands over your nose, and inhale throughout the day as needed.

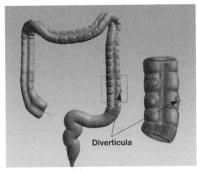

Diverticula

Large Intestine

- Put 8-10 drops of oil on a cotton ball or tissue and put it in an air vent in your house, vehicle, hotel room, etc.
- If diffusing while sleeping, set your timer for the desired length of time for automatic shut off.

Topical

You may apply single oils or blends neat or diluted, depending on the oil or oils being used. Please see the instructions at the beginning of this chapter for more information on applying oils to the skin.

- Dilute 50:50 and apply on lower abdomen 2 times daily.
- Massage 2-4 drops on the intestinal Vita Flex points on the feet 2-3 times daily.
- Retention: Rectal, nightly before retiring, retain overnight.

Ingestion and Oral

The amount of oil ingested varies with different oils. Whether putting the oils in a capsule or drinking them in a liquid, please refer to the instructions at the beginning of this chapter.

- Take 1 capsule with desired oil 2 times daily.
- Put 2-3 drops of oil in a spoonful of Blue Agave, Yacon Syrup, maple syrup, coconut oil, milk, etc.
- Put the desired amount of oils in a glass of

rice milk, almond milk, goat milk, carrot juice, NingXia Red, or even water and then drink it.

Dysentery

Dysentery is a serious disorder of the digestive tract that commonly occurs throughout the world. It can be caused by viruses, bacteria, protozoa, parasitic worms, or chemical irritation of the intestines.

It is one of the oldest known gastrointestinal disorders, often called the "bloody flux," that frequently occurred in army camps, walled cities, aboard sailing vessels, and where large groups of people lived together with poor sanitation.

In the modern world, dysentery is most likely to affect people who live in less developed countries and travelers who visit those countries. It also affects immigrants from developing countries, people who live in housing with poor sanitation, military personnel serving in developing countries, people in nursing homes, and children in day care centers.

Recommendations

Singles: Peppermint, Lemon, Myrrh, Mountain Savory, Oregano

Blends: Thieves, DiGize, JuvaCleanse, JuvaFlex, ParaFree

Nutritionals: Inner Defense, Detoxzyme, Essentialzymes-4, ImmuPro, ICP, ComforTone, Essentialzyme, Mineral Essence

Dysentery Blend

- 5 drops Thieves
- 5 drops Peppermint

Application and Usage

Inhalation

- Diffuse your choice of oils for ½ hour every 4-6 hours or as desired.
- Put 2-3 drops of your chosen oil in your hands and rub them together, cup your hands over your nose, and inhale throughout the day as needed.
- Put 8-10 drops of oil on a cotton ball or tissue and put it in an air vent in your house, vehicle, hotel room, etc.
- If diffusing while sleeping, set your timer for the desired length of time for automatic shut off.

Topical

You may apply single oils or blends neat or diluted, depending on the oil or oils being used. Please see the instructions at the beginning of this chapter for more information on applying oils to the skin.

Ingestion and Oral

The amount of oil ingested varies with different oils. Whether putting the oils in a capsule or drinking them in a liquid, please refer to the instructions at the beginning of this chapter.

- Take 1 capsule with desired oil 3 times daily.
- Put 2-3 drops of oil in a spoonful of Blue Agave, Yacon Syrup, maple syrup, coconut oil, milk, etc.
- Put the desired amount of oils in a glass of rice milk, almond milk, goat milk, carrot juice, NingXia Red, or even water and then drink it.

Gas (Flatulence)

Gas (flatulence) can be caused by a lack of digestive enzymes and the consumption of indigestible starches that promote bifid bacteria production in the colon.

Although increasing bifid bacteria production can lead to gas, it is highly beneficial to long-term health, as the increase of beneficial flora crowds out disease-causing microorganisms such as *Clostridium perfringens*.

Consumption of FOS (fructooligosaccharides), an indigestible sugar, can create short-term flatulence, even as it drastically improves bifidobacteria production in the small and large intestine and increases mineral absorption.

Recommendations

Singles: Peppermint, Nutmeg, Oregano, Plectranthus Oregano, Thyme, Clove, Ginger, Cumin, Anise, Fennel

Blends: DiGize, Thieves, Longevity

Nutritionals: AlkaLime, Detoxzyme, Life 5, Digest & Cleanse, ICP, ComforTone, Essentialzyme, Essentialzymes-4, Inner Defense, JuvaPower, Longevity Softgels

Application and Usage

Inhalation

- Diffuse your choice of oils for ½ hour every 4-6 hours or as desired.
- Applying a single drop under the nose is helpful and refreshing.
- Put 2-3 drops of your chosen oil in your hands and rub them together, cup your hands over your nose, and inhale throughout the day as needed.
- Put 8-10 drops of oil on a cotton ball or tissue and put it in an air vent in your house, vehicle, hotel room, etc.
- If diffusing while sleeping, set your timer for the desired length of time for automatic shut off.

Topical

You may apply single oils or blends neat or diluted, depending on the oil or oils being used. Please see the instructions at the beginning of this chapter for more information on applying oils to the skin.

Ingestion and Oral

The amount of oil ingested varies with different oils. Whether putting the oils in a capsule or drinking them in a liquid, please refer to the instructions at the beginning of this chapter.

- Take 1 capsule with desired oil 2 times daily.
- Put 2-3 drops of oil in a spoonful of Blue Agave, Yacon Syrup, maple syrup, coconut oil, milk, etc.
- Put the desired amount of oils in a glass of rice milk, almond milk, goat milk, carrot juice, NingXia Red, or even water and then drink it.
- Take suggested supplements as directed.

....

Giardia

Giardia is a microscopic parasite found on surfaces or in soil, water, or food that has been contaminated with feces from infected animals or humans. It is most commonly transmitted in water.

Recommendations

Singles: Basil, Patchouli, Peppermint, Spearmint

Blends: DiGize, JuvaCleanse, Melrose, Purification

Nutritionals: Detoxzyme, Essentialzyme, Digest & Cleanse, Mineral Essence, ParaFree

Application and Usage

Ingestion and Oral

The amount of oil ingested varies with different oils. Whether putting the oils in a capsule or drinking them in a liquid, please refer to the instructions at the beginning of this chapter.

- Take 1 capsule with desired oil 2 times daily.
- Take 10 drops of Basil, Peppermint, DiGize, or other oils desired diluted 50:50 in a capsule every 2 hours.
- Put 2-3 drops of oil in a spoonful of Blue Agave, Yacon Syrup, maple syrup, coconut oil, milk, etc.
- Put the desired amount of oils in a glass of rice milk, almond milk, goat milk, carrot juice, NingXia Red, or even water and then drink it.

Heartburn

Heartburn is a burning feeling or pain in the center of the chest that may extend into your back or neck during or after eating.

Lemon juice is one of the best remedies for heartburn. Mix the juice of ½ of a squeezed lemon in 8 oz. of water and sip slowly upon awakening each morning.

Lemon juice helps the stomach stop making digestive acids, therefore alleviating heartburn or other stomach ailments.

Recommendations

Singles: Spearmint, Ginger, Lemon, Cypress, Tarragon, Fennel

Blends: DiGize, JuvaCleanse

Nutritionals: AlkaLime, ICP, ComforTone, Essentialzymes-4, Detoxzyme

Heartburn Blend

- 8 drops Sage
- 3 drops Sandalwood
- 2 drops Basil
- 1 drop Idaho Tansy

Application and Usage
Inhalation

- Diffuse your choice of oils for ½ hour every 4-6 hours or as desired.
- Put 2-3 drops of your chosen oil in your hands and rub them together, cup your hands over your nose, and inhale throughout the day as needed.
- Put 8-10 drops of oil on a cotton ball or tissue and put it in an air vent in your house, vehicle, hotel room, etc.
- If diffusing while sleeping, set your timer for the desired length of time for automatic shut off.

Topical

You may apply single oils or blends neat or diluted, depending on the oils being used. Please refer to the information at the beginning of this chapter for more information on applying oils to the skin.

- Dilute 50:50 and apply on location 3-6 times daily.
- Place a warm compress with 1-3 drops of recommended oils over stomach.
- Apply recommended oils to the Vita Flex points of the feet.

Ingestion and Oral

The amount of oil ingested varies with different oils. Whether putting the oils in a capsule or drinking them in a liquid, please refer to the instructions at the beginning of this chapter.

- Take 1 capsule with desired oil 2 times daily.
- Put 2-3 drops of oil in a spoonful of Blue Agave, Yacon Syrup, maple syrup, coconut oil, milk, etc.
- Put the desired amount of oils in a glass of rice milk, almond milk, goat milk, carrot juice, NingXia Red, or even water and then drink it.

Indigestion (Bloating)

Indigestion causes discomfort in the upper abdomen, resulting in bloating, belching, and nausea. It often occurs during or right after eating and is medically known as dyspepsia.

Recommendations

Singles: Peppermint, Nutmeg, Fennel, Ginger, Cumin, Spearmint, Grapefruit, Copaiba, Wintergreen

Blends: DiGize, JuvaCleanse

Nutritionals: AlkaLime, Detoxzyme, ICP, ComforTone, JuvaPower, Essentialzyme, Essentialzymes-4, Mineral Essence

Application and Usage
Topical

You may apply single oils or blends neat or diluted, depending on the oil or oils being used. Please see the instructions at the beginning of this chapter for more information on applying oils to the skin.

- Dilute 50:50 and apply on location 3-6 times daily.
- Place a warm compress with 1-3 drops of recommended oil over the stomach.

Ingestion and Oral

The amount of oil ingested varies with different oils. Whether putting the oils in a capsule or drinking them in a liquid, please refer to the instructions at the beginning of this chapter.

- Take 1 capsule with desired oil 2 times daily.
- Put 2-3 drops of oil in a spoonful of Blue Agave, Yacon Syrup, maple syrup, coconut oil, milk, etc.
- Put the desired amount of oils in a glass of rice milk, almond milk, goat milk, carrot juice, NingXia Red, or even water and then drink it.
- Take 2-4 capsules of Essentialzymes-4, Essentialzyme, or Detoxzyme before eating to help with digestion and upset stomach.
- When the stomach feels "heavy" from eating meat, Essentialzymes-4 is a beneficial companion to DiGize.

....

Spastic Colon Syndrome/ Irritable Bowel Syndrome

Spastic colon syndrome, often called irritable bowel syndrome, is a functional disorder where the bowel does not work as it should. It is characterized by constipation, diarrhea, gas, bloating, lower abdominal pain or discomfort, and nausea.

Singles: Fennel, Anise
Blends: DiGize
Nutritionals: AlkaLime, Essentialzymes-4, Life 5, Mineral Essence, NingXia Red, Slique Tea

Inhalation

- Diffuse your choice of oils for ½ hour every 4-6 hours or as desired.
- Put 2-3 drops of your chosen oil in your

hands and rub them together, cup your hands over your nose, and inhale throughout the day as needed.
- Put 8-10 drops of oil on a cotton ball or tissue and put it in an air vent in your house, vehicle, hotel room, etc.
- If diffusing while sleeping, set your timer for the desired length of time for automatic shut off.

Topical

You may apply single oils or blends neat or diluted, depending on the oils being used. Please refer to the information at the beginning of this chapter for more information on applying oils to the skin.

- Dilute 50:50 and apply on location 3-6 times daily.
- Place a warm compress with 1-3 drops of recommended oils over stomach.
- Apply recommended oils to the Vita Flex points of the feet.

Ingestion and Oral

The amount of oil ingested varies with different oils. Whether putting the oils in a capsule or drinking them in a liquid, please refer to the instructions at the beginning of this chapter.

- Take 1 capsule with desired oil 2 times daily.
- Put 2-3 drops of oil in a spoonful of Blue Agave, Yacon Syrup, maple syrup, coconut oil, milk, etc.
- Put the desired amount of oils in a glass of rice milk, almond milk, goat milk, carrot juice, NingXia Red, or even water and then drink it.

....

Stomachache

The term "stomachache" is used for many types of stomach or other abdominal discomfort. Some of the following symptoms may occur: pain before or after eating, bloating, heartburn, flatulence, feeling full, vomiting, loss of appetite, etc.

Recommendations

Singles: Peppermint, Roman Chamomile, Lavender, Blue Tansy, Cedarwood, Marjoram, Rose, Sandalwood, Sacred Frankincense, Frankincense, Valerian

Blends: Trauma Life, Humility, Harmony, RutaVaLa, RutaVaLa Roll-On, Valor, Valor Roll-On, Peace & Calming, Tranquil Roll-On

Nutritionals: Super B, Super C, MultiGreens, MegaCal, Mineral Essence, OmegaGize³, AlkaLime, Life 5

Application and Usage
Inhalation

- Diffuse your choice of oils for ½ hour every 4-6 hours or as desired.
- Put 2-3 drops of your chosen oil in your hands and rub them together, cup your hands over your nose, and inhale throughout the day as needed.
- Put 8-10 drops of oil on a cotton ball or tissue and put it in an air vent in your house, vehicle, hotel room, etc.
- If diffusing while sleeping, set your timer for the desired length of time for automatic shut off.

Topical

You may apply single oils or blends neat or diluted, depending on the oil or oils being used. Please see the instructions at the beginning of this chapter for more information on applying oils to the skin.

- Apply any of the desired oils diluted 50:50 on temples, neck, and shoulders 2 times daily or as needed.
- Add desired oil to bath salts and incorporate into daily bathing.

Ingestion and Oral

The amount of oil ingested varies with different oils. Whether putting the oils in a capsule or drinking them in a liquid, please refer to the instructions at the beginning of this chapter.

- Take 1 capsule with desired oil 2 times daily.
- Put 2-3 drops of oil in a spoonful of Blue Agave, Yacon Syrup, maple syrup, coconut oil, milk, etc.
- Put the desired amount of oils in a glass of rice milk, almond milk, goat milk, carrot juice, NingXia Red, or even water and then drink it.

....

Stomach Ulcers

Ulcers may be caused by several gastro-duodenal diseases such as gastritis or gastric or peptic ulcers caused by the *Helicobacter pylori* bacteria.

Recommendations

Singles: Lemongrass, Copaiba, Lemon, Myrtle, German Chamomile, Myrrh, Patchouli, Peppermint

Blends: Thieves, DiGize, Melrose

Nutritionals: Digest & Cleanse, Inner Defense, ICP, JuvaPower, AlkaLime, Essentialzymes-4

Application and Usage
Inhalation

- Diffuse your choice of oils for ½ hour every 4-6 hours or as desired.
- Put 2-3 drops of your chosen oil in your hands and rub them together, cup your hands over your nose, and inhale throughout the day as needed.
- Put 8-10 drops of oil on a cotton ball or tissue and put it in an air vent in your house, vehicle, hotel room, etc.
- If diffusing while sleeping, set your timer for the desired length of time for automatic shut off.

Topical

You may apply single oils or blends neat or diluted, depending on the oil or oils being used. Please see the instructions at the beginning of this chapter for more information on applying oils to the skin.

Any calming oil applied through massage may help to decrease stress and bring a relaxing atmosphere: Dream Catcher, Gathering, Egyptian Gold, The Gift, Harmony, Inner Child, White Angelica, etc.

Ingestion and Oral

The amount of oil ingested varies with different oils. Whether putting the oils in a capsule or drinking them in a liquid, please refer to the instructions at the beginning of this chapter.

- Take 1 capsule with desired oil 3 times daily for 20 days.
- Put 2-3 drops of oil in a spoonful of Blue Agave, Yacon Syrup, maple syrup, coconut oil, milk, etc.
- Put the desired amount of oils in a glass of rice milk, almond milk, goat milk, carrot juice, NingXia Red, or even water and then drink it.

DIPHTHERIA

Diphtheria is an acute infectious disease caused by toxigenic strains of *Corynebacterium diphtheriae*, acquired by contact with an infected person or carrier. It is usually confined to the upper respiratory tract and characterized by the formation of a tough, false membrane attached firmly to the underlying tissue that will bleed if forcibly removed.

In the most serious infections, the membrane begins in the tonsil area and may spread to the uvula, soft palate, and pharyngeal wall, followed by the larynx, trachea, and bronchial tree, where it may cause life-threatening bronchial obstructions. See your physician.

Recommendations

Singles: Oregano, Plectranthus Oregano, Thyme, Clove, Mountain Savory, Eucalyptus Radiata, Palo Santo, Sacred Frankincense, Frankincense, Eucalyptus Blue, Spearmint, Ravintsara, Peppermint, Dorado Azul

Blends: Thieves, Melrose, Exodus II, Raven, R.C., DiGize

Nutritionals: Inner Defense, Essentialzyme, ICP, JuvaPower

Oral: Thieves Fresh Essence Plus Mouthwash, Thieves Spray, Thieves Lozenges (Hard/Soft)

Application and Usage

Inhalation

- Diffuse your choice of oils for ½ hour every 4-6 hours or as desired.
- Put 2-3 drops of your chosen oil in your hands and rub them together, cup your hands over your nose, and inhale throughout the day as needed.
- Put 8-10 drops of oil on a cotton ball or tissue and put it in an air vent in your house, vehicle, hotel room, etc.
- If diffusing while sleeping, set your timer for the desired length of time for automatic shut off.

Topical

You may apply single oils or blends neat or diluted, depending on the oil or oils being used. Please see the instructions at the beginning of this chapter for more information on applying oils to the skin.

- Applying a single drop under the nose is helpful and refreshing.
- Apply 2-3 drops over neck and lung areas several times daily.

Ingestion and Oral

The amount of oil ingested varies with different oils. Whether putting the oils in a capsule or drinking them in a liquid, please refer to the instructions at the beginning of this chapter.

- Take 1 capsule with desired oil 2 times daily.
- Put 2-3 drops of oil in a spoonful of Blue Agave, Yacon Syrup, maple syrup, coconut oil, milk, etc.
- Put the desired amount of oils in a glass of rice milk, almond milk, goat milk, carrot juice, NingXia Red, or even water and then

drink it.

- Gargle with Thieves Fresh Essence Plus Mouthwash several times daily.
- Spray throat as desired with Thieves Spray.
- Use throat lozenges as desired.

DIZZINESS

Feeling dizzy is not an illness but a symptom of something else. Lightheadedness is often caused by a decrease in blood supply to the brain, while vertigo may be caused by an imbalance in the inner ear or brain. Dizziness may also be caused by dehydration or heat stroke.

Recommendations

Singles: Peppermint, Ocotea, Eucalyptus Blue, Dorado Azul, Tangerine, Basil, Cardamom, Niaouli, Sandalwood, Sacred Frankincense, Frankincense, Idaho Blue Spruce

Blends: Clarity, R.C., Brain Power, Common Sense, M-Grain, Grounding, Citrus Fresh, Harmony

Nutritionals: NingXia Red, MultiGreens, Master Formula HIS or HERS, MegaCal, Mineral Essence

Application and Usage

Inhalation

- Diffuse your choice of oils for ½ hour every 4-6 hours or as desired.
- Put 2-3 drops of your chosen oil in your hands and rub them together, cup your hands over your nose, and inhale throughout the day as needed.
- Put 8-10 drops of oil on a cotton ball or tissue and put it in an air vent in your house, vehicle, hotel room, etc.
- If diffusing while sleeping, set your timer for the desired length of time for automatic shut off.

Topical

You may apply single oils or blends neat or diluted, depending on the oil or oils being used.

Please see the instructions at the beginning of this chapter for more information on applying oils to the skin.

- Apply 1-2 drops neat (undiluted) on temples and back of neck, as desired.
- Applying a single drop under the nose is helpful and refreshing.
- Massage 2-4 drops of oil neat on the soles of the feet just before bedtime.

Ingestion and Oral

The amount of oil ingested varies with different oils. Whether putting the oils in a capsule or drinking them in a liquid, please refer to the instructions at the beginning of this chapter.

- Take 1 capsule with desired oil 2 times daily.
- Put 2-3 drops of oil in a spoonful of Blue Agave, Yacon Syrup, maple syrup, coconut oil, milk, etc.
- Put the desired amount of oils in a glass of rice milk, almond milk, goat milk, carrot juice, NingXia Red, or even water and then drink it.

EAR PROBLEMS

Although ear problems are often caused by infections, other conditions may also cause ear pain or discomfort.

....

Earache

Earaches result from inflammation and swelling of the structures that make up the ear and have a multitude of causes and a variety of symptoms.

Recommendations

Singles: Helichrysum, Lavender, Melaleuca Alternifolia, Roman Chamomile, Ravintsara, Peppermint, Eucalyptus Radiata

Blends: Purification, PanAway, ImmuPower, Melrose

Nutritionals: ImmuPro, Super C, Super C Chewable

Spray: Thieves Spray

Application and Usage

Inhalation

- Diffuse your choice of oils for ½ hour every 4-6 hours or as desired.
- Put 2-3 drops of your chosen oil in your hands and rub them together, cup your hands over your nose, and inhale throughout the day as needed.
- Put 8-10 drops of oil on a cotton ball or tissue and put it in an air vent in your house, vehicle, hotel room, etc.
- If diffusing while sleeping, set your timer for the desired length of time for automatic shut off.

Topical

You may apply single oils or blends neat or diluted, depending on the oil or oils being used. Please see the instructions at the beginning of this chapter for more information on applying oils to the skin.

- Apply 2 drops of oil diluted 50:50 in warm olive or fractionated coconut oil to a cotton swab. Using the swab, apply traces to the skin around the opening of the ear, but not in it. Put 2-3 drops of the diluted essential oil on a piece of cotton and place it carefully over the ear opening. Leave in overnight.
- Additional relief may be obtained by placing a warm compress over the ear.
- Massage 1-2 drops on ears and ear lobes using the Vita Flex Technique and on the Vita Flex points for the ear on the feet.

CAUTION: Never put essential oils directly into the ear canal. Ear pain can be very serious. Always seek medical attention if pain persists.

Ingestion and Oral

The amount of oil ingested varies with different oils. Whether putting the oils in a capsule or drinking them in a liquid, please refer to the instructions at the beginning of this chapter.

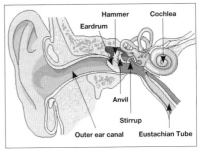

Ear

- Take 1 capsule with desired oil 2 times daily.
- Put 2-3 drops of oil in a spoonful of Blue Agave, Yacon Syrup, maple syrup, coconut oil, milk, etc.
- Put the desired amount of oils in a glass of rice milk, almond milk, goat milk, carrot juice, NingXia Red, or even water and then drink it.
- Gargle up to 8 times daily with Thieves Fresh Essence Plus Mouthwash.
- Spray Thieves Spray into the throat up to 5 times daily.

....

Ear Infection

An ear infection often occurs in conjunction with other symptoms, which may vary in character and intensity in different individuals.

Recommendations

Singles: Myrrh, Thyme, Wintergreen, Helichrysum, Mountain Savory, Basil

Blends: ImmuPower, Melrose, Thieves, Purification, Exodus II

Nutritionals: ImmuPro, Inner Defense

Application and Usage

Inhalation

- Diffuse your choice of oils for ½ hour every 4-6 hours or as desired.
- Put 2-3 drops of your chosen oil in your hands and rub them together, cup your hands

over your nose, and inhale throughout the day as needed.

- Put 8-10 drops of oil on a cotton ball or tissue and put it in an air vent in your house, vehicle, hotel room, etc.
- If diffusing while sleeping, set your timer for the desired length of time for automatic shut off.

Topical

You may apply single oils or blends neat or diluted, depending on the oil or oils being used. Please see the instructions at the beginning of this chapter for more information on applying oils to the skin.

- Apply 2 drops of oil diluted 50:50 in warm olive oil to a cotton swab. Using the swab, apply traces to the skin around the opening of the ear, but not in it.
- Put 2-3 drops of the diluted essential oil on a piece of cotton and place it carefully over the ear opening. Leave in overnight.

CAUTION: Never put essential oils directly into the ear. Ear pain can be very serious. Always seek medical attention if pain persists.

Hearing Impairment

Hearing impairment refers to people with either partial or full hearing loss.

Recommendations

Singles: Helichrysum, Juniper, Geranium, Peppermint, Lavender, Basil

Blends: Purification, Surrender, Awaken, Magnify Your Purpose

Application and Usage

Inhalation

- Diffuse your choice of oils for ½ hour every 4-6 hours or as desired.
- Put 2-3 drops of your chosen oil in your hands and rub them together, cup your hands over your nose, and inhale throughout the day as needed.

- Put 8-10 drops of oil on a cotton ball or tissue and put it in an air vent in your house, vehicle, hotel room, etc.
- If diffusing while sleeping, set your timer for the desired length of time for automatic shut off.

Topical

You may apply single oils or blends neat or diluted, depending on the oil or oils being used. Please see the instructions at the beginning of this chapter for more information on applying oils to the skin.

- Apply single oils or blends neat or diluted, depending on the oils that are used.
- Apply 1 drop neat on a cotton ball and place it carefully in the opening of the ear canal. Retain overnight. **DO NOT place oils directly in the ear canal.**
- Massage 1-2 drops of oil neat on each ear lobe, behind the ears, and down the jaw line along the Eustachian tube.

Hearing Vita Flex Regimen

- Apply 1-2 drops neat of Helichrysum to the area **outside** the opening to the ear canal with fingertip or cotton swab. **DO NOT** put oil inside the ear canal.
- After applying the Helichrysum, hold ear lobes firmly and pull in a circular motion 10 times to help stimulate absorption and circulation in the ear canal.

Tinnitus (Ringing in the Ears)

Tinnitus is a sound in one or both ears like buzzing, whistling, or ringing and occurs without an external stimulus.

Recommendations

Singles: Helichrysum, Juniper, Geranium, Rose, Peppermint, Lavender, Basil

Blends: Purification

Nutritionals: NingXia Red, Detoxzyme, Sulfurzyme

Application and Usage
Inhalation

- Diffuse your choice of oils for ½ hour every 4-6 hours or as desired.
- Put 2-3 drops of your chosen oil in your hands and rub them together, cup your hands over your nose, and inhale throughout the day as needed.
- Put 8-10 drops of oil on a cotton ball or tissue and put it in an air vent in your house, vehicle, hotel room, etc.
- If diffusing while sleeping, set your timer for the desired length of time for automatic shut off.

Topical

You may apply single oils or blends neat or diluted, depending on the oil or oils being used. Please see the instructions at the beginning of this chapter for more information on applying oils to the skin.

- Massage 1-2 drops neat on temples, forehead, and back of neck.
- Apply one drop each on tips of the toes and fingers so that the oils get into the Vita Flex pathways.
- Hearing Vita Flex Regimen:
- Apply 1-2 drops neat of Helichrysum to the area **outside** the opening to the ear canal with fingertip or cotton swab. **DO NOT** put oil inside the ear canal.
- After applying the Helichrysum, hold ear lobes firmly and pull in a circular motion 10 times to help stimulate absorption and circulation in the ear canal.

EATING DISORDERS
(See also ADDICTIONS)

Eating disorders are serious psychological conditions that generally involve negative, self-critical feelings and thoughts about body weight, size, and shape. They involve eating habits that disrupt daily activities and normal body functions.

Anorexia Nervosa

Anorexia nervosa is an eating disorder characterized by total avoidance of food and virtual self-starvation. It may or may not be accompanied by bulimia (binge-purge behavior).

While psychotherapy remains indispensable, the inhalation of essential oils may alter emotions enough to effect a change in the underlying psychology or disturbed-thinking patterns that support this self-destructive behavior. This is accomplished by the ability of aroma to directly stimulate the amygdala gland, which is part of the emotional center of the brain known as the limbic system.

Many essential oils such as Lemon and Ginger when inhaled regularly can combat the emotional addiction that leads anorexics to premature death.

Many people with anorexia believe they do not deserve to be healthy or loved unless they are "slender."

Many people who are anorexic suffer life-threatening nutrient and mineral deficiencies. The lack of magnesium and potassium can actually trigger heart rhythm abnormalities and cardiac arrest. It is absolutely essential that calcium, magnesium, potassium, and other mineral deficiencies are replenished.

Recommendations

Singles: Lemon, Tangerine, Ginger, Mandarin
Blends: Valor, Valor Roll-On, Motivation, Brain Power, Stress Away Roll-On
Nutritionals: Mineral Essence, Balance Complete, MegaCal, Power Meal, Essentialzyme, Essentialzymes-4, OmegaGize^3, Slique Bars

Application and Usage
Inhalation

- Diffuse your choice of oils for ½ hour every 4-6 hours or as desired.
- Put 2-3 drops of your chosen oil in your hands and rub them together, cup your hands

over your nose, and inhale throughout the day as needed.

- Put 8-10 drops of oil on a cotton ball or tissue and put it in an air vent in your house, vehicle, hotel room, etc.
- If diffusing while sleeping, set your timer for the desired length of time for automatic shut off.

Topical

You may apply single oils or blends neat or diluted, depending on the oil or oils being used. Please see the instructions at the beginning of this chapter for more information on applying oils to the skin.

Ingestion and Oral

The amount of oil ingested varies with different oils. Whether putting the oils in a capsule or drinking them in a liquid, please refer to the instructions at the beginning of this chapter.

- Take 1 capsule with desired oil 2 times daily.
- Put 2-3 drops of oil in a spoonful of Blue Agave, Yacon Syrup, maple syrup, coconut oil, milk, etc.
- Put the desired amount of oils in a glass of rice milk, almond milk, goat milk, carrot juice, NingXia Red, or even water and then drink it.

....

Appetite, Loss of

Ginger has been shown to stimulate digestion and improve appetite.

Recommendations

Singles: Ginger, Spearmint, Orange, Nutmeg, Peppermint

Blends: Citrus Fresh, Christmas Spirit, RutaVaLa, RutaVaLa Roll-On, DiGize

Nutritionals: Essentialzyme, Essentialzymes-4, ComforTone, MegaCal, Mineral Essence, NingXia Red, Slique Bars, Wolfberry Crisp

Application and Usage
Inhalation

- Diffuse your choice of oils for ½ hour every 4-6 hours or as desired.
- Put 2-3 drops of your chosen oil in your hands and rub them together, cup your hands over your nose, and inhale throughout the day as needed.
- Put 8-10 drops of oil on a cotton ball or tissue and put it in an air vent in your house, vehicle, hotel room, etc.
- If diffusing while sleeping, set your timer for the desired length of time for automatic shut off.

Topical

You may apply single oils or blends neat or diluted, depending on the oil or oils being used. Please see the instructions at the beginning of this chapter for more information on applying oils to the skin.

- Apply 5-6 drops with massage oil 3-5 times daily or as needed.
- You may also apply 2-3 drops on the Vita Flex points on the feet.
- Applying a single drop under the nose is helpful and refreshing.

Ingestion and Oral

The amount of oil ingested varies with different oils. Whether putting the oils in a capsule or drinking them in a liquid, please refer to the instructions at the beginning of this chapter.

- Take 1 capsule with DiGize or other desired oil 2 times daily.
- Put 2-3 drops of oil in a spoonful of Blue Agave, Yacon Syrup, maple syrup, coconut oil, milk, etc.
- Put the desired amount of oils in a glass of rice milk, almond milk, goat milk, carrot juice, NingXia Red, or even water and then drink it.

Binge Eating Disorder

Binge eating disorder is characterized by the binge eater consuming unnaturally large amounts of food in a short period of time, which acts as a psychological release for excessive emotional stress. However, unlike a bulimic, the binge eater does not usually engage in excessive exercise, vomiting, or taking laxatives to reduce weight.

Singles: Sacred Frankincense, Frankincense, Peppermint

Blends: Slique Essence, 3 Wise Men

Nutritionals: Slique Tea, Slique Slim Caps, Slique Bars, Slique Gum, NingXia Red

Inhalation

- Diffuse your choice of oils for ½ hour every 4-6 hours or as desired.
- Put 2-3 drops of your chosen oil in your hands and rub them together, cup your hands over your nose, and inhale throughout the day as needed.
- Put 8-10 drops of oil on a cotton ball or tissue and put it in an air vent in your house, vehicle, hotel room, etc.
- If diffusing while sleeping, set your timer for the desired length of time for automatic shut off.

Topical

You may apply single oils or blends neat or diluted, depending on the oil or oils being used. Please see the instructions at the beginning of this chapter for more information on applying oils to the skin.

Ingestion and Oral

The amount of oil ingested varies with different oils. Whether putting the oils in a capsule or drinking them in a liquid, please refer to the instructions at the beginning of this chapter.

- Take 1 capsule with desired oil 2 times daily.
- Put 2-3 drops of oil in a spoonful of Blue Agave, Yacon Syrup, maple syrup, coconut oil, milk, etc.
- Put the desired amount of oils in a glass of rice milk, almond milk, goat milk, carrot juice, NingXia Red, or even water and then drink it.

Bulimia

Bulimia is characterized by habitual binge eating and then purging.

Singles: Idaho Balsam Fir, Fennel, Nutmeg

Blends: Slique Essence, Common Sense, DiGize, Forgiveness

Nutritionals: Slique Tea, Slique Slim Caps, Slique Bars, Slique Gum, NingXia Red

Inhalation

- Diffuse your choice of oils for ½ hour every 4-6 hours or as desired.
- Put 2-3 drops of your chosen oil in your hands and rub them together, cup your hands over your nose, and inhale throughout the day as needed.
- Put 8-10 drops of oil on a cotton ball or tissue and put it in an air vent in your house, vehicle, hotel room, etc.
- If diffusing while sleeping, set your timer for the desired length of time for automatic shut off.

Topical

You may apply single oils or blends neat or diluted, depending on the oil or oils being used. Please see the instructions at the beginning of this chapter for more information on applying oils to the skin.

Ingestion

The amount of oil ingested varies with different oils. Whether putting the oils in a capsule or drinking them in a liquid, please refer to the instructions at the beginning of this chapter.

- Take 1 capsule with desired oil 2 times daily.
- Put 2-3 drops of oil in a spoonful of Blue Agave, Yacon Syrup, maple syrup, coconut oil, milk, etc.

- Put the desired amount of oils in a glass of rice milk, almond milk, goat milk, carrot juice, NingXia Red, or even water and then drink it.

EDEMA (SWELLING)
(See also PHLEBITIS)

Swelling, particularly around the ankles, is noticeable when fluids accumulate in the tissue. This puffiness under the skin and around the ankles is more apparent at the end of the day when fluids settle to the lowest part of the body. A potassium deficiency can make swelling worse, so the first recourse is to increase potassium intake.

Recommendations

Singles: German Chamomile, Peppermint, Lavender, Grapefruit, Helichrysum, Tangerine, Geranium, Cypress

Blends: Aroma Life, EndoFlex, DiGize

Nutritionals: Digest & Cleanse, Super C, Super C Chewable, ICP, JuvaPower, Essentialzyme, Detoxzyme, Life 5, MegaCal, Balance Complete

Edema Blend (General)
- 10 drops Wintergreen
- 8 drops Tangerine
- 6 drops Fennel
- 4 drops Juniper
- 3 drops Patchouli

Edema Blend (Morning)
- 10 drops Tangerine
- 10 drops Cypress

Edema Blend (Evening)
- 8 drops Geranium
- 5 drops Cypress
- 5 drops Helichrysum or Grapefruit

Application and Usage
Topical

You may apply single oils or blends neat or diluted, depending on the oil or oils being used. Please see the instructions at the beginning of

this chapter for more information on applying oils to the skin.

- Apply 1-3 drops diluted 50:50 on affected area 2-3 times daily.
- Place a cold compress with 1-2 drops of chosen oil 1-2 times daily on the area.
- Massage 1-3 drops on bladder Vita Flex point on foot.
- Massage 15-20 drops of the General Edema Blend diluted 60:40 in V-6 Vegetable Oil Complex or other massage oil on legs, working from the feet up to the thighs. Do this for 1 week.
- Massage 15-20 drops of Morning Edema Blend diluted 60:40 in V-6 Vegetable Oil Complex or other massage oil on legs, working from the feet up to the thighs. Do this in the morning for 1 week. Repeat the same process in the evening with the Evening Edema Blend.

Ingestion and Oral

The amount of oil ingested varies with different oils. Whether putting the oils in a capsule or drinking them in a liquid, please refer to the instructions at the beginning of this chapter.

- Take 1 capsule with desired oil 2 times daily.
- Put 2-3 drops of oil in a spoonful of Blue Agave, Yacon Syrup, maple syrup, coconut oil, milk, etc.
- Put the desired amount of oils in a glass of rice milk, almond milk, goat milk, carrot juice, NingXia Red, or even water and then drink it.

EMOTIONAL TRAUMA

The effect of heavy emotional trauma can disrupt the stomach and digestive system.

Recommendations

Singles: Sacred Frankincense, Frankincense, Idaho Blue Spruce, Idaho Balsam Fir, Lemon, German Chamomile, Rose, Galbanum,

Lavender, Valerian, Vetiver

Blends: Trauma Life, Hope, Present Time, Valor, Valor Roll-On, Release, Sacred Mountain, Christmas Spirit, 3 Wise Men, Tranquil Roll-On, Stress Away Roll-On, Harmony, Forgiveness, Peace & Calming, White Angelica, The Gift, Oola Balance, Oola Grow, Grounding

Nutritionals: Thyromin, Ultra Young Plus, Master HIS or HERS, EndoGize, PD 80/20

Emotional Pain Relief Blend No. 1
- 10 drops Idaho Blue Spruce
- 5 drops Idaho Balsam Fir
- 5 drops Sacred Frankincense

Emotional Pain Relief Blend No. 2
- 8 drops Lavender
- 6 drops Marjoram
- 3 drops Spearmint
- 2 drops Peppermint

Application and Usage
Inhalation
- Diffuse your choice of oils for ½ hour every 4-6 hours or as desired.
- Put 2-3 drops of your chosen oil in your hands and rub them together, cup your hands over your nose, and inhale throughout the day as needed.
- Put 8-10 drops of oil on a cotton ball or tissue and put it in an air vent in your house, vehicle, hotel room, etc.
- If diffusing while sleeping, set your timer for the desired length of time for automatic shut off.

Topical
You may apply single oils or blends neat or diluted, depending on the oil or oils being used. Please see the instructions at the beginning of this chapter for more information on applying oils to the skin.
- Place 1-3 drops of Release over the thymus and rub in gently. Apply up to 3 times daily as needed.

- Blend equal parts Frankincense and Valor and apply 1-2 drops neat on temples, forehead, crown, and back of neck before retiring. Use for 3 nights.
- Apply 1-2 drops neat to the crown of head and forehead as needed. It is best if it is applied in a quiet, darkened room.
- Massage 1-3 drops on heart Vita Flex points 2-3 times daily.
- Rub 1-2 drops of oil on the temples and back of neck several times daily.

Ingestion and Oral
The amount of oil ingested varies with different oils. Whether putting the oils in a capsule or drinking them in a liquid, please refer to the instructions at the beginning of this chapter.
- Take 1 capsule with desired oil 2 times daily.
- Put 2-3 drops of oil in a spoonful of Blue Agave, Yacon Syrup, maple syrup, coconut oil, milk, etc.
- Put the desired amount of oils in a glass of rice milk, almond milk, goat milk, carrot juice, NingXia Red, or even water and then drink it.

ENDOCRINE SYSTEM
(See also THYROID PROBLEMS, CUSHING'S SYNDROME (DISEASE), MALE HORMONE IMBALANCE, MENSTRUAL AND FEMALE HORMONE CONDITIONS)

The endocrine system encompasses the hormone-producing glands of the body. These glands cluster around blood vessels and release their hormones directly into the bloodstream. The pituitary gland exerts a wide range of control over the hormonal (endocrine) system and is often called the master gland. Other glands include the pancreas, adrenals, thyroid and parathyroid, ovaries, and testes.

The limbic system lies along the margin of the cerebral cortex (brain) and is the hormone-

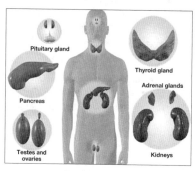

Endocrine System

producing system of the brain. It includes the amygdala, hippocampus, pineal, pituitary, thalamus, and hypothalamus.

Essential oils increase circulation to the brain and enable the pituitary and other glands to better secrete neural transmitters and hormones that support the endocrine and immune systems.

The thyroid is one of the most important glands for regulating the body systems. The hypothalamus plays an even more important role, since it regulates not only the thyroid but also the adrenals and the pituitary gland.

Singles: Canadian Fleabane (Conyza), Myrtle, Sacred Frankincense, Fennel, Idaho Blue Spruce

Blends: EndoFlex, Harmony, The Gift

Nutritionals: Ultra Young, Thyromin, CortiStop Women's, Super B, NingXia Red, Master Formula HIS or HERS

EPILEPSY

Note: Epileptics should consult their healthcare professional before using essential oils. Use extreme caution with high ketone oils such as Basil, Rosemary, Sage, and Idaho Tansy.

Recommendations

Singles: Clary Sage, Sandalwood, Cedarwood, Sacred Frankincense, Frankincense, Lavender

Blends: Valor, Valor Roll-On, Brain Power, RutaVaLa, RutaVaLa Roll-On, Common Sense, Peace & Calming

Nutritionals: ICP, ComforTone, Essentialzyme, NingXia Red, JuvaPower, Master Formula HIS or HERS, Super B

Application and Usage
Inhalation

- Diffuse your choice of oils for ½ hour every 4-6 hours or as desired.
- Put 2-3 drops of your chosen oil in your hands and rub them together, cup your hands over your nose, and inhale throughout the day as needed.
- Put 8-10 drops of oil on a cotton ball or tissue and put it in an air vent in your house, vehicle, hotel room, etc.
- If diffusing while sleeping, set your timer for the desired length of time for automatic shut off.

Topical

You may apply single oils or blends neat or diluted, depending on the oil or oils being used. Please see the instructions at the beginning of this chapter for more information on applying oils to the skin.

- Massage 2-4 drops on brain Vita Flex points on feet 2-3 times daily.

EPSTEIN-BARR VIRUS

Epstein-Barr virus is a type of herpes virus that also causes mononucleosis.

Symptoms include indigestion, upper and lower gas, poor assimilation, poor electrolyte balance, allergic reaction to foods and other substances, emotional mood swings, fatigue, irritability, and a lack of motivation, discipline, and creativity.

Hypoglycemia is a precursor and can render the body susceptible to the Epstein-Barr virus. Treat the hypoglycemia, and the symptoms of the Epstein-Barr virus may begin to disappear.

Recommendations

Singles: Palo Santo, Mountain Savory, Oregano, Plectranthus Oregano, Rosemary, Thyme, Clove, Sandalwood, Grapefruit, Nutmeg, Melaleuca Alternifolia

Blends: Thieves, ImmuPower, EndoFlex, Longevity, DiGize, Exodus II

Nutritionals: Inner Defense, Super C, Super C Chewable, ImmuPro, Thyromin, Detoxzyme, Digest & Cleanse, ICP, JuvaPower, Comfor-Tone, Essentialzyme, Allerzyme, Life 5, Essentialzymes-4, Master Formula HIS or HERS

Application and Usage

Inhalation

- Diffuse your choice of oils for ½ hour every 4-6 hours or as desired.
- Put 2-3 drops of your chosen oil in your hands and rub them together, cup your hands over your nose, and inhale throughout the day as needed.
- Put 8-10 drops of oil on a cotton ball or tissue and put it in an air vent in your house, vehicle, hotel room, etc.
- If diffusing while sleeping, set your timer for the desired length of time for automatic shut off.

Topical

You may apply single oils or blends neat or diluted, depending on the oil or oils being used. Please see the instructions at the beginning of this chapter for more information on applying oils to the skin.

- Receive a Raindrop Technique weekly with ImmuPower, Thieves, Exodus II, and the oils of Raindrop Technique.
- Massage 2-4 drops of oil neat on the soles of the feet just before bedtime.

Ingestion and Oral

The amount of oil ingested varies with different oils. Whether putting the oils in a capsule or drinking them in a liquid, please refer to the instructions at the beginning of this chapter.

- Take 1 capsule with desired oil 3 times daily.
- Put 2-3 drops of oil in a spoonful of Blue Agave, Yacon Syrup, maple syrup, coconut oil, milk, etc.
- Put the desired amount of oils in a glass of rice milk, almond milk, goat milk, carrot juice, NingXia Red, or even water and then drink it.

Mononucleosis

Infectious mononucleosis is a disease caused by the Epstein-Barr virus (EBV), which is a type of herpes virus. The symptoms usually last for four weeks or more. The spleen enlarges and may even rupture in severe cases.

Recommendations

Singles: Ravintsara, Hyssop, Thyme, Sacred Frankincense, Frankincense, Palo Santo, Mountain Savory, Ocotea

Blends: Thieves, Inner Defense, R.C., Breathe Again Roll-On, Raven, Exodus II, ImmuPower

Nutritionals: ImmuPro, Super C, Super C Chewable, Longevity Softgels, ICP, Comfor-Tone, Essentialzyme, Detoxzyme, Life 5

Mononucleosis Blend

3 drops Thieves
3 drops Thyme
3 drops Mountain Savory
2 drops Ravintsara

Application and Usage

Inhalation

- Diffuse your choice of oils for ½ hour every 4-6 hours or as desired.
- Put 2-3 drops of your chosen oil in your

hands and rub them together, cup your hands over your nose, and inhale throughout the day as needed.

- Put 8-10 drops of oil on a cotton ball or tissue and put it in an air vent in your house, vehicle, hotel room, etc.
- If diffusing while sleeping, set your timer for the desired length of time for automatic shut off.

Topical

You may apply single oils or blends neat or diluted, depending on the oil or oils being used. Please see the instructions at the beginning of this chapter for more information on applying oils to the skin.

- Receive a Raindrop Technique 2 times weekly.
- Massage 3-6 drops using the Vita Flex technique on the bottoms of feet 2 times daily.

Ingestion and Oral

The amount of oil ingested varies with different oils. Whether putting the oils in a capsule or drinking them in a liquid, please refer to the instructions at the beginning of this chapter.

- Take 1 capsule with desired oil 3 times daily.
- Put 2-3 drops of oil in a spoonful of Blue Agave, Yacon Syrup, maple syrup, coconut oil, milk, etc.
- Put the desired amount of oils in a glass of rice milk, almond milk, goat milk, carrot juice, NingXia Red, or even water and then drink it.

EYE DISORDERS

In 1997 Dr. Terry Friedmann, MD, eliminated his need for glasses after applying Sandalwood and Juniper on the areas around his eyes, above the eyebrows, and on the cheeks, being careful never to get oil into his eyes. He also used the supplements of MultiGreens, ICP, ComforTone, Essentialzyme, JuvaTone, and JuvaPower for a complete colon and liver cleanse.

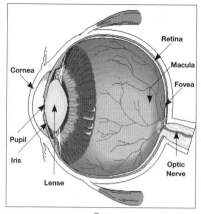

Eye

Caution: Never put any essential oils in the eyes or on the eyelids.

....

Age-Related Macular Degeneration (AMD)

AMD is one of the most common causes of blindness among people over 60 years of age. In fact 30 percent of all people over 70 years of age suffer to some degree from this disease. The most common form of the disease is called "dry" when macular cells degenerate irreversibly.

The "wet" form of the disease is when there is abnormal blood vessel growth that results in macula-damaging blood leaks. The disease results in a steady loss of central vision until eyesight is totally impaired.

For dry AMD, the best prevention will be foods rich in antioxidants and carotenoids. The Ningxia wolfberry, the highest known antioxidant food, is also extremely high in lutein and zeazanthin, which are vital for preserving eye health. Other foods rich in carotenoids that are also powerful antioxidants include blueberries and spinach.

For dry AMD, Lemon oil may be helpful as

a dietary supplement.

Clove oil, the highest known antioxidant nutrient, may be a good nutritional defense for wet AMD only.

Recommendations
Singles: Sacred Frankincense, Lemon (dry AMD only) as a dietary supplement, Clove (wet AMD only) as a dietary supplement
Blends: Longevity
Nutritionals: NingXia Red, OmegaGize³, Longevity Softgels, Power Meal, MultiGreens, Essentialzyme, Essentialzymes-4, Super C, Super C Chewable, Ningxia Wolfberries (Dried), Master Formula HIS or HERS

Application and Usage
Inhalation
- Diffuse your choice of oils for ½ hour every 4-6 hours or as desired.
- Put 2-3 drops of your chosen oil in your hands and rub them together, cup your hands over your nose, and inhale throughout the day as needed.
- Put 8-10 drops of oil on a cotton ball or tissue and put it in an air vent in your house, vehicle, hotel room, etc.
- If diffusing while sleeping, set your timer for the desired length of time for automatic shut off.

Topical
You may apply single oils or blends neat or diluted, depending on the oil or oils being used. Please see the instructions at the beginning of this chapter for more information on applying oils to the skin.
- Receive a Raindrop Technique 2 times weekly.
- Massage 3-6 drops using the Vita Flex technique on the bottoms of feet 2 times daily.

Ingestion and Oral
The amount of oil ingested varies with different oils. Whether putting the oils in a capsule or drinking them in a liquid, please refer to the instructions at the beginning of this chapter.
- Take 1 capsule with desired oil 2 times daily.
- Put 2-3 drops of oil in a spoonful of Blue Agave, Yacon Syrup, maple syrup, coconut oil, milk, etc.
- Put the desired amount of oils in a glass of rice milk, almond milk, goat milk, carrot juice, NingXia Red, or even water and then drink it.

Blocked Tear Ducts
A blocked tear duct is a partial or complete blockage in the system that carries tears away from the eye into the nose.

Recommendations
Singles: Lavender, Sacred Frankincense, Frankincense, Cypress, Idaho Blue Spruce
Blends: Inner Child, Sacred Mountain
Nutritionals: NingXia Red, OmegaGize3, Longevity Softgels, Essentialzyme, Essentialzymes-4, Master Formula HIS or HERS

Application and Usage
Inhalation
- Diffuse your choice of oils for ½ hour every 4-6 hours or as desired.
- Put 2-3 drops of your chosen oil in your hands and rub them together, cup your hands over your nose, and inhale throughout the day as needed.
- Put 8-10 drops of oil on a cotton ball or tissue and put it in an air vent in your house, vehicle, hotel room, etc.
- If diffusing while sleeping, set your timer for the desired length of time for automatic shut off.

Topical
You may apply single oils or blends neat or diluted, depending on the oil or oils being used. Please see the instructions at the beginning of

this chapter for more information on applying oils to the skin.

- Rubbing 1 drop of Lavender oil over the bridge of the nose 2 times daily has been reported to help in some cases.
- Receive a Raindrop Technique 2 times weekly.
- Massage 3-6 drops using the Vita Flex technique on the bottoms of feet 2 times daily.

Ingestion and Oral

The amount of oil ingested varies with different oils. Whether putting the oils in a capsule or drinking them in a liquid, please refer to the instructions at the beginning of this chapter.

- Take 1 capsule with desired oil 3 times daily.
- Put 2-3 drops of oil in a spoonful of Blue Agave, Yacon Syrup, maple syrup, coconut oil, milk, etc.
- Put the desired amount of oils in a glass of rice milk, almond milk, goat milk, carrot juice, NingXia Red, or even water and then drink it.

· ·

Cataracts

Cataracts are a clouding of the eye lens that often comes with aging.

Recommendations

Singles: Lavender, Sacred Frankincense, Frankincense, Lemon

Blends: Longevity, Melrose, En-R-Gee, Purification

Nutritionals: JuvaPower, OmegaGize[3], Mineral Essence, Essentialzyme, ImmuPro (at bedtime), NingXia Red (2-6 ounces daily or more if desired), Ningxia Wolfberries (Dried)

Eye Blend
- 10 drops Lemongrass
- 5 drops Cypress
- 3 drops Eucalyptus Radiata
- 2 drops Sacred Frankincense or Frankincense

Mix this blend with a little V-6 Vegetable Oil Complex and apply around the eyes, being careful not to touch the eyes. It is best at night because the eyes could water, just like when you cut onions.

Note: If essential oils should ever accidentally get into the eyes, dilute with V-6 Vegetable Oil Complex or other pure vegetable oil. **Never rinse with water.** However, the essential oils will not cause any damage and will slowly stop burning.

Application and Usage

Inhalation

- Diffuse your choice of oils for ½ hour every 4-6 hours or as desired.
- Put 2-3 drops of your chosen oil in your hands and rub them together, cup your hands over your nose, and inhale throughout the day as needed.
- Put 8-10 drops of oil on a cotton ball or tissue and put it in an air vent in your house, vehicle, hotel room, etc.
- If diffusing while sleeping, set your timer for the desired length of time for automatic shut off.

Topical

You may apply single oils or blends neat or diluted, depending on the oil or oils being used. Please see the instructions at the beginning of this chapter for more information on applying oils to the skin.

- Apply 2-4 drops diluted 20:80 in a wide circle around the eye 1-3 times daily, being careful not to get any oil in the eyes or on the eyelids. This may also help with puffiness.
- Apply on temples and eye Vita Flex points on the feet and hands (the undersides of your two largest toes and your index and middle fingers).

Note: If essential oils should ever accidentally get into the eyes, dilute with V-6 Vegetable Oil Complex or other pure vegetable oil. **Never rinse with water.** However, the essential oils will not cause any damage and will slowly stop burning.

Ingestion and Oral

The amount of oil ingested varies with different oils. Whether putting the oils in a capsule or drinking them in a liquid, please refer to the instructions at the beginning of this chapter.

- Take 1 capsule with desired oil 2 times daily.
- Put 2-3 drops of oil in a spoonful of Blue Agave, Yacon Syrup, maple syrup, coconut oil, milk, etc.
- Put the desired amount of oils in a glass of rice milk, almond milk, goat milk, carrot juice, NingXia Red, or even water and then drink it.
- Clove oil is the most powerful known antioxidant, and when taken internally, it can slow or prevent both cataracts and AMD.

....

Conjunctivitis / Pink Eye

Conjunctivitis (also called pink eye) is inflammation of the outermost layer of the eye and the inner surface of the eyelids. It has many causes, which may be infectious or noninfectious.

Recommendations

Singles: Myrrh, Lavender, Vetiver
Nutritionals: NingXia Red, Ningxia Wolfberries (Dried), OmegaGize[3], ImmuPro (at bedtime), Exodus II, Raindrop

Application and Usage

Inhalation

- Diffuse your choice of oils for ½ hour every 4-6 hours or as desired.
- Put 2-3 drops of your chosen oil in your hands and rub them together, cup your hands over your nose, and inhale throughout the day as needed.

- Put 8-10 drops of oil on a cotton ball or tissue and put it in an air vent in your house, vehicle, hotel room, etc.
- If diffusing while sleeping, set your timer for the desired length of time for automatic shut off.

Topical

You may apply single oils or blends neat or diluted, depending on the oil or oils being used. Please see the instructions at the beginning of this chapter for more information on applying oils to the skin.

- Apply 2-4 drops diluted 20:80 in a wide circle around the eye 1-3 times daily, being careful not to get any oil in the eyes or on the eyelids. This may also help with puffiness.
- Apply on temples and eye Vita Flex points on the feet and hands (the undersides of your two largest toes and your index and middle fingers).
  Note: If essential oils should ever accidentally get into the eyes, dilute with V-6 Vegetable Oil Complex or other pure vegetable oil. **Never rinse with water.** However, the essential oils will not cause any damage and will slowly stop burning.

Ingestion and Oral

The amount of oil ingested varies with different oils. Whether putting the oils in a capsule or drinking them in a liquid, please refer to the instructions at the beginning of this chapter.

- Take 1 capsule with desired oil 3 times daily.
- Put 2-3 drops of oil in a spoonful of Blue Agave, Yacon Syrup, maple syrup, coconut oil, milk, etc.
- Put the desired amount of oils in a glass of rice milk, almond milk, goat milk, carrot juice, NingXia Red, or even water and then drink it.

FAINTING
(See also SHOCK)

Fainting happens when your brain does not get enough oxygen and you lose consciousness for a brief time. It can be caused by many different things.

Recommendations

Singles: Idaho Blue Spruce, Melissa, Peppermint, Sandalwood, Cardamom, Spearmint, Sacred Frankincense, Frankincense

Blends: Clarity, Trauma Life, Brain Power, R.C., Awaken

Application and Usage
Inhalation

- Open an oil bottle and wave it under the nose of the person who fainted.
- If you are feeling faint, open the oil bottle and inhale or put 2-3 drops of your chosen oil in your hands and rub them together, cup your hands over your nose, and inhale.

Topical

You may apply single oils or blends neat or diluted, depending on the oil or oils being used. Please see the instructions at the beginning of this chapter for more information on applying oils to the skin.

FATIGUE

Hormone imbalances may play a large role in fatigue as well as in latent viral infections (herpes virus and/or Epstein-Barr virus). Also, mineral deficiencies (especially magnesium) can play a large part in low energy.

Natural progesterone for women and DHEA for men can be instrumental in helping combat the fatigue that comes with age and declining hormone levels. Because pregnenolone is a precursor for all male and female hormones, both men and women can benefit from its supplementation.

Mental Fatigue

Mental fatigue is excessive mental tiredness and may manifest itself in difficulty concentrating and solving problems, irritability, loss of passion for work, anxiety, sleeplessness, confusion, or frustration.

Recommendations

Singles: Idaho Blue Spruce, Peppermint, Spearmint, Idaho Balsam Fir, Sacred Frankincense, Frankincense, Frereana Frankincense, Black Pepper, Sage, Nutmeg, Pine

Blends: Envision, Valor, Oola Balance, Oola Grow, Motivation, En-R-Gee, Clarity, Common Sense

Nutritionals: Power Meal, Balance Complete, MultiGreens, Mineral Essence, Longevity Softgels, NingXia Red, NingXia Nitro, Pure Protein, Essentialzymes-4, Ultra Young Plus, Super B, EndoGize, Sleep Essence, Slique Bars

Application and Usage
Inhalation

- Diffuse your choice of oils for ½ hour every 2 hours or as desired.
- Put 2-3 drops of your chosen oil in your hands and rub them together, cup your hands over your nose, and inhale throughout the day as needed.
- Put 8-10 drops of oil on a cotton ball or tissue and put it in an air vent in your house, vehicle, hotel room, etc.
- If diffusing while sleeping, set your timer for the desired length of time for automatic shut off.

Topical

You may apply single oils or blends neat or diluted, depending on the oil or oils being used. Please see the instructions at the beginning of this chapter for more information on applying oils to the skin.

- Apply 2-4 drops diluted 50:50 at base of throat, temples, and back of neck as needed.

- Massage 1-3 drops on corresponding Vita Flex points on feet 1-3 times daily.

Ingestion and Oral

The amount of oil ingested varies with different oils. Whether putting the oils in a capsule or drinking them in a liquid, please refer to the instructions at the beginning of this chapter.

- Take 1 capsule with desired oil 2 times daily.
- Put 2-3 drops of oil in a spoonful of Blue Agave, Yacon Syrup, maple syrup, coconut oil, milk, etc.
- Put the desired amount of oils in a glass of rice milk, almond milk, goat milk, carrot juice, NingXia Red, or even water and then drink it.

....

Physical Fatigue

Physical fatigue is a lack of energy that can be caused by a host of factors, including poor thyroid function, adrenal imbalance, diabetes, cancer, and other conditions.

MultiGreens is a plant-derived, high-protein energy formula that athletes use to boost endurance. Longevity Softgels increase energy and endurance. Digestion and colon problems may cause fatigue. A colon and liver cleanse unburdens the digestive system and increases energy.

Recommendations

Singles: Peppermint, Nutmeg, Lemongrass, Eucalyptus Blue, Dorado Azul, Juniper, Basil, Lemon, Rosemary, Thyme, Cypress,

Blends: Awaken, Motivation, Valor, Valor Roll-On, En-R-Gee, Oola Balance, Oola Grow, Hope, EndoFlex

Nutritionals: Thyromin, MultiGreens, Power Meal, EndoGize, Longevity Softgels, Super B, NingXia Red, Ningxia Wolfberries (Dried), Digest & Cleanse, Life 5, NingXia Nitro, ImmuPro (at bedtime)

Application and Usage
Inhalation

- Diffuse your choice of oils for 10 minutes 3 times daily.
- Put 2-3 drops of your chosen oil in your hands and rub them together, cup your hands over your nose, and inhale throughout the day as needed.
- Put 8-10 drops of oil on a cotton ball or tissue and put it in an air vent in your house, vehicle, hotel room, etc.
- If diffusing while sleeping, set your timer for the desired length of time for automatic shut off.

Topical

You may apply single oils or blends neat or diluted, depending on the oil or oils being used. Please see the instructions at the beginning of this chapter for more information on applying oils to the skin.

- Apply 2-4 drops diluted 50:50 on temples, in clavicle notch (over thyroid), and behind ears 2-4 times daily as needed.
- Place a warm compress with 1-2 drops of chosen oil on the back.

Ingestion and Oral

The amount of oil ingested varies with different oils. Whether putting the oils in a capsule or drinking them in a liquid, please refer to the instructions at the beginning of this chapter.

- Take 1 capsule with desired oil 3 times daily.
- Put 2-3 drops of oil in a spoonful of Blue Agave, Yacon Syrup, maple syrup, coconut oil, milk, etc.
- Put the desired amount of oils in a glass of rice milk, almond milk, goat milk, carrot juice, NingXia Red, or even water and then drink it.

FEVER

Fevers are one of the most powerful healing responses of the human body and are an indication that the body is fighting an infectious disease. However, if the fever raises body temperature excessively (over 104° F), then neurological damage can occur.

Reducing the fever is best accomplished by using anti-inflammatory essential oils internally and topically.

Recommendations

Singles: Peppermint, Eucalyptus Blue, Nutmeg, German Chamomile, Idaho Balsam Fir, Copaiba, Myrrh, Dorado Azul

Blends: ImmuPower, Melrose, Raven, Clarity, M-Grain, RutaVaLa, RutaVaLa Roll-On

Nutritionals: Super C, Super C Chewable, ImmuPro, Longevity Softgels, Thieves Spray

Lip Balm: Cinnamint Lip Balm, Lavender Lip Balm, Grapefruit Lip Balm

Application and Usage

Inhalation

- Diffuse your choice of oils for ½ hour every 4-6 hours or as desired.
- Put 2-3 drops of your chosen oil in your hands and rub them together, cup your hands over your nose, and inhale throughout the day as needed.
- Put 8-10 drops of oil on a cotton ball or tissue and put it in an air vent in your house, vehicle, hotel room, etc.
- If diffusing while sleeping, set your timer for the desired length of time for automatic shut off.

Topical

You may apply single oils or blends neat or diluted, depending on the oil or oils being used. Please see the instructions at the beginning of this chapter for more information on applying oils to the skin.

- Apply 2-3 drops diluted 50:50 to forehead, temples, and back of neck.
- You may also apply 2-3 drops on the Vita Flex liver point of the right foot.

Ingestion and Oral

The amount of oil ingested varies with different oils. Whether putting the oils in a capsule or drinking them in a liquid, please refer to the instructions at the beginning of this chapter.

- Take 1 capsule with desired oil 2 times daily.
- Put 2-3 drops of oil in a spoonful of Blue Agave, Yacon Syrup, maple syrup, coconut oil, milk, etc.
- Put the desired amount of oils in a glass of rice milk, almond milk, goat milk, carrot juice, NingXia Red, or even water and then drink it.

FIBROIDS
(See Also MENSTRUAL AND FEMALE HORMONE CONDITIONS)

Fibroids are fairly common benign tumors of the female pelvis that are composed of smooth muscle cells and fibrous connective tissue. Fibroids are not cancerous and neither develop into cancer nor increase a woman's cancer risk in the uterus.

Fibroids can have a diameter as small as 1 mm or as large as 8 inches. They can develop in clusters or alone as a single knot or nodule.

Fibroids frequently occur in premenopausal women and are seldom seen in young women who have not begun menstruation. Fibroids usually stabilize or even regress in women who have been through menopause.

Recommendations

Singles: Sacred Frankincense, Frankincense, Idaho Tansy, Oregano, Plectranthus Oregano, Pine, Cistus, Helichrysum, Lavender, Geranium

Blends: Valor, Valor Roll-On, EndoFlex

Nutritionals: MultiGreens, Power Meal, Balance Complete, PD 80/20, Essentialzyme, Life 5

Massage Oil: Cel-Lite Magic Massage Oil

Application and Usage

Inhalation

- Diffuse your choice of oils for ½ hour every 4-6 hours or as desired.
- Put 2-3 drops of your chosen oil in your hands and rub them together, cup your hands over your nose, and inhale throughout the day as needed.
- Put 8-10 drops of oil on a cotton ball or tissue and put it in an air vent in your house, vehicle, hotel room, etc.
- If diffusing while sleeping, set your timer for the desired length of time for automatic shut off.

Topical

You may apply single oils or blends neat or diluted, depending on the oil or oils being used. Please see the instructions at the beginning of this chapter for more information on applying oils to the skin.

- Place a warm compress with 1-2 drops of chosen oil on the back.
- Applying a single drop under the nose is helpful and refreshing.
- Dilute 50:50 and apply on location 3-6 times daily.
- Massage 2-4 drops of oil neat on the soles of the feet just before bedtime.

Ingestion and Oral

The amount of oil ingested varies with different oils. Whether putting the oils in a capsule or drinking them in a liquid, please refer to the instructions at the beginning of this chapter.

- Take 1 capsule with desired oil 2 times daily.
- Put 2-3 drops of oil in a spoonful of Blue Agave, Yacon Syrup, maple syrup, coconut oil, milk, etc.

- Put the desired amount of oils in a glass of rice milk, almond milk, goat milk, carrot juice, NingXia Red, or even water and then drink it.

FIBROMYALGIA

Fibromyalgia is an autoimmune disorder of the soft tissues and appears to include problems within the pain-signaling pathways of the brain and the spinal cord. By contrast, arthritis occurs in the joints.

The symptoms of fibromyalgia include general body pain, in some places worse than others, and are usually brought on by short periods of exercise or low levels of stimulation. Diagnosis includes tenderness or pain in at least 11 of 18 specific points in muscles, tendons, and bones.

The pain is generally continuous and interrupts sleep patterns so that the fourth stage of sleep is never attained, and the body cannot rejuvenate and heal. Fibromyalgia is an acid condition in which the liver is toxic (See Liver Disorders).

The best natural remedy for fibromyalgia is to consume supplements such as flax seed and omegas, proteolytic enzymes such as bromelain and pancreatin, and MSM.

According to UCLA researcher Ronald Lawrence, MD, PhD, supplementation with MSM often offers a breakthrough in the treatment of fibromyalgia.

Recommendations

Singles: Sacred Frankincense, Frankincense, Wintergreen, Idaho Blue Spruce, Copaiba, German Chamomile, Nutmeg, Idaho Balsam Fir

Blends: PanAway, Relieve It, ImmuPower, Ortho Ease, Deep Relief Roll-On, Stress Away Roll-On, EndoFlex

Nutritionals: AlkaLime, Sulfurzyme, Life 5, Essentialzyme, Super C, Super C Chewable,

MultiGreens, ICP, ComforTone, SuperCal, Thyromin, SleepEssence, Essentialzymes-4, OmegaGize³, EndoGize

Resin: Frankincense Gum Resin

Application and Usage
Inhalation

- Diffuse your choice of oils for ½ hour every 4-6 hours or as desired.
- Put 2-3 drops of your chosen oil in your hands and rub them together, cup your hands over your nose, and inhale throughout the day as needed.
- Put 8-10 drops of oil on a cotton ball or tissue and put it in an air vent in your house, vehicle, hotel room, etc.
- If diffusing while sleeping, set your timer for the desired length of time for automatic shut off.

Topical

You may apply single oils or blends neat or diluted, depending on the oil or oils being used. Please see the instructions at the beginning of this chapter for more information on applying oils to the skin.

- Apply a warm compress on location 3 times weekly.
- Massage into muscle tissue in a full-body massage weekly.
- Receive a Raindrop Technique and add an immune blend weekly.

Ingestion and Oral

The amount of oil ingested varies with different oils. Whether putting the oils in a capsule or drinking them in a liquid, please refer to the instructions at the beginning of this chapter.

- Take 1-2 capsules with desired oil 2 times daily.
- Put 2-3 drops of oil in a spoonful of Blue Agave, Yacon Syrup, maple syrup, coconut oil, milk, etc.
- Put the desired amount of oils in a glass of rice milk, almond milk, goat milk, carrot juice, NingXia Red, or even water and then drink it.

FOOD POISONING
(See also Giardia under DIGESTIVE PROBLEMS)

Food poisoning symptoms vary with the source and type of contamination and may include nausea, diarrhea, vomiting, congestion, coughing, abdominal pain, cramps, sore throat, and fever.

Recommendations

Singles: Oregano, Plectranthus Oregano, Thyme, Clove, Ginger

Blends: Thieves, DiGize

Nutritionals: Essentialzymes-4, Inner Defense, ComforTone, Digest & Cleanse, Detoxzyme, Essentialzyme, AlkaLime

Application and Usage
Ingestion and Oral

The amount of oil ingested varies with different oils. Whether putting the oils in a capsule or drinking them in a liquid, please refer to the instructions at the beginning of this chapter.

- Take 2 capsules with desired oil 2-3 times daily.
- Put 2-3 drops of oil in a spoonful of Blue Agave, Yacon Syrup, maple syrup, coconut oil, milk, etc.
- Put the desired amount of oils in a glass of rice milk, almond milk, goat milk, carrot juice, NingXia Red, or even water and then drink it.

FOOT CONDITIONS AND PROBLEMS

Foot problems can occur due to a variety of reasons such as injuries, medical conditions such as fungal and bacterial conditions or spurs, poorly fit shoes, or age.

Recommendations

Singles: Peppermint, White Fir, Lavender, Patchouli, Myrrh, Sacred Frankincense, Frankincense, Sandalwood, Vetiver

Blends: Melrose, PanAway, Relieve It

Application and Usage

Inhalation

- Diffuse your choice of oils for ½ hour every 4-6 hours or as desired.
- Put 2-3 drops of your chosen oil in your hands and rub them together, cup your hands over your nose, and inhale throughout the day as needed.
- Put 8-10 drops of oil on a cotton ball or tissue and put it in an air vent in your house, vehicle, hotel room, etc.
- If diffusing while sleeping, set your timer for the desired length of time for automatic shut off.

Topical

You may apply single oils or blends neat or diluted, depending on the oil or oils being used. Please see the instructions at the beginning of this chapter for more information on applying oils to the skin.

- Dilute any of the recommended oils 50:50 and massage 6-9 drops onto each foot at night.
- Create a warm, oil-infused compress for added effect and penetration.
- Add any of the recommended oils to bath salts, mix 10 drops of essential oils per 1 tablespoon of Epsom salts, and add to hot water.

....

Athlete's Foot

Athlete's foot *(Tinea pedis)* is a fungal infection of the feet. It is identical to ringworm that infects the skin elsewhere on the body (See Ringworm). This fungus thrives in a warm, moist environment.

The best remedy is to keep feet cool and dry and avoid wearing tight-fitting shoes or heavy, natural-fiber socks such as cotton. It is helpful to wear sandals, shoes, and socks woven from a light, breathable fabric.

Essential oils with antifungal properties such as Melaleuca Alternifolia, Melaleuca Ericifolia, and Melaleuca Quinquenervia or Melrose (a blend Melaleuca Alternifolia and Melaleuca Quinquenervia, combined with Clove and Rosemary) can be added to bath water or to Epsom salts and used in specially designed showerheads to help add antifungal protection to the water.

Recommendations

Singles: Patchouli, Melaleuca Alternifolia, Melaleuca Ericifolia, Blue Cypress, Lemongrass (usually diluted), Lavender, Ocotea, Peppermint, Thyme, Mountain Savory, Melissa, Hinoki, Rosemary

Blends: Melrose, Thieves, Purification

Nutritionals: Detoxzyme, Digest & Cleanse

Body Care Massage Oils, Creams, and Sprays: ClaraDerm, Thieves Spray, Ortho Ease Massage Oil, Thieves Fresh Essence Plus Mouthwash

Athlete's Foot Blend

- 8 drops Melaleuca Alternifolia
- 4 drops Peppermint
- 2 drops Mountain Savory
- 1 drop Myrrh

Application and Usage

Topical

You may apply single oils or blends neat or diluted, depending on the oil or oils being used. Please see the instructions at the beginning of this chapter for more information on applying oils to the skin.

- Pour ½ cup of Thieves Fresh Essence Plus Mouthwash into a pan of water for soaking the feet. It works amazingly well.

315

Blisters
(See Blisters under SKIN DISORDERS)

Bunions
(See also BURSITIS)

Bunions are caused from bursitis at the base of a toe and develop when the joints in the big toe no longer fit together as they should and become tender and swollen.

Recommendations
Singles: Eucalyptus Radiata, Raven, Lemon, Wintergreen, Vetiver, Idaho Blue Spruce, Hinoki

Blends: PanAway, Deep Relief, Relieve It

Bunion Blend
- 6 drops Eucalyptus Radiata
- 4 drops Raven
- 3 drops Lemon
- 1 drop Wintergreen
- 1 drop Vetiver

Application and Usage
Topical

You may apply single oils or blends neat or diluted, depending on the oil or oils being used. Please see the instructions at the beginning of this chapter for more information on applying oils to the skin.
- Apply 2-4 drops neat or diluted 50:50 over bunion area 2-3 times daily.

Corns and Calluses

Corns and calluses are caused by friction and pressure when the bony parts of the feet rub against the shoes.

Recommendations
Singles: Lavender, Helichrysum, Idaho Blue Spruce

Blends: PanAway, Deep Relief, Relieve It

Corns Blend
- 4 drops Basil
- 2 drops Myrrh
- 2 drops Cypress
- 1 drop Oregano
- 1 drop Hinoki

Application and Usage
Topical

You may apply single oils or blends neat or diluted, depending on the oil or oils being used. Please see the instructions at the beginning of this chapter for more information on applying oils to the skin.
- Apply 1 drop neat directly on the corn 2-3 times daily.

Sore Feet

Having sore feet is very common and is usually a symptom of an underlying problem or condition. Some causes are simple and require simple fixes, while others are more complicated and require more complex treatment.

Recommendations
Single Oils: Peppermint, White Fir, Lavender, Patchouli, Myrrh, Sacred Frankincense, Frankincense, Sandalwood, Vetiver, Wintergreen, German Chamomile, Orange

Blends: Melrose, PanAway, Relieve It

Massage Oil: Ortho Ease Massage Oil

Sore Feet Blend
- 5 drops Wintergreen
- 3 drops Peppermint
- 2 drops German Chamomile
- 2 drops Idaho Blue Spruce
- 1 drop Copaiba
- 1 drop Sandalwood

Application and Usage
Topical

You may apply single oils or blends neat or diluted, depending on the oil or oils being used. Please see the instructions at the beginning of this chapter for more information on applying oils to the skin.
- Dilute 50:50 and massage 6-9 drops onto

each foot at night.
- Apply a warm compress for added effect and penetration.
- Mix 10 drops essential oils in 1 tablespoon Epsom salts and add to hot water in a basin large enough for a footbath.

FUNGAL INFECTIONS

Fungi and yeast feed on decomposing or dead tissues and exist inside our stomachs, on our skin, out on the lawn, and just about everywhere. When kept under control, the yeast and fungi populating our bodies are harmless and digest what our bodies cannot or do not use.

When we feed the naturally occurring fungi in our bodies too many simple sugars, the fungal populations can grow out of control. This condition is known as systemic candidiasis and is marked by fungi invading the blood, gastrointestinal tract, and tissues.

Reducing or eliminating simple sugars from the diet is essential to combating all fungal infections. Antibiotics should also be avoided, and alcohol is deadly.

Fungal cultures such as candida excrete large amounts of poisons called mycotoxins as part of their life cycles. These poisons in the blood flow through the liver and hopefully are digested and eliminated from the body. If there is too much poison creating a toxic overload, the body eventually weakens. These toxins can wreak enormous damage on the tissues and organs and can be an aggravating factor in many degenerative diseases such as cancer, arteriosclerosis, and diabetes.

Insufficient intake of minerals and trace minerals like magnesium, potassium, and zinc may also stimulate candida and fungal overgrowth in the body.

Symptoms of Systemic Fungal Infection
- Fatigue/low energy
- Overweight
- Low resistance to illness
- Allergies
- Unbalanced blood sugar
- Headaches
- Irritability
- Mood swings
- Indigestion
- Colitis and ulcers
- Diarrhea/constipation
- Urinary tract infections
- Rectal or vaginal itch

Recommendations
Singles: Melaleuca Ericifolia, Blue Cypress, Lemongrass (always dilute), Lavender, Mastrante, Thyme, Mountain Savory, Idaho Ponderosa Pine, Melissa, Myrrh, Hinoki

Blends: Melrose, Thieves, Purification, DiGize, Exodus II

Nutritionals: Mineral Essence, Essentialzyme, Detoxzyme, AlkaLime

Sprays and Oral Application: ClaraDerm, Thieves Spray on the skin, Thieves Fresh Essence Plus Mouthwash on the feet

Massage Oils: Ortho Ease Massage Oil or V-6 Vegetable Oil Complex mixed with your choice of singles or blends

Application and Usage
Topical
- You may apply single oils or blends neat or diluted, depending on the oil or oils being used. Please see the instructions at the beginning of this chapter for more information on applying oils to the skin.
- Apply any of the recommended oils neat or diluted 50:50. Always dilute Lemongrass.
- Apply 5-7 drops to affected areas between toes and around toenails.
- Add any of the recommended oils to bath salts and soak affected area daily.

Athlete's Foot
(See Athlete's Foot under FOOT CONDITIONS AND PROBLEMS; see also RINGWORM in this section).

Candida Albicans (Candidiasis)

Two of the most powerful weapons for fighting intestinal fungal infections such as candida are FOS (fructooligosaccharides) and *L. acidophilus* cultures.

FOS has been clinically documented in dozens of peer-reviewed studies for its ability to build up the healthy intestinal flora in the colon and combat the overgrowth of negative bacteria and fungi.

Acidophilus cultures have also been shown to combat fungus overgrowth in the gastrointestinal tract.

Recommendations
Singles: Lemongrass, Geranium, Melaleuca Alternifolia, Mastrante, Niaouli, Ravintsara, Thyme, Peppermint, Lavender, Rosemary, Palmarosa, Idaho Ponderosa Pine
Blends: Melrose, Raven, R.C., ImmuPower, Breathe Again Roll-On
Nutritionals: Detoxzyme, Life 5, Essentialzyme, ImmuPro, MultiGreens, Digest & Cleanse, Super C, Super C Chewable, AlkaLime

Candida Blend
* 5 drops Lemongrass
* 4 drops Thyme
* 4 drops Melaleuca Alternifolia
* 2 drops Geranium

(**Note:** This blend is not recommended for those with estrogen-sensitive cancers.)

Application and Usage
Inhalation
* Diffuse your choice of oils for ½ hour every 4-6 hours or as desired.

* Put 2-3 drops of your chosen oil in your hands and rub them together, cup your hands over your nose, and inhale throughout the day as needed.
* Put 8-10 drops of oil on a cotton ball or tissue and put it in an air vent in your house, vehicle, hotel room, etc.
* If diffusing while sleeping, set your timer for the desired length of time for automatic shut off.

Topical
You may apply single oils or blends neat or diluted, depending on the oil or oils being used. Please see the instructions at the beginning of this chapter for more information on applying oils to the skin.
* Dilute 50:50 or 20:80, as needed, and massage 3-4 drops on thymus (at clavicle notch, center of collarbone at base of throat) to stimulate the immune system. Also apply 3-6 drops on bottoms of the feet and on the chest. Also apply 5-10 drops on stomach. Do these applications 2 times daily.
* Massage 2-4 drops on relevant Vita Flex points on feet 2-4 times daily.
* Use bath salts daily.

Ingestion and Oral
The amount of oil ingested varies with different oils. Whether putting the oils in a capsule or drinking them in a liquid, please refer to the instructions at the beginning of this chapter.
* Take 1 capsule with desired oil 2 times daily.
* Put 2-3 drops of oil in a spoonful of Blue Agave, Yacon Syrup, maple syrup, coconut oil, milk, etc.
* Put the desired amount of oils in a glass of rice milk, almond milk, goat milk, carrot juice, NingXia Red, or even water and then drink it.

Ringworm and Skin Candida

The ringworm fungus infects the skin, causing scaly, round, itchy patches. It is infectious and can be spread from an animal or human host alike. Skin candida is a fungal infection that can erupt almost anywhere on the skin. It shows up in various places such as behind the knees, inside the elbows, behind the ears, on temple area, and between the breasts.

Recommendations

Singles: Melaleuca Ericifolia, Geranium, Melaleuca Alternifolia, Melaleuca Quinquenervia (Niaouli), Cypress, Lavender, Rosemary, Mastrante, Rosewood, Lemongrass, Lemon Myrtle

Blends: Melrose, Raven, R.C., Ortho Ease, Breathe Again Roll-On

Massage Oil and Spray: Thieves Spray, Ortho Sport Massage Oil

Ringworm Blend
- 3 drops Melaleuca Alternifolia
- 3 drops Spearmint
- 1 drop Peppermint
- 1 drop Rosemary

Skin Candida Blend
- 10 drops Melaleuca Alternifolia
- 4 drops Lavender
- 2 drops Geranium
- 1 drop Oregano

Application and Usage
Topical

You may apply single oils or blends neat or diluted, depending on the oil or oils being used. Please see the instructions at the beginning of this chapter for more information on applying oils to the skin.

- Dilute 50:50 and massage 2-4 drops over affected area 2-4 times daily. In severe cases, use 35 percent food-grade hydrogen peroxide to clean infected areas before applying essential oils. Saturate a gauze pad with essential oils, apply to affected area, and wrap to hold in place.

Thrush

Thrush is a fungal infection of the mouth and throat marked by creamy, curd-like patches in the oral cavity. Even though it appears in the mouth, thrush is usually a sign of systemic fungal overgrowth throughout the body. Thrush can usually be treated locally through the use of antifungal essential oils such as Clove, Cinnamon, Rosemary, Peppermint, and Rosewood.

Recommendations

Singles: Clove, Cinnamon, Peppermint, Rosemary, Mastrante, Geranium, Rosewood, Orange, Lavender

Blends: Melrose, Thieves, Inner Defense, Purification

Oral Hygiene: Thieves Lozenges (Hard/Soft), Thieves Fresh Essence Plus Mouthwash, Thieves Spray

Application and Usage
Inhalation

- Diffuse your choice of oils for ½ hour every 4-6 hours or as desired.
- Put 2-3 drops of your chosen oil in your hands and rub them together, cup your hands over your nose, and inhale throughout the day as needed.
- Put 8-10 drops of oil on a cotton ball or tissue and put it in an air vent in your house, vehicle, hotel room, etc.
- If diffusing while sleeping, set your timer for the desired length of time for automatic shut off.

Topical

You may apply single oils or blends neat or diluted, depending on the oil or oils being used. Please see the instructions at the beginning of this chapter for more information on applying oils to the skin.

- Dilute 50:50 or 20:80 as needed and massage 3-4 drops on thymus (at clavicle notch, center of collarbone at base of throat) to stimulate the immune system. Also apply 3-6 drops on bottoms of the feet and on the chest. Also apply 5-10 drops on stomach. Do these applications 2 times daily.

- Massage 2-4 drops on relevant Vita Flex points on feet 2-4 times daily.

Ingestion and Oral

The amount of oil ingested varies with different oils. Whether putting the oils in a capsule or drinking them in a liquid, please refer to the instructions at the beginning of this chapter.

- Take 1 capsule with desired oil 2-3 times daily between meals.
- Put 2-3 drops of oil in a spoonful of Blue Agave, Yacon Syrup, maple syrup, coconut oil, milk, etc.
- Put the desired amount of oils in a glass of rice milk, almond milk, goat milk, carrot juice, NingXia Red, or even water and then drink it.
- Gargle 3-5 times daily with Thieves Fresh Essence Plus Mouthwash.

    Note: These applications are for adults, not infants. In cases of infants with thrush, consult a medical professional first.

....

Vaginal Yeast Infection

Vaginal yeast infections are usually caused from overgrowth of fungi like *Candida albicans*. These naturally occurring intestinal yeast and fungi are normally kept under control by the immune system, but when excess sucrose is consumed or antibiotics are used, these organisms convert from relatively harmless yeast into an invasive, harmful fungus that secretes toxins as part of its life cycle.

Vaginal yeast infections are just one symptom of systemic fungal infestation. While the yeast infection can be treated locally, the underlying problem of systemic candidiasis may still remain, unless specific dietary and health practices are used.

Diet and cleansing are two major factors in overcoming this problem. Sugar, milk products, breads, and medications such as antibiotics all contribute to the growth of candida. A cleansing program should be considered with various supplements and essential oils.

Recommendations

Singles: Melaleuca Alternifolia, Myrrh, Melissa, Oregano, Plectranthus Oregano, Thyme, Mastrante, Rosemary, Palo Santo, Mountain Savory, Idaho Blue Spruce, Hinoki

Blends: Melrose, Thieves, Exodus II, Purification, 3 Wise Men, Inspiration

Nutritionals: ICP (a.m.), JuvaPower (p.m.), ComforTone, Detoxzyme, Essentialzymes-4, Life 5 (for 60 days)

Sprays: ClaraDerm

Vaginal Yeast Infection Blend

- 7 drops Melaleuca Alternifolia
- 5 drops Mountain Savory
- 2 drops Myrrh

Application and Usage

Retention:

- Mix an 80:20 ratio (8 parts chosen essential oil to 2 parts V-6 Vegetable Oil Complex), put 1-2 tablespoons on a tampon, and insert into the vagina daily for internal infection.
- Alternate approach: Douche with 1 tablespoon Thieves Fresh Essence Plus Mouthwash overnight 3 times a week. If it stings a little, dilute with a little V-6 Vegetable Oil Complex.

Oral:

- Stop sugar intake.

GALLBLADDER INFECTION (CHOLECYSTITIS)

The gallbladder stores the bile created by the liver and releases it through the biliary ducts into the duodenum to promote digestion. Bile is extremely important for fat digestion and the absorption of vitamins A, D, and E.

When the bile flow is obstructed due to gallstones or inflamed due to infection, serious consequences can ensue, including poor digestion, jaundice, and severe abdominal pain.

Recommendations

Singles: Lemon, Cistus, Myrrh, Ledum, Hyssop, Juniper, German Chamomile, Oregano, Plectranthus Oregano, Cumin

Blends: GLF, Thieves, Citrus Fresh, JuvaFlex, JuvaCleanse, PanAway, DiGize

Nutritionals: Inner Defense, Sulfurzyme, JuvaTone, Essentialzyme, Essentialzymes-4, Longevity Softgels, Life 5

Application and Usage

Topical

You may apply single oils or blends neat or diluted, depending on the oil or oils being used. Please see the instructions at the beginning of this chapter for more information on applying oils to the skin.

- Apply 6-10 drops of any of the recommended oils or oil blends over gallbladder area 2-3 times daily.
- Apply a warm, oil-infused compress over gallbladder area 2-3 times daily.
- Apply 1-3 drops of suggested oils over liver and use Vita Flex massage.
- Use Vita Flex massage on the feet 2-3 times daily.

GALLSTONES

When bile contains excessive cholesterol, bilirubin, or bile salts, gallstones can form. Stones made from hardened cholesterol account for the vast majority of gallstones, while stones made from bilirubin, the brownish pigment in bile, constitute only about 20 percent of gallstones.

Gallstones can block both bile flow and the passage of pancreatic enzymes. This can result in inflammation in the gallbladder (cholecystitis), pancreas (pancreatitis), and jaundice. In some cases, gallstones can be life threatening, depending on where they are lodged.

Several Japanese studies show that limonene, a key constituent in Orange, Lemon, and Tangerine oils, can effectively dissolve gallstones with no negative side effects.[22, 23]

Recommendations

Singles: Lemon, Helichrysum, Sacred Frankincense, Frankincense, Orange, Grapefruit, Mandarin, Tangerine, Juniper, Rosemary, Idaho Balsam Fir

Blends: GLF, Citrus Fresh, JuvaCleanse

Nutritionals: Essentialzyme, JuvaPower, ComforTone, ICP, JuvaTone

Application and Usage

Topical

You may apply single oils or blends neat or diluted, depending on the oil or oils being used. Please see the instructions at the beginning of this chapter for more information on applying oils to the skin.

- Dilute 50:50 and massage 6-10 drops over gallbladder 2 times daily.
- Apply a compress 2-3 times daily.
- You may also apply 1-3 drops on the Vita Flex liver and digestive points of the right foot 2-3 times daily.

Ingestion and Oral

The amount of oil ingested varies with different oils. Whether putting the oils in a capsule or drinking them in a liquid, please refer to the instructions at the beginning of this chapter.

- Take 1 capsule with desired oil 2 times daily for 2 weeks.
- Put 2-3 drops of oil in a spoonful of Blue Agave, Yacon Syrup, maple syrup, coconut oil, milk, etc.
- Put the desired amount of oils in a glass of rice milk, almond milk, goat milk, carrot juice, NingXia Red, or even water and then drink it.

GANGRENE

Note: As with all serious medical conditions, consult your health-care professional immediately if you suspect gangrene.

Gangrene is the death or decay of living tissue caused by a lack of blood supply. A shortage of blood can result from a blood clot, arteriosclerosis, frostbite, diabetes, infection, or some other obstruction in the arterial blood supply. Gas gangrene, also known as acute or moist gangrene, occurs when tissues are infected with clostridium bacteria. Unless the body is given antibiotics to treat the disease or the limb is amputated, gangrene can be fatal.

The part of the body affected by gangrene displays the following symptoms:

- Coldness
- Dark in color or even black
- Looks rotten or decomposed
- Putrid smell
- Fever
- Anemia

Dr. René Gattefossé suffered gas gangrene as a result of burns from a chemical explosion at the turn of the century. He successfully engineered his own recovery solely with the use of pure lavender oil.

Recommendations
Singles: Myrrh, Lavender, Thyme, Peppermint, Oregano, Plectranthus Oregano, Rosemary, Sacred Frankincense, Frankincense, Mountain Savory, Cistus, Cypress, Vetiver, Copaiba

Blends: Exodus II, Thieves, ImmuPower, Melrose

Nutritionals: Super C, Super C Chewable, Inner Defense, Mineral Essence, Essentialzyme, Detoxzyme

Application and Usage
Topical

You may apply single oils or blends neat or diluted, depending on the oils being used. Please see the instructions at the beginning of this chapter for more information on applying oils to the skin.

- Apply 2-4 drops diluted 20:80 on the affected area 3-5 times daily.
- Apply a warm compress 3 times daily every other day.

GASTRITIS

Gastritis occurs when the stomach's mucosal lining becomes inflamed and the cells become eroded. This can lead to bleeding ulcers and severe digestive disturbances. Gastritis is caused by excess acid production in the stomach, alcohol consumption, stress, and fungal or bacterial infections.

Symptoms of gastritis are weight loss, abdominal pain, and cramping.

Recommendations
Singles: Peppermint, Lemon, Fennel, Patchouli, Tarragon, Spearmint

Blends: DiGize, Purification, JuvaCleanse, Slique Essence

Nutritionals: AlkaLime, Essentialzymes-4, Essentialzyme, Detoxzyme, Life 5, Digest & Cleanse, Balance Complete

Application and Usage
Ingestion and Oral

The amount of oil ingested varies with different oils. Whether putting the oils in a capsule or drinking them in a liquid, please refer to the instructions at the beginning of this chapter.

- Take 1 capsule with desired oil 2 times daily.
- Put 2-3 drops of oil in a spoonful of Blue Agave, Yacon Syrup, maple syrup, coconut oil, milk, etc.
- Put the desired amount of oils in a glass of rice milk, almond milk, goat milk, carrot juice, NingXia Red, or even water and then drink it.

Supplementation regimen for gastritis:
- **AlkaLime:** Take ½ teaspoon each morning.
- **Essentialzymes-4:** Take 3-4 yellow capsules 3 times daily.
- **ComforTone and ICP:** Begin after 2 weeks of using the products listed above.
- **MegaCal:** Take 1 tablespoon each morning in 8 oz. warm water.

GOUT
(See Also JOINT STIFFNESS/PAIN)

Gout is a disease marked by abrupt, temporary bouts of joint pain and swelling that are most evident in the joint of the big toe. It can also affect the wrist, elbow, knee, ankle, hand, and foot. As the disease progresses, pain and swelling in the joints become more frequent and chronic, with deposits called tophi appearing over many joints, including on the elbows and on the ears.

Gout is characterized by accumulation of uric acid crystals in the joints caused by excess uric acid in the blood. Uric acid is a byproduct of the breakdown of protein that is normally excreted by the kidneys into the urine. To reduce uric acid concentrations, it is necessary to support the kidneys, adrenals, and immune functions. It is also necessary to detoxify by cleansing and drinking plenty of fluids.

Excess alcohol, allergy-producing foods, or strict diets can cause outbreaks of gout. Foods rich in purines, such as wine, anchovies, and animal liver, can also cause gout.

Recommendations
Singles: Juniper, Lemon, Idaho Blue Spruce, Sacred Frankincense, Frankincense
Blend: GLF, JuvaCleanse
Nutritionals: AlkaLime, MultiGreens, ICP (a.m.), ComforTone, Essentialzyme, JuvaPower (p.m.), JuvaTone
Massage Oils: Ortho Ease Massage Oil, Ortho Sport Massage Oil

Gout Blend
- 10 drops Lemon
- 5 drops Idaho Blue Spruce
- 4 drops Juniper
- 3 drops Melaleuca Alternifolia
- 2 drops Roman Chamomile

Application and Usage
Topical
You may apply single oils or blends neat or diluted, depending on the oil or oils being used. Please see the instructions at the beginning of this chapter for more information on applying oils to the skin.
- Gently massage 1-3 drops neat on affected joints 2-3 times daily.

Ingestion and Oral
The amount of oil ingested varies with different oils. Whether putting the oils in a capsule or drinking them in a liquid, please refer to the instructions at the beginning of this chapter.
- Take 1 capsule with desired oil 1 time daily for 10 days, rest 4 days, repeat as needed.
- Put 2-3 drops of oil in a spoonful of Blue Agave, Yacon Syrup, maple syrup, coconut oil, milk, etc.
- Put the desired amount of oils in a glass of rice milk, almond milk, goat milk, carrot juice, NingXia Red, or even water and then drink it.

HAIR AND SCALP PROBLEMS

Sulfur is the single most important mineral for maintaining the strength and integrity of the hair and hair follicle.

Recommendations

Singles: Lavender, Cedarwood (dry scalp), Peppermint (oily scalp), Rosemary, Clary Sage, Sage, Basil, Juniper, Ylang Ylang, Amazonian Ylang Ylang, Sandalwood, Lemon, Cypress, Rosewood

Blends: Melrose, Thieves, Citrus Fresh, Purification, Inspiration, The Gift

Nutritionals: Sulfurzyme, AlkaLime, Super B, Pure Protein Complete, Essentialzymes-4, Balance Complete

Shampoos and Rinses: Lavender Mint Daily Shampoo and Conditioner, Copaiba Vanilla Moisturizing Shampoo and Conditioner, Lavender Shampoo and Conditioner

Dry Scalp Blend
- 6 drops Cedarwood
- 4 drops Lavender
- 2 drops Sandalwood or Geranium
- 2 drops Patchouli

Oily Scalp Blend
- 6 drops Peppermint
- 4 drops Lemon
- 2 drops Lavender

Scalp Rinse Blend to Restore Acid Mantle
- 1 drop Rosemary
- 1 teaspoon pure apple cider vinegar
- 8 oz. water

Rub 1-2 drops of oil on hair to prevent static electricity.

Application and Usage
Topical

You may apply single oils or blends neat or diluted, depending on the oils being used. Please see the instructions at the beginning of this chapter for more information on applying oils to the skin.

- Apply 1 teaspoon diluted 20:80 onto the scalp and rub vigorously for 2-3 minutes. Leave on scalp for 60-90 minutes.
- Mix 2-4 drops of essential oils with 1-2 teaspoons of shampoo to wash hair after exercising.

Ingestion and Oral

The amount of oil ingested varies with different oils. Whether putting the oils in a capsule or drinking them in a liquid, please refer to the instructions at the beginning of this chapter.

- Take 1 capsule with desired oil 2 times daily.
- Put 2-3 drops of oil in a spoonful of Blue Agave, Yacon Syrup, maple syrup, coconut oil, milk, etc.
- Put the desired amount of oils in a glass of rice milk, almond milk, goat milk, carrot juice, NingXia Red, or even water and then drink it.

....

Baldness/Hair Loss (Alopecia Areata)

Male pattern baldness is often a result of hormonal imbalances such as excess conversion of testosterone to dihydrotestosterone through the enzyme 5-alpha reductase. It can also be caused by an inflammatory condition called alopecia areata.

Alopecia is an inflammatory hair loss disease that is the second-leading cause of baldness in the U.S. A double-blind study that was conducted at the Aberdeen Royal Infirmary in Scotland found that certain essential oils were extremely effective in combating this disease.[24]

Essential oils are excellent for cleansing, nourishing, and strengthening the hair follicle and shaft. Rosemary (cineole chemotype) encourages hair growth. The Arabian people for centuries have used frankincense resin water to rinse their hair and massage their scalp to maintain a healthy head of hair and stimulate regrowth.

Thyroid balance also prevents hair loss.

Recommendations

Singles: Lavender, Sacred Frankincense, Frankincense, Peppermint, Canadian Fleabane (Conyza), Black Pepper, Rosemary, Thyme, Cedarwood, Eucalyptus Blue, Palo Santo

Blends: Melrose, Longevity, Mister, M-Grain, Transformation, JuvaCleanse

Nutritionals: Prostate Health, PD 80/20, EndoGize, Master Formula HIS or HERS, Sulfurzyme, Balance Complete, Mineral Essence, Essentialzyme, Allerzyme, Thyromin

Hair Loss Prevention Blend No. 1

- 10 drops Cedarwood
- 10 drops Sandalwood
- 10 drops Lavender
- 8 drops Rosemary
- 1 drop Juniper

Hair Loss Prevention Blend No. 2

- 5 drops Lavender
- 4 drops Cypress
- 3 drops Rosemary
- 2 drops Clary sage
- 2 drops Palo Santo

Hair Loss Prevention Blend No. 3

- 5 drops Lavender
- 5 drops Sacred Frankincense or Frankincense
- 2 drops Clary Sage
- 3 drops Eucalyptus Blue
- 1 drop Peppermint

Hair Loss Prevention Blend No. 4

- 4 drops Rosemary
- 4 drops Thyme
- 4 drops Lavender
- 4 drops Cedarwood
- 2 drops Sacred Frankincense or Frankincense

Application and Usage
Topical

You may apply single oils or blends neat or diluted, depending on the oil or oils being used. Please see the instructions at the beginning of this chapter for more information on applying oils to the skin.

- Dilute 50:50 oil of choice and V-6 Vegetable Oil Complex and massage 1 teaspoon into scalp vigorously and thoroughly for 2-3 minutes before retiring.
- Dilute 5 drops of your essential oil in 20 drops of V-6 Vegetable Oil Complex, grape seed oil, or coconut oil and massage into scalp before going to bed.
- Add 10 drops of any of the above blends to 1 teaspoon of coconut oil and massage into the scalp where it is balding; then rub gently into the remainder of the scalp. This works best when done at night. It may also help to alternate blends.
- Mix 2-4 drops of essential oils with 1-2 teaspoons of shampoo. Massage into the scalp vigorously and thoroughly for 2-3 minutes, then leave the shampoo on the scalp for 15 minutes. This is an excellent time to do an exercise routine. Rinse hair afterward.

Ingestion and Oral

The amount of oil ingested varies with different oils. Whether putting the oils in a capsule or drinking them in a liquid, please refer to the instructions at the beginning of this chapter.

- Take 1 capsule with desired oil 2 times daily.
- Put 2-3 drops of oil in a spoonful of Blue Agave, Yacon Syrup, maple syrup, coconut oil, milk, etc.
- Put the desired amount of oils in a glass of rice milk, almond milk, goat milk, carrot juice, NingXia Red, or even water and then drink it.

Dandruff

Dandruff may be caused by allergies, parasites (fungal), and/or chemicals. The mineral selenium has been shown to help prevent dandruff.

Melaleuca Alternifolia has been shown to be effective in treating dandruff and other fungal infections.[25]

Recommendations

Singles: Melaleuca Alternifolia, Cedarwood, Lavender, Rosemary, Peppermint, Copaiba, Eucalyptus Blue, Sacred Frankincense, Frankincense, Vetiver, Dorado Azul

Blends: Citrus Fresh, Melrose, Thieves, The Gift

Shampoos and Rinses: Lavender Mint Daily Shampoo and Conditioner, Copaiba Vanilla Moisturizing Shampoo and Conditioner, Lavender Shampoo and Conditioner

Dandruff Blend

- 5 drops Lemon
- 2 drops Lavender
- 2 drops Peppermint
- 1 drop Rosemary

Application and Usage

Topical

You may apply single oils or blends neat or diluted, depending on the oil or oils being used. Please see the instructions at the beginning of this chapter for more information on applying oils to the skin.

- Add a few drops of a single oil or blend to your shampoo and massage it into your scalp or add a few drops of the oils of your choice to the Bath & Shower Gel Base for your own custom shampoo.
- Apply 1 teaspoon of the shampoo mixture to the scalp and rub vigorously for 2-3 minutes and then leave shampoo on scalp for 15 minutes. Mix 2-4 drops of the essential oils with 1 teaspoon shampoo to wash hair afterward.

HALITOSIS (BAD BREATH) (See also ORAL CARE, TEETH AND GUMS; CANDIDA; FUNGAL INFECTIONS)

Persistent bad breath or gum disease may be a sign of poor digestion, candida, yeast infestation, or other health problems.

Recommendations

Singles: Clove, Peppermint, Lemon, Melaleuca Alternifolia, Spearmint, Mandarin, Cinnamon Bark, Rosemary, Wintergreen, Ocotea

Blends: Thieves, Melrose, Purification, DiGize, Slique Essence

Nutritionals: Detoxzyme, Allerzyme, Digest & Cleanse, Mineral Essence, Life 5, ICP, ComforTone, Slique Gum

Oral Care: Thieves AromaBright Toothpaste, Thieves Spray, Thieves Lozenges (Hard/Soft), KidScents Slique Toothpaste, Thieves Dentarome Plus Toothpaste, Thieves Dentarome Ultra Toothpaste, Thieves Dental Floss

Bad Breath Blend No. 1

- 3 drops Peppermint
- 2 drops Lemon
- 2 drops Clove
- 1 drop Melaleuca Alternifolia

Bad Breath Blend No. 2

- 4 drops Spearmint
- 2 drops Mandarin
- 2 drops Cinnamon

Application and Usage

Topical

You may apply single oils or blends neat or diluted, depending on the oil or oils being used. Please see the instructions at the beginning of this chapter for more information on applying oils to the skin.

- Swab 4-8 drops of the singles or blends above diluted 50:50 inside cheeks and on tongue, gums, and teeth 2-4 times daily as needed.

Ingestion and Oral

The amount of oil ingested varies with different oils. Whether putting the oils in a capsule or drinking them in a liquid, please refer to the instructions at the beginning of this chapter.

- Take 1 capsule with desired oil 2 times daily.
- Put 2-3 drops of oil in a spoonful of Blue Agave, Yacon Syrup, maple syrup, coconut oil, milk, etc.

- Put the desired amount of oils in a glass of rice milk, almond milk, goat milk, carrot juice, NingXia Red, or even water and then drink it.
- Dilute essential oils and blends in 2 teaspoons of Blue Agave nectar and 4 oz. of hot water. Gargle as needed (2-4 times daily).

HEADACHE
(See also STRESS, HYPOGLYCEMIA, LIVER DISORDERS, MENSTRUAL AND FEMALE HORMONE CONDITIONS)

Headaches are usually caused by hormone imbalances, circulatory problems, stress, sugar imbalance (hypoglycemia), structural (spinal) misalignments, and blood pressure concerns.

Placebo-controlled, double-blind, crossover studies at the Christian-Albrecht University in Kiel, Germany, found that essential oils were just as effective in blocking pain from tension-type headaches as acetaminophen (i.e., Tylenol®). [26, 27]

Essential oils also promote circulation, reduce muscle spasms, and decrease inflammatory response.

Recommendations
Singles: Peppermint, Clove, Copaiba, Eucalyptus Globulus, Eucalyptus Blue, Dorado Azul, Mastrante, German Chamomile, Lavender, Myrrh, Roman Chamomile, Rosemary, Spearmint, Valerian, Wintergreen

Blends: Brain Power, Clarity, Deep Relief Roll-On, M-Grain, PanAway, Stress Away Roll-On, Relieve It, R.C., Raven, Tranquil Roll-On

Creams and Serums: Prenolone Plus Body Cream, Progessence Plus

General Headache Blend No. 1
- 4 drops Wintergreen
- 3 drops German Chamomile
- 2 drops Lavender
- 2 drops Copaiba
- 1 drop Clove

General Headache Blend No. 2
- 6 drops Peppermint
- 4 drops Eucalyptus Globulus
- 2 drops Myrrh

Application and Usage
Inhalation
Diffuse your choice of oils for ½ hour every 4-6 hours or as desired.
- Put 2-3 drops of your chosen oil in your hands and rub them together, cup your hands over your nose, and inhale throughout the day as needed.
- Put 8-10 drops of oil on a cotton ball or tissue and put it in an air vent in your house, vehicle, hotel room, etc.
- If diffusing while sleeping, set your timer for the desired length of time for automatic shut off.

Topical
You may apply single oils or blends neat or diluted, depending on the oil or oils being used. Please see the instructions at the beginning of this chapter for more information on applying oils to the skin.
- Dilute 50:50 and apply 1-3 drops on the back of the neck, behind the ears, on the temples, on the forehead, and under the nose. Be careful to keep away from eyes and eyelids.
- Massage 2-4 drops of oil neat on the soles of the feet just before bedtime. Children love it.
- Place a warm compress with 1-2 drops of chosen oil on the back.

Ingestion and Oral
The amount of oil ingested varies with different oils. Whether putting the oils in a capsule or drinking them in a liquid, please refer to the instructions at the beginning of this chapter.
- Take 1 capsule with desired oil 2 times daily.
- Place 1 drop on the tongue and then push it against the roof of the mouth.
- Put 2-3 drops of oil in a spoonful of Blue

Agave, Yacon Syrup, maple syrup, coconut oil, milk, etc.

- Put the desired amount of oils in a glass of rice milk, almond milk, goat milk, carrot juice, NingXia Red, or even water and then drink it.

. . . .

Migraine (Vascular-type Headache)

The vast majority of migraine headaches may be due to colon congestion or poor digestion. The combination of ICP, ComforTone, and Essentialzyme is most important for cleansing the colon. Eyestrain and decreased vision can accompany migraine headaches. Dried wolfberries contain large amounts of lutein and zeaxanthin, which are vital for healthy vision.

Recommendations

Singles: Basil, Copaiba, Eucalyptus Globulus, Mastrante, German Chamomile, Helichrysum, Lavender, Marjoram, Peppermint, Rosemary, Wintergreen

Blends: M-Grain, Thieves, Clarity, PanAway, The Gift, R.C., Raven, Stress Away Roll-On, Tranquil Roll-On

Nutritionals: Essentialzyme, Essentialzymes-4, NingXia Red, Balance Complete, ComforTone, Ningxia Wolfberries (Dried), ICP, MegaCal

Application and Usage
Inhalation

- Diffuse your choice of oils for ½ hour every 4-6 hours or as desired.
- Put 2-3 drops of your chosen oil in your hands and rub them together, cup your hands over your nose, and inhale throughout the day as needed.
- Put 8-10 drops of oil on a cotton ball or tissue and put it in an air vent in your house, vehicle, hotel room, etc.
- If diffusing while sleeping, set your timer for the desired length of time for automatic shut off.

Topical

You may apply single oils or blends neat or diluted, depending on the oil or oils being used. Please see the instructions at the beginning of this chapter for more information on applying oils to the skin.

- Apply 1-2 drops neat to temples, at the base of the neck, in the center of the forehead, and at the nostril openings. Also massage on thumbs and big toes.
- Place a warm compress with 1-2 drops of chosen oil on the back of the neck or on the back.

. . . .

Sinus Headache
(See also Sinus Infections)

Signs and symptoms of migraines and sinus headaches can be confused. With both kinds, the pain often gets worse when you bend forward and can be accompanied by various nasal signs and symptoms. However, sinus headaches are usually not associated with nausea or vomiting or aggravated by bright light or noise, which are common features of migraines.

Recommendations

Singles: Dorado Azul, Eucalyptus Blue, Eucalyptus Radiata, Mastrante, Geranium, Lavender, Peppermint, Rosemary

Blends: R.C., Breathe Again Roll-On, Melrose, Purification, Raven, RutaVaLa, RutaVaLa Roll-On, Stress Away Roll-On

Nutritionals: Super C, Super C Chewable, ImmuPro, Mineral Essence, Detoxzyme

Sinus Headache Blend

- 9 drops Rosemary
- 5 drops Melaleuca Alternifolia
- 4 drops Geranium
- 3 drops Peppermint
- 2 drops Eucalyptus Blue
- 2 drops Lavender

Application and Usage
Inhalation

- Diffuse your choice of oils for 10 minutes at a time throughout the day or as desired.
- Put 2-3 drops of your chosen oil in your hands and rub them together, cup your hands over your nose, and inhale throughout the day as needed.
- Put 8-10 drops of oil on a cotton ball or tissue and put it in an air vent in your house, vehicle, hotel room, etc.
- If diffusing while sleeping, set your timer for the desired length of time for automatic shut off.

Topical

You may apply single oils or blends neat or diluted, depending on the oil or oils being used. Please see the instructions at the beginning of this chapter for more information on applying oils to the skin.

- Apply 1-2 drops neat or diluted 2-5 times daily or as needed.
- Massage 2-4 drops neat on the soles of the feet just before bedtime.

....

Tension (Stress) Headache (See also STRESS)

Tension headaches are the most common type of headaches among adults and are commonly referred to as stress headaches. They are usually triggered by some type of internal or environmental stress. In some people tension headaches are caused by tightened muscles in the scalp and in the back of the neck and may be caused by anxiety, fatigue, overexertion, hunger, inadequate rest, poor posture, mental or emotional stress, or depression.

Recommendations

Singles: Valerian, Cardamom, Tangerine, Jasmine, Palmarosa, Mastrante, Geranium, Sacred Frankincense, Frankincense, Peppermint, Lavender, Roman Chamomile

Blends: Valor, Aroma Siez, M-Grain, Peace & Calming, Hope, Sacred Mountain, Trauma Life, PanAway, Stress Away Roll-On, RutaVaLa, RutaVaLa Roll-On, Tranquil Roll-On, Valor, Valor Roll-On

Nutritionals: MegaCal, Essentialzymes-4, Balance Complete, NingXia Red, Mineral Essence, ICP, ComforTone, Essentialzyme

Application and Usage
Inhalation

- Diffuse your choice of oils for ½ hour every 4-6 hours or as desired.
- Put 2-3 drops of your chosen oil in your hands and rub them together, cup your hands over your nose, and inhale throughout the day as needed.
- Put 8-10 drops of oil on a cotton ball or tissue and put it in an air vent in your house, vehicle, hotel room, etc.
- If diffusing while sleeping, set your timer for the desired length of time for automatic shut off.

Topical

You may apply single oils or blends neat or diluted, depending on the oil or oils being used. Please see the instructions at the beginning of this chapter for more information on applying oils to the skin.

- Apply 1-2 drops diluted 50:50 around the hairline, on the back of the neck, and across the forehead. Be careful not to use too much, as it will burn if any oil drips near the eyes. If this should occur, dilute with a pure vegetable oil—never with water.

HEAVY METALS

We absorb heavy metals from air, water, food, skin care products, mercury fillings in teeth, etc. These chemicals lodge in the fatty tissues of the body, which, in turn, give off toxic gases that may cause allergic symptoms. Cleansing the body of these heavy metals is extremely important to have a healthy immune function, especially if one has amalgam fillings. Drink at least 64 ounces of distilled water daily to flush toxins and chemicals out of the body (see Circulation).

Recommendations
Singles: Helichrysum, Lemon, Orange, Tangerine, Clove, Patchouli
Blends: GLF, Thieves, JuvaCleanse, DiGize
Nutritionals: MultiGreens, Detoxzyme, Essentialzyme, ComforTone, MegaCal, JuvaPower, Super C, Super C Chewable, Mineral Essence, Life 5, ICP

....

Aluminum Toxicity
Aluminum is a very toxic metal that can cause serious neurological damage in the human body—even in minute amounts. Aluminum has been implicated as a possible cause of many maladies in the body, especially Alzheimer's disease.

People unwittingly ingest aluminum from their cookware, beverage cans, antacids, and even deodorants and other cosmetic compounds. The first step toward reducing aluminum toxicity in the body is to avoid these types of aluminum-based products. Start reading the labels and see for yourself.

Recommendations
Singles: Helichrysum, Lemon, Orange, Tangerine, Clove, Patchouli
Blends: GLF, Thieves, JuvaCleanse, DiGize
Nutritionals: JuvaTone, ICP (a.m.), Detoxzyme, Essentialzyme, MegaCal, ComforTone, JuvaPower (p.m.)

Application and Usage
Inhalation
- Diffuse your choice of oils for ½ hour every 4-6 hours or as desired.
- Put 2-3 drops of your chosen oil in your hands and rub them together, cup your hands over your nose, and inhale throughout the day as needed.
- Put 8-10 drops of oil on a cotton ball or tissue and put it in an air vent in your house, vehicle, hotel room, etc.
- If diffusing while sleeping, set your timer for the desired length of time for automatic shut off.

Topical
•You may apply single oils or blends neat or diluted, depending on the oil or oils being used. Please see the instructions at the beginning of this chapter for more information on applying oils to the skin.

Ingestion
- Begin by cleansing the liver, blood, and colon to rid the body of toxins and waste.

The amount of oil ingested varies with different oils. Whether putting the oils in a capsule or drinking them in a liquid, please refer to the instructions at the beginning of this chapter.

- Take 1 capsule with desired oil 2 times daily.
- Put 2-3 drops of oil in a spoonful of Blue Agave, Yacon Syrup, maple syrup, coconut oil, milk, etc.
- Put the desired amount of oils in a glass of rice milk, almond milk, goat milk, carrot juice, NingXia Red, or even water and then drink it.

HEMORRHOIDS
Symptoms of hemorrhoids are bleeding during bowel movements, rectal pain, and itching.

Recommendations
Singles: Myrrh, Helichrysum, Cypress, Cistus, Lemon, Spikenard, Peppermint
Blends: Deep Relief, Melrose, Purification, Aroma Siez, Aroma Life, PanAway
Nutritionals: Essentialzymes-4, MultiGreens, Longevity Softgels, MegaCal, Digest &

Cleanse, ICP, ComforTone, Essentialzyme,
JuvaPower

Creams, Salves: Rose Ointment, KidScents
Tender Tush

Hemorrhoid Blend No. 1

- 4 drops Basil
- 1 drop Cistus
- 1 drop Cypress
- 1 drop Helichrysum
  Mix with Rose Ointment for dilution and
  easier application.

Hemorrhoid Blend No. 2

- 4 drops Myrrh
- 3 drops Cypress
- 2 drops Helichrysum
  Mix with Rose Ointment for dilution and
  easier application.

Application and Usage
Topical

You may apply single oils or blends neat or
diluted, depending on the oil or oils being used.
Please see the instructions at the beginning of
this chapter for more information on applying
oils to the skin.

- Apply single oils or blends neat or diluted,
  depending on the oils that are used.
- Use a rectal implant of your choice of the
  above formulas; place in rectum with a small
  syringe 1 time every other day for 6 days. It is
  best done at night to be able to retain as long
  as possible.
- Apply 3-5 drops diluted 50:50 on location.
  This may sting but usually brings relief with
  1 or 2 applications.

Ingestion and Oral

The amount of oil ingested varies with different oils. Whether putting the oils in a capsule
or drinking them in a liquid, please refer to the
instructions at the beginning of this chapter.

- Take 1 capsule with desired oil 2 times daily.
- Put 2-3 drops of oil in a spoonful of Blue
  Agave, Yacon Syrup, maple syrup, coconut
  oil, milk, etc.
- Put the desired amount of oils in a glass of
  rice milk, almond milk, goat milk, carrot
  juice, NingXia Red, or even water and then
  drink it.

HICCUPS

People have been curious about the cause
of hiccups for years. There are many ideas, but
scientifically, everyone is still waiting for an
explanation. Some say hiccups are caused by
irritated nerves of the diaphragm, possibly from
eating too much or from indigestion.

One technique that often works for stopping
hiccups is to put 1 drop of Cypress and 1 drop
of Tarragon on the end of the index finger and
then place that finger on the neck against the
esophagus in the clavicle notch in the center,
curl inward and down like you are curling
down inside the throat, and release.

Tarragon or Cypress applied topically or
taken as a dietary supplement may relax intestinal spasms, nervous digestion, and hiccups. It's
worth a try.

Recommendations

Singles: Tarragon, Cypress, Spearmint, Pep-
permint
Blends: DiGize, JuvaFlex
Nutritionals: AlkaLime, Digest & Cleanse,
MegaCal

Application and Usage
Topical

You may apply single oils or blends neat or
diluted, depending on the oil or oils being used.
Please see the instructions at the beginning of
this chapter for more information on applying
oils to the skin.

Follow the suggestions above.

- Apply 3-5 drops diluted 50:50 to chest and
  stomach areas.

Ingestion and Oral

The amount of oil ingested varies with different oils. Whether putting the oils in a capsule or drinking them in a liquid, please refer to the instructions at the beginning of this chapter.

- Take 1 capsule with desired oil 2 times daily.
- Put 2-3 drops of oil in a spoonful of Blue Agave, Yacon Syrup, maple syrup, coconut oil, milk, etc.
- Put the desired amount of oils in a glass of rice milk, almond milk, goat milk, carrot juice, NingXia Red, or even water and then drink it.

HIVES

Hives are a generalized itching or dermatitis that can be due to allergies, damaged liver, chemicals, or other factors.

Recommendations

Singles: Myrrh, German Chamomile, Roman Chamomile, Ravintsara, Lavender, Eucalyptus Radiata, Melaleuca Alternifolia, Peppermint, Myrrh

Blends: RutaVaLa, RutaVaLa Roll-On, Stress Away Roll-On, Tranquil Roll-On, Peace & Calming

Nutritionals: SuperCal, MegaCal, Mineral Essence, Sulfurzyme, Master Formula HIS or HERS, MultiGreens, Super B

Ointments: KidScents Tender Tush, Rose Ointment

Application and Usage
Inhalation

- Diffuse your choice of oils for ½ hour every 4-6 hours or as desired.
- Put 2-3 drops of your chosen oil in your hands and rub them together, cup your hands over your nose, and inhale throughout the day as needed.
- Put 8-10 drops of oil on a cotton ball or tissue and put it in an air vent in your house, vehicle, hotel room, etc.

- If diffusing while sleeping, set your timer for the desired length of time for automatic shut off.

Topical

You may apply single oils or blends neat or diluted, depending on the oil or oils being used. Please see the instructions at the beginning of this chapter for more information on applying oils to the skin.

- Apply 2-4 drops diluted 50:50 on location as needed.
- Place a cold compress on location as needed.

HYPERACTIVITY
(See also ATTENTION DEFICIT DISORDER)

Hyperactivity behavior usually refers to a group of characteristics, including inability to concentrate, being easily distracted, being impulsive, being aggressive, fidgeting, constant moving, too much talking, and difficulty participating in quiet activities.

Recommendations

Singles: Lavender, Vetiver, Hinoki, Idaho Blue Spruce, Roman Chamomile, Peppermint, Ocotea, Valerian, Cedarwood

Blends: RutaVaLa, RutaVaLa Roll-On, Peace & Calming, Stress Away Roll-On, Tranquil Roll-On, Sacred Mountain, Grounding, Gathering

Nutritionals: Super B, Master Formula HIS or HERS, MegaCal, Ultra Young Plus

Application and Usage
Inhalation

- Diffuse 5 times daily for up to 30 days, stop for 5 days, and then repeat, if necessary.
- Put 2-3 drops of your chosen oil in your hands and rub them together, cup your hands over your nose, and inhale throughout the day as needed.
- Put 8-10 drops of oil on a cotton ball or tissue and put it in an air vent in your house,

vehicle, hotel room, etc.
- If diffusing while sleeping, set your timer for the desired length of time for automatic shut off.

Topical

You may apply single oils or blends neat or diluted, depending on the oil or oils being used. Please see the instructions at the beginning of this chapter for more information on applying oils to the skin.

- Apply 2-4 drops neat on toes and balls of feet as needed.

INFECTION (BACTERIAL AND VIRAL)

Diffusing essential oils is one of the best ways to prevent the spread of airborne bacteria and viruses. Many essential oils, such as Oregano, Plectranthus Oregano, Mountain Savory, and Rosemary, exert highly antimicrobial effects and can effectively eliminate many kinds of pathogens.

Viruses and bacteria have a tendency to hibernate along the spine. The body may hold a virus in a suspended state for a long period of time. When the immune system is compromised, these viruses may be released and then manifest as illness.

Raindrop Technique along the spine using Oregano and Thyme helps reduce inflammation and kill the microorganisms. However, other oils may also be used, which also have strong antiviral and antibacterial properties. Immu-Power, R.C., and Purification all work well in the Raindrop Technique application method.

Mountain Savory, Ravintsara, Eucalyptus Blue, Palo Santo, Sacred Frankincense or Frankincense, and Thyme, etc., applied along the spine through the Raindrop Technique application may be beneficial for many infections, particularly chest-related (See Colds, Lung, Sinus, and Throat Infection).

Recommendations

Singles: Palo Santo, Ocotea, Sacred Frankincense, Frankincense, Mountain Savory, Rosemary, Lemongrass, Clove, Idaho Ponderosa Pine, Rosewood, Melaleuca Alternifolia, Oregano, Plectranthus Oregano, Thyme, Geranium, Dorado Azul

Blends: Thieves, Purification, Melrose, R.C., ImmuPower, Exodus II, Raven, The Gift, Breathe Again Roll-On

Nutritionals: Inner Defense, Super C, Super C Chewable, NingXia Red, Longevity Softgels, MultiGreens, ImmuPro, OmegaGize^3, Life 5, Ningxia Wolfberries (Dried)

Application and Usage

Inhalation

- Diffuse your choice of oils for ½ hour every 4-6 hours or as desired.
- Put 2-3 drops of your chosen oil in your hands and rub them together, cup your hands over your nose, and inhale throughout the day as needed.
- Put 8-10 drops of oil on a cotton ball or tissue and put it in an air vent in your house, vehicle, hotel room, etc.
- If diffusing while sleeping, set your timer for the desired length of time for automatic shut off.

Topical

You may apply single oils or blends neat or diluted, depending on the oil or oils being used. Please see the instructions at the beginning of this chapter for more information on applying oils to the skin.

- Apply 4-6 drops on location diluted 20:80 2-3 times daily.
- Receive a Raindrop Technique treatment 1-2 times weekly.

Ingestion and Oral

The amount of oil ingested varies with different oils. Whether putting the oils in a capsule or drinking them in a liquid, please

refer to the instructions at the beginning of this chapter.

- Take 1 capsule with desired oil 2 times daily.
- Put 2-3 drops of oil in a spoonful of Blue Agave, Yacon Syrup, maple syrup, coconut oil, milk, etc.
- Put the desired amount of oils in a glass of rice milk, almond milk, goat milk, carrot juice, NingXia Red, or even water and then drink it.

INFLAMMATION
(See also MUSCLES)

Inflammation can be caused by a variety of conditions, including bacterial infection, poor diet, chemicals, hormonal imbalance, and physical injury.

Certain essential oils have been documented to be excellent for reducing inflammation such as German Chamomile, which contains azulene, a blue compound with highly anti-inflammatory properties. Other oils with anti-inflammatory properties include Peppermint, Melaleuca Alternifolia, Clove, Mountain Savory, Palo Santo, Dorado Azul, and Wintergreen.

Some oils are better suited for certain types of inflammation, for example:

- Myrrh, Vetiver, Cistus, and Helichrysum work well for inflammation due to tissue and capillary damage and bruising.
- German Chamomile and Melaleuca Alternifolia are helpful with inflammation due to bacterial infection.
- Ravintsara, Hyssop, Myrrh, and Thyme are appropriate for inflammation caused by viral infection.

Recommendations

Singles: Wintergreen, Vetiver, German Chamomile, Idaho Blue Spruce, Myrrh, Ravintsara, Hinoki, Copaiba, Palo Santo, Clove, Nutmeg, Lavender, Thyme, Frereana Frankincense, Roman Chamomile, Hyssop, Peppermint, Melaleuca Alternifolia,

Blends: Purification, PanAway, Aroma Siez, Melrose, Relieve It, Deep Relief Roll-On

Nutritionals: ImmuPro, Super C, Super C Chewable, Power Meal

Body Care Massage Oils: Ortho Ease Massage Oil, Ortho Sport Massage Oil

Anti-inflammation Blend No. 1

- 6 drops Eucalyptus Blue
- 6 drops Melaleuca Alternifolia
- 4 drops German Chamomile
- 2 drops Peppermint
- 2 drops Idaho Blue Spruce

Anti-inflammation Blend No. 2

- 6 drops Myrrh
- 6 drops Eucalyptus Globulus
- 4 drops Clove
- 3 drops Palo Santo
- 1 drop Vetiver

Application and Usage
Topical

You may apply single oils or blends neat or diluted, depending on the oil or oils being used. Please see the instructions at the beginning of this chapter for more information on applying oils to the skin.

- Apply 2-4 drops diluted 50:50 2 times daily.
- Place a cold compress 1-3 times daily as needed.

Ingestion and Oral

The amount of oil ingested varies with different oils. Whether putting the oils in a capsule or drinking them in a liquid, please refer to the instructions at the beginning of this chapter.

- Take 1 capsule with desired oil 2 times daily.
- Put 2-3 drops of oil in a spoonful of Blue Agave, Yacon Syrup, maple syrup, coconut oil, milk, etc.
- Put the desired amount of oils in a glass of rice milk, almond milk, goat milk, carrot juice, NingXia Red, or even water and then drink it.

INFLUENZA

Having the flu may seem like just having a cold with a sore throat, runny nose, and sneezing. However, colds usually develop slowly, whereas the flu generally comes on suddenly. Although a cold can be a nuisance, you usually feel much worse with the flu.

Common symptoms of the flu include nasal congestion, headache, dry cough, fatigue and weakness, aching muscles, chills and sweats, and high fever.

Recommendations

Singles: Mountain Savory, Oregano, Plectranthus Oregano, Eucalyptus Radiata, Peppermint, Clove, Melaleuca Alternifolia, Eucalyptus Blue, Dorado Azul, Idaho Ponderosa Pine

Blends: ImmuPower, DiGize, Exodus II, Thieves, Raven, R.C., Breathe Again Roll-On

Nutritionals: Digest & Cleanse, Inner Defense, AlkaLime, Life 5, Essentialzyme, Essentialzymes-4, Detoxzyme, ICP, JuvaPower

Application and Usage

Inhalation

- Diffuse your choice of oils for ½ hour every 4-6 hours or as desired.
- Put 2-3 drops of your chosen oil in your hands and rub them together, cup your hands over your nose, and inhale throughout the day as needed.
- Put 8-10 drops of oil on a cotton ball or tissue and put it in an air vent in your house, vehicle, hotel room, etc.
- If diffusing while sleeping, set your timer for the desired length of time for automatic shut off.

Topical

You may apply single oils or blends neat or diluted, depending on the oil or oils being used. Please see the instructions at the beginning of this chapter for more information on applying oils to the skin.

- Apply 2-4 drops diluted 50:50 on chest, stomach, or lower back 2 times daily or as needed.
- Receive Raindrop Technique 1-2 times weekly.
- Place a warm compress on lower abdomen 1-2 times daily.
- Take a warm bath with custom bath salts using the following influenza blend:

Blend for Influenza or Colds

- 15 drops Ravintsara
- 6 drops Sacred Frankincense or Frankincense
- 6 drops Idaho Blue Spruce
- 3 drops Dorado Azul
- 2 drops Eucalyptus Radiata
- 1 drop Wintergreen
  Stir above essential oils thoroughly into ¼ cup Epsom salt or baking soda, and then add salt and oil mixture to hot bath water while tub is filling. Soak in hot bath for 20 to 30 minutes or until water cools.

Ingestion and Oral

The amount of oil ingested varies with different oils. Whether putting the oils in a capsule or drinking them in a liquid, please refer to the instructions at the beginning of this chapter.

- Take 1 capsule with desired oil 3 times daily.
- Put 2-3 drops of oil in a spoonful of Blue Agave, Yacon Syrup, maple syrup, coconut oil, milk, etc.
- Put the desired amount of oils in a glass of rice milk, almond milk, goat milk, carrot juice, NingXia Red, or even water and then drink it.

INSECT BITES AND STINGS

Essential oils are ideal for treating most kinds of insect bites because of their outstanding antiseptic and oil-soluble properties. Essential oils such as Lavender and Peppermint reduce insect-bite-induced itching and infection.

Recommendations

Singles: Lavender, Citronella, Eucalyptus Globulus, Melaleuca Alternifolia, Peppermint, Rosemary, Copaiba, Dorado Azul, Idaho Tansy, Palo Santo

Blends: PanAway, Purification, Melrose, Thieves

Stings and Bites Blend No. 1

- 10 drops Lavender
- 4 drops Eucalyptus Radiata
- 3 drops German Chamomile
- 2 drops Thyme

  Spray sheets and clothing to kill any insects that might be imbedded in the cloth.

Insect Bite Blend No. 2

- 20 drops Palo Santo
- 20 drops Idaho Tansy
- 10 drops Eucalyptus Blue

  Rub a small amount on skin or use in spray bottle.

Application and Usage
Topical

You may apply single oils or blends neat or diluted, depending on the oil or oils being used. Please see the instructions at the beginning of this chapter for more information on applying oils to the skin.

- Apply 1-2 drops of the sting and bite blends neat or diluted 50:50 on location 2-4 times daily.

....

Bee Stings

Bee stings can be painful and annoying, but they rarely cause problems, unless you are allergic to the venom—then they can be fatal.

Recommendations

Singles: Lavender, Idaho Tansy, Peppermint, Palo Santo, Spikenard, Idaho Balsam Fir

Blends: Purification, PanAway, Melrose, Deep Relief Roll-On

Bee Sting Blend

- 2 drops Lavender
- 1 drop Peppermint
- 1 drop German Chamomile
- 1 drop Vetiver

Bee Sting Regimen

- Flick or scrape stinger out with a knife or hard plastic like a credit card, taking care not to squeeze the venom sack.
- Apply 1-2 drops of the Bee Sting Blend on location. Repeat every 15 minutes for 1 hour.
- Apply any of the recommended blends 2-3 times daily until redness abates.

....

Bites

Essential oils are ideal for treating most kinds of insect bites because of their outstanding antiseptic and oil-soluble properties. Essential oils such as Lavender and Peppermint reduce insect bite-induced itching and infection.

Recommendations

Singles: Lavender, Citronella, Eucalyptus Globulus, Melaleuca Alternifolia, Peppermint, Rosemary, Copaiba, Dorado Azul

Blends: PanAway, Purification, Melrose

Stings and Bites Blend No. 1

- 10 drops Lavender
- 4 drops Eucalyptus Radiata
- 3 drops German Chamomile
- 2 drops Thyme

Application and Usage
Topical

You may apply single oils or blends neat or diluted, depending on the oil or oils being used. Please see the instructions at the beginning of this chapter for more information on applying oils to the skin.

- Apply 1-2 drops of the Stings and Bites Blend neat or diluted 50:50 on location 2-4 times daily.

Bedbug Bites

Bedbug bites can be difficult to distinguish from other insect bites. However, bedbug bites are usually:

- Found on the face, neck, arms, and hands
- Arranged in a rough line or in a cluster
- Itchy
- Red, often with a darker red spot in the middle

Singles: Idaho Tansy, Palo Santo, Eucalyptus Blue

Blends: Purification, Thieves

Insect Bite Blend No. 2

- 20 drops Palo Santo
- 20 drops Idaho Tansy
- 10 drops Eucalyptus Blue

Black Widow Spider Bite

A bite from a female black widow spider can cause pain and affect the victim's nervous system, but it is rarely fatal. If you know you have been bitten by a black widow spider, seek emergency medical treatment immediately.

Singles: Myrrh, Lemon

Blends: Purification, Thieves, Melrose, Pan-Away, The Gift

Nutritionals: Inner Defense

Topical

You may apply single oils or blends neat or diluted, depending on the oil or oils being used. Please see the instructions at the beginning of this chapter for more information on applying oils to the skin.

- Put on 1 drop of any oil you have such as Purification, Melrose, The Gift, Lemon, etc.

Brown Recluse Spider Bite

The bite of this spider causes a painful redness and blistering, which progresses to a gangrenous slough of the affected area. Seek immediate medical attention.

Singles: Myrrh, Sacred Frankincense, Frankincense, Rosemary, Ocotea, Idaho Tansy

Blends: Purification, Thieves, PanAway

Nutritionals: Inner Defense

Spider Bite Blend

- 1 drop Sacred Frankincense or Frankincense
- 1 drop Myrrh
- 1 drop Melrose

Topical

You may apply single oils or blends neat or diluted, depending on the oil or oils being used. Please see the instructions at the beginning of this chapter for more information on applying oils to the skin.

- Apply 1 drop of any of the above blends every 10 minutes until you reach professional medical treatment.
- Put on 1 drop of any oil you have such as Purification, Melrose, The Gift, Lemon, etc.

Chigger and Tick Bites

It is important that ticks and chiggers be removed before treating the bite. People have tried many different ways of getting rid of these invaders. Sometimes chiggers can be removed or killed by covering the bite with clear fingernail polish.

A common method for removing ticks is to touch them gently with a recently blown-out match head. The heat often causes ticks to let go so that they can just be brushed off.

Essential oils work quickly to remove ticks and chiggers. Mix Thyme or Oregano in a 50:50 dilution and apply 1-2 drops over the bite area. The phenols in these oils will usually cause them to let go and squirm to get away from the oil. When they do, they can be brushed off and killed.

Applying a single drop of Peppermint, Abundance, Exodus II, or any other oil or blend that is considered to be "hot" will cause the tick or chigger to come out of the skin. A "hot" oil is one that is high in phenols that can burn the skin when applied neat. In this case, the objective is to "get the critter out."

For most people, a little stinging does not matter. After the tick or chigger is removed, apply 1-2 drops of any of the oils listed below on the bite location.

Recommendations

Singles: Peppermint, Oregano, Plectranthus Oregano, Clove, Melaleuca Alternifolia, Lavender, Rosemary, Myrrh, Sacred Frankincense, Frankincense, Idaho Balsam Fir

Blends: Purification, Exodus II, Abundance, Melrose, Thieves, R.C., The Gift

Application and Usage
Topical

You may apply single oils or blends neat or diluted, depending on the oil or oils being used. Please see the instructions at the beginning of this chapter for more information on applying oils to the skin.

- Apply 1-6 drops neat or diluted, depending on size of affected area 3-5 times daily.

Mosquito Bites

For most people, a mosquito bite causes minor irritation. For those who are allergic to bites, their skin breaks out in hives, the chest and throat feel tight, they develop a dry cough, their eyes itch, and they often have nausea, vomiting, abdominal pain, and dizziness.

If you suspect you have a mosquito bite allergy, let your health-care professional see your red, swollen bite.

Recommendations

Singles: Peppermint, Melaleuca Alternifolia, Lavender, Rosemary, Myrrh, Sacred Frankincense, Frankincense, Idaho Balsam Fir, Idaho Tansy

Blends: Purification, Melrose, Thieves, R.C., The Gift

Application and Usage
Topical

You may apply single oils or blends neat or diluted, depending on the oil or oils being used. Please see the instructions at the beginning of this chapter for more information on applying oils to the skin.

- Apply 1-6 drops neat or diluted, depending on size of affected area 3-5 times daily.

West Nile Virus

Most people infected with West Nile virus have no signs or symptoms, and mild symptoms usually go away in a few days. However, if you experience symptoms or signs of a serious infection like a high fever, severe headache, stiff neck, or an altered mental state, see your health professional immediately. A serious West Nile virus infection generally requires hospitalization.

Recommendations

Singles: Peppermint, Melaleuca Alternifolia, Lavender, Rosemary, Myrrh, Sacred Frankincense, Frankincense, Idaho Balsam Fir, Oregano, Plectranthus Oregano, Thyme, Idaho Tansy

Blends: Purification, Melrose, Thieves, R.C., The Gift

Application and Usage
Topical

You may apply single oils or blends neat or diluted, depending on the oil or oils being used. Please see the instructions at the beginning of this chapter for more information on applying oils to the skin.

- Apply 1-6 drops neat or diluted, depending on size of affected area, 3-5 times daily.

Scorpion Sting

Several species of scorpions are found in the United States and Canada, but most do not produce a significant toxicity by stinging and are not as toxic as those found in South America and other parts of the world. A sting may cause swelling and a lot of discomfort but is rarely fatal.

However, a person who has been stung by a scorpion should see a doctor as soon as possible. Follow these first-aid measures:

- If breathing and heartbeat stop, start CPR immediately.
- Apply an ice pack or cold water to the bite area to help slow the spread of the venom.
- Seek medical care.

Recommendations
Singles: Lemongrass, Sacred Frankincense, Frankincense
Blends: Purification

Application and Usage
Topical
You may apply single oils or blends neat or diluted, depending on the oil or oils being used. Please see the instructions at the beginning of this chapter for more information on applying oils to the skin.

- Apply 1-6 drops neat or diluted 50:50, depending on size of affected area, 3-5 times daily.

INSECT REPELLENT
An insect repellent is a substance applied to skin, clothing, or other surfaces that discourages insects from landing on those surfaces. Repellents help prevent the outbreak of insect-borne diseases such as West Nile fever, Lyme disease, dengue fever, bubonic plague, and malaria.

Recommendations
Singles: Idaho Tansy, Palo Santo, Peppermint, Melaleuca Alternifolia, Geranium, Lemon, Rosemary, Lemongrass, Thyme, Spearmint, Citronella
Blends: Purification, Melrose, Thieves

Insect Repellents

- **Mosquito-repellent:** Palo Santo, Lemon, Idaho Tansy, Citronella
- **Moth repellent:** Patchouli, Palo Santo
- **Horse-fly repellent:** Idaho Tansy, Citronella
- **Aphids repellent:** Mix 10 drops Spearmint and 15 drops Orange essential oils in 2 quarts salt water, shake well, and spray on plants.
- **Cockroach repellent:** Mix 10 drops Peppermint and 5 drops Cypress in ½ cup salt water. Shake well and spray where roaches live.
- **Silverfish repellent:** Eucalyptus Radiata, Thieves
- To repel insects, essential oils can be diffused or put on cotton balls or cedar chips (for use in closets or drawers).
- Experiment with your own combination of oils and make new discoveries.

Insect Repellent Blend No. 1
- 9 drops Idaho Tansy
- 6 drops Peppermint
- 6 drops Citronella

Insect Repellent Blend No. 2
- 6 drops Idaho Tansy
- 6 drops Palo Santo
  Mix together and use undiluted or diluted with a little water.

Ed & Steven Geiger's Bug Spray
- 1 gallon distilled water
- 1 ounce organic catnip made into a tea, strained, and cooled
- 1 teaspoon Bath Gel Base
- 40 drops Purification
- 40 drops Idaho Tansy
- 40 drops DiGize

- 20 drops Rosemary
- 8 drops Peppermint
  Optional: Add Lemongrass and/or Oregano

Chérie Ross's Formula for Flea, Tick, and Insect Repellent

- 1 gallon distilled or pure water
- 4 heaping tablespoons organic dried catnip
- 2½ tablespoons organic Neem oil
- 2 teaspoons Thieves Household Cleaner or Bath Gel Base
- 80 drops Purification
- 80 drops Lemongrass
- 40 drops Idaho Tansy
- 40 drops Palo Santo
- 40 drops Ocotea or Basil
- 20 drops Peppermint (optional for high temperatures)

Steep the catnip in the gallon of water for 20-30 minutes. Cool to room temperature. Strain if needed. Add all remaining ingredients into Thieves Household Cleaner or Bath Gel Base. Then mix together and put into spray bottle. Use as needed.

Application and Usage
Topical

You may apply single oils or blends neat or diluted, depending on the oil or oils being used. Please see the instructions at the beginning of this chapter for more information on applying oils to the skin.

- Apply 1-6 drops neat or diluted, depending on size of affected area, 3-5 times daily.

INSOMNIA
(See also DEPRESSION, THYROID PROBLEMS)

After age 40, sleep quality and quantity deteriorate noticeably as melatonin production in the brain declines. Supplemental melatonin has been researched to dramatically improve sleep/wake cycles and combat age-related insomnia.

Insomnia may also be caused by bowel or liver toxicity, poor heart function, negative memories and trauma, depression, mineral deficiencies, hormone imbalance, or underactive thyroid.

The fragrance of many essential oils can exert a powerful, calming effect on the mind through their influence on the limbic region of the brain. Historically, lavender sachets or pillows were used for babies, children, and adults alike.

Recommendations

Singles: Lavender, Valerian, Cedarwood, Orange, Roman Chamomile

Blends: RutaVaLa, RutaVaLa Roll-On, Peace & Calming, Harmony, Dream Catcher, Valor, Valor Roll-On, Gentle Baby, Tranquil Roll-On, Trauma Life, Stress Away Roll-On

Nutritionals: ImmuPro, MegaCal, PD 80/20, Power Meal, Life 5, NingXia Red, Omega-Gize³, SleepEssence, Stress Away

Body Care Serums and Creams: Progessence Plus, Prenolone Plus Body Cream

Insomnia Blend

- 12 drops Orange
- 8 drops Lavender
- 4 drops Dorado Azul
- 3 drops Valerian
- 2 drops Roman Chamomile

Application and Usage
Inhalation

- Diffuse 30-60 minutes at bedtime.
- Apply 1-3 drops on a cotton ball and place on or near your pillow.
- Put 2-3 drops of your chosen oil in your hands and rub them together, cup your hands over your nose, and inhale as needed.
- Put 8-10 drops of oil on a cotton ball or tissue and put it in an air vent in your house, vehicle, hotel room, etc.
- If diffusing while sleeping, set your timer for the desired length of time for automatic shut off.

Topical

You may apply single oils or blends neat or diluted, depending on the oil or oils being used. Please see the instructions at the beginning of this chapter for more information on applying oils to the skin.

- Apply 1-3 drops neat to shoulders, stomach, and on bottoms of feet.
- Mix 6-8 drops of oils with ¼ cup Epsom salt or baking soda in hot water and add to hot bath water while tub is filling. Soak in bathtub for 20 to 30 minutes or until water cools.
- Rub 1-2 drops of oil on the temples and back of neck several times daily.
- Place a warm compress with 1-2 drops of chosen oil on the back.

Ingestion and Oral

The amount of oil ingested varies with different oils. Whether putting the oils in a capsule or drinking them in a liquid, please refer to the instructions at the beginning of this chapter.

- Take 1 capsule with desired oil 2 times daily.
- Take 1 capsule of Lavender oil or any desired oil undiluted or diluted 50:50 1 hour before bedtime.
- Put 2-3 drops of oil in a spoonful of Blue Agave, Yacon Syrup, maple syrup, coconut oil, milk, etc.
- Put the desired amount of oils in a glass of rice milk, almond milk, goat milk, carrot juice, NingXia Red, or even water and then drink it.

IRRITABLE BOWEL SYNDROME

Irritable bowel syndrome (IBS) is a common disorder of the intestines marked by the following symptoms:

- Cramps
- Gas and bloating
- Constipation
- Diarrhea and loose stools

It may be caused by a combination of stress and a high-fat diet. Fatty foods increase the intensity of the contractions in the colon, thereby increasing symptoms. Chocolate and milk products, in particular, seem to have the most negative effects on those suffering.

Irritable bowel syndrome is not the same as colitis, mucous colitis, spastic colon, and spastic bowel. Unlike colitis, it does not involve any inflammation and is actually called "functional disorder" because it presents no obvious, outward signs of disease.

A number of medical studies have documented that Peppermint oil, in capsules, is beneficial in treating irritable bowel syndrome and decreasing pain.[28, 29, 30]

Recommendations

Singles: Tarragon, Peppermint, Fennel, Nutmeg, Juniper, Ocotea

Blends: DiGize, JuvaFlex

Nutritionals: Detoxzyme, OmegaGize³, Digest & Cleanse, Life 5, AlkaLime, JuvaPower. After symptoms stop, then start Essentialzymes-4, Essentialzyme, and ICP.

Application and Usage

Inhalation

- Diffuse your choice of oils for ½ hour every 4-6 hours or as desired.
- Put 2-3 drops of your chosen oil in your hands and rub them together, cup your hands over your nose, and inhale throughout the day as needed.
- Put 8-10 drops of oil on a cotton ball or tissue and put it in an air vent in your house, vehicle, hotel room, etc.
- If diffusing while sleeping, set your timer for the desired length of time for automatic shut off.

Topical

- You may apply single oils or blends neat or diluted, depending on the oil or oils being used.

Please see the instructions at the beginning of this chapter for more information on applying oils to the skin.

Ingestion and Oral

The amount of oil ingested varies with different oils. Whether putting the oils in a capsule or drinking them in a liquid, please refer to the instructions at the beginning of this chapter.

- Take 1 capsule with desired oil 3 times daily.
- Put 2-3 drops of oil in a spoonful of Blue Agave, Yacon Syrup, maple syrup, coconut oil, milk, etc.
- Put the desired amount of oils in a glass of rice milk, almond milk, goat milk, carrot juice, NingXia Red, or even water and then drink it.

JOINT STIFFNESS OR PAIN

Joint stiffness is caused by inflammation in the lining of the joint. Specific causes may be rheumatoid arthritis, osteoarthritis, bone diseases, cancer, joint trauma, or overuse of the joint. However, no matter what causes it, joint pain and stiffness can be very bothersome.

Recommendations

Singles: Wintergreen, Palo Santo, Idaho Blue Spruce, Douglas Fir, Elemi, Idaho Balsam Fir, German Chamomile, Peppermint, Pine, Idaho Tansy

Blends: PanAway, Aroma Siez, Relieve It, Deep Relief Roll-On

Nutritionals: BLM, MegaCal, Sulfurzyme, OmegaGize[3]

Resins: Myrrh or Frankincense Gum Resin (ingest 2 crystals 2 times daily)

Body Care Massage Oils and Creams: Regenolone Moisturizing Cream, Ortho Ease Massage Oil, Ortho Sport Massage Oil

Joint Pain Blend No. 1
- 10 drops Black Pepper
- 5 drops Marjoram
- 5 drops Idaho Blue Spruce
- 2 drops Rosemary

Joint Pain Blend No. 2
- 7 drops Idaho Balsam Fir
- 4 drops Wintergreen
- 3 drops Vetiver
- 2 drops Blue Chamomile

Application and Usage
Topical

You may apply single oils or blends neat or diluted, depending on the oil or oils being used. Please see the instructions at the beginning of this chapter for more information on applying oils to the skin.

- Massage 3-6 drops diluted 50:50 on location. Repeat as needed to control pain.
- Apply to appropriate Vita Flex points on the feet. Repeat as needed.

KIDNEY DISORDERS

The kidneys remove waste products from the blood and help control blood pressure. They filter over 200 quarts of blood each day and remove over 2 quarts of waste products and water that flow into the bladder as urine through tubes called ureters.

Strong kidneys are essential for good health. Inefficient or damaged kidneys can result in waste accumulating in the blood and causing serious damage.

High blood pressure can be a cause and a result of chronic kidney failure, since kidneys are central to blood regulation (See Blood Pressure, High).

Symptoms of poor kidney function:
- Infrequent or inefficient urinations
- Swelling, especially around the ankles
- Labored breathing due to fluid accumulation in the chest

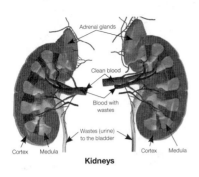

Kidneys

Recommendations
Singles: Grapefruit, Lemon, Geranium, Juniper
Blends: DiGize, GLF, JuvaFlex
Nutritionals: K&B, Digest & Cleanse

Application and Usage
Inhalation
- Diffuse your choice of oils for ½ hour every 4-6 hours or as desired.
- Put 2-3 drops of your chosen oil in your hands and rub them together, cup your hands over your nose, and inhale throughout the day as needed.
- Put 8-10 drops of oil on a cotton ball or tissue and put it in an air vent in your house, vehicle, hotel room, etc.
- If diffusing while sleeping, set your timer for the desired length of time for automatic shut off.

Topical
You may apply single oils or blends neat or diluted, depending on the oil or oils being used. Please see the instructions at the beginning of this chapter for more information on applying oils to the skin.
- Apply 6-8 drops diluted 50:50 on the back over the kidney area as needed.
- Applying a single drop under the nose is helpful and refreshing.

- Massage 2-4 drops of oil neat on the soles of the feet just before bedtime. Children with kidney disorders may especially benefit from this application.
- Place a warm compress with 1-2 drops of chosen oil on the back 1-2 times daily.

Ingestion and Oral
The amount of oil ingested varies with different oils. Whether putting the oils in a capsule or drinking them in a liquid, please refer to the instructions at the beginning of this chapter.
- Take 1 capsule with desired oil 2 times daily.
- Put 2-3 drops of oil in a spoonful of Blue Agave, Yacon Syrup, maple syrup, coconut oil, milk, etc.
- Put the desired amount of oils in a glass of rice milk, almond milk, goat milk, carrot juice, NingXia Red, or even water and then drink it.

....

Kidney Inflammation/Infection (Nephritis)
Kidney inflammation can be caused by structural defects, poor diet, or bacterial infection from *Escherichia coli, Staphylococcus aureus, Enterobacter,* and *Klebsiella* bacteria. Abnormal proteins trapped in the glomeruli (tiny filtering units in the kidneys), called glomerulonephritis, can also cause inflammation and damage to these tiny filtering units.

This disease can be acute (flaring up in a few days) or chronic (taking months or years to develop). The mildest forms may not show any symptoms except through a urine test. At more advanced stages, urine appears smoky as small amounts of blood are passed and eventually turn red as more blood is excreted—the signs of impending kidney failure.

As with all serious conditions, you should immediately consult a health-care professional if you suspect a kidney infection of any kind.

Symptoms may include the following:
- Feeling of discomfort in lower back
- Drowsiness
- Nausea
- Smokey or red-colored urine

Damage to the glomeruli caused by bacterial infections is called pyelonephritis. To reduce infection, drink a gallon of water mixed with 8 oz. of unsweetened cranberry juice daily and use the products listed below.

Recommendations

Singles: Cumin, Cistus, Sacred Frankincense, Frankincense, Juniper, Myrrh, Helichrysum, Lemongrass, Rosemary, Geranium, Thyme

Blends: Melrose, Purification, Longevity, Thieves, 3 Wise Men

Nutritionals: Mineral Essence, ICP, JuvaPower, Inner Defense, Super C, Super C Chewable, Life 5, Digest & Cleanse, K&B

Application and Usage
Inhalation

- Diffuse your choice of oils for ½ hour every 4-6 hours or as desired.
- Put 2-3 drops of your chosen oil in your hands and rub them together, cup your hands over your nose, and inhale throughout the day as needed.
- Put 8-10 drops of oil on a cotton ball or tissue and put it in an air vent in your house, vehicle, hotel room, etc.
- If diffusing while sleeping, set your timer for the desired length of time for automatic shut off.

Topical

You may apply single oils or blends neat or diluted, depending on the oil or oils being used. Please see the instructions at the beginning of this chapter for more information on applying oils to the skin.

- Massage 2-4 drops of oil neat on the soles of the feet Vita Flex points just before bedtime.
- Place a cold compress with 1-2 drops of chosen oil over the kidney area 1-2 times daily.

Ingestion and Oral

The amount of oil ingested varies with different oils. Whether putting the oils in a capsule or drinking them in a liquid, please refer to the instructions at the beginning of this chapter.

- Take 2 capsules with desired oil 2 times daily for 10 days.
- Put 2-3 drops of oil in a spoonful of Blue Agave, Yacon Syrup, maple syrup, coconut oil, milk, etc.
- Put the desired amount of oils in a glass of rice milk, almond milk, goat milk, carrot juice, NingXia Red, or even water and then drink it.

Kidney Stones
(See BLADDER / Urinary Tract Infection)

Kidney stones can create intense pain and dangerous infection. You should always consult a qualified health-care professional before beginning any treatment for kidney stones.

A kidney stone is a solid piece of material that forms in the kidney from mineral or protein-breakdown products in the urine. Occasionally, larger stones can become trapped in a ureter, bladder, or urethra, which can block urine flow, causing intense pain.

There are four types of kidney stones:
- Stones made from calcium (the most common type)
- Stones made from magnesium and ammonia (a struvite stone)
- Stones made from uric acid
- Stones made from cystine (the rarest)

Symptoms may include the following:
- Persistent, penetrating pain in side or lower back
- Blood in the urine
- Fainting
- It is important to drink plenty of water (at least six 8 oz. glasses daily) to help pass a kidney stone.

Recommendations

Singles: Helichrysum, Lemon, Sacred Frankincense, Frankincense, Geranium, Juniper, Orange, Lemon

Blends: Citrus Fresh, Purification

Nutritionals: K&B, Essentialzymes-4, Essentialzyme, Detoxzyme

Liquids: Apple Cider Vinegar

Application and Usage

Inhalation
- Diffuse your choice of oils for ½ hour every 4-6 hours or as desired.
- Put 2-3 drops of your chosen oil in your hands and rub them together, cup your hands over your nose, and inhale throughout the day as needed.
- Put 8-10 drops of oil on a cotton ball or tissue and put it in an air vent in your house, vehicle, hotel room, etc.
- If diffusing while sleeping, set your timer for the desired length of time for automatic shut off.

Topical
You may apply single oils or blends neat or diluted, depending on the oil or oils being used. Please see the instructions at the beginning of

---

Detoxifying the Kidneys

The Chinese wolfberry has been used in China for centuries as a kidney tonic and detoxifier. Essential oils can also assist in the detoxification due to various chemical constituents and unique, lipid-soluble properties.

Kidney Detoxifying Recipe:
- 6 drops German chamomile
- 6 drops juniper
- 2 drops fennel

Put 5 drops of the recipe in a gel capsule and then fill the capsule with V-6 Vegetable Oil Complex; take 2 times daily. You may also apply the recipe neat in a compress over the kidneys.

Supplements:
K&B, MultiGreens, Sulfurzyme, Detoxzyme, Essentialzyme, ICP, JuvaPower

---

this chapter for more information on applying oils to the skin.
- Massage 2-4 drops neat to the kidney Vita Flex points of the feet just before bedtime.
- Apply 6-10 drops of recommended oils neat over kidney area 1-2 times daily.
- Place a warm compress with 1-2 drops of chosen oil over the back.

Ingestion and Oral
The amount of oil ingested varies with different oils. Whether putting the oils in a capsule or drinking them in a liquid, please refer to the instructions at the beginning of this chapter.
- Take 2 capsules with desired oil 2 times daily.
- Put 2-3 drops of oil in a spoonful of Blue Agave, Yacon Syrup, maple syrup, coconut oil, milk, etc.
- Put the desired amount of oils in a glass of rice milk, almond milk, goat milk, carrot juice, NingXia Red, or even water and then drink it.

LICE

The most common remedy for lice (pediculosis) and their eggs (nits) is lindane (gamma benzene hexachloride), a highly toxic polychlorinated chemical that is structurally very similar to hazardous banned pesticides such as DDT and chlordane. It is so dangerous that Dr. Guy Sansfacon, head of the Quebec Poison Control Centre in Canada, has requested that lindane be banned.

Essential oils offer a safe, effective alternative. A 1996 study by researchers in Iceland showed the effectiveness against head lice of the essential oils of anise seed, cinnamon leaf, thyme, Melaleuca Alternifolia, peppermint, and nutmeg in shampoo and rinse solutions.[31]

Recommendations

Singles: Melaleuca Alternifolia, Palo Santo, Idaho Tansy, Lavender, Peppermint, Thyme, Geranium, Nutmeg, Rosemary, Cinnamon

Blends: Purification, Thieves

Head Lice Blend
- 4 drops Thyme
- 2 drops Lavender
- 2 drops Geranium

Application and Usage

Topical

You may apply single oils or blends neat or diluted, depending on the oil or oils being used. Please see the instructions at the beginning of this chapter for more information on applying oils to the skin.

- Add 1 teaspoon of oil diluted 50:50 to shampoo and massage onto entire scalp.
- Cover with a disposable shower cap and leave on for at least ½ hour.
- Rinse well using 1 cup of Thieves Fresh Essence Plus Mouthwash massaged into hair and scalp. Leave on for 10 minutes before rinsing out.

LIVER DISEASES AND DISORDERS

The liver is one of the most important organs, playing a major role in detoxifying the body. When the liver is damaged, frequently due to excess alcohol consumption, viral hepatitis, or poor diet, an excess of toxins can build up in the blood and tissues that can result in degenerative disease and death.

Jaundice (abnormal yellow color of the skin), may be the only visible sign of liver disease. Symptoms of a stressed or diseased liver:
- Nausea
- Loss of appetite
- Dark-colored urine
- Yellowish or gray-colored bowel movements
- Abdominal pain or ascites, an unusual swelling of the abdomen caused by an accumulation of fluid, itching, dermatitis, or hives
- Disturbed sleep caused by the buildup of unfiltered toxins in the blood
- General fatigue and loss of energy
- Lack of sex drive

....

Hepatitis

Viral hepatitis is a serious, life-threatening disease of the liver that can result in scarring (cirrhosis) and eventual organ destruction and death. A qualified health professional should be seen immediately if you suspect hepatitis.

There are several different kinds of hepatitis: Hepatitis A (spread by contaminated food, water, or feces) and Hepatitis B and C (spread by contaminated blood or semen).

An unpublished 2003 study conducted by Roger Lewis, MD, at the Young Life Research Clinic in Springville, Utah, evaluated the efficacy of Helichrysum, Ledum, and Celery Seed in treating cases of advanced Hepatitis C. In one case a 20-year-old male diagnosed with Hepatitis C had a viral count of 13,200. After taking 2 capsules (approximately 750 milligrams each) of GLF, a blend of Helichrysum, Ledum, Celery

Seed, and JuvaCleanse daily for one month with no other intervention, the patient's viral count dropped more than 80 percent to 2,580.

Symptoms include jaundice, weakness, loss of appetite, nausea, brownish or tea colored urine, abdominal discomfort, fever, and whitish bowel movements.

Recommendations

Singles: German Chamomile, Helichrysum, Ledum, Celery Seed, Ravintsara, Peppermint, Myrrh

Blends: GLF, JuvaCleanse, JuvaFlex

Nutritionals: ImmuPro, MultiGreens, JuvaPower, JuvaSpice (for salads and cooking), JuvaTone, Essentialzymes-4, Detoxzyme, Life 5, ICP, ComforTone, Essentialzyme, Master Formula HIS or HERS

Note: Avoid grapefruit juice and any medications that stress the liver.

Application and Usage

Inhalation

- Diffuse your choice of oils for ½ hour every 4-6 hours or as desired.
- Put 2-3 drops of your chosen oil in your hands and rub them together, cup your hands over your nose, and inhale throughout the day as needed.
- Put 8-10 drops of oil on a cotton ball or tissue and put it in an air vent in your house, vehicle, hotel room, etc.
- If diffusing while sleeping, set your timer for the desired length of time for automatic shut off.

Topical

You may apply single oils or blends neat or diluted, depending on the oil or oils being used. Please see the instructions at the beginning of this chapter for more information on applying oils to the skin.

- Apply 1-3 drops diluted 50:50 on carotid arteries on the right and left side of the throat

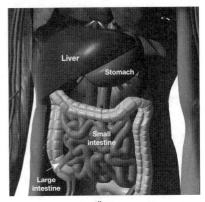

liver

just under the jaw bone on either side 2-5 times daily. Carotid arteries are an excellent place to apply oils for fast absorption.

- Apply 1-3 drops on the Vita Flex liver point of the right foot 1-3 times daily.
- Receive a Raindrop Technique 2-3 times weekly.
- Place a warm compress with 1-2 drops of chosen oil over the liver 1-2 times daily.

Ingestion and Oral

The amount of oil ingested varies with different oils. Whether putting the oils in a capsule or drinking them in a liquid, please refer to the instructions at the beginning of this chapter.

- Take 2 capsules with desired oil 3 times daily.
- Put 2-3 drops of oil in a spoonful of Blue Agave, Yacon Syrup, maple syrup, coconut oil, milk, etc.
- Put the desired amount of oils in a glass of rice milk, almond milk, goat milk, carrot juice, NingXia Red, or even water and then drink it.

Daily hepatitis regimen

- Begin with a colon cleanse using ICP, ComforTone, and Essentialzyme.
- After 3 days, add 1-2 tablets of JuvaTone 3 times daily.

Protecting Your Liver

- Avoid alcoholic beverages.

- Avoid unnecessary use of prescription drugs. Even over-the-counter pain relievers can have toxic effects on the liver in moderately high doses.

- Consume a diet high in selenium found in plant food, Brazil nuts, tuna, meat, eggs, etc. Selenium helps proteins make important antioxidant enzymes that prevent cellular damage from free radicals.

- Avoid mixing pharmaceutical drugs, especially with alcohol.

- Avoid exposure to industrial chemicals whenever possible.

- Eat a healthy diet of vegetables and fruits; fruits are naturally cleansing.

- Nutritionals: Detoxzyme, Essentialzyme, and Ningxia wolfberry, which is widely used in China as a liver tonic and detoxifier.

- ImmuPro: Take 4 tablets at night, 1-2 tablets morning and afternoon.
- MultiGreens: Take 1-3 capsules 3 times daily.

....

Jaundice

Jaundice is the yellowish staining of the skin and the whites of the eyes that is caused by too much bilirubin being produced for the liver to remove it from the blood.

Recommendations

Singles: German Chamomile, Ledum, Celery Seed, Ravintsara, Peppermint, Myrrh

Blends: JuvaCleanse, JuvaFlex, GLF

Nutritionals: JuvaPower, JuvaSpice (for salads and cooking), MultiGreens, JuvaTone, ImmuPro, Essentialzymes-4, Detoxzyme, Life 5, ICP, ComforTone, Essentialzyme, Master Formula HIS or HERS

Note: Avoid grapefruit juice and any medications that stress the liver.

Application and Usage

Inhalation

- Diffuse your choice of oils for ½ hour every 4-6 hours or as desired.
- Put 2-3 drops of your chosen oil in your hands and rub them together, cup your hands over your nose, and inhale throughout the day as needed.
- Put 8-10 drops of oil on a cotton ball or tissue and put it in an air vent in your house, vehicle, hotel room, etc.
- If diffusing while sleeping, set your timer for the desired length of time for automatic shut off.

Topical

You may apply single oils or blends neat or diluted, depending on the oil or oils being used. Please see the instructions at the beginning of this chapter for more information on applying oils to the skin.

- Apply 1-3 drops diluted 50:50 on carotid arteries on the right and left side of the throat just under the jaw bone on either side 2-5 times daily. Carotid arteries are an excellent place to apply oils for fast absorption.
- Apply 1-3 drops on the Vita Flex liver point of the right foot 1-3 times daily.
- Receive a Raindrop Technique 2-3 times weekly.
- Place a warm compress with 1-2 drops of chosen oil over the liver 1-2 times daily.

Ingestion and Oral

The amount of oil ingested varies with different oils. Whether putting the oils in a capsule or drinking them in a liquid, please refer to the instructions at the beginning of this chapter.

- Take 2 capsules with desired oil 3 times daily.
- Put 2-3 drops of oil in a spoonful of Blue Agave, Yacon Syrup, maple syrup, coconut oil, milk, etc.

• Put the desired amount of oils in a glass of rice milk, almond milk, goat milk, carrot juice, NingXia Red, or even water and then drink it.

....

Toxic Liver

The liver is important in transforming and eliminating chemicals and is susceptible to becoming toxic from these substances.

Recommendations

Singles: Orange, Ledum, Celery Seed, Lemon, Cardamom, Geranium, Carrot Seed, German Chamomile, Rosemary

Blends: GLF, JuvaFlex, Release, JuvaCleanse

Nutritionals: JuvaTone, JuvaPower, JuvaSpice (for salads and cooking), Longevity Softgels, Sulfurzyme, Digest & Cleanse, ICP, Comfor-Tone, Essentialzyme, Life 5, K&B

Liver Support Blend

• 10 drops Orange
• 5 drops Rosemary
• 3 drops Celery Seed
• 2 drops German Chamomile

Application and Usage

Inhalation

• Diffuse your choice of oils for ½ hour every 4-6 hours or as desired.
• Put 2-3 drops of your chosen oil in your hands and rub them together, cup your hands over your nose, and inhale throughout the day as needed.
• Put 8-10 drops of oil on a cotton ball or tissue and put it in an air vent in your house, vehicle, hotel room, etc.
• If diffusing while sleeping, set your timer for the desired length of time for automatic shut off.

Topical

You may apply single oils or blends neat or diluted, depending on the oil or oils being used. Please see the instructions at the beginning of this chapter for more information on applying oils to the skin.

• Apply 1-3 drops on the liver Vita Flex point of the right foot.
• Massage 2-4 drops of oil neat on the soles of the feet just before bedtime.
• Place a warm compress with 1-2 drops of chosen oil over the liver 1-2 times daily.
• Have Raindrop Technique 1-2 times weekly.

Ingestion and Oral

The amount of oil ingested varies with different oils. Whether putting the oils in a capsule or drinking them in a liquid, please refer to the instructions at the beginning of this chapter.

• Take 1 capsule with desired oil 2 times daily.
• Put 2-3 drops of oil in a spoonful of Blue Agave, Yacon Syrup, maple syrup, coconut oil, milk, etc.
• Put the desired amount of oils in a glass of rice milk, almond milk, goat milk, carrot juice, NingXia Red, or even water and then drink it 2-4 times daily.

LIVER SPOTS (SOLAR LENTIGINES)

Liver spots (also called age spots and solar lentigines) are flat brown, gray, or black spots and vary in size. They usually are found on the face, arms, shoulders, and hands—the areas that receive the greatest exposure to the sun.

Recommendations

Singles: Idaho Tansy, Sandalwood, Blue Cypress, Lavender, Nutmeg

Blends: DiGize, GLF

Liver Spot Blend

• 20 drops Avocado Oil
• 6 drops Sandalwood
• 4 drops Blue Cypress
• 4 drops Lavender
• 4 drops Nutmeg

Application and Usage

Topical

You may apply single oils or blends neat or

diluted, depending on the oil or oils being used. Please see the instructions at the beginning of this chapter for more information on applying oils to the skin.

- Apply 2-4 drops neat of the liver spot blend over affected area 3 times daily for 2 weeks.

LUNG INFECTIONS AND PROBLEMS

The lungs provide us with oxygen and remove carbon dioxide through respiration. Breathing brings irritants and contaminants into the lungs, making them susceptible to damage and infection.

....

Asthma
(See also ALLERGIES)

During an asthma attack, the bronchial air tubes in the lungs become swollen and clogged with thick, sticky mucus. The muscles of the air tubes will also begin to constrict or tighten.

This results in very difficult or labored breathing. If an attack is severe, it can actually be life-threatening.

Many asthma attacks are triggered by an allergic reaction to pollen, skin particles, dandruff, cat and dog dander, dust mites, as well as from foods such as eggs, milk, flavorings, dyes, preservatives, and other chemicals. Asthma can also be triggered by respiratory infection, exercise, stress, and psychological factors.

Recommendations

Singles: Dorado Azul, Eucalyptus Radiata, Sacred Frankincense, Frankincense, Eucalyptus Blue, Ravintsara, Palo Santo, Idaho Ponderosa Pine

Blends: R.C., Breathe Again Roll-On, Valor, Raven, Inspiration, Sacred Mountain

Nutritionals: Detoxzyme, ICP, JuvaPower, MultiGreens, ImmuPro, Essentialzyme, Essentialzymes-4

Application and Usage
Inhalation

- Diffuse your choice of oils for 3-5 minutes or as often as it is comfortable.
- Put 2-3 drops of your chosen oil in your hands and rub them together, cup your hands over your nose, and inhale throughout the day as needed.
- Put 8-10 drops of oil on a cotton ball or tissue and put it in an air vent in your house, vehicle, hotel room, etc.
- If diffusing while sleeping, set your timer for the desired length of time for automatic shut off.

Topical

You may apply single oils or blends neat or diluted, depending on the oil or oils being used. Please see the instructions at the beginning of this chapter for more information on applying oils to the skin.

- Apply 1-2 drops mixed with Ortho Ease, Relaxation, or Sensation massage oils on temples and back of neck as desired.
- You may also apply 2-3 drops on the Vita Flex points on the feet.

Ingestion and Oral

The amount of oil ingested varies with different oils. Whether putting the oils in a capsule or drinking them in a liquid, please refer to the instructions at the beginning of this chapter.

- Take 1 capsule of Dorado Azul or other desired oil 2 times daily.
- Put 2-3 drops of oil in a spoonful of Blue Agave, Yacon Syrup, maple syrup, coconut oil, milk, etc.
- Put the desired amount of oils in a glass of rice milk, almond milk, goat milk, carrot juice, NingXia Red, or even water and then drink it.
- Take 1-2 capsules daily of Dorado Azul, Eucalyptus Blue, or other oil you might like.

Bronchitis
(See also ASTHMA)

Bronchitis is characterized by inflammation of the bronchial tube lining accompanied by a heavy mucus discharge. Bronchitis can be caused by an infection or exposure to dust, chemicals, air pollution, or cigarette smoke.

When bronchitis occurs regularly over long periods (i.e., 3 months out of the year for several years), it is known as chronic bronchitis. It can eventually lead to emphysema.

Symptoms may include the following:
- Persistent, hacking cough
- Mucus discharge from the lungs
- Difficulty breathing

Avoiding air pollution is an easy way to reduce bronchitis symptoms. In cases where bronchitis is caused by a bacteria or virus, the inhalation of high antimicrobial essential oils may help combat the infection. Heavy mucus may increase after eating foods containing processed sugar or flour or high levels of fat.

Recommendations

Singles: Dorado Azul, Myrtle, Ravintsara, Eucalyptus Blue, Palo Santo, Rosemary, Eucalyptus Radiata, Eucalyptus Globulus, Thyme, Idaho Ponderosa Pine, Wintergreen, Pine, Oregano, Plectranthus Oregano, Melaleuca Alternifolia, Idaho Balsam Fir, Bay Laurel, Copaiba

Blends: Raven, Melrose, Purification, PanAway, R.C., Thieves, Breathe Again Roll-On, Exodus II

Nutritionals: Super C, Super C Chewable, Life 5, Longevity Softgels, Digest & Cleanse, Inner Defense

Oral: Thieves Fresh Essence Plus Mouthwash

Bronchitis Blend No. 1
- 6 drops Ravintsara
- 5 drops Clove
- 4 drops Myrrh
- 2 drops Palo Santo

Bronchitis Blend No. 2
- 10 drops Dorado Azul
- 6 drops Eucalyptus Blue
- 5 drops Lavender
- 3 drops Eucalyptus Globulus

Note: Essential oil blends work especially well in respiratory applications.

Application and Usage
Inhalation
- Diffuse your choice of oils, alternating between singles and blends, for ½ hour every 4-6 hours or as desired.
- Put 2-3 drops of your chosen oil in your hands and rub them together, cup your hands over your nose, and inhale throughout the day as needed.
- Put 8-10 drops of oil on a cotton ball or tissue and put it in an air vent in your house, vehicle, hotel room, etc.
- If diffusing while sleeping, set your timer for the desired length of time for automatic shut off.
- Add a few drops of oil to a bowl of boiling water. Position the face above the bowl and drape a towel over the head to create a vaporizing effect. Repeat 2-3 times daily.

Topical
You may apply single oils or blends neat or diluted, depending on the oil or oils being used. Please see the instructions at the beginning of this chapter for more information on applying oils to the skin.

- Apply 2-6 drops neat or diluted 50:50 to the neck and chest as needed.
- Massage 2-3 drops on the lung Vita Flex points of the feet 2-4 times daily.
- Place a warm compress with 1-2 drops of chosen oil on the neck, chest, and upper back areas 1-3 times daily.
- Rectal: Using any of the recommended blends, combine 20 drops with 1 tablespoon olive oil. Insert into rectum with bulb syringe

and retain throughout the night. Repeat nightly for 2-3 days.

Ingestion and Oral

The amount of oil ingested varies with different oils. Whether putting the oils in a capsule or drinking them in a liquid, please refer to the instructions at the beginning of this chapter.

- Take 1 capsule with desired oil 2 times daily.
- Put 2-3 drops of oil in a spoonful of Blue Agave, Yacon Syrup, maple syrup, coconut oil, milk, etc.
- Put the desired amount of oils in a glass of rice milk, almond milk, goat milk, carrot juice, NingXia Red, or even water and then drink it.
- Gargle a mixture of essential oils and water 4-8 times daily.

....

Pleurisy

This is an inflammation of the pleura, the outer membranes covering the lungs and the thoracic cavity.

Recommendations

Singles: Ravintsara, Eucalyptus Blue, Dorado Azul, Eucalyptus Radiata, Wintergreen, Myrrh, German Chamomile

Blends: PanAway, Raven, Exodus II, Thieves

Nutritionals: Sulfurzyme, Super C, Super C Chewable, OmegaGize^3, Mineral Essence, Essentialzyme, Digest & Cleanse, ICP, JuvaPower

Application and Usage

Inhalation

- Diffuse your choice of oils for ½ hour every 4-6 hours or as desired.
- Put 2-3 drops of your chosen oil in your hands and rub them together, cup your hands over your nose, and inhale throughout the day as needed.
- Put 8-10 drops of oil on a cotton ball or tissue and put it in an air vent in your house, vehicle, hotel room, etc.

- If diffusing while sleeping, set your timer for the desired length of time for automatic shut off.

Topical

You may apply single oils or blends neat or diluted, depending on the oil or oils being used. Please see the instructions at the beginning of this chapter for more information on applying oils to the skin.

- Massage 5-7 drops of oil diluted 20:80 on neck and chest 2-3 times daily.
- Place a warm compress with 1-2 drops of oil on the neck, chest, and upper back areas daily.
- Apply 1-3 drops on the lung Vita Flex points on the feet daily.
- Receive a Raindrop Technique 1-2 times weekly.

....

Pneumonia

Pneumonia is a lung infection caused by bacteria or viruses. It starts when you breathe germs into your lungs and is likely to occur after having a cold or the flu.

Recommendations

Singles: Thyme, Ravintsara, Eucalyptus Radiata, Eucalyptus Globulus, Mountain Savory, Clove, Oregano, Plectranthus Oregano, Melaleuca Alternifolia, Eucalyptus Blue, Dorado Azul

Blends: Raven, Melrose, R.C., Thieves, Breathe Again Roll-On

Nutritionals: Inner Defense, Super C, Super C Chewable, Longevity Softgels, MultiGreens, ImmuPro, Digest & Cleanse, Life 5

Oral Care: Thieves Spray, Thieves Lozenges (Hard/Soft), Thieves Fresh Essence Plus Mouthwash

Pneumonia Blend

- 10 drops Eucalyptus Globulus
- 8 drops Ravintsara
- 2 drops Oregano
- 2 drops Dorado Azul

Application and Usage

Inhalation

- Diffuse your choice of oils, alternating between singles and blends, for ½ hour every 4-6 hours or as desired. If diffusing at night while sleeping, set your timer for the desired length of time for automatic shut off.
- Put 2-3 drops of your chosen oil in your hands and rub them together, cup your hands over your nose, and inhale throughout the day as needed.
- Put 8-10 drops of oil on a cotton ball or tissue and put it in an air vent in your house, vehicle, hotel room, etc.
- If diffusing while sleeping, set your timer for the desired length of time for automatic shut off.
- Add a few drops of oil to a bowl of boiling water. Position your face above the bowl and drape a towel over your head to create a vaporizing effect. Repeat 2-3 times daily.

Topical

You may apply single oils or blends neat or diluted, depending on the oil or oils being used. Please see the instructions at the beginning of this chapter for more information on applying oils to the skin.

- Apply 2-6 drops neat or diluted 50:50 to the neck and chest as needed.
- Massage 2-3 drops on the lung Vita Flex points of the feet 2-4 times daily.
- Place a warm compress with 1-2 drops of chosen oil on the neck, chest, and upper back areas 1-3 times daily.
- Rectal: Using any of the recommended blends, combine 20 drops with 1 tablespoon olive oil. Insert into rectum with bulb syringe and retain throughout the night. Repeat nightly for 5-6 days.

Ingestion and Oral

The amount of oil ingested varies with different oils. Whether putting the oils in a capsule or drinking them in a liquid, please refer to the instructions at the beginning of this chapter.

- Take 1 capsule with desired oil 2 times daily.
- Put 2-3 drops of oil in a spoonful of Blue Agave, Yacon Syrup, maple syrup, coconut oil, milk, etc.
- Put the desired amount of oils in a glass of rice milk, almond milk, goat milk, carrot juice, NingXia Red, or even water and then drink it.
- Gargle a mixture of essential oils and water 4-8 times daily.

Tuberculosis

Tuberculosis (TB) is a highly contagious lung disease caused by Mycobacterium tuberculosis. The germs are spread via coughs, sneezes, and physical contact.

The most worrisome aspect of this disease is its latency. Those infected may harbor the germ for years, yet display no outward or visible signs of infection. However, when the immune system becomes challenged or weakened due to stress, candida, diabetes, corticosteroid use, or other factors, the bacteria can become activated and develop into full-blown TB.

Because many essential oils have broad-spectrum, antimicrobial properties, they can be diffused to prevent the spread of airborne bacteria like Mycobacterium tuberculosis. Essential oils and blends like Thieves, Purification, Raven, R.C., and Sacred Mountain are extremely effective for killing this type of germ.

Many essential oils have also been shown to stimulate the immune system. Lemon oil has been shown to increase lymphocyte production—a pivotal part of the immune system.

Recommendations

Singles: Melissa, Oregano, Plectranthus Oregano, Thyme, Eucalyptus Blue, Dorado Azul, Sacred Frankincense, Frankincense, Palo

Santo, Ravintsara, Rosemary, Cinnamon, Eucalyptus Radiata, Clove, Mountain Savory, Peppermint, Spearmint, Myrtle, Idaho Balsam Fir

Blends: Exodus II, Thieves, Raven, Melrose, R.C., ImmuPower, Purification, Sacred Mountain, Breathe Again Roll-On

Nutritionals: Inner Defense, ImmuPro, Super C, Super C Chewable, Longevity Softgels, MultiGreens, ICP, ComforTone, Essentialzyme, Essentialzymes-4, NingXia Red

Application and Usage

Inhalation

- Diffuse your choice of oils 1 hour, 2 times daily at night.
- Put 2-3 drops of your chosen oil in your hands and rub them together, cup your hands over your nose, and inhale throughout the day as needed.
- Put 8-10 drops of oil on a cotton ball or tissue and put it in an air vent in your house, vehicle, hotel room, etc.
- If diffusing while sleeping, set your timer for the desired length of time for automatic shut off.

Topical

You may apply single oils or blends neat or diluted, depending on the oil or oils being used. Please see the instructions at the beginning of this chapter for more information on applying oils to the skin.

- Apply 6-10 drops of oil, diluted 50:50, on chest and upper back 1-3 times daily.
- Apply a warm compress with chosen oils on chest and upper back 2 times daily.

Ingestion and Oral

The amount of oil ingested varies with different oils. Whether putting the oils in a capsule or drinking them in a liquid, please refer to the instructions at the beginning of this chapter.

- Take 1 capsule with desired oil 2 times daily.
- Put 2-3 drops of oil in a spoonful of Blue

Agave, Yacon Syrup, maple syrup, coconut oil, milk, etc.

- Put the desired amount of oils in a glass of rice milk, almond milk, goat milk, carrot juice, NingXia Red, or even water and then drink it.

Tuberculosis-Specific Regimen

- Alternate diffusing Raven and R.C. combined with Eucalyptus Globulus as often as possible during the day.

Retention Blend No. 1

- 15 drops Sacred Frankincense or Frankincense
- 5 drops Clove
- 4 drops Myrrh
- 2 drops Oregano

Retention Blend No. 2

- 10 drops Dorado Azul
- 5 drops Eucalyptus Blue
- 5 drops Myrrh
- 2 drops Oregano

  Mix blend with 2 tablespoons of V-6 Vegetable Oil Complex. Using a bulb syringe, insert into rectum and retain overnight. Do this nightly for 7 nights, rest for 4 nights, and then repeat.
- Take 2 Inner Defense 3 times daily for 10 days.
- Rub 4-6 drops Thieves on the bottoms of the feet nightly.
- Massage Melrose (15 drops) up the spine daily. Apply compress on back and chest 2 times daily.
- Receive a Raindrop Technique weekly.
- **For cough:** Mix 10 drops Myrrh and 1 drop Peppermint in water and gargle.

....

Whooping Cough

Whooping cough is a contagious disease affecting the respiratory system, particularly in children. The lungs become infected as the air passages become clogged with thick mucus. Over the course of several days, the condition worsens, resulting in long coughing bouts (up to 1 minute). The continual coughing makes breathing difficult and labored. Watch carefully and seek medical attention if needed.

Whooping cough usually affects children, so always dilute the essential oils in V-6 Vegetable Oil Complex or other cold-pressed vegetable oil before topically applying. Start with low concentrations until response is observed. Diffuse intermittently and observe reaction.

Recommendations

Singles: Rosemary, Lavender, Basil, Wintergreen, Idaho Ponderosa Pine, Thyme, Oregano, Mastrante, Plectranthus Oregano, Melaleuca Alternifolia, Nutmeg, Peppermint, Eucalyptus Blue, Dorado Azul

Blends: Thieves, Melrose, Raven, R.C., Breathe Again Roll-On

Nutritionals: Super C, Super C Chewable, Longevity Softgels, Essentialzyme, Detoxzyme, MultiGreens, ImmuPro, Sulfurzyme, Digest & Cleanse, Inner Defense, Master Formula HIS or HERS

Oral Care: Thieves Spray, Thieves Fresh Essence Plus Mouthwash, Thieves Lozenges (Hard/Soft)

Application and Usage

Inhalation

- Diffuse your choice of oils for 15 minutes, alternating between singles and blends 3-10 times daily as needed.
- Put 2-3 drops of your chosen oil in your hands and rub them together, cup your hands over your nose, and inhale throughout the day as needed.
- Put 8-10 drops of oil on a cotton ball or tissue and put it in an air vent in your house, vehicle, hotel room, etc.
- If diffusing while sleeping, set your timer for the desired length of time for automatic shut off.

- Add a few drops of oil to a bowl of boiling water. Position the face above the bowl and drape a towel over the head to create a vaporizing effect. Repeat 2-4 times daily.

Topical

You may apply single oils or blends neat or diluted, depending on the oil or oils being used. Please see the instructions at the beginning of this chapter for more information on applying oils to the skin.

- Apply 2-4 drops diluted 50:50 on neck and chest as needed.
- Massage 2-4 drops of oil neat on the soles of the feet and on Vita Flex points just before bedtime. Children may especially benefit from this application.
- Place a warm compress with 1-2 drops of chosen oil on the neck, chest, and upper back area 1-3 times daily.

LUPUS
(See also MIXED CONNECTIVE TISSUE DISEASE)

Lupus is an autoimmune disease that has several different varieties:

Lupus vulgaris is characterized by brownish lesions that may form on skin and/or face and become ulcerous and form scars.

Discoid *Lupus erythematosus* is characterized by scaly, red patches on the skin or butterfly-shaped lesions on the face. It is milder than the systemic type.

Systemic *Lupus erythematosus* is more serious—and more common—than discoid lupus. It inflames the connective tissue in any part of the body, including the joints, muscles, skin, blood vessels, membranes surrounding the lungs and heart, and occasionally the kidneys and brain.

Because lupus is an autoimmune disease, it has been successfully treated using MSM, a form of organic sulfur, which can be found in Sulfurzyme.

Recommendations

Singles: Myrrh, Wintergreen, Basil, Eucalyptus Globulus, Thyme, Nutmeg

Blends: Valor, Valor Roll-On, PanAway, R.C., Breathe Again Roll-On, EndoFlex

Nutritionals: Thyromin, Sulfurzyme, Essentialzyme, Essentialzymes-4, MultiGreens, Master HIS or HERS

Lupus Blend

- 10 drops Lavender
- 4 drops Eucalyptus Globulus
- 3 drops Myrrh
- 3 drops Nutmeg

Application and Usage

Inhalation

- Diffuse your choice of oils for ½ hour every 4-6 hours or as desired.
- Put 2-3 drops of your chosen oil in your hands and rub them together, cup your hands over your nose, and inhale throughout the day as needed.
- Put 8-10 drops of oil on a cotton ball or tissue and put it in an air vent in your house, vehicle, hotel room, etc.
- If diffusing while sleeping, set your timer for the desired length of time for automatic shut off.

Topical

You may apply single oils or blends neat or diluted, depending on the oil or oils being used. Please see the instructions at the beginning of this chapter for more information on applying oils to the skin.

- Apply 1-2 drops neat on temples and back of neck as desired.
- Have Raindrop Technique 1-2 times weekly.
- Have body massage using desired essential oils once every other day.

Ingestion and Oral

The amount of oil ingested varies with different oils. Whether putting the oils in a capsule or drinking them in a liquid, please refer to the instructions at the beginning of this chapter.

- Take 1 capsule with 5 drops of desired oil 2 times daily.
- Put 2-3 drops of oil in a spoonful of Blue Agave, Yacon Syrup, maple syrup, coconut oil, milk, etc.
- Put the desired amount of oils in a glass of rice milk, almond milk, goat milk, carrot juice, NingXia Red, or even water and then drink it.

Lupus Daily Regimen

1. **Bath Salts:** Using lupus blend above, add 30 drops to ½ cup Epsom salt or baking soda and add to hot bath. Soak for 20-30 minutes or until water cools.
2. **Vita Flex:** Massage PanAway on bottoms of the feet and follow 2 hours later with a foot massage using Thieves.
3. **Topical:** Massage 10-15 drops Basil over liver and on feet 2-3 times daily.
4. **Sulfurzyme:** Take 1-2 tablespoons of powder or 5 capsules 1-2 times daily.
5. **Essentialzyme:** Take 2-6 tablets 2 times daily.
6. **MultiGreens:** Take 2-4 capsules 2 times daily.

LYME DISEASE / ROCKY MOUNTAIN SPOTTED FEVER

Lyme disease is a bacterial infection caused by the bite of an infected tick. It is caused by the microorganism *Borrelia burgdorferi*. Some researchers believe that "stealth viruses" may also be involved in Lyme disease. While the suggested oils of Eucalyptus Blue and Dorado Azul are antibacterial, all other oils listed are both antibacterial and antiviral, which will fight either type of infection.

Rocky Mountain Spotted Fever is caused by the bacterium *Rickettsia rickettsii* and is also transmitted to humans by the bite of an infected tick.

Typical symptoms are headache, fever, muscle pain, abdominal pain, and vomiting. A rash may develop after a few days. Both illnesses can be severe or even fatal if not treated in the first few days of symptoms. Seek medical attention as soon as possible after being bitten by a tick.

Recommendations

Singles: Melissa, Oregano, Plectranthus Oregano, Myrrh, Eucalyptus Blue, Dorado Azul, Thyme, Clove

Blends: PanAway, Melrose, Thieves, Exodus II

Nutritionals: Inner Defense, Power Meal, Essentialzymes-4, Detoxzyme

Application and Usage

Inhalation

- Diffuse your choice of oils for ½ hour every 4-6 hours or as desired.
- Put 2-3 drops of your chosen oil in your hands and rub them together, cup your hands over your nose, and inhale throughout the day as needed.
- Put 8-10 drops of oil on a cotton ball or tissue and put it in an air vent in your house, vehicle, hotel room, etc.
- If diffusing while sleeping, set your timer for the desired length of time for automatic shut off.

Topical

You may apply single oils or blends neat or diluted, depending on the oil or oils being used. Please see the instructions at the beginning of this chapter for more information on applying oils to the skin.

- Apply 1-2 drops neat on temples and back of neck, as desired.
- Massage 2-4 drops of oil neat on the soles of the feet just before bedtime.

Ingestion and Oral

The amount of oil ingested varies with different oils. Whether putting the oils in a capsule or drinking them in a liquid, please refer to the instructions at the beginning of this chapter.

- Take 1 capsule with desired oil 3 times daily.
- Put 2-3 drops of oil in a spoonful of Blue Agave, Yacon Syrup, maple syrup, coconut oil, milk, etc.
- Put the desired amount of oils in a glass of rice milk, almond milk, goat milk, carrot juice, NingXia Red, or even water and then drink it.

LYMPHATIC SYSTEM

Essential oils have long been known to aid in stimulating and detoxifying the lymphatic system, which filters lymph, fights infection, recycles plasma proteins, and drains fluid back into the circulatory system from the tissues in order to prevent dehydration. It plays a crucial role in maintaining good health.

Recommendations

Singles: Myrtle, Grapefruit, Lemongrass, Tangerine, Orange, Rosemary, Cypress, Hyssop, Myrrh

Blends: DiGize, Aroma Life, En-R-Gee, Citrus Fresh

Nutritionals: ImmuPro, Super C, Super C Chewable, Longevity Softgels, MultiGreens, Digest & Cleanse, Life 5

Body Care Massage Oils and Creams: Cel-Lite Magic Massage Oil, Regenolone Moisturizing Cream

Lymphatic System Blend

- 3 drops Cypress
- 2 drops Grapefruit
- 1 drop Orange

Application and Usage

Inhalation

- Diffuse your choice of oils for ½ hour every 4-6 hours or as desired.
- Put 2-3 drops of your chosen oil in your hands and rub them together, cup your hands

over your nose, and inhale throughout the day as needed.

- Put 8-10 drops of oil on a cotton ball or tissue and put it in an air vent in your house, vehicle, hotel room, etc.
- If diffusing while sleeping, set your timer for the desired length of time for automatic shut off.

Topical

You may apply single oils or blends neat or diluted, depending on the oil or oils being used. Please see the instructions at the beginning of this chapter for more information on applying oils to the skin.

- Apply 2-4 drops of lymphatic system blend above or other recommended oils diluted 50:50 on sore lymph glands and under arms 2-3 times daily.
- Have Raindrop Technique weekly or as needed.
- Place a warm compress with 1-2 drops of chosen oil over affected areas 1-2 times daily.
- Massage lymphatic system blend above over lymph gland areas and then apply Cel-Lite Magic Massage Oil and Grapefruit or Cypress oil that help detoxify chemicals stored in body fat.

Ingestion and Oral

The amount of oil ingested varies with different oils. Whether putting the oils in a capsule or drinking them in a liquid, please refer to the instructions at the beginning of this chapter.

- Take 1 capsule with 5 drops of Lymphatic System Blend 2 times daily.
- Put 2-3 drops of oil in a spoonful of Blue Agave, Yacon Syrup, maple syrup, coconut oil, milk, etc.
- Put the desired amount of oils in a glass of rice milk, almond milk, goat milk, carrot juice, NingXia Red, or even water and then drink it.

MCT (MIXED CONNECTIVE TISSUE DISEASE)
(See also LUPUS)

MCT is an autoimmune disease similar to lupus in which the connective tissue in the body becomes inflamed and painful. This condition is usually due to poor assimilation of protein and mineral deficiencies.

Recommendations

Singles: Rosemary, Nutmeg, Clove, Basil, Marjoram, Peppermint, Wintergreen

Blends: Relieve It, Valor, Valor Roll-On, ImmuPower

Nutritionals: Sulfurzyme, Essentialzyme, Detoxzyme, JuvaPower, ICP, MultiGreens, MegaCal, OmegaGize[3]

MCT Blend for Aches and Discomfort

- 10 drops Basil
- 8 drops Wintergreen
- 6 drops Cypress
- 3 drops Peppermint

Application and Usage
Inhalation

- Diffuse your choice of oils for ½ hour every 4-6 hours or as desired.
- Put 2-3 drops of your chosen oil in your hands and rub them together, cup your hands over your nose, and inhale throughout the day as needed.
- Put 8-10 drops of oil on a cotton ball or tissue and put it in an air vent in your house, vehicle, hotel room, etc.
- If diffusing while sleeping, set your timer for the desired length of time for automatic shut off.

Topical

You may apply single oils or blends neat or diluted, depending on the oil or oils being used. Please see the instructions at the beginning of this chapter for more information on applying oils to the skin.

- Massage 4-8 drops diluted 50:50 on affected locations 2-3 times daily.
- Apply 1-3 drops on the Vita Flex points of the feet.
- Have Raindrop Technique weekly or as needed.

MCT/Lupus Regimen
- Rub 2-4 drops of ImmuPower over the liver and on the liver Vita Flex Points on the bottom of the right foot 2-3 times daily. This has been reported to help fight lupus, which is similar to MCT.

MALARIA

Malaria is a serious disease contracted from several species of Anopheles mosquitoes. While malaria is largely confined to the continents of Asia and Africa, an increasing number of cases have arisen in North and South America. If not treated, malaria can be fatal. If malaria is suspected, seek medical attention.

Symptoms are fever, chills, and anemia.

The best defense against malaria is to use insect repellents effective against Anopheles mosquitoes. Once a person has contracted the disease, one of the few natural aids to healing it is natural quinine. Essential oils such as Melaleuca Quinquenervia (Niaouli) can help amplify immune response.

Recommendations

Singles: Ocotea, Melaleuca Quinquenervia (Niaouli), Lemon, Thyme, Sacred Frankincense, Frankincense, Rosemary, Sage, Fennel, Geranium, Yarrow

Blends: Thieves, Melrose, ImmuPower

Nutritionals: Inner Defense, Digest & Cleanse, MultiGreens, JuvaPower

Body Care Creams and Sprays: Prenolone Plus Body Cream, Thieves Spray (for protection from nerve damage)

Application and Usage

Inhalation
- Diffuse your choice of oils for ½ hour every 4-6 hours or as desired.
- Put 2-3 drops of your chosen oil in your hands and rub them together, cup your hands over your nose, and inhale throughout the day as needed.
- Put 8-10 drops of oil on a cotton ball or tissue and put it in an air vent in your house, vehicle, hotel room, etc.
- If diffusing while sleeping, set your timer for the desired length of time for automatic shut off.

Topical
You may apply single oils or blends neat or diluted, depending on the oil or oils being used. Please see the instructions at the beginning of this chapter for more information on applying oils to the skin.
- Apply 1-2 drops neat or diluted 50:50 on temples and back of neck, as desired.
- Applying a single drop under the nose is helpful and refreshing.
- Massage 2-4 drops of oil neat on the soles of the feet just before bedtime.

Ingestion and Oral
The amount of oil ingested varies with different oils. Whether putting the oils in a capsule or drinking them in a liquid, please refer to the instructions at the beginning of this chapter.
- Take 1 capsule with desired oil 2 times daily.
- Put 2-3 drops of oil in a spoonful of Blue Agave, Yacon Syrup, maple syrup, coconut oil, milk, etc.
- Put the desired amount of oils in a glass of rice milk, almond milk, goat milk, carrot juice, NingXia Red, or even water and then drink it.
- Mix 3-6 drops Lemon oil in 1 teaspoon Blue Agave or Yacon Syrup and 8 oz. of water, shake, and sip regularly to build the immune system.

MALE HORMONE IMBALANCE

As men age, their DHEA and testosterone levels decline. Conversely, levels of dihydrotestosterone (DHT) increase, contributing to prostate enlargement and hair loss.

Because pregnenolone is the master hormone from which all hormones are created. Men can directly benefit from transdermal pregnenolone creams as a way of jump-starting sagging DHEA levels.

Herbs such as saw palmetto and *Pygeum africanum* can prevent the conversion of testosterone into DHT, thereby reducing prostate enlargement and slowing hair loss.

Recommendations

Singles: Idaho Blue Spruce, Rosemary, Sage, Fennel, Geranium, Clary Sage, Yarrow, Sacred Frankincense, Frankincense

Blends: Mister, SclarEssence

Nutritionals: EndoGize, Prostate Health, Protec

Body Care Creams, Lotions, and Serums: Prenolone Plus Body Cream

Application and Usage

Inhalation

- Diffuse your choice of oils for ½ hour every 4-6 hours or as desired.
- Put 2-3 drops of your chosen oil in your hands and rub them together, cup your hands over your nose, and inhale throughout the day as needed.
- Put 8-10 drops of oil on a cotton ball or tissue and put it in an air vent in your house, vehicle, hotel room, etc.
- If diffusing while sleeping, set your timer for the desired length of time for automatic shut off.

Topical

You may apply single oils or blends neat or diluted, depending on the oil or oils being used. Please see the instructions at the beginning of this chapter for more information on applying oils to the skin.

- Applying a single drop under the nose is helpful and refreshing.
- Dilute 50:50 and apply on location 3-6 times daily.
- Massage 2-4 drops of oil neat on the soles of the feet just before bedtime.

Ingestion and Oral

The amount of oil ingested varies with different oils. Whether putting the oils in a capsule or drinking them in a liquid, please refer to the instructions at the beginning of this chapter.

- Take 1 capsule with desired oil 2 times daily.
- Put 2-3 drops of oil in a spoonful of Blue Agave, Yacon Syrup, maple syrup, coconut oil, milk, etc.
- Put the desired amount of oils in a glass of rice milk, almond milk, goat milk, carrot juice, NingXia Red, or even water and then drink it.
- Take 1 capsule with recommended oils 1 time daily.

MEASLES

Measles, also called rubella, is a highly contagious—but rare—respiratory infection caused by a virus. It causes a total-body skin rash and flu-like symptoms, including a fever, cough, and runny nose.

Since measles is caused by a virus, symptoms typically go away on their own without medical treatment once the virus has run its course. A person with measles should get plenty of fluids and rest and avoid spreading the infection to others.

The first symptoms of the infection are sometimes a hacking cough, runny nose, high fever, and watery, red eyes. Another indicator is Koplik's spots, small red spots with blue-white centers inside the mouth.

The measles rash typically has a red or reddish brown, blotchy appearance and first usually shows up on the forehead, then spreads downward over the face, neck, and body and then down to the feet.

Recommendations

Singles: Lavender, Roman Chamomile, Melaleuca Alternifolia, Clove, Thyme, German Chamomile, Ravintsara

Blends: Thieves, Melrose

Nutritionals: ImmuPro, Super C, Super C Chewable, Longevity Softgels, Life 5, Digest & Cleanse, Inner Defense

Measles Blend

- 10 drops Lavender
- 10 drops German Chamomile
- 5 drops Ravintsara
- 5 drops Melaleuca Alternifolia

Application and Usage

Inhalation

- Diffuse your choice of oils for ½ hour every 4-6 hours or as desired.
- Put 2-3 drops of your chosen oil in your hands and rub them together, cup your hands over your nose, and inhale throughout the day as needed.
- Put 8-10 drops of oil on a cotton ball or tissue and put it in an air vent in your house, vehicle, hotel room, etc.
- If diffusing while sleeping, set your timer for the desired length of time for automatic shut off.

Topical

You may apply single oils or blends neat or diluted, depending on the oil or oils being used. Please see the instructions at the beginning of this chapter for more information on applying oils to the skin.

- Apply 2-3 drops diluted 50:50 on location 3-5 times daily or as needed.
- Mix 6-9 drops of any of the recommended oils in bath salts and soak at least 30 minutes daily.
- Mix 6-9 drops of any of the recommended oils in 8 oz. water, shake well, and use to sponge down the patient 1-2 times daily.

Ingestion and Oral

The amount of oil ingested varies with different oils. Whether putting the oils in a capsule or drinking them in a liquid, please refer to the instructions at the beginning of this chapter.

- Take 1 capsule with 5 drops of desired oil 2-3 times daily.
- Put 2-3 drops of oil in a spoonful of Blue Agave, Yacon Syrup, maple syrup, coconut oil, milk, etc.
- Put the desired amount of oils in a glass of rice milk, almond milk, goat milk, carrot juice, NingXia Red, or even water and then drink it.

MENSTRUAL AND FEMALE HORMONE CONDITIONS (See also OVARIAN AND UTERINE CYSTS)

Natural hormones such as natural progesterone and pregnenolone are the most effective treatment for menstrual difficulties and irregularities. The most effective method of administration is transdermal delivery in a cream. Just 20 mg applied to the skin twice daily is equivalent to 1,000 mg taken internally.

As women reach menopause, progesterone production declines, and a state of estrogen dominance often arises. The most commonly prescribed drugs are conjugated estrogens (from horse urine) or synthetic medroxyprogesterone. The molecules in these synthetic hormones are foreign to the human body and can dramatically increase the risk for ovarian and breast cancer with time.

Endometriosis

This occurs when the uterine lining develops on the outer wall of the uterus, ovaries, fallopian tubes, vagina, intestines, or on the abdominal wall. These fragments cannot escape like the normal uterine lining that is shed during menstruation.

Because of this, fibrous cysts often form around the misplaced uterine tissue. Symptoms can include abdominal or back pain during menstruation or pain that often increases after the period is over. Other symptoms may include heavy periods and pain during intercourse.

Recommendations

Singles: Fennel, Clary Sage, Sage

Blends: Thieves, Melrose, SclarEssence, Lady Sclareol

Nutritionals: ImmuPro, EndoGize, FemiGen, Super C, Super C Chewable, PD 80/20, ICP, Estro, ComforTone, Essentialzyme

Body Care Creams, Lotions, and Serums: Prenolone Plus Body Cream, Progessence Plus

Application and Usage

Inhalation

- Diffuse your choice of oils for ½ hour every 4-6 hours or as desired.
- Put 2-3 drops of your chosen oil in your hands and rub them together, cup your hands over your nose, and inhale throughout the day as needed.
- Put 8-10 drops of oil on a cotton ball or tissue and put it in an air vent in your house, vehicle, hotel room, etc.
- If diffusing while sleeping, set your timer for the desired length of time for automatic shut off.

Topical

You may apply single oils or blends neat or diluted, depending on the oil or oils being used. Please see the instructions at the beginning of this chapter for more information on applying oils to the skin.

- Apply a hot compress containing Melrose on the stomach.
- Massage 2-4 drops of Thieves blend neat on the soles of the feet.

Ingestion and Oral

The amount of oil ingested varies with different oils. Whether putting the oils in a capsule or drinking them in a liquid, please refer to the instructions at the beginning of this chapter.

- Take 1 capsule with desired oil 2 times daily.
- Put 2-3 drops of oil in a spoonful of Blue Agave, Yacon Syrup, maple syrup, coconut oil, milk, etc.
- Put the desired amount of oils in a glass of rice milk, almond milk, goat milk, carrot juice, NingXia Red, or even water and then drink it.
- Colon and liver cleanse: ICP, ComforTone, Detoxzyme, Essentialzyme, JuvaPower

Excessive Bleeding

The most common causes of heavy menstrual bleeding are hormonal imbalances, uterine fibroids or polyps, lack of ovulation, use of an intrauterine device, miscarriage, use of anticoagulants, or endometriosis.

Recommendations

Singles: Helichrysum, Cistus

Blends: PanAway, Deep Relief Roll-On, Relieve It

Nutritionals: OmegaGize³, JuvaTone, Rehemogen

Body Care Creams, Lotions, and Serums: Progessence Plus, Prenolone Plus Body Cream

Excessive Bleeding Blend

- 10 drops Cypress
- 5 drops Helichrysum
- 5 drops Cistus

Application and Usage
Inhalation
- Diffuse your choice of oils for ½ hour every 4-6 hours or as desired.
- Put 2-3 drops of your chosen oil in your hands and rub them together, cup your hands over your nose, and inhale throughout the day as needed.
- Put 8-10 drops of oil on a cotton ball or tissue and put it in an air vent in your house, vehicle, hotel room, etc.
- If diffusing while sleeping, set your timer for the desired length of time for automatic shut off.

Topical
You may apply single oils or blends neat or diluted, depending on the oil or oils being used. Please see the instructions at the beginning of this chapter for more information on applying oils to the skin.
- Apply 4-6 drops diluted 50:50 to the forehead, crown of the head, soles of the feet, lower abdomen, and lower back 1-3 times daily.
- Place a warm compress with 1-2 drops of chosen oil on lower back and abdomen.

Ingestion and Oral
The amount of oil ingested varies with different oils. Whether putting the oils in a capsule or drinking them in a liquid, please refer to the instructions at the beginning of this chapter.
- Take 1 capsule with desired oil 2 times daily.
- Put 2-3 drops of oil in a spoonful of Blue Agave, Yacon Syrup, maple syrup, coconut oil, milk, etc.
- Put the desired amount of oils in a glass of rice milk, almond milk, goat milk, carrot juice, NingXia Red, or even water and then drink it.
- Drink 1/10 teaspoon cayenne in 8 oz. warm water to help regulate bleeding during periods.

Hormonal Edema (Cyclic)
This type of edema usually fluctuates with the female menstrual cycle. A good progesterone hormone cream might be the way to begin; however, before starting any hormone therapy, you should see your doctor or health-care professional and ask for a hormone blood panel to evaluate your needs.

Recommendations
Singles: Clary Sage, Sage, Geranium, Tangerine
Blends: SclarEssence, Lady Sclareol, Dragon Time, EndoFlex
Nutritionals: Thyromin, PD 80/20, Ultra Young Plus, FemiGen, EndoGize
Body Care Creams, Lotions, and Serums: Progessence Plus, Prenolone Plus Body Cream

Hysterectomy
A hysterectomy is a surgical removal of all or part of a woman's uterus.

Recommendations
Singles: Sage, Clary Sage
Blends: Dragon Time, Lady Sclareol, SclarEssence
Nutritionals: PD 80/20, EndoGize, FemiGen
Body Care Creams, Lotions, and Serums: Progessence Plus, Prenolone Plus Body Cream

Application and Usage
Inhalation
- Diffuse your choice of oils for ½ hour every 4-6 hours or as desired.
- Put 2-3 drops of your chosen oil in your hands and rub them together, cup your hands over your nose, and inhale throughout the day as needed.
- Put 8-10 drops of oil on a cotton ball or tissue and put it in an air vent in your house, vehicle, hotel room, etc.
- If diffusing while sleeping, set your timer for the desired length of time for automatic shut off.

Topical

You may apply single oils or blends neat or diluted, depending on the oil or oils being used. Please see the instructions at the beginning of this chapter for more information on applying oils to the skin.

- Massage 2-4 drops of oil neat on the soles of the feet just before bedtime.
- Place a warm compress with 1-2 drops of chosen oil over the lower back and abdomen.

....

Irregular Periods

Menstrual cycles that vary more than a few days in length from month to month are considered to be irregular. All women have variations occasionally, but true irregularity persists over several months.

Recommendations

Singles: Peppermint, Clary Sage, Sage, Roman Chamomile, Fennel, Jasmine

Blends: EndoFlex, SclarEssence, Inner Child, Peace & Calming

Body Care Creams, Lotions, and Serums: Progessence Plus, Prenolone Plus Body Cream

Period Regulator Blend No. 1
- 16 drops Clary Sage
- 11 drops Sage
- 9 drops Canadian Fleabane (Conyza)
- 5 drops Peppermint
- 5 drops Jasmine

Period Regulator Blend No. 2
- 10 drops Roman Chamomile
- 10 drops Fennel

Application and Usage
Inhalation
- Diffuse your choice of oils for ½ hour every 4-6 hours or as desired.
- Put 2-3 drops of your chosen oil in your hands and rub them together, cup your hands over your nose, and inhale throughout the day as needed.

- Put 8-10 drops of oil on a cotton ball or tissue and put it in an air vent in your house, vehicle, hotel room, etc.
- If diffusing while sleeping, set your timer for the desired length of time for automatic shut off.

Topical

You may apply single oils or blends neat or diluted, depending on the oil or oils being used. Please see the instructions at the beginning of this chapter for more information on applying oils to the skin.

- Apply 4-6 drops diluted 50:50 to forehead, crown of the head, soles of the feet, lower abdomen, and lower back 1-3 times daily.
- Massage 3-6 drops on the reproductive Vita Flex points of the feet 2-3 times daily.
- Place a warm compress on the lower back and lower abdomen daily.

....

Menopause

As women age, their levels of progesterone decline and contribute to osteoporosis, increased risk of breast and uterine cancers, mood swings, depression, and many other conditions. Estrogen levels can also decline and increase women's risk of heart disease.

Between the ages of 45 and 55, these hormones decline to a point where menstruation ceases. Replacing these declining levels using topically applied progesterone or pregnenolone creams may be the most effective way to replace and boost declining hormone levels.

Pregnenolone may be especially effective as it is the precursor hormone from which the body creates both progesterone and estrogens.

Recommendations

Singles: Geranium, Clary Sage, Sage

Blends: Dragon Time, Lady Sclareol, Transformation, SclarEssence

Nutritionals: PD 80/20, EndoGize

Body Care Creams, Lotions, and Serums:
Progessence Plus, Prenolone Plus Body
Cream

Application and Usage
Inhalation
- Diffuse your choice of oils for ½ hour every
4-6 hours or as desired.
- Put 2-3 drops of your chosen oil in your
hands and rub them together, cup your hands
over your nose, and inhale throughout the
day as needed.
- Put 8-10 drops of oil on a cotton ball or tissue and put it in an air vent in your house,
vehicle, hotel room, etc.
- If diffusing while sleeping, set your timer for
the desired length of time for automatic shut
off.

Topical
You may apply single oils or blends neat or
diluted, depending on the oil or oils being used.
Please see the instructions at the beginning of
this chapter for more information on applying
oils to the skin.
- Apply 4-6 drops diluted 50:50 to forehead,
crown of the head, soles of the feet, lower
abdomen, and lower back 1-3 times daily.
- Massage 3-6 drops on the reproductive Vita
Flex points of the feet.
- Place a warm compress on the lower back and
lower abdomen daily.

....

Menstrual Cramps

Menstrual cramps (dysmenorrhea) are throb-
bing, dull, or cramping pains in the lower abdomen that many women experience just before
and during their menstrual periods. The pain
may be just annoying, or it may be severe enough
to interfere with daily activities. Treating the underlying cause is important to reducing pain.

Recommendations
Singles: Valerian, Lavender, Clary Sage, Basil,
Rosemary, Sage, Roman Chamomile, Cy-
press, Tarragon, Vetiver, Idaho Blue Spruce
Blends: Dragon Time, EndoFlex
Nutritionals: PD 80/20, EndoGize, Deep Re-
lief Roll-On, Relieve It, PanAway, NingXia
Red
Body Care Creams, Lotions, and Serums:
Prenolone Plus Body Cream, Regenolone
Moisturizing Cream
Menstrual Cramp Relief Blend
- 10 drops Dragon Time
- 5 drops Hops (*Humulus lupulus*)

Application and Usage
Inhalation
- Diffuse your choice of oils for ½ hour every
4-6 hours or as desired.
- Put 2-3 drops of your chosen oil in your
hands and rub them together, cup your hands
over your nose, and inhale throughout the
day as needed.
- Put 8-10 drops of oil on a cotton ball or tissue and put it in an air vent in your house,
vehicle, hotel room, etc.
- If diffusing while sleeping, set your timer for
the desired length of time for automatic shut
off.

Topical
You may apply single oils or blends neat or
diluted, depending on the oil or oils being used.
Please see the instructions at the beginning of
this chapter for more information on applying
oils to the skin.
- Place a warm compress over the uterus area
2-3 times weekly.
- Massage 2-4 drops on the reproductive Vita
Flex points of the feet.
- Apply 2-3 drops of the recommended oils
above to the lower back and stomach area
several times daily as needed.

Ingestion and Oral

The amount of oil ingested varies with different oils. Whether putting the oils in a capsule or drinking them in a liquid, please refer to the instructions at the beginning of this chapter.

- Take 1 capsule with desired oil 2 times daily for 2 weeks prior to menses.
- Put 2-3 drops of oil in a spoonful of Blue Agave, Yacon Syrup, maple syrup, coconut oil, milk, etc.
- Put the desired amount of oils in a glass of rice milk, almond milk, goat milk, carrot juice, NingXia Red, or even water and then drink it.
- If migraine headaches accompany periods, a colon and liver cleanse may reduce symptoms.

....

Premenstrual Syndrome (PMS)

PMS is one of the most common hormone-related conditions in otherwise healthy women.

Women can experience a wide range of symptoms for 10 to 14 days before menstruation and even 2 to 3 days into menstruation. These symptoms include mood swings, fatigue, headaches, breast tenderness, abdominal bloating, anxiety, depression, confusion, memory loss, sugar cravings, cramps, low back pain, irritability, weight gain, acne, and oily skin and hair.

Causes are hormonal, nutritional, and psychological. The stress of the Western culture can also be a cause.

Recommendations

Singles: Rose, Clary Sage, Idaho Blue Spruce, Sage, Anise, Fennel, Ylang Ylang, Amazonian Ylang Ylang, Neroli, Bergamot

Blends: SclarEssence, Dragon Time, Mister, EndoFlex, Acceptance, Aroma Siez, Lady Sclareol, Transformation

Nutritionals: MultiGreens, Super B, Sulfurzyme, Mineral Essence, ImmuPro, PD 80/20, Thyromin, EndoGize

Body Care Creams, Lotions, and Serums: Prenolone Plus Body Cream, Progessence Plus

Application and Usage
Inhalation

- Diffuse your choice of oils for ½ hour every 4-6 hours or as desired.
- Put 2-3 drops of your chosen oil in your hands and rub them together, cup your hands over your nose, and inhale throughout the day as needed.
- Put 8-10 drops of oil on a cotton ball or tissue and put it in an air vent in your house, vehicle, hotel room, etc.
- If diffusing while sleeping, set your timer for the desired length of time for automatic shut off.

Topical

You may apply single oils or blends neat or diluted, depending on the oil or oils being used. Please see the instructions at the beginning of this chapter for more information on applying oils to the skin.

- Apply 4-6 drops diluted 50:50 to forehead, crown of the head, soles of the feet, lower abdomen, and lower back 1-3 times daily.
- Massage 2-4 drops on reproductive Vita Flex points of the feet.
- Place a warm compress on the lower back and lower abdomen daily.

Ingestion and Oral

The amount of oil ingested varies with different oils. Whether putting the oils in a capsule or drinking them in a liquid, please refer to the instructions at the beginning of this chapter.

- Take 1 capsule with desired oil 2 times daily.
- Put 2-3 drops of oil in a spoonful of Blue Agave, Yacon Syrup, maple syrup, coconut oil, milk, etc.
- Put the desired amount of oils in a glass of rice milk, almond milk, goat milk, carrot

juice, NingXia Red, or even water and then drink it.

- Place 1 drop of EndoFlex on the tongue and then hold the tongue on the roof of the mouth 2-4 times daily.

MUCUS (EXCESS)

Many oils are natural expectorants, helping tissues discharge mucus, soft and hard plaque, and toxins.

Recommendations

Singles: Lavender, Lemon, Cypress, Peppermint, Melaleuca Alternifolia, Pine, Thyme, Eucalyptus Globulus, Rosemary

Blends: DiGize, Raven, 3 Wise Men, Purification, R.C., Breathe Again Roll-On

Nutritionals: Allerzyme, Detoxzyme, Essentialzyme, Essentialzymes-4, ImmuPro, Inner Defense, Life 5

Expectorant Blend

- 3 drops Lemon
- 3 drops Eucalyptus Globulus
- 2 drops Pine

Application and Usage

Inhalation

Note: Some studies conclude that the expectorant effect of essential oils is obtained faster and stronger through inhalation than through ingestion.

- Diffuse your choice of oils for ½ hour every 4-6 hours or as desired.
- Put 2-3 drops of your chosen oil in your hands and rub them together, cup your hands over your nose, and inhale throughout the day as needed.
- Put 8-10 drops of oil on a cotton ball or tissue and put it in an air vent in your house, vehicle, hotel room, etc.
- If diffusing while sleeping, set your timer for the desired length of time for automatic shut off.

Topical

You may apply single oils or blends neat or diluted, depending on the oil or oils being used. Please see the instructions at the beginning of this chapter for more information on applying oils to the skin.

- Apply 2-4 drops, diluted 50:50, on the T4 and T5 thoracic vertebrae at the neck to the shoulder intersection 3-5 times daily.
- Massage recommended oils on Vita Flex points of the feet 2-4 times daily.

Ingestion and Oral

The amount of oil ingested varies with different oils. Whether putting the oils in a capsule or drinking them in a liquid, please refer to the instructions at the beginning of this chapter.

- Take 1 capsule with desired oil 2 times daily.
- Put 2-3 drops of oil in a spoonful of Blue Agave, Yacon Syrup, maple syrup, coconut oil, milk, etc.
- Put the desired amount of oils in a glass of rice milk, almond milk, goat milk, carrot juice, NingXia Red, or even water and then drink it.

MUMPS (INFECTIOUS PAROTITIS)

Mumps is an acute, contagious, viral disease marked by painful swelling and inflammation of the salivary glands. The causative agent is a paramyxovirus that is spread by direct contact, airborne droplets, and urine.

Recommendations

Singles: Dorado Azul, Thyme, Melaleuca Alternifolia, Ravintsara, Melissa, Myrrh, Blue Cypress, Wintergreen

Blends: R.C., Raven, Breathe Again Roll-On, Thieves, Deep Relief Roll-On, JuvaCleanse

Nutritionals: ImmuPro, Super C, Super C Chewable, Exodus II, Inner Defense, Essentialzyme, Detoxzyme, JuvaPower, Sulfurzyme, Power Meal

Application and Usage
Inhalation
- Diffuse your choice of oils for ½ hour every 4-6 hours or as desired.
- Put 2-3 drops of your chosen oil in your hands and rub them together, cup your hands over your nose, and inhale throughout the day as needed.
- Put 8-10 drops of oil on a cotton ball or tissue and put it in an air vent in your house, vehicle, hotel room, etc.
- If diffusing while sleeping, set your timer for the desired length of time for automatic shut off.

Topical
You may apply single oils or blends neat or diluted, depending on the oil or oils being used. Please see the instructions at the beginning of this chapter for more information on applying oils to the skin.
- Apply 2-4 drops diluted 50:50 behind the ears 4 times daily.
- Receive a Raindrop Technique 1-2 times weekly.
- Place a warm compress 1-3 times daily around the throat and jaw.

Ingestion and Oral
The amount of oil ingested varies with different oils. Whether putting the oils in a capsule or drinking them in a liquid, please refer to the instructions at the beginning of this chapter.
- Take 1 capsule with desired oil 2 times daily.
- Put 2-3 drops of oil in a spoonful of Blue Agave, Yacon Syrup, maple syrup, coconut oil, milk, etc.
- Put the desired amount of oils in a glass of rice milk, almond milk, goat milk, carrot juice, NingXia Red, or even water and then drink it.

MUSCLES
The body has more than 600 muscles that are grouped into three categories: smooth, cardiac, and skeletal and are all made of a type of elastic tissue.

....

Bruised Muscles
(See also BRUISING)
A bruise is a skin discoloration and occurs when small blood vessels break and leak their contents into the tissue beneath the skin. The main symptoms of a bruise are pain, skin discoloration, and swelling.

Recommendations
Singles: Helichrysum, Copaiba, German Chamomile, Wintergreen, Peppermint, Geranium, Lavender

Blends: Aroma Siez, PanAway, Peace & Calming, Deep Relief Roll-On, Relieve It

Nutritionals: MegaCal, Mineral Essence, NingXia Red, Sulfurzyme, Balance Complete, Power Meal, BLM, Super B

Body Massage Oils: Ortho Ease Massage Oil, Ortho Sport Massage Oil, Relaxation Massage Oil

Application and Usage
Topical
You may apply single oils or blends neat or diluted, depending on the oil or oils being used. Please see the instructions at the beginning of this chapter for more information on applying oils to the skin.
- Apply 2-4 drops diluted 50:50 to bruised area 3 times daily.
- Sequence of application for bruising:
- When a bruise displays black and blue discoloration and pain, start with Helichrysum, Geranium, or Wintergreen.
- When the pain and inflammation decrease, use Cypress, then Basil, and then Aroma Siez to help the muscle relax.

- Follow with Peppermint to stimulate nerve response and reduce inflammation.
- Finish with cold packs.

....

Inflammation Due to Infection

Inflammation is the first response of the immune system to irritation or infection and is characterized by swelling, heat, redness, pain, and dysfunction of the organs involved. Treatment depends on the type of infection.

Recommendations

Singles: Ravintsara, Thyme, Myrrh, Hyssop, Blue Cypress

Nutritionals: Longevity Softgels, Immu-Pro, Detoxzyme, Essentialzyme, Digest & Cleanse, BLM

Application and Usage
Topical

You may apply single oils or blends neat or diluted, depending on the oil or oils being used. Please see the instructions at the beginning of this chapter for more information on applying oils to the skin.

- Massage 2-4 drops diluted 50:50 on inflamed muscle 3 times daily.
- Place a cold compress on location up to 1-3 times daily.

....

Inflammation Due to Injury

Tissue damage is usually accompanied by inflammation. Reduce inflammation by massaging with anti-inflammatory oils to minimize further tissue damage and speed healing.

Recommendations

Singles: Wintergreen, German Chamomile, Nutmeg, Palo Santo, Peppermint, Frereana Frankincense, Lavender, Idaho Ponderosa Pine, Myrrh, Marjoram, Clove, Thyme, Copaiba, Vetiver

Blends: PanAway, Aroma Siez, Deep Relief Roll-On

Tired and Fatigued Muscles

Tired muscles may be lacking in minerals such as calcium and magnesium. Mega Cal and Mineral Essence are excellent sources of both trace and macro minerals and are good for all muscle conditions. Enzymes including Essentialzyme, Essentialzymes-4, and Allerzyme all help with the needed enzymatic conversion of minerals for absorption.

Nutritionals: Mineral Essence, MegaCal, Sulfurzyme, Detoxzyme, Allerzyme, Multi-Greens, Life 5, BLM

Muscle Injury Blend
- 10 drops German Chamomile
- 8 drops Lavender
- 6 drops Marjoram
- 3 drops Yarrow
- 2 drops Peppermint

Application and Usage
Topical

You may apply single oils or blends neat or diluted, depending on the oil or oils being used. Please see the instructions at the beginning of this chapter for more information on applying oils to the skin.

- Massage 2-4 drops diluted 50:50 on inflamed muscle 3 times daily.

....

Muscle Spasms, Cramps, and Charley Horses

Magnesium and calcium deficiency may contribute to muscle cramps.

Recommendations

Singles: Idaho Blue Spruce, Idaho Balsam Fir, Dorado Azul, Wintergreen, Ravintsara, Basil, Rosemary, Fennel, Marjoram, Elemi, Nutmeg, Copaiba, Palo Santo

Blends: PanAway, Relieve It, Aroma Siez, Deep Relief Roll-On

Nutritionals: MegaCal, Mineral Essence, BLM, Sulfurzyme, Life 5

Body Care Massage Oils, Creams: Ortho Sport Massage Oil, Ortho Ease Massage Oil, Relaxation Massage Oil, Regenolone Moisturizing Cream

Application and Usage

Inhalation

- Diffuse your choice of oils for ½ hour every 4-6 hours or as desired.
- Put 2-3 drops of your chosen oil in your hands and rub them together, cup your hands over your nose, and inhale throughout the day as needed.
- Put 8-10 drops of oil on a cotton ball or tissue and put it in an air vent in your house, vehicle, hotel room, etc.
- If diffusing while sleeping, set your timer for the desired length of time for automatic shut off.

Topical

You may apply single oils or blends neat or diluted, depending on the oil or oils being used. Please see the instructions at the beginning of this chapter for more information on applying oils to the skin.

Blend for Muscle Spasms

- 2 drops Ravintsara
- 5 drops Aroma Siez
- 2 drops Black Pepper

Apply 2-4 drops diluted 50:50 on cramped muscle 3 times daily.

Alternate with cold and hot packs when applying the blend for muscle spasms.

....

Muscle Weakness

To overcome temporary muscle weakness, eat a balanced diet, replace lost fluids, engage in only light activities, and slowly start exercising again. However, muscles that slowly become weaker for no apparent reason could indicate a disease or condition in the body.

Make Your Own High-powered Massage Oil

Add either of these recipes to 4 oz. of V-6 Vegetable Oil Complex to create a custom, muscle-toning formula.

Massage Oil Recipe No. 1:
- 10 drops Eucalyptus Blue
- 10 drops Idaho Balsam Fir
- 10 drops Marjoram
- 8 drops Elemi
- 8 drops Vetiver
- 5 drops Helichrysum
- 5 drops Cypress
- 5 drops Peppermint

Massage Oil Recipe No. 2:
- 20 drops Eucalyptus Blue
- 15 drops Marjoram
- 10 drops Juniper
- 10 drops Cypress
- 6 drops Dorado Azul

Recommendations

Singles: Idaho Balsam Fir, Ravintsara, Dorado Azul, Palo Santo, Douglas Fir, Juniper, Nutmeg

Blends: En-R-Gee, The Gift, Sacred Mountain

Nutritionals: BLM, Power Meal, MultiGreens, Balance Complete, Protein Complete, MegaCal, JuvaPower, JuvaSpice (for salads and cooking)

Application and Usage

Topical

You may apply single oils or blends neat or diluted, depending on the oil or oils being used. Please see the instructions at the beginning of this chapter for more information on applying oils to the skin.

- Massage 4-6 drops diluted 50:50 into weak muscles 3 times daily.

Sore Muscles

Whenever you engage in a more strenuous activity than you normally do, you may create microscopic tears in your muscle tissue. The more tears you create, the more soreness you feel later on as the muscles are being repaired. The soreness is a result of both the damage to the muscles and the chemical waste products produced by the muscles when they are being used.

Recommendations

Singles: Rosemary, Wintergreen, Black Pepper, Eucalyptus Blue, Ginger, Spruce, Pine, Marjoram, Peppermint

Blends: PanAway, Deep Relief Roll-On, Peace & Calming, M-Grain, Aroma Siez

Nutritionals: MegaCal, Mineral Essence, Power Meal, Sulfurzyme

Sore Muscle Blend No. 1
- 5 drops Idaho Balsam Fir
- 4 drops Marjoram
- 4 drops Basil
- 2 drops Rosemary

Sore Muscle Blend No. 2
- 5 drops Pine
- 4 drops Rosemary
- 4 drops Ginger
- 1 drop Vetiver

Application and Usage
Topical

You may apply single oils or blends neat or diluted, depending on the oil or oils being used. Please see the instructions at the beginning of this chapter for more information on applying oils to the skin.

- Massage 4-6 drops diluted 50:50 into sore muscles up to 3 times daily.
- Place a warm compress on location up to 1-3 times daily.

MUSCULAR DYSTROPHY

Muscular dystrophy is a group of disorders that involve loss of muscle tissue and muscle weakness that get progressively worse. All or only specific groups of muscles may be affected.

Recommendations

Singles: Palo Santo, Pine, Lavender, Marjoram, Lemongrass, Vetiver, Idaho Balsam Fir

Blends: PanAway, Aroma Siez, Relieve It, Deep Relief Roll-On

Nutritionals: BLM, Sulfurzyme, Essentialzymes-4, Power Meal, Pure Protein, MultiGreens, Mineral Essence, Essentialzyme, Super B

Body Care Massage Oils: Ortho Ease Massage Oil, Ortho Sport Massage Oil

Application and Usage
Topical

You may apply single oils or blends neat or diluted, depending on the oil or oils being used. Please see the instructions at the beginning of this chapter for more information on applying oils to the skin.

- Massage 4-6 drops diluted 50:50 along spine 3 times daily.

NAILS, BRITTLE OR WEAK

Poor or weak nails, often containing ridges, indicate a sulfur, calcium, and/or vitamin A deficiency; disease; infection; trauma; unhealthy diet; use of nail polish and remover; use of detergents; or excessive exposure to water.

Recommendations

Singles: Myrrh, Lemon, Sacred Frankincense, Frankincense, Idaho Balsam Fir

Blends: Citrus Fresh, DiGize, GLF, Super B

Nutritionals: Sulfurzyme, MegaCal, Mineral Essence, Master Formula HIS or HERS, Essentialzyme, NingXia Red

Nail Strengthening Blend
- 4 drops Wheat Germ Oil
- 2 drops Sacred Frankincense or Frankincense
- 2 drops Myrrh
- 2 drops Lemon
- 1 drop Wintergreen

Application and Usage
Topical
You may apply single oils or blends neat or diluted, depending on the oil or oils being used. Please see the instructions at the beginning of this chapter for more information on applying oils to the skin.
- Apply 1-3 drops neat on nails and at base of nails daily for 30 days.
- Apply 1 drop of the blend on each nail 2-3 times daily for 30 days.

NARCOLEPSY
(See also THYROID PROBLEMS)
Narcolepsy is a chronic ailment consisting of uncontrollable, recurrent attacks of drowsiness and sleep during the daytime. Narcolepsy may be aggravated by hypothalamus dysregulation or thyroid hormone deficiency.

Recommendations
Singles: Peppermint, Lemon, Canadian Fleabane (Conyza), Rosemary, Black Pepper
Blends: Clarity, Brain Power, Awaken, Common Sense, Motivation, M-Grain
Nutritionals: Thyromin, MultiGreens, Mineral Essence, Essentialzyme, Sulfurzyme, JuvaPower, Power Meal

Application and Usage
Inhalation
- Diffuse your choice of oils for ½ hour every 4-6 hours or as desired.
- Put 2-3 drops of your chosen oil in your hands and rub them together, cup your hands over your nose, and inhale throughout the day as needed.

- Put 8-10 drops of oil on a cotton ball or tissue and put it in an air vent in your house, vehicle, hotel room, etc.
- If diffusing while sleeping, set your timer for the desired length of time for automatic shut off.

Topical
You may apply single oils or blends neat or diluted, depending on the oil or oils being used. Please see the instructions at the beginning of this chapter for more information on applying oils to the skin.
- Apply 1-2 drops diluted 50:50 on temples, behind ears, back of neck, on forehead, and under nostrils as needed.

NAUSEA
Patchouli oil contains compounds that are extremely effective in preventing vomiting due to their ability to reduce the gastrointestinal muscle contractions associated with vomiting.[24] Peppermint has also been found to be effective in many kinds of stomach upset, including nausea.

Recommendations
Singles: Peppermint, Ginger, Nutmeg, Ocotea
Blends: DiGize, JuvaCleanse, GLF
Nutritionals: AlkaLime, Detoxzyme, Essentialzymes-4, Essentialzyme, Digest & Cleanse, MegaCal, Life 5

Application and Usage
Inhalation
- Diffuse your choice of oils for ½ hour every 4-6 hours or as desired.
- Put 2-3 drops of your chosen oil in your hands and rub them together, cup your hands over your nose, and inhale throughout the day as needed.
- Put 8-10 drops of oil on a cotton ball or tissue and put it in an air vent in your house, vehicle, hotel room, etc.

- If diffusing while sleeping, set your timer for the desired length of time for automatic shut off.

Topical

You may apply single oils or blends neat or diluted, depending on the oil or oils being used. Please see the instructions at the beginning of this chapter for more information on applying oils to the skin.

- Massage 1-3 drops diluted 50:50 behind each ear (mastoids) and over navel 2-3 times hourly.
- Place a warm compress with 1-2 drops of chosen oil over the back or the stomach as needed.
- Rub 1-2 drops of oil on the temples and back of neck several times daily.

Ingestion and Oral

The amount of oil ingested varies with different oils. Whether putting the oils in a capsule or drinking them in a liquid, please refer to the instructions at the beginning of this chapter.

- Take 1 capsule with desired oil 2 times daily.
- Place a few drops of oil on the tongue 1-4 times as needed.
- Put 2-3 drops of oil in a spoonful of Blue Agave, Yacon Syrup, maple syrup, coconut oil, milk, etc.
- Put the desired amount of oils in a glass of rice milk, almond milk, goat milk, carrot juice, NingXia Red, or even water and then drink it.

....

Morning Sickness

The medical definition for "morning sickness" is "nausea and vomiting of pregnancy." Sometimes the symptoms are worse in the morning, but they can strike at any time; and for many women, they last all day long. The intensity varies from woman to woman.

Recommendations

Singles: Peppermint, Ginger, Spearmint, Lavender, Lemon

Blends: DiGize, Gentle Baby

Nutritionals: Essentialzymes-4, Essentialzyme, Life 5, Detoxzyme, AlkaLime, Power Meal, MegaCal

Application and Usage

Inhalation

- Diffuse your choice of oils for ½ hour every 4-6 hours or as desired.
- Put 2-3 drops of your chosen oil in your hands and rub them together, cup your hands over your nose, and inhale throughout the day as needed.
- Put 8-10 drops of oil on a cotton ball or tissue and put it in an air vent in your house, vehicle, hotel room, etc.
- If diffusing while sleeping, set your timer for the desired length of time for automatic shut off.

Topical

You may apply single oils or blends neat or diluted, depending on the oil or oils being used. Please see the instructions at the beginning of this chapter for more information on applying oils to the skin.

- Massage 1-3 drops diluted 50:50 behind each ear (mastoids) and over navel 2-3 times hourly.
- Place a warm compress on stomach as needed.

Ingestion and Oral

The amount of oil ingested varies with different oils. Whether putting the oils in a capsule or drinking them in a liquid, please refer to the instructions at the beginning of this chapter.

- Take 1 capsule with desired oil 2 times daily.
- Place a few drops of oil on the tongue 1-4 times as needed.

- Put 2-3 drops of oil in a spoonful of Blue Agave, Yacon Syrup, maple syrup, coconut oil, milk, etc.
- Put the desired amount of oils in a glass of rice milk, almond milk, goat milk, carrot juice, NingXia Red, or even water and then drink it.

....

Motion Sickness

Motion sickness is a bodily response to real or perceived movement. The inner ear senses movement, while your eyes tell you that you are standing still. This confuses the brain and causes dopamine levels to increase, which causes motion sickness. Common symptoms are nausea, vomiting, dizziness, and fatigue.

Recommendations

Singles: Peppermint, Ginger, Patchouli, Spearmint, Lavender, Rose, Sacred Frankincense, Frankincense, Palo Santo

Blends: Valor, Valor Roll-On, Harmony, DiGize, Tranquil Roll-On, Peace & Calming

Nutritionals: Essentialzymes-4, Essentialzyme, Detoxzyme, MegaCal, Mineral Essence, EndoGize

Motion Sickness Preventative Blend

- 2 drops Peppermint
- 2 drops Ginger
- 2 drops Patchouli
- 5 drops V-6 Vegetable Oil Complex

Application and Usage

Inhalation

- Diffuse your choice of oils for ½ hour every 4-6 hours or as desired.
- Put 2-3 drops of your chosen oil in your hands and rub them together, cup your hands over your nose, and inhale throughout the day as needed.
- Put 8-10 drops of oil on a cotton ball or tissue and put it in an air vent in your house, vehicle, hotel room, etc.

- If diffusing while sleeping, set your timer for the desired length of time for automatic shut off.

Topical

You may apply single oils or blends neat or diluted, depending on the oil or oils being used. Please see the instructions at the beginning of this chapter for more information on applying oils to the skin.

- Massage 1-3 drops diluted 50:50 behind each ear (mastoids) and over navel 2-3 times hourly.
- Place a warm compress on stomach as needed.
- Rub 6-10 drops of the blend on chest and stomach 1 hour before traveling.

Ingestion and Oral

The amount of oil ingested varies with different oils. Whether putting the oils in a capsule or drinking them in a liquid, please refer to the instructions at the beginning of this chapter.

- Take 1 capsule with desired oil 2 times daily.
- Place a few drops of oil on the tongue 1-4 times as needed.
- Put 2-3 drops of oil in a spoonful of Blue Agave, Yacon Syrup, maple syrup, coconut oil, milk, etc.
- Put the desired amount of oils in a glass of rice milk, almond milk, goat milk, carrot juice, NingXia Red, or even water and then drink it.

NERVE DISORDERS
(See also NEUROLOGICAL DISEASES)

Nerve disorders usually involve peripheral or surface nerves and include Bell's palsy, carpal tunnel syndrome, neuralgia, neuritis, and neuropathy. In contrast, neurological diseases are usually associated with deep neurological disturbances in the brain. These conditions include ALS (Lou Gehrig's disease), MS, and

Parkinson's disease.

MegaCal and Mineral Essence used with OmegaGize³ help provide calcium, magnesium, and natural lipids necessary to maintain nerve signal transmissions along neurological pathways.

Sulfur deficiency is often present in nerve problems. Sulfur requires calcium and vitamins B and C for the body to metabolize. Super B, Super C, and Sulfurzyme work well together to help repair nerve damage and the myelin sheath.

CAUTION: Never use hot packs for neurological problems. Always use cold packs to reduce pain and inflammation.

....

Bell's Palsy

This is a type of neuritis, marked by paralysis on one side of the face and inability to open or close the eyelid.

Recommendations

Singles: Peppermint, Rosemary, Vetiver, Cypress, Sandalwood, Helichrysum, Pine

Blends: Aroma Siez, RutaVaLa, RutaVaLa Roll-On, Deep Relief Roll-On, PanAway, Relieve It

Nutritionals: MultiGreens, Sulfurzyme, MegaCal, Ultra Young Plus, OmegaGize³

Application and Usage
Inhalation

- Diffuse your choice of oils for ½ hour every 4-6 hours or as desired.
- Put 2-3 drops of your chosen oil in your hands and rub them together, cup your hands over your nose, and inhale throughout the day as needed.
- Put 8-10 drops of oil on a cotton ball or tissue and put it in an air vent in your house, vehicle, hotel room, etc.
- If diffusing while sleeping, set your timer for the desired length of time for automatic shut off.

Topical

You may apply single oils or blends neat or diluted, depending on the oil or oils being used. Please see the instructions at the beginning of this chapter for more information on applying oils to the skin.

Use 1-2 drops neat to massage on the facial nerve in front and behind the ears and on any areas of pain 3-5 times daily until symptoms end.

....

Carpal Tunnel Syndrome

Nerves pass through a tunnel formed by wrist bones (known as carpals) and a tough membrane on the underside of the wrist that binds the bones together. The tunnel is rigid, so if the tissues within it swell, they press and pinch the nerves and create a painful condition known as carpal tunnel syndrome, which is often the result of a combination of factors that increase pressure on the median nerve and tendons in the carpal tunnel, rather than a problem with the nerve itself.

Often the problem is due to a genetic factor in which the carpal tunnel is smaller in some people than in others. Other possible factors are trauma or injury to the wrist that causes swelling, such as a fracture or sprain; overactivity of the pituitary gland; work stress; hypothyroidism; rheumatoid arthritis; repeated use of vibrating hand tools; fluid retention during pregnancy or menopause; mechanical problems in the wrist joint; or the development of a cyst or tumor in the canal. Sometimes other causes or no causes can be identified.

Repeated motions can result in repetitive motion disorders such as tendonitis or bursitis, but there is little clinical data to prove that such repetitive or forceful movements of the hand and wrist during leisure activities or work can cause carpal tunnel syndrome.

A similar, but less common condition can occur in the ankle (tarsal tunnel syndrome) or elbow.

Recommendations

Singles: Wintergreen, Marjoram, Peppermint, Vetiver, Basil, Cypress, Lemongrass, Myrrh

Blends: PanAway, Relieve It, Aroma Siez, Deep Relief Roll-On

Nutritionals: Sulfurzyme, MegaCal, Mineral Essence, Ultra Young Plus, PD 80/20, BLM

Creams and Massage Oils: Regenolone Moisturizing Cream, Ortho Ease Massage Oil, Ortho Sport Massage Oil

Carpal Tunnel Blend

- 5 drops Wintergreen
- 3 drops Cypress
- 3 drops Myrrh
- 2 drops Marjoram
- 1 drop Peppermint

Application and Usage
Topical

You may apply single oils or blends neat or diluted, depending on the oil or oils being used. Please see the instructions at the beginning of this chapter for more information on applying oils to the skin.

- Apply 2-4 drops neat or diluted 50:50 to affected area 3-5 times daily, as needed.
- Place a cold compress on location 2-3 times daily.

....

Neuralgia

Neuralgia is pain from a damaged nerve. It can occur in the face, spine, or elsewhere. This recurring pain can be traced along a nerve pathway. Carpal tunnel syndrome is a specific type of neuralgia. The primary symptom is temporary sharp pain in the peripheral nerve(s).

Recommendations

Singles: Wintergreen, Peppermint, Marjoram, Helichrysum, Nutmeg, Melaleuca Alternifolia, Roman Chamomile, Rosemary

Blends: RutaVaLa, RutaVaLa Roll-On, Relieve It, Peace & Calming, Deep Relief Roll-On,

PanAway

Nutritionals: PD 80/20, BLM, Sulfurzyme, Super B, Super C, Super C Chewable, OmegaGize[3]

Creams and Massage Oils: Regenolone Moisturizing Cream, Prenolone Plus Body Cream, Ortho Ease Massage Oil, Ortho Sport Massage Oil

Application and Usage
Topical

You may apply single oils or blends neat or diluted, depending on the oil or oils being used. Please see the instructions at the beginning of this chapter for more information on applying oils to the skin.

- Apply 2-4 oil drops neat or diluted 50:50 to affected area 3-5 times daily, as needed.
- Place a cold compress on location 2-3 times daily.

....

Neuritis

Neuritis is a painful inflammation of the peripheral nerves. It is usually caused by prolonged exposure to cold temperature, heavy-metal poisoning, diabetes, vitamin deficiencies (beriberi and pellagra), and infectious diseases such as typhoid fever and malaria.

Symptoms may include pain, burning, numbness, tingling, muscle weakness, or paralysis.

Recommendations

Singles: Lavender, Nutmeg, Copaiba, Juniper, Vetiver, Valerian, Thyme, Yarrow, Clove

Blends: Valor, Valor Roll-On, Aroma Siez, Deep Relief Roll-On, RutaVaLa, RutaVaLa Roll-On

Nutritionals: Sulfurzyme, Super B, Super C, Super C Chewable, PD 80/20, OmegaGize[3], Ultra Young Plus

Creams or Lotions: Regenolone Moisturizing Cream, Prenolone Plus Body Cream

Application and Usage

Inhalation

- Diffuse your choice of oils for ½ hour every 4-6 hours or as desired.
- Put 2-3 drops of your chosen oil in your hands and rub them together, cup your hands over your nose, and inhale throughout the day as needed.
- Put 8-10 drops of oil on a cotton ball or tissue and put it in an air vent in your house, vehicle, hotel room, etc.
- If diffusing while sleeping, set your timer for the desired length of time for automatic shut off.

Topical

You may apply single oils or blends neat or diluted, depending on the oil or oils being used. Please see the instructions at the beginning of this chapter for more information on applying oils to the skin.

- Apply 2-4 drops neat or diluted 50:50 to affected area 3-5 times daily as required.
- Place a cold compress on location 2-3 times daily.

....

Neuropathy

Neuropathy refers to actual damage to the peripheral nerves, usually from an autoimmune condition.

Damage to these peripheral nerves (other than spinal or those in the brain) generally starts as tingling in hands and feet and slowly spreads along limbs to the trunk.

Numbness, sensitive skin, neuralgic pain, and weakening of muscle power can all develop in varying degrees. Most common causes include complications from diabetes (diabetic neuropathy), alcoholism, vitamin B12 deficiency, tumors, too many painkillers, exposure to and absorption of chemicals, metals, pesticides, etc.

B vitamins and minerals such as magnesium, calcium, potassium, and organic sulfur are important in repairing nerve damage and quenching pain from inflamed nerves.

Canadian Fleabane (Conyza) may boost production of pregnenolone and human growth hormone. Pregnenolone aids in repairing damage to the myelin sheath.[25] Juniper also may help in supporting nerve repair.

If paralysis is a problem, a regeneration of up to 60 percent may be possible. If, however, the nerve damage is too severe, treatment may not help. If the damage starts to reverse, there will be pain. Apply a few drops of PanAway neat on location.

Symptoms include tingling or numbness, gangrene.

Recommendations

Singles: Sacred Frankincense, Frankincense, Lavender, Cedarwood, Idaho Blue Spruce, Peppermint, Roman Chamomile, Vetiver, Valerian, Geranium, Yarrow, Goldenrod, Helichrysum, Canadian Fleabane (Conyza), Nutmeg

Blends: Aroma Siez, Peace & Calming, PanAway, RutaVaLa, RutaVaLa Roll-On, Deep Relief Roll-On

Nutritionals: Ultra Young Plus, Super B, OmegaGize³, Sulfurzyme, Longevity Softgels, Mineral Essence, MegaCal, Super C, Super C Chewable, MultiGreens, PD 80/20

Body Care Creams: Prenolone Plus Body Cream

Neuropathy Blend No. 1

- 3 drops Sacred Frankincense or Frankincense
- 3 drops Geranium
- 3 drops Lavender

Neuropathy Blend No. 2

- 3 drops Geranium
- 3 drops Canadian Fleabane (Conyza)
- 3 drops Cedarwood
- 2 drops Peppermint

Application and Usage
Inhalation

- Diffuse or inhale Peace & Calming 2-4 times daily.
- Put 2-3 drops of your chosen oil in your hands and rub them together, cup your hands over your nose, and inhale throughout the day as needed.
- Put 8-10 drops of oil on a cotton ball or tissue and put it in an air vent in your house, vehicle, hotel room, etc.
- If diffusing while sleeping, set your timer for the desired length of time for automatic shut off.

Topical

You may apply single oils or blends neat or diluted, depending on the oil or oils being used. Please see the instructions at the beginning of this chapter for more information on applying oils to the skin.

- Apply 2-4 drops neat or diluted 50:50 to affected area 3-5 times daily, as required.
- Place a cold compress on location 2-3 times daily.

NERVOUS SYSTEM, AUTONOMIC

The autonomic nervous system controls involuntary activities such as heartbeat, breathing, digestion, glandular activity, and contraction and dilation of blood vessels.

The autonomic nervous system is composed of two parts that balance and complement each other: the parasympathetic and sympathetic nervous systems.

....

To Stimulate Parasympathetic Nervous System

The parasympathetic nervous system has relaxing effects and is responsible for secreting acetylcholine, which slows the heart and speeds digestion.

Recommendations

Singles: Lavender, Valerian, Patchouli, Marjoram, Ylang Ylang, Amazonian Ylang Ylang, Rose, Vetiver, Idaho Blue Spruce

Blends: Peace & Calming, Harmony, Valor, Valor Roll-On, RutaVaLa, RutaVaLa Roll-On

Nutritionals: NingXia Red, MegaCal, Sulfurzyme, Mineral Essence, Super B, Super C, Super C Chewable

Application and Usage
Inhalation

- Diffuse your choice of oils for ½ hour every 4-6 hours or as desired.
- Put 2-3 drops of your chosen oil in your hands and rub them together, cup your hands over your nose, and inhale throughout the day as needed.
- Put 8-10 drops of oil on a cotton ball or tissue and put it in an air vent in your house, vehicle, hotel room, etc.
- If diffusing while sleeping, set your timer for the desired length of time for automatic shut off.

Topical

You may apply single oils or blends neat or diluted, depending on the oil or oils being used. Please see the instructions at the beginning of this chapter for more information on applying oils to the skin.

- Have Raindrop Technique 2 times a week.

Ingestion and Oral

The amount of oil ingested varies with different oils. Whether putting the oils in a capsule or drinking them in a liquid, please refer to the instructions at the beginning of this chapter.

- Take 1 capsule with desired oil 2 times daily.
- Put 2-3 drops of oil in a spoonful of Blue Agave, Yacon Syrup, maple syrup, coconut oil, milk, etc.
- Put the desired amount of oils in a glass of rice milk, almond milk, goat milk, carrot

juice, NingXia Red, or even water and then drink it.

....

To Stimulate Sympathetic Nervous System

The sympathetic nervous system has stimulatory effects and is responsible for secreting stress hormones like adrenaline and noradrenaline.

Recommendations

Singles: Fennel, Ginger, Eucalyptus Radiata, Peppermint, Rosemary, Black Pepper

Blends: Clarity, Brain Power

Nutritionals: Super B, Super C, Super C Chewable, Sulfurzyme, Mineral Essence, Essentialzymes-4, Essentialzyme, MegaCal

Application and Usage

Inhalation

- Diffuse your choice of oils for ½ hour every 4-6 hours or as desired.
- Put 2-3 drops of your chosen oil in your hands and rub them together, cup your hands over your nose, and inhale throughout the day as needed.
- Put 8-10 drops of oil on a cotton ball or tissue and put it in an air vent in your house, vehicle, hotel room, etc.
- If diffusing while sleeping, set your timer for the desired length of time for automatic shut off.

Topical

You may apply single oils or blends neat or diluted, depending on the oil or oils being used. Please see the instructions at the beginning of this chapter for more information on applying oils to the skin.

- Have Raindrop Technique 2 times a week.

Ingestion and Oral

The amount of oil ingested varies with different oils. Whether putting the oils in a capsule or drinking them in a liquid, please refer to the instructions at the beginning of this chapter.

- Take 1 capsule with desired oil 2 times daily.
- Put 2-3 drops of oil in a spoonful of Blue Agave, Yacon Syrup, maple syrup, coconut oil, milk, etc.
- Put the desired amount of oils in a glass of rice milk, almond milk, goat milk, carrot juice, NingXia Red, or even water and then drink it.

NEUROLOGIC DISEASES (See also NERVE DISORDERS)

Neurologic diseases are disorders of the spinal cord, brain, and nerves throughout your body. Together they control all of the functions of the body. There are more than 600 neurologic diseases.

CAUTION: Never use hot packs for neurological problems. Always use cold packs to reduce pain and inflammation. In other words, reduce the temperature of the damaged site.

....

ALS (Lou Gehrig's Disease)

Lou Gehrig's disease is another name for Amyotrophic Lateral Sclerosis (ALS), a degenerative nerve disorder. ALS affects the nerve fibers in the spinal cord that control voluntary movement.

Muscles require continuous stimulation by their associated nerves to maintain their tone. Removal or deadening of these nerves results in muscular atrophy. The lack of control forces the muscles to spasm, resulting in twitching and cramps. The sensory pathways are unaffected, so feeling is never lost in the afflicted muscles.

Juniper may support nerve function. Frankincense may help clear the emotions of fear and anger, which is common with people who have these neurologic diseases. When these diseases are contracted, people often become suicidal.

Hope, Joy, Gathering, and Forgiveness will help individuals work through the psychological and emotional aspects of the disease.

Sulfur deficiency is often prevalent in neurological diseases. Sulfur requires calcium and vitamin C for the body to metabolize. Super B and Sulfurzyme work well together to help repair nerve damage and the myelin sheath.

Recommendations

Singles: Rosemary, Sandalwood, Sacred Frankincense, Frankincense, Helichrysum, Cypress, Sage, Juniper, Clove, Cardamom

Blends: Hope, Joy, Gathering, Brain Power, Clarity, Forgiveness, Common Sense

Nutritionals: PD 80/20, Sulfurzyme, MultiGreens, MegaCal, Super C, Super C Chewable, Super B, Longevity Softgels, Omega-Gize[3]

Body Care Creams: Prenolone Plus Body Cream

ALS Blend

- 3 drops Rosemary
- 2 drops Clove
- 1 drop Eucalyptus Blue
- 1 drop Ylang Ylang (or Amazonian Ylang Ylang)
- 1 drop Sacred Frankincense or Frankincense

Application and Usage

Inhalation

- Diffuse your choice of oils for ½ hour every 4-6 hours or as desired.
- Put 2-3 drops of your chosen oil in your hands and rub them together, cup your hands over your nose, and inhale throughout the day as needed.
- Put 8-10 drops of oil on a cotton ball or tissue and put it in an air vent in your house, vehicle, hotel room, etc.
- If diffusing while sleeping, set your timer for the desired length of time for automatic shut off.

Topical

You may apply single oils or blends neat or diluted, depending on the oil or oils being used. Please see the instructions at the beginning of this chapter for more information on applying oils to the skin.

- Apply 1-3 drops diluted 50:50 on the brain reflex points on the forehead, temples, and mastoids (just behind ears).
- Use a direct pressure application and massage 6-10 drops diluted 50:50 from the base of the skull, down the neck, and down the spine.
- Place a few drops of oil on a loofah brush and rub along the spine vigorously. (Always use a natural bristle brush, since the oils may dissolve plastic bristles.)
- Receive a Raindrop Technique 3 times monthly.

....

Huntington's Chorea

Huntington's chorea is a degenerative nerve disease that generally becomes manifest in middle age. It is marked by uncontrollable body movements, which are followed—and occasionally preceded—by mental deterioration.

Note: Huntington's chorea should not be confused with Sydenham's chorea, often called St. Vitus Dance, chorea minor, or juvenile chorea that affects children, especially females, usually appearing between the ages of 7 and 14. The jerking symptoms eventually disappear.

Recommendations

Singles: Peppermint, Ocotea, Juniper, Basil, Sandalwood, Sacred Frankincense, Frankincense, Geranium, Palo Santo, Eucalyptus Blue

Blends: Aroma Siez, RutaVaLa, RutaVaLa Roll-On, EndoFlex, Awaken, Christmas Spirit, Citrus Fresh, Tranquil Roll-On

Nutritionals: Sulfurzyme, MultiGreens, Power Meal, Super C, Super C Chewable, Super B, MegaCal, OmegaGize[3], Master Formula HIS or HERS, Balance Complete, Mineral Essence, Essentialzyme, Allerzyme

Nerve Blend
- 5 drops Juniper
- 3 drops Aroma Siez
- 2 drops Peppermint
- 1 drop Basil

Application and Usage

Inhalation
- Diffuse your choice of oils for ½ hour every 4-6 hours or as desired.
- Put 2-3 drops of your chosen oil in your hands and rub them together, cup your hands over your nose, and inhale throughout the day as needed.
- Put 8-10 drops of oil on a cotton ball or tissue and put it in an air vent in your house, vehicle, hotel room, etc.
- If diffusing while sleeping, set your timer for the desired length of time for automatic shut off.

Topical
You may apply single oils or blends neat or diluted, depending on the oil or oils being used. Please see the instructions at the beginning of this chapter for more information on applying oils to the skin.
- Apply 1-3 drops diluted 50:50 on the brain reflex points on the forehead, temples, and mastoids just behind ears.
- Use a direct pressure application and massage 6-10 drops diluted 50:50 from the base of the skull, down the neck, and down the spine.
- Place a few drops of oil on a loofah brush and rub along the spine vigorously. Always use a natural bristle brush, since the oils may dissolve plastic bristles.
- Receive a Raindrop Technique 3 times monthly.

Multiple Sclerosis (MS)

Multiple sclerosis is a progressive, disabling autoimmune disease of the nervous system, brain, and spinal cord in which inflammation occurs in the central nervous system. Eventually, the myelin sheaths protecting the nerves are destroyed, resulting in a slowing or blocking of nerve transmission.

MS is an autoimmune disease in which the body's own immune system attacks the nerves. Some researchers believe that MS is triggered by a virus, while others make a case that it has a strong genetic or environmental component.

Symptoms
- Muscle weakness in extremities
- Deteriorating coordination and balance
- Numbness or prickling sensations
- Poor attention or memory
- Speech impediments
- Incontinence
- Tremors
- Dizziness
- Hearing loss

Recommendations
Singles: Juniper, Geranium, Sacred Frankincense, Frankincense, Rosemary, Basil, Helichrysum, Peppermint, Thyme, Marjoram

Blends: PanAway, Valor, Valor Roll-On, Aroma Siez, RutaVaLa, RutaVaLa Roll-On, Acceptance, Awaken

Nutritionals: OmegaGize[3], Sulfurzyme, Multi-Greens, Power Meal, Essentialzyme, Mineral Essence, MegaCal, Super C, Super C Chewable, Super B, NingXia Red

Body Creams and Serums: Progessence Plus, Regenolone Moisturizing Cream

MS Blend
- 4 drops Geranium
- 4 drops Rosemary
- 2 drops Helichrysum
- 2 drops Juniper

Application and Usage

Inhalation

- Diffuse your choice of oils for ½ hour every 4-6 hours or as desired.
- Put 2-3 drops of your chosen oil in your hands and rub them together, cup your hands over your nose, and inhale throughout the day as needed.
- Put 8-10 drops of oil on a cotton ball or tissue and put it in an air vent in your house, vehicle, hotel room, etc.
- If diffusing while sleeping, set your timer for the desired length of time for automatic shut off.

Topical

You may apply single oils or blends neat or diluted, depending on the oil or oils being used. Please see the instructions at the beginning of this chapter for more information on applying oils to the skin.

- Apply 1-3 drops diluted 50:50 on the brain reflex points on the forehead, temples, and mastoids just behind the ears.
- Apply direct pressure and massage 6-10 drops diluted 50:50 from the base of the skull, down the neck, and down the spine.
- Place a few drops of oil on a loofah brush and rub along the spine vigorously. Always use a natural bristle brush, since the oils may dissolve plastic bristles.
- Receive a Raindrop Technique 3-4 times monthly.

MS Daily Regimen

1. Apply neat 4-6 drops of Helichrysum, Geranium, Juniper, Sandalwood, Rosemary, and Peppermint Raindrop-style along the spine. Lightly massage oils in the direction of the MS paralysis. For example, if it is in the lower part of the spine, massage down; if it is in the upper part of the spine, massage up. Follow the application with 30 minutes of cold packs (change cold packs as needed).
2. Apply 4-6 drops of Valor on the spine. If the MS affects the legs, rub down the spine; if it affects the neck, rub up the spine.
3. Apply 2-3 drops each of Cypress, Sandalwood, and Marjoram to the back of the neck and then cover with 2-3 drops of Aroma Siez. To give additional emotional support to the person with MS symptoms, use Acceptance and Awaken. Be patient. Overcoming MS is a long-term endeavor.

....

Parkinson's Disease

Parkinson's disease is a deterioration of specific nerve centers in the brain that affects more men than women by a ratio of 3:2.

Symptoms

- Tremors, an involuntary shaking of hands, head, or both

- Rigidity, slowed movement, and loss of balance
- Stooped posture

- Continuous rubbing together of thumb and forefinger
- Mask-like face

- Trouble swallowing
- Depression
- Difficulty performing simple tasks

These symptoms may all be seen at different stages of the disease. The tremors are most severe when the affected part of the body is not in use. There is no pain or other sensation, other than a decreased ability to move. Symptoms appear slowly in no particular order and may end before they interfere with normal activities.

Restoring dopamine levels in the brain can reduce symptoms of Parkinson's. Sulfurzyme provides a source of organic sulfur, a vital nutrient for nerve and myelin sheath formation.

Recommendations

Singles: Helichrysum, Lavender, Peppermint, Cedarwood, Myrrh, Basil, Sandalwood, Rosewood

Blends: GLF, Peace & Calming, Valor, Valor Roll-On, Brain Power

Nutritionals: Sulfurzyme, Super B, PD 80/20, BLM, Mineral Essence, Power Meal, JuvaPower, Super C, Super C Chewable, Life 5, OmegaGize[3]

Application and Usage
Inhalation
- Diffuse your choice of oils for ½ hour every 4-6 hours or as desired.
- Put 2-3 drops of your chosen oil in your hands and rub them together, cup your hands over your nose, and inhale throughout the day as needed.
- Put 8-10 drops of oil on a cotton ball or tissue and put it in an air vent in your house, vehicle, hotel room, etc.
- If diffusing while sleeping, set your timer for the desired length of time for automatic shut off.

Topical
You may apply single oils or blends neat or diluted, depending on the oil or oils being used. Please see the instructions at the beginning of this chapter for more information on applying oils to the skin.
- Apply 1-3 drops diluted 50:50 on the brain reflex points on the forehead, temples, and mastoids just behind the ears.
- Use a direct pressure application and massage 6-10 drops diluted 50:50 from the base of the skull, down the neck, and down the spine.
- Place a few drops of oil on a loofah brush and rub along the spine vigorously. Always use a natural bristle brush, since the oils may dissolve plastic bristles.
- Receive a Raindrop Technique 3 times monthly.

CAUTION: Never use hot packs for neurological problems. Always use cold packs to reduce pain and inflammation. In other words, reduce the temperature of the affected area.

....

Restless Legs Syndrome (See also ATTENTION DEFICIT DISORDER)
Restless legs syndrome (Willis-Ekbom disease) is a neurologic disorder characterized by an irresistible urge to move the body to stop odd or uncomfortable sensations. It commonly affects the legs but can also affect the torso, arms, and even phantom limbs.

Recommendations
Singles: Valerian, Lavender, Basil, Marjoram, Cypress, Roman Chamomile

Blends: RutaVaLa, RutaVaLa Roll-On, Aroma Siez, Peace & Calming, Tranquil Roll-On, Stress Away Roll-On, Valor, Valor Roll-On

Nutritionals: ImmuPro, Mineral Essence, MultiGreens, MegaCal, OmegaGize[3], SleepEssence, Thyromin

Application and Usage
Inhalation
- Diffuse your choice of oils for 20 minutes 4 times daily.
- Put 2-3 drops of your chosen oil in your hands and rub them together, cup your hands over your nose, and inhale throughout the day as needed.
- Put 8-10 drops of oil on a cotton ball or tissue and put it in an air vent in your house, vehicle, hotel room, etc.
- If diffusing while sleeping, set your timer for the desired length of time for automatic shut off.

Topical
You may apply single oils or blends neat or diluted, depending on the oil or oils being used. Please see the instructions at the beginning of this chapter for more information on applying oils to the skin.
- Apply 2-4 drops neat as desired.
- Massage 2-4 drops of oil on the Vita Flex points of the feet before retiring.
- Receive a Raindrop Technique 1 time a week.

....

Schizophrenia
This is a neurologic disease that involves identity confusion. Onset is typically between the late teens and early 30's. Abnormal neurological findings may show a broad range of dysfunction, including slow reaction time, poor coordination, abnormalities in eye tracking, and impaired sensory gating.

Typically, schizophrenia involves dysfunction in one or more areas such as interpersonal relations, work, education, or self-care. Some cases are believed to be caused by viral infection.

Recommendations
Singles: Cardamom, Cedarwood, Rosewood, Vetiver, Melissa, Rosemary, Valerian, Peppermint, Sacred Frankincense, Frankincense

Blends: Brain Power, Valor, Valor Roll-On, M-Grain, Clarity, Common Sense

Nutritionals: Mineral Essence, MegaCal, NingXia Red, Super B, Power Meal, JuvaPower, Master HIS or HERS, Ningxia Wolfberries (Dried)

Application and Usage
Inhalation
- Diffuse your choice of oils for ½ hour every 4-6 hours or as desired.
- Put 2-3 drops of your chosen oil in your hands and rub them together, cup your hands over your nose, and inhale throughout the day as needed.
- Put 8-10 drops of oil on a cotton ball or tissue and put it in an air vent in your house, vehicle, hotel room, etc.
- If diffusing while sleeping, set your timer for the desired length of time for automatic shut off.

Topical
You may apply single oils or blends neat or diluted, depending on the oil or oils being used. Please see the instructions at the beginning of this chapter for more information on applying oils to the skin.
- Receive a Raindrop Technique treatment 1 time a week.

NOSE AND SINUS PROBLEMS
Millions of people have chronic sinus troubles, and millions more suffer from rhinitis, a term for stuffy nose. One of the most effective treatments for nasal and sinus problems is a saltwater nose rinse.

....

Dry Nose
Dry nose refers to a lack of moisture in the nasal passage, which can occasionally cause the skin inside the nose to itch, crack, and bleed.

Recommendations

Singles: Myrrh, Lavender, Lemon, Peppermint

Blends: R.C., Raven, Breathe Again Roll-On

Ointments: Boswellia Wrinkle Cream, Rose Ointment

Dry Nose Blend

- 2 drops Lavender
- 1 drop Myrrh

Application and Usage

Inhalation

- Diffuse your choice of oils for ½ hour every 4-6 hours or as desired, especially before retiring.
- Put 2-3 drops of your chosen oil in your hands and rub them together, cup your hands over your nose, and inhale throughout the day as needed.
- Put 8-10 drops of oil on a cotton ball or tissue and put it in an air vent in your house, vehicle, hotel room, etc.
- If diffusing while sleeping, set your timer for the desired length of time for automatic shut off.

Topical

You may apply single oils or blends neat or diluted, depending on the oil or oils being used. Please see the instructions at the beginning of this chapter for more information on applying oils to the skin.

- Apply 1-2 drops diluted 50:50 to the nostril walls with a cotton swab 2 times daily.
- Massage 2-4 drops of oil neat on the soles on the Vita Flex points of the feet just before bedtime. Children love it.

....

Loss of Smell

The senses of smell and taste are strongly connected. Some of the common causes of loss of smell and taste are cigarette smoke, medications like antibiotics and blood pressure medicines, the common cold, pollutants, allergies,

---

Nasal Irrigation Regimen:

Rosemary and Melaleuca Alternifolia oils can be used in a saline solution for very effective nasal irrigation that clears and decongests sinuses. As recommended by Daniel Pénoël, MD, the saline solution is prepared as follows:

- 10 drops Rosemary
- 6 drops Thyme
- 2 drops Cypress
- 8 tablespoons ultra-fine salt

The essential oils are mixed thoroughly in the fine salt and stored in a sealed container. For each nasal irrigation session, 1 teaspoon of this salt mixture is dissolved into 1½ cups distilled water.

This solution is then placed in the tank of an oral irrigator or neti pot to irrigate the nasal cavities, which is done while bending over a sink. This application has brought surprisingly positive results in treating latent sinusitis and other nasal congestion problems.

---

blocked nasal passages, tooth and gum diseases, chemotherapy, Alzheimer's disease, surgery, tumors, Parkinson's disease, polyps, or even a head injury.

Recommendations

Singles: Peppermint, Thyme, Myrtle, Eucalyptus Globulus

Blends: R.C., Raven, Exodus II, Joy, Highest Potential, The Gift, Sensation

Nutritionals: NingXia Red

Application and Usage

Inhalation

- Diffuse your choice of oils for ½ hour every 4-6 hours or as desired.
- Put 2-3 drops of your chosen oil in your hands and rub them together, cup your hands over your nose, and inhale throughout the

day as needed.
- Put 8-10 drops of oil on a cotton ball or tissue and put it in an air vent in your house, vehicle, hotel room, etc.
- If diffusing while sleeping, set your timer for the desired length of time for automatic shut off.

Topical

You may apply single oils or blends neat or diluted, depending on the oil or oils being used. Please see the instructions at the beginning of this chapter for more information on applying oils to the skin.

....

Nosebleeds

Nosebleeds usually are not serious. However, if bleeding does not stop in a short time or is excessive or frequent, consult your doctor.

Recommendations

Singles: Helichrysum, Cistus, Cypress, Dorado Azul, Geranium
Blends: GLF, JuvaCleanse
Nutritionals: Mineral Essence, Sulfurzyme, Master Formula HIS or HERS

Nosebleed Blend
- 3 drops Helichrysum or Geranium
- 2 drops Cistus
- 2 drops Cypress

Application and Usage
Topical

You may apply single oils or blends neat or diluted, depending on the oil or oils being used. Please see the instructions at the beginning of this chapter for more information on applying oils to the skin.
- Apply 2-4 drops neat to the bridge and sides of the nose and back of the neck. Repeat as needed.
- Applying a single drop under the nose is helpful and refreshing.

- Dilute 50:50 and apply on location 3-6 times daily.
- Massage 2-4 drops of oil neat on the soles on the Vita Flex points of the feet just before bedtime. Children love it.

Nosebleed Regimen
- Put 1 drop of Geranium on a tissue paper and wrap the paper around a chip of ice about the size of a thumb nail, push it up under the top lip in the center to the base of the nose. Hold from the outside with lip pressure. This usually will stop bleeding in a very short time.

....

Polyps, Nasal

Nasal polyps are soft, painless, noncancerous growths on the lining of the nasal passages or sinuses. They hang down like grapes or teardrops and result from chronic inflammation due to allergies, asthma, recurring infection, drug sensitivity, or certain immune disorders.

Small polyps may not cause problems, but larger growths or groups of polyps can block the nasal passages, lead to breathing problems, cause frequent infections, or cause a lost sense of smell.

Recommendations

Singles: Citronella, Helichrysum, Sacred Frankincense, Frankincense
Blend: Purification, Citrus Fresh, Melrose

Application and Usage
Topical

You may apply single oils or blends neat or diluted, depending on the oil or oils being used. Please see the instructions at the beginning of this chapter for more information on applying oils to the skin.
- Apply 1-2 drops diluted 50:50 on a cotton swab and carefully apply on the inside nostrils 1-3 times daily.

OBESITY
(See also DEPRESSION)

Hormone treatments using natural progesterone (for women) and testosterone (for men) may be one of the most powerful treatments for obesity. In women, progesterone levels drop dramatically after menopause, and this can result in substantial weight gain, particularly around the hips and thighs. Using transdermal creams or serums to replace declining progesterone can result in a substantial decline in body fat.

Diffusing or directly inhaling essential oils can have an immediate positive impact on moods and appetites. Olfaction is the only sense that can have a direct effect on the limbic region of the brain. Studies at the University of Vienna have shown that some essential oils and their primary constituents can stimulate blood flow and activity in the emotional centers of the brain.[32]

Fragrance influences can penetrate the amygdala in the center of the brain in such a manner that frequent inhalation of pleasing aromas can significantly reduce appetite. Dr. Alan Hirsch, in his landmark studies, showed dramatic weight loss in research subjects using aromas from peppermint oil and vanilla absolute to curb food cravings.[33]

Recommendations

Singles: Peppermint, Roman Chamomile, Nutmeg, Clove, Grapefruit, Fennel, Cinnamon, Lavender, Sacred Frankincense, Frankincense, Vanilla Absolute

Blends: Valor, Valor Roll-On, JuvaCleanse, Slique Essence, Oola Balance, Joy, The Gift, 3 Wise Men, Sacred Mountain, White Angelica, Gathering

Nutritionals: JuvaPower, Thyromin, Detoxzyme, OmegaGize³, Slique Slim Caps, Slique Bar, Slique Gum, Balance Complete, Digest & Cleanse, Chocolessence

Body Creams and Serums: Progessence Plus, Prenolone Plus Body Cream

Application and Usage
Inhalation

- Diffuse your choice of oils for ½ hour every 4-6 hours or as desired.
- Put 2-3 drops of your chosen oil in your hands and rub them together, cup your hands over your nose, and inhale throughout the day as needed.
- Put 8-10 drops of oil on a cotton ball or tissue and put it in an air vent in your house, vehicle, hotel room, etc.
- If diffusing while sleeping, set your timer for the desired length of time for automatic shut off.

Topical

You may apply single oils or blends neat or diluted, depending on the oil or oils being used. Please see the instructions at the beginning of this chapter for more information on applying oils to the skin.

- Applying a single drop under the nose is helpful and refreshing.
- Massage 2-4 drops of oil neat on the soles of the feet just before bedtime. Children love it.

ORAL CARE, TEETH AND GUMS

Poor oral hygiene has not only been linked to bad breath (halitosis) but also to cardiovascular disease. Some of the same bacteria that populate the mouth have now been implicated in arteriosclerosis.

Essential oils make excellent oral antiseptics, analgesics, and anti-inflammatories. Clove essential oil has been used in mainstream dentistry for decades to numb the gums and help prevent infections. Similarly, menthol (found in Peppermint oil), methyl salicylate (found in Wintergreen oil), thymol (found in Thyme essential oil), and eucalyptol (found in Eucalyptus and Rosemary essential oils) are approved OTC drug products for combating gingivitis and periodontal disease.

Bleeding Gums

Bleeding gums can be a sign that you have, or are at risk for, gum disease. However, persistent gum bleeding may be caused by serious medical conditions such as leukemia or bleeding and platelet disorders. Bleeding gums are mainly due to inadequate plaque removal from the teeth at the gum line, which will lead to gingivitis, or inflamed gums.

Recommendations

Singles: Clove, Sacred Frankincense, Frankincense, Helichrysum, Wintergreen, Cinnamon, Mountain Savory, Myrrh

Blends: Thieves, Melrose, PanAway, Relieve It, Slique Essence

Nutritionals: Slique Gum, KidScents Slique Toothpaste, Super C

Blend for Combating Gum Bleeding

- 2 drops Myrrh
- 2 drops Helichrysum
- 1 drop Thieves
- 1 drop Sacred Frankincense or Frankincense

Application and Usage

Topical

You may apply single oils or blends neat or diluted, depending on the oil or oils being used. Please see the instructions at the beginning of this chapter for more information on applying oils to the skin.

- Apply 1-2 drops diluted 50:50 on gums 2-3 times daily.

Ingestion and Oral

The amount of oil ingested varies with different oils. Whether putting the oils in a capsule or drinking them in a liquid, please refer to the instructions at the beginning of this chapter.

- Take 1 capsule with desired oil 2 times daily.
- Put 2-3 drops of oil in a spoonful of Blue Agave, Yacon Syrup, maple syrup, coconut oil, milk, etc.

- Put the desired amount of oils in a glass of rice milk, almond milk, goat milk, carrot juice, NingXia Red, or even water and then drink it.
- Gargle 3-10 times daily with Thieves Fresh Essence Plus Mouthwash or as needed.
- Brush teeth and gums after every meal with Thieves AromaBright Toothpaste.

Dental Visits

Prior to visiting the dentist, rub 1 drop each of Helichrysum, Clove, and PanAway on gums and jaw. Clove may interfere with bonding of crowns, so keep it off the teeth if this procedure is planned.

General Oral Infection:

For general oral infection of any kind, roll a piece of gauze tightly into a string about ¼ inch thick. Put drops of Thieves blend on it; if it feels too "hot," add V-6. Put the string between the teeth and the lip and leave it all night, allowing it to "wick up," or absorb, the infection. Change as often as needed.

Gingivitis and Periodontitis

Periodontal diseases are infections of the gum and bone that hold the teeth in place. Gingivitis affects the upper areas of the gum where it bonds to the visible enamel, while periodontitis is a more internal infection affecting the gum at the root level of the tooth. In advanced stages, these diseases can lead to painful chewing problems and even tooth loss.

Oils such as Peppermint, Wintergreen, Clove, Thyme, and Eucalyptus can kill bacteria and effectively combat a variety of gum infections.

Recommendations

Singles: Clove, Melaleuca Alternifolia, Thyme, Mountain Savory, Wintergreen, Peppermint, Oregano, Plectranthus Oregano, Eucalyptus Globulus

Blends: Thieves, Exodus II, PanAway, Slique Essence

Nutritionals: Super C, Super C Chewable, Longevity Softgels, OmegaGize³, Inner Defense

Oral Care: Thieves AromaBright Toothpaste, KidScents Slique Toothpaste, Thieves Dentarome Plus Toothpaste, Thieves Dentarome Ultra Toothpaste, Thieves Fresh Essence Plus Mouthwash, Thieves Lozenges (Hard/Soft), Thieves Spray, Thieves Dental Floss, Slique Gum

Application and Usage
Ingestion and Oral
The amount of oil ingested varies with different oils. Whether putting the oils in a capsule or drinking them in a liquid, please refer to the instructions at the beginning of this chapter.

- Take 1 capsule with desired oil 2 times daily.
- Put 2-3 drops of oil in a spoonful of Blue Agave, Yacon Syrup, maple syrup, coconut oil, milk, etc.
- Put the desired amount of oils in a glass of rice milk, almond milk, goat milk, carrot juice, NingXia Red, or even water and then drink it.
- Gargle up to 10 times daily as needed with Thieves Fresh Essence Plus Mouthwash.
- Brush teeth and gums after every meal with Thieves AromaBright Toothpaste or Kid-Scents Slique Toothpaste.

Topical
You may apply single oils or blends neat or diluted, depending on the oil or oils being used. Please see the instructions at the beginning of this chapter for more information on applying oils to the skin.

Ingestion and Oral
The amount of oil ingested varies with different oils. Whether putting the oils in a capsule or drinking them in a liquid, please refer to the instructions at the beginning of this chapter.

- Take 1 capsule with desired oil 2 times daily.
- Put 2-3 drops of oil in a spoonful of Blue Agave, Yacon Syrup, maple syrup, coconut oil, milk, etc.
- Put the desired amount of oils in a glass of rice milk, almond milk, goat milk, carrot juice, NingXia Red, or even water and then drink it.

....

Mouth Ulcers
(See Canker Sores)
Mouth ulcers are sores or open lesions in the mouth and are caused by many disorders such as canker sores, oral cancer, thrush, fever blisters, or gingivostomatitis.

Recommendations
Singles: Melaleuca Alternifolia, Thyme, Myrrh, Lavender, Peppermint, Ocotea, Oregano

Blends: Thieves, Exodus II

Nutritionals: AlkaLime

Oral Care: Thieves AromaBright Toothpaste, KidScents Slique Toothpaste, Thieves Dentarome Plus Toothpaste, Thieves Dentarome Ultra Toothpaste, Thieves Fresh Essence Plus Mouthwash, Thieves Lozenges (Hard/Soft), Thieves Spray, Slique Gum

Application and Usage
Topical
You may apply single oils or blends neat or diluted, depending on the oil or oils being used. Please see the instructions at the beginning of this chapter for more information on applying oils to the skin.

- Apply 1-2 drops diluted 50:50 on gums 2 times daily.

Ingestion and Oral
The amount of oil ingested varies with different oils. Whether putting the oils in a capsule or drinking them in a liquid, please

refer to the instructions at the beginning of this chapter.

- Take 1 capsule with desired oil 2 times daily.
- Put 2-3 drops of oil in a spoonful of Blue Agave, Yacon Syrup, maple syrup, coconut oil, milk, etc.
- Put the desired amount of oils in a glass of rice milk, almond milk, goat milk, carrot juice, NingXia Red, or even water and then drink it.
- Gargle 3-10 times daily as needed.
- Gargle with Thieves Fresh Essence Plus Mouthwash or Thieves Spray and add 1-2 drops of Thieves, Clove, and Exodus II to strengthen the therapeutic action.

....

Oral Infection Control

Oral infection control procedures are precautions taken in dental offices and other health-care settings to prevent the spread of disease.

Recommendations

Singles: Clove, Myrrh, Oregano, Plectranthus Oregano, Thyme, Helichrysum, Eucalyptus Radiata

Blends: PanAway, Thieves, R.C., Slique Essence

Oral Care: Fresh Essence Plus Mouthwash, Thieves Spray, Thieves, Thieves AromaBright Toothpaste, KidScents Slique Toothpaste, Thieves Dentarome Plus Toothpaste, Thieves Dentarome Ultra Toothpaste, Thieves Lozenges (Hard/Soft), Slique Gum

Application and Usage
Topical

You may apply single oils or blends neat or diluted, depending on the oil or oils being used. Please see the instructions at the beginning of this chapter for more information on applying oils to the skin.

- Apply 1-2 drops diluted 50:50 on gums and around teeth. Repeat as needed.

- Just before a tooth extraction, rub 1-2 drops of Helichrysum, Thieves, and R.C. around the gum area.
- Rubbing R.C. on gums may also help to bring back feeling after numbness from anesthesia.

....

Pyorrhea

Essential oils are some of the best treatments against gum diseases such as gingivitis and pyorrhea. For example: The active principle in clove oil is eugenol, which is used as a dental disinfectant and is one of the best-studied germ killers available.

Recommendations

Singles: Clove (diluted 50:50), Thyme (diluted 50:50), Oregano (diluted 50:50), Wintergreen

Blends: Thieves (diluted if desired), Exodus II (diluted if desired)

Oral Care: Thieves Fresh Essence Plus Mouthwash, Thieves Spray, Thieves AromaBright Toothpaste, KidScents Slique Toothpaste, Thieves Dentarome Ultra Toothpaste, Thieves Dentarome Plus Toothpaste, Thieves Lozenges (Hard/Soft), Thieves Dental Floss

Nutritionals: BLM, Mineral Essence, Essentialzyme, Detoxzyme, MegaCal, Power Meal, Inner Defense

Application and Usage
Topical

You may apply single oils or blends neat or diluted, depending on the oil or oils being used. Please see the instructions at the beginning of this chapter for more information on applying oils to the skin.

- Put 1-2 drops of Thieves on your toothbrush directly or put 1-2 drops of Thieves on your Dentarome toothpaste.
- Put 1 drop of Thieves directly on affected tooth and gum area, as needed.

- Use any of the recommended single oils or blends with toothpaste on toothbrush or alone. Generally, 1-2 drops are very sufficient. For some people, the recommended oils will seem very "hot." Even one drop mixed with toothpaste may seem very strong, but within a minute the "hot" feeling is gone, and the mouth feels very clean and refreshed. Many people like using one drop of Slique Essence or Thieves directly on the toothbrush without using any toothpaste.

Oral
- Gargle 4-6 times daily with Thieves Fresh Essence Plus Mouthwash or as needed.
- Mix 1-2 drops of Clove or any other recommended oil of choice in a glass of water and gargle.
- Spray mouth several times daily with Thieves Spray.

....

Teeth Grinding
Teeth grinding (bruxism) is a condition in which you grind, clench, or gnash your teeth, consciously or unconsciously. If it is frequent and severe enough, it can lead to jaw disorders, headaches, damaged teeth, and other problems.

Recommendations
Singles: Valerian, Lavender, Roman Chamomile

Blends: Peace & Calming, RutaVaLa, RutaVaLa Roll-On, Stress Away Roll-On, Tranquil Roll-On

Nutritionals: Mineral Essence, MegaCal, ImmuPro, SleepEssence

Oral Care: Thieves Spray, Thieves AromaBright Toothpaste, KidScents Slique Toothpaste, Thieves Dentarome Plus Toothpaste, Thieves Dentarome Ultra Toothpaste, Thieves Fresh Essence Plus Mouthwash, Slique Gum

Application and Usage
Inhalation
- Diffuse your choice of oils for ½ hour every 4-6 hours or as desired, especially before retiring.
- Put 2-3 drops of your chosen oil in your hands and rub them together, cup your hands over your nose, and inhale throughout the day as needed.
- Put 8-10 drops of oil on a cotton ball or tissue and put it in an air vent in your house, vehicle, hotel room, etc.
- If diffusing while sleeping, set your timer for the desired length of time for automatic shut off.

Topical
You may apply single oils or blends neat or diluted, depending on the oil or oils being used. Please see the instructions at the beginning of this chapter for more information on applying oils to the skin.
- Massage 1-3 drops neat of Lavender, RutaVaLa, and Valerian on bottoms of feet each night before retiring.

....

Toothache and Teething Pain
A toothache is a pain in or around a tooth, and treatment for a toothache depends on the cause.

Recommendations
Singles: Clove, Sacred Frankincense, Frankincense, German Chamomile, Melaleuca Alternifolia, Idaho Tansy

Blends: Thieves, PanAway, Slique Essence

Oral Care: Thieves Spray, Thieves AromaBright Toothpaste, KidScents Slique Toothpaste, Thieves Dentarome Plus Toothpaste, Thieves Dentarome Ultra Toothpaste, Thieves Fresh Essence Plus Mouthwash, Slique Gum

Application and Usage
Topical
You may apply single oils or blends neat or diluted, depending on the oil or oils being used. Please see the instructions at the beginning of this chapter for more information on applying oils to the skin.

- Apply oil neat or diluted 50:50 on affected tooth and gum area as needed.

Ingestion and Oral
The amount of oil ingested varies with different oils. Whether putting the oils in a capsule or drinking them in a liquid, please refer to the instructions at the beginning of this chapter.

- Take 1 capsule with desired oil 2 times daily.
- Put 2-3 drops of oil in a spoonful of Blue Agave, Yacon Syrup, maple syrup, coconut oil, milk, etc.
- Put the desired amount of oils in a glass of rice milk, almond milk, goat milk, carrot juice, NingXia Red, or even water and then drink it.
- Gargle 4-6 times daily or as needed with Thieves Fresh Essence Plus Mouthwash.

Note: All essential oils should be diluted 20:80 before being used orally on small children.

PAIN
One of the most effective essential oils for blocking pain is Helichrysum. A study in 1994 showed that Peppermint is extremely effective in blocking calcium channels and substance P, important factors in the transmission of pain signals.[34] Other essential oils also have unique pain-relieving properties, including Helichrysum, Sacred Frankincense, Frankincense, Eucalyptus Blue, Vetiver, Dorado Azul, Palo Santo, Valerian, Idaho Balsam Fir, and Douglas Fir.

MSM, a source of organic sulfur, has also been proven to be extremely effective for al-

---

How MSM Works to Control Pain
When fluid pressure inside cells is higher than outside, pain is experienced. MSM, found in Sulfurzyme, equalizes fluid pressure inside cells and helps balance the protein envelope of the cell so that water transfers freely in and out.

---

leviating pain, especially tissue and joint pain. The subject of a best-selling book by Dr. Ronald Lawrence and Dr. Stanley Jacobs, MSM is redefining the treatment of pain, especially associated with arthritis and fibromyalgia. Sulfurzyme is an excellent source of MSM.

Natural pregnenolone can also blunt pain.

....

Bone-related Pain
Bone pain emanates from the bone tissue and occurs as a result of disease and/or physical conditions. Each type of bone pain has many potential sources or causes.

Recommendations
Singles: Helichrysum, Wintergreen, Idaho Balsam Fir, Copaiba, Peppermint, Vetiver, Dorado Azul, Palo Santo, Idaho Blue Spruce, Pine

Blends: PanAway, Relieve It, Deep Relief Roll-On

Nutritionals: Sulfurzyme, MegaCal, BLM, Mineral Essence, Master HIS or HERS, MultiGreens, Super B, Super C, Super C Chewable

Body Care Massage Oils and Creams: Ortho Ease Massage Oil, Ortho Sport Massage Oil, Regenolone Moisturizing Cream

Application and Usage
Topical
You may apply single oils or blends neat or diluted, depending on the oil or oils being used.

Please see the instructions at the beginning of this chapter for more information on applying oils to the skin.

- Apply 2-4 drops diluted 50:50 on location, as needed.
- Massage several drops onto the Vita Flex points of the feet and repeat as needed.

....

Chronic Pain

To pinpoint the most effective essential oil for quenching pain, it may be necessary to try each of the essential oils in these categories in order to find the one that is most effective for your particular pain situation.

Recommendations

Singles: Helichrysum, Wintergreen, Clove, Peppermint, Dorado Azul, Palo Santo, Idaho Blue Spruce, Elemi, Oregano, Plectranthus Oregano, Douglas Fir, Idaho Balsam Fir, Copaiba, Sacred Frankincense, Frankincense

Blends: PanAway, Deep Relief Roll-On, Relieve It, Aroma Siez, Release, Sacred Mountain

Nutritionals: Sulfurzyme, SuperCal, MegaCal, BLM, Sacred Frankincense or Frankincense (1 capsule daily)

Application and Usage

Topical

You may apply single oils or blends neat or diluted, depending on the oil or oils being used.

Please see the instructions at the beginning of this chapter for more information on applying oils to the skin.

- Apply 2-4 drops diluted 50:50 on location, as needed.
- Place 1-2 drops oil with a warm compress on location, as needed.
- Sacred Frankincense or Frankincense: Take 1 capsule daily.

PANCREATITIS

Pancreatitis is an inflammation of the pancreas that can be either acute or chronic.

Acute pancreatitis can be brought on by a sudden blockage in the main pancreatic duct caused by enzymes unable to function properly with pancreas function and literally begin digesting the pancreas unless remedied. If there is not good flow of the enzymatic process whereby nutrients are able to be absorbed and waste eliminated, the enzymes begin to fight against that blockage.

Chronic pancreatitis occurs more gradually, with attacks recurring over weeks or months.

Symptoms

- Abdominal pain
- Muscle aches
- Vomiting
- Jaundice
- Abdominal swelling
- Sudden hypertension
- Rapid weight loss
- Fever

In the case of acute pancreatitis, a total fast for at least 4-5 days is one of the safest and most effective methods of alleviating the problem. In the case of infection, fasting should be combined with immune stimulation by using Exodus II combined with vitamin C and Super B vitamin complex.

Recommendations

Singles: Geranium, Peppermint, Oregano, Plectranthus Oregano, Vetiver, Mountain Savory, Orange

Blends: DiGize, Exodus II, Thieves, Immu-Power

Nutritionals: MultiGreens, Super B, Digest & Cleanse, OmegaGize³, Super C, Super C Chewable, Essentialzyme, Essentialzymes-4, Detoxzyme

Application and Usage
Topical

You may apply single oils or blends neat or diluted, depending on the oil or oils being used. Please see the instructions at the beginning of this chapter for more information on applying oils to the skin.

- Receive a Raindrop Technique 2 times a week.
- Retention: Use an enema with the recommended oils 3 times per week.

Ingestion and Oral

The amount of oil ingested varies with different oils. Whether putting the oils in a capsule or drinking them in a liquid, please refer to the instructions at the beginning of this chapter.

- Take 1 capsule with desired oil 3 times weekly.
- Put 2-3 drops of oil in a spoonful of Blue Agave, Yacon Syrup, maple syrup, coconut oil, milk, etc.
- Put the desired amount of oils in a glass of rice milk, almond milk, goat milk, carrot juice, NingXia Red, or even water and then drink it.

PARASITES, INTESTINAL (WORMS)

Many types of parasites use up nutrients while giving off toxins; this can leave the body depleted, nutritionally deficient, and susceptible to infectious disease.

Di-Gize and ParaFree for Parasite Control

The essential oil blend Di-Gize and ParaFree softgel capsules are excellent for parasite removal.

Di-Gize: Add 6 drops to 1 tsp. V-6 Vegetable Oil Complex or to 4 oz. rice, soy, almond, or goat milk and take as a dietary supplement 2 times a day, or take 15 drops in a capsule 3 times a day for 7 days. Di-Gize can also be diluted in massage oil and applied on abdomen.

ParaFree: Take 5 softgels, 2-3 times daily for 21 days, then rest for 7 days. Repeat up to 3 times to achieve desired results.

Occasionally, parasites can lie dormant in the body and then become active due to ingestion of a particular food or drink. This can result in the appearance and disappearance of symptoms, even though parasites are always present.

The parasite *Cryptosporidium parvum* may be present in many municipal or tap waters. To remove this parasite, the water must be distilled or filtered using a 0.3 micron filter.

Symptoms

- Fatigue
- Weakness
- Diarrhea
- Blood in stools
- Chronic pain
- Weight loss
- Gas and bloating
- Cramping
- Nausea
- Irregular bowel movements

The first step to controlling parasites is beginning a fasting and cleansing program. A colon cleanse is particularly important.

Recommendations

Singles: Tarragon, Fennel, Idaho Tansy, Basil, Peppermint, Ginger, Nutmeg, Melaleuca Alternifolia, Rosemary, Cumin

Blends: Thieves, DiGize, JuvaFlex, JuvaCleanse

Nutritionals: ParaFree, Digest & Cleanse, Inner Defense, Life 5, ICP, ComforTone, Detoxzyme, JuvaPower, Essentialzyme, Essentialzymes-4

Retention Blend for Parasite Killing

- 4 drops Ginger
- 4 drops DiGize
- 16 drops V-6 Vegetable Oil Complex

Application and Usage

Topical

You may apply single oils or blends neat or diluted, depending on the oil or oils being used. Please see the instructions at the beginning of this chapter for more information on applying oils to the skin.

- Place a warm compress with recommended oils over intestinal area 2 times weekly.
- Massage up to 6 drops on the small intestine and colon Vita Flex points of the feet daily (instep area on both feet).
- Retention: Add the blend for parasite killing to an enema and insert nightly for 7 nights; then rest for 7 nights. Repeat this cycle 3 times to eliminate all stages of parasite development.

Ingestion and Oral

The amount of oil ingested varies with different oils. Whether putting the oils in a capsule or drinking them in a liquid, please refer to the instructions at the beginning of this chapter.

- Take 1 capsule with desired oil 2 times daily.
- Put 2-3 drops of oil in a spoonful of Blue Agave, Yacon Syrup, maple syrup, coconut oil, milk, etc.
- Put the desired amount of oils in a glass of rice milk, almond milk, goat milk, carrot juice, NingXia Red, or even water and then drink it.

POLIO

Polio (poliomyelitis) is an acute, infectious disease, usually manifested in epidemics and caused by a virus. It creates an inflammation of the gray matter of the spinal cord and is characterized by fever, sore throat, headache, vomiting, and sometimes stiffness of the neck and back. If it develops into the major illness, it can involve paralysis and atrophy of groups of muscles, ending in contraction and permanent deformity.

If polio is suspected, seek medical attention.

Recommendations

Singles: Sacred Frankincense, Frankincense, Ravintsara, Blue Cypress, Wintergreen, Melaleuca Alternifolia, Melissa, Peppermint, Sandalwood, Palo Santo, Oregano, Plectranthus Oregano, Thyme, Mountain Savory

Blends: The Gift, Aroma Siez, Valor, Valor Roll-On

Nutritionals: ImmuPro, Life 5

Polio Blend

- 15 drops Myrrh
- 10 drops Ravintsara
- 10 drops Wintergreen
- 7 drops Sacred Frankincense or Frankincense
- 8 drops Blue Cypress
- 6 drops Lemon

Application and Usage

Inhalation

- Diffuse your choice of oils for ½ hour every 4-6 hours or as desired.
- Put 2-3 drops of your chosen oil in your hands and rub them together, cup your hands over your nose, and inhale throughout the day as needed.
- Put 8-10 drops of oil on a cotton ball or tissue and put it in an air vent in your house, vehicle, hotel room, etc.
- If diffusing while sleeping, set your timer for the desired length of time for automatic shut off.

Topical

You may apply single oils or blends neat or diluted, depending on the oil or oils being used. Please see the instructions at the beginning of this chapter for more information on applying oils to the skin.

- Apply 1-2 drops neat or undiluted as desired.
- Applying a single drop under the nose is helpful and refreshing.
- Receive a Raindrop Technique 3 times weekly.

Ingestion and Oral

The amount of oil ingested varies with different oils. Whether putting the oils in a capsule or drinking them in a liquid, please refer to the instructions at the beginning of this chapter.

- Take 1 capsule with desired oil 2 times daily.
- Put 2-3 drops of oil in a spoonful of Blue Agave, Yacon Syrup, maple syrup, coconut oil, milk, etc.
- Put the desired amount of oils in a glass of rice milk, almond milk, goat milk, carrot juice, NingXia Red, or even water and then drink it.

PREGNANCY

Essential oils can be invaluable companions during pregnancy. Oils like Lavender and Myrrh may help reduce stretch marks and improve the elasticity of the skin. Geranium and Gentle Baby have similar effects and can be massaged on the perineum (tissue between vagina and rectum) to lower the risk of tearing or the need for an episiotomy (an incision in the perineum) during birth.

Recommendations

Singles: Lavender, Myrrh, Rose, Geranium, Helichrysum, German Chamomile, Neroli, Sandalwood

Essential Oils and Pregnancy

As always, when using essential oils, common sense is most important when deciding how to use them.

During pregnancy most oils are safe and bring peace and contentment. When rubbing them over the stomach, many women have said that they have felt a positive response from the unborn infant. Energy sensitivity is very high during this time and is something to be aware of and enjoyed. Gentle Baby, Valor, White Angelica, RutaVaLa, Magnify Your Purpose, Joy, Harmony, Highest Potential, Gathering, Di-Gize, and Dream Catcher are just a few that are enjoyable for both mother and baby throughout the pregnancy.

Oils such as Basil, Clary Sage, Fennel, Hyssop, Nutmeg, Rosemary, Sage, Tansy, and Tarragon should be used carefully with a good understanding as to their benefits and how to use them.

Some essential oils such as Fennel and Clary Sage may help to accelerate labor once it has begun. Take 1-2 capsules 2 times daily when labor is imminent. Always consult a health professional before using essential oils during pregnancy, other than the ones recommended in this book.

A few drops of Vetiver and Valerian mixed together with 1 tablespoon of V-6 Vegetable Oil Complex may help reduce the pain of contractions when applied on the lower back.

Blends: Gentle Baby, Forgiveness, Valor, Valor Roll-On, Grounding, Peace & Calming, Highest Potential, Joy, Sacred Mountain, White Angelica

Ointments and Sprays: ClaraDerm, Tender Tush

Labor Blend (Use only after labor has started.)
- 5 drops Ylang Ylang (or Amazonian Ylang Ylang)
- 4 drops Helichrysum
- 2 drops Fennel
- 2 drops Peppermint
- 2 drops Clary Sage

Application and Usage
Inhalation
- Diffuse your choice of oils for ½ hour every 4-6 hours or as desired.
- Put 2-3 drops of your chosen oil in your hands and rub them together, cup your hands over your nose, and inhale throughout the day as needed.
- Put 8-10 drops of oil on a cotton ball or tissue and put it in an air vent in your house, vehicle, hotel room, etc.
- If diffusing while sleeping, set your timer for the desired length of time for automatic shut off.
- Diffuse Gentle Baby, Joy, or Valor to reduce stress before and after the birth. Expectant fathers will also find this helps to reduce anxiety during delivery.

Topical
You may apply single oils or blends neat or diluted, depending on the oil or oils being used. Please see the instructions at the beginning of this chapter for more information on applying oils to the skin.
- Massage 2-4 drops Labor Blend from above diluted 50:50 on reproductive Vita Flex points on the sides of the ankles. Apply **ONLY** after labor has started.
- Massage 2-4 drops Labor Blend from above on lower stomach and lower back.

PROSTATE PROBLEMS

Natural progesterone is one of the best natural remedies for prostate inflammation (BPH) that can obstruct urinary flow and lead to impotence. Transdermal creams are the most effective means of hormone delivery.

Scientists are tracing the higher incidence of hormone-dependent cancers, including cancer of the breast, prostate, and testes, to exposure to endocrine disrupters in the environment. Contamination from 39 petrochemicals like DDT, PCB, pesticides, the phthalate DBP, recombinant bovine growth hormone (rBGH) in milk, and synthetic steroids in meat are all implicated in interfering with hormone receptors, rendering them unable to function properly, eventually leading to cancer.

For prostate problems, Peppermint acts as an anti-inflammatory to the prostate. Saw palmetto, *Pygeum africanum*, and pumpkin seed oil also help reduce prostate swelling.

Recommendations
Singles: Myrrh, Idaho Balsam Fir, Oregano, Plectranthus Oregano, Sage, Yarrow, Thyme, Wintergreen

Blends: Mister, EndoFlex, Australian Blue

Nutritionals: Prostate Health (a good source of zinc that helps reduce prostate swelling), Master Formula HIS, Longevity Softgels, PD 80/20

Retention Oils and Creams: Protec, Prenolone Plus Body Cream

Application and Usage
Inhalation
- Diffuse your choice of oils for ½ hour every 4-6 hours or as desired.
- Put 2-3 drops of your chosen oil in your hands and rub them together, cup your hands over your nose, and inhale throughout the day as needed.
- Put 8-10 drops of oil on a cotton ball or tis-

sue and put it in an air vent in your house, vehicle, hotel room, etc.

- If diffusing while sleeping, set your timer for the desired length of time for automatic shut off.

Topical

You may apply single oils or blends neat or diluted, depending on the oil or oils being used. Please see the instructions at the beginning of this chapter for more information on applying oils to the skin.

- Apply 2-4 drops diluted 20:80 between the rectum and scrotum 2 times daily. Mister works especially well applied there.
- Massage 4-6 drops on the Vita Flex reproductive points on the feet 2 times daily.
- Retention: Rectal, nightly for 7 days, rest 7 days, then repeat.

....

Benign Prostate Hyperplasia (BPH)

Almost all males over age 50 have some degree of prostate hyperplasia, a condition that worsens with age. BPH can severely restrict urine flow and result in frequent, small urinations.

Three herbs that are extremely effective for treating this condition are saw palmetto, pumpkin seed oil, and *Pygeum africanum*. The mineral zinc is also important for normal prostate function and prostate health. The hormone-like activity of some essential oils can support a nutritional regimen to reduce BPH swelling.

Recommendations

Singles: Sacred Frankincense, Frankincense, Myrrh, Idaho Balsam Fir, Blue Cypress

Blends: Mister, EndoFlex, Australian Blue, Chivalry

Nutritionals: Prostate Health (a good source of zinc that helps reduce prostate swelling), Master Formula HIS, Longevity Softgels, Mineral Essence

Retention Oils and Body Creams: Protec, Prenolone Plus Body Cream

BPH Blend

- 10 drops Sacred Frankincense or Frankincense
- 5 drops Myrrh
- 3 drops Sage

Application and Usage

Inhalation

- Diffuse your choice of oils for ½ hour every 4-6 hours or as desired.
- Put 2-3 drops of your chosen oil in your hands and rub them together, cup your hands over your nose, and inhale throughout the day as needed.
- Put 8-10 drops of oil on a cotton ball or tissue and put it in an air vent in your house, vehicle, hotel room, etc.
- If diffusing while sleeping, set your timer for the desired length of time for automatic shut off.

Topical

You may apply single oils or blends neat or diluted, depending on the oil or oils being used. Please see the instructions at the beginning of this chapter for more information on applying oils to the skin.

- PSA counts typically rise when BPH occurs. The following regimen reduced PSA (prostate specific antigen) counts 70 percent in 2 months. Use the following applications simultaneously:
- Mix the BPH Blend found above with 1 tablespoon olive oil and use 3 times weekly as an overnight rectal retention enema.
- Apply 2-4 drops of the BPH Blend diluted 50:50 between the rectum and scrotum 1-3 times daily.
- Massage 1-3 drops of the BPH Blend on the reproductive Vita Flex points on the feet 2 times daily.

Ingestion and Oral

The amount of oil ingested varies with different oils. Whether putting the oils in a capsule

or drinking them in a liquid, please refer to the instructions at the beginning of this chapter.
- Take 1 capsule with desired oil 3 times daily.
- Put 2-3 drops of oil in a spoonful of Blue Agave, Yacon Syrup, maple syrup, coconut oil, milk, etc.
- Put the desired amount of oils in a glass of rice milk, almond milk, goat milk, carrot juice, NingXia Red, or even water and then drink it.

....

Prostatitis

Prostatitis is an inflammation of the prostate that can present symptoms similar to benign prostate hyperplasia: frequent urinations, restricted flow, etc.

Recommendations

Singles: Peppermint, Clary Sage, Palo Santo, Yarrow, German Chamomile, Wintergreen, Rosemary, Myrtle, Thyme, Tsuga, Blue Cypress

Blends: Australian Blue, Mister, Aroma Siez, DiGize

Nutritionals: Prostate Health (a good source of zinc that helps reduce prostate swelling), Longevity Softgels, ImmuPro, Mineral Essence, JuvaPower, ICP

Retention Oils and Body Creams: Protec, Prenolone Plus Body Cream

Application and Usage
Topical

You may apply single oils or blends neat or diluted, depending on the oil or oils being used. Please see the instructions at the beginning of this chapter for more information on applying oils to the skin.
- Apply 1-3 drops diluted 20:80 to the area between the rectum and the scrotum daily.
- Massage 4-6 drops on the reproductive Vita Flex points on the feet daily.
- Retention: Rectal 3 times per week at night.

Ingestion and Oral

The amount of oil ingested varies with different oils. Whether putting the oils in a capsule or drinking them in a liquid, please refer to the instructions at the beginning of this chapter.
- Take 1 capsule with desired oil 2 times daily.
- Put 2-3 drops of oil in a spoonful of Blue Agave, Yacon Syrup, maple syrup, coconut oil, milk, etc.
- Put the desired amount of oils in a glass of rice milk, almond milk, goat milk, carrot juice, NingXia Red, or even water and then drink it.

RADIATION EXPOSURE DAMAGE

Many cancer treatments use radiation therapy that can severely damage both the skin and vital organs. Using gentle, antioxidant essential oils topically, as well as proper nutrients internally, is helpful in minimizing radiation damage.

Daily radiation from cell phones, computers, air travel, televisions, all types of electronic equipment, and kitchen appliances bombards us constantly. The more we can do to protect ourselves as well as cleanse on a regular basis, the better health we can maintain.

....

Environmental Protection Kits

QuadShield and EndoShield are two kits for environmental protection:

QuadShield™

The QuadShield kit combines four powerful products to help individuals take precautionary and prudent steps against potential radiation effects that bombard us daily. It contains the essential oil blends Longevity and Melrose and the nutritional supplements Super C (or Chewable) and Thyromin.

A suggested daily regimen could include:
- **Longevity Softgels**. The essential oils in

Longevity Softgels increase the oxygen and ATP (adenosine triphosphate) cellular fuel for increasing cell life and immunity for stronger resistance against damage from environmental pollution and potential daily radiation exposure.

Children and teens ages 10–18: 1–2 capsules daily

Adults: 2–4 capsules daily

• **Melrose** (essential oil blend) is formulated with two species of Melaleuca oil, *M. alternifolia* and *M. quinquenervia*, also known as niaouli, that were found through research by Daniel Pénoël, MD, and Pierre Franchomme, PhD, to prevent cellular damage from environmental pollution and potential daily radiation exposure.

Children ages 1–3: 1 drop in yogurt or other liquid

Children ages 4–7: 2 drops in yogurt or other liquid

Children 8 and older: 6 drops per capsule 1–3 times daily or in yogurt or other liquid

Adults: 20 drops per capsule, 1–2 capsules, 1–3 times daily or in yogurt or other liquid

• **Super C (or Chewable)** provides the body with 2,166 percent of the recommended dietary intake of the powerful antioxidant vitamin C and is enhanced with minerals, bioflavonoids, and pure Orange, Lemon, and other essential oils. It is a natural antioxidant and free radical scavenger that supports the immune system and protects healthy cells from becoming damaged by the effects of environmental pollution and potential daily radiation exposure.

Children ages 1–3: MightyMist Oral Spray: 3 squirts 2 times daily or 1–2 MightyVites daily

Children ages 4–7: 2–3 MightyVites or Super C Chewable daily

Children 8 and older: 3–4 MightyVites or Super C Chewable daily

Adults: 4–6 tablets daily

• **Thyromin** contains potassium iodide and kelp, researched and proven to protect the thyroid from environmental radiation. Other ingredients give support and nutrition to both the thyroid and adrenal glands for a healthier glandular system.

Children: Continue to use MightyMist Oral Spray: 3 squirts 2 times daily or MightyVites: 2–4 daily

Adults: only 1 capsule, 3 times daily

• **NingXia Red** — Drink 4–6 oz. of NingXia Red for a delicious and healthy addition to your diet.

EndoShield™

The EndoShield kit combines four powerful essential oil blends of Longevity Softgels, Melrose, EndoFlex, and Citrus Fresh to help one take precautionary and prudent steps against environmental pollution and potential radiation effects that bombard us daily.

A suggested daily regimen could include:

• **Longevity Softgels**. The essential oils in Longevity Softgels increase the oxygen and ATP (adenosine triphosphate) cellular fuel for increasing cell life and immunity for stronger resistance against damage from environmental pollution and possible daily radiation exposure.

Children and teens ages 10–18: 1–2 capsules daily

Adults: 2–4 capsules daily

• **Melrose** (essential oil blend) is formulated with two species of Melaleuca oil, *M. alternifolia* and *M. quinquenervia*, also known as niaouli, that were found through research by Daniel Pénoël, MD, and Pierre Franchomme, PhD, to prevent cellular damage from environmental pollution and potential daily radiation exposure.

Children ages 1–3: 1 drop 1–3 times daily

or in yogurt or other liquid

Children ages 4–7: 2 drops in yogurt or other liquid

Children 8 and older: 6 drops per capsule 2 times daily or in yogurt or other liquid

Adults: 20 drops per capsule, 1–2 capsules, 1–3 times daily or in yogurt or other liquid

- **EndoFlex** contains oils very specific to the thyroid while at the same time addressing the entire endocrine system.

  Myrtle oil stimulates and promotes good thyroid health when combined with Spearmint, encouraging better circulation, stronger metabolism, and production of digestive enzymes.

  Geranium contains esters that protect the thyroid, which may explain why it is so heralded in French publications as a general tonic for the body. It supports the thyroid in being able to uptake iodine from food.

  Children ages 1–3: 1 drop in yogurt or other liquid

  Children ages 4–7: 2 drops in yogurt or other liquid

  Children 8 and older: 6 drops per capsule 2 times daily or in yogurt or other liquid

  Adults: 20 drops per capsule, 1–2 capsules, 1–3 times daily or in yogurt or other liquid

- **Citrus Fresh** combines six citrus oils that are naturally antioxidant, antibacterial, and increase the uptake of vitamin C.

  Children ages 1–3: 1 drop in yogurt or other liquid

  Children ages 4–7: 2 drops in yogurt or other liquid

  Children 8 and older: 6 drops per capsule 2 times daily or in yogurt or other liquid

  Adults: 20 drops per capsule, 1–2 capsules, 1–3 times daily or in yogurt or other liquid

- **NingXia Red** — Drink 4–6 oz. of NingXia Red for a delicious and healthy addition to your diet.

Recommendations

Singles: Sacred Frankincense, Frankincense, Idaho Balsam Fir, Blue Cypress, Sandalwood, Hyssop, Oregano, Plectranthus Oregano, Melaleuca Alternifolia, Melaleuca Quinquenervia

Blends: Melrose, Longevity, Valor, Stress Away Roll-On

Nutritionals: QuadShield or EndoShield products, Super C, Super C Chewable, Power Meal, ImmuPro, NingXia Red, Mineral Essence, Essentialzyme, Longevity Softgels, OmegaGize^3, Ultra Young Plus, Ningxia Wolfberries (Dried)

Application and Usage
Inhalation

- Diffuse your choice of oils for ½ hour every 4-6 hours or as desired.
- Put 2-3 drops of your chosen oil in your hands and rub them together, cup your hands over your nose, and inhale throughout the day as needed.
- Put 8-10 drops of oil on a cotton ball or tissue and put it in an air vent in your house, vehicle, hotel room, etc.
- If diffusing while sleeping, set your timer for the desired length of time for automatic shut off.

Topical

You may apply single oils or blends neat or diluted, depending on the oil or oils being used. Please see the instructions at the beginning of this chapter for more information on applying oils to the skin.

- Apply 1-2 drops diluted 50:50 on affected area 1-2 times daily.
- Massage 2-4 drops of oil neat on the soles of the feet just before bedtime.

Ingestion and Oral

The amount of oil ingested varies with different oils. Whether putting the oils in a capsule or drinking them in a liquid, please

refer to the instructions at the beginning of this chapter.

- Take 1 capsule with desired oil 2 times daily.
- Put 2-3 drops of oil in a spoonful of Blue Agave, Yacon Syrup, maple syrup, coconut oil, milk, etc.
- Put the desired amount of oils in a glass of rice milk, almond milk, goat milk, carrot juice, NingXia Red, or even water and then drink it.

RHEUMATIC FEVER

Rheumatic fever results from a streptococcus infection that primarily strikes children (usually before age 14). It can lead to inflammation that damages the heart muscle and valve.

Rheumatic fever is caused by the same genus of bacteria that causes strep throat and scarlet fever. Diffusing essential oils can help reduce the likelihood of contracting the disease. Essential oils such as Mountain Savory, Rosemary, Melaleuca Alternifolia, Thyme, Palo Santo, Sacred Frankincense, Frankincense, Eucalyptus Blue, and Oregano have powerful antimicrobial effects.

In cases where a person is already infected, the use of essential oils in the Raindrop Technique may be appropriate.

Recommendations

Singles: Oregano, Plectranthus Oregano, Clove, Melaleuca Alternifolia, Mountain Savory, Peppermint, Thyme, Rosemary, Black Pepper, Eucalyptus Blue, Sacred Frankincense, Frankincense, Palo Santo, Cistus

Blends: Thieves, Melrose, Exodus II, ImmuPower

Nutritionals: Inner Defense, ImmuPro, Super C, Super C Chewable, Sulfurzyme, Longevity Softgels, Master Formula HIS or HERS, NingXia Red, Essentialzyme, Mineral Essence

Application and Usage
Inhalation

- Diffuse your choice of oils for 1 hour 3 times daily.
- Put 2-3 drops of your chosen oil in your hands and rub them together, cup your hands over your nose, and inhale throughout the day as needed.
- Put 8-10 drops of oil on a cotton ball or tissue and put it in an air vent in your house, vehicle, hotel room, etc.
- If diffusing while sleeping, set your timer for the desired length of time for automatic shut off.

Topical

You may apply single oils or blends neat or diluted, depending on the oil or oils being used. Please see the instructions at the beginning of this chapter for more information on applying oils to the skin.

- Apply 3-5 drops diluted 50:50 on the bottoms of the feet and on carotid artery spots under the earlobes.
- Receive a Raindrop Technique 1 time weekly.

ROCKY MOUNTAIN SPOTTED FEVER (See LYME DISEASE / ROCKY MOUNTAIN SPOTTED FEVER)

SCAR TISSUE

Scar tissue is the fibrous connective tissue that forms a scar and can be found on any tissue on the body where an injury, surgery, cut, or disease has taken place and then healed. It is thicker, paler, and denser than the surrounding tissue because it has a limited blood supply.

Recommendations

Singles: Sacred Frankincense, Frankincense, Sandalwood, Cypress, Elemi, Yarrow, Rose, Cistus, Myrrh, Helichrysum, Lavender

Blends: Gentle Baby, Australian Blue, 3 Wise Men

Nutritionals: Super C, Super C Chewable, Sulfurzyme, Power Meal, MegaCal, Mineral Essence, Essentialzyme

Body Care Ointments: KidScents Tender Tush, Regenolone Body Cream, Rose Ointment, Boswellia Wrinkle Cream

Scar Prevention Blend
- 4 drops Myrrh
- 3 drops Lavender
- 2 drops Helichrysum
- 1 drop Sandalwood

Application and Usage
Topical

You may apply single oils or blends neat or diluted, depending on the oil or oils being used. Please see the instructions at the beginning of this chapter for more information on applying oils to the skin.

- Apply 2-6 drops neat of the scar prevention blend around and over the wound daily until healed.

SCURVY

This condition is due to a deficiency of vitamin C in the diet and marked by weakness, anemia, spongy gums, bleeding of the gums and nose, and a hardening of the muscles of the calves and legs.

Recommendations
Singles: Orange, Lemon, Spearmint, Lavender
Blends: Thieves, GLF, Deep Relief
Nutritionals: Super C Chewable, Super C, Power Meal, Balance Complete, NingXia Red, Mineral Essence, Essentialzyme,Essentialzymes-4, Detoxzyme, Super B, Master Formula HIS or HERS

SEIZURES

Many seizures can be reduced or alleviated by removing all forms of sugar, artificial colors and flavors, and processed food from the diet and chemicals of all types. Avoid using personal care products with ammonia-based compounds such as quaterniums and polyquaterniums.

Recommendations
Singles: Peppermint, Sacred Frankincense, Frankincense, Sandalwood, Melissa, Jasmine, Basil
Blends: RutaVaLa, RutaVaLa Roll-On, R.C., Valor, Valor Roll-On, Breathe Again Roll-On, Aroma Siez, Exodus II, Peace & Calming, Trauma Life, Stress Away Roll-On
Nutritionals: Mineral Essence, MultiGreens, Essentialzyme, BLM, Super B, Longevity Softgels, Power Meal, Sulfurzyme, Omega-Gize[3], Balance Complete, Master Formula HIS or HERS, and Blue Agave, Yacon Syrup, or Stevia Extract in place of sugars

Application and Usage
Inhalation
- Diffuse your choice of oils for ½ hour every 4-6 hours or as desired.
- Put 2-3 drops of your chosen oil in your hands and rub them together, cup your hands over your nose, and inhale throughout the day as needed.
- Put 8-10 drops of oil on a cotton ball or tissue and put it in an air vent in your house, vehicle, hotel room, etc.
- If diffusing while sleeping, set your timer for the desired length of time for automatic shut off.

Topical

You may apply single oils or blends neat or diluted, depending on the oil or oils being used. Please see the instructions at the beginning of this chapter for more information on applying oils to the skin.

- Massage 10 drops into scalp diluted 50:50 up to 3 times daily to help reduce risk of seizure.
- Supplement with Inhalation therapy below.

Seizure Regimen (do all of the following)

- Massage 4-6 drops Valor on bottoms of feet daily.
- Diffuse Peace & Calming for 30 minutes 3-4 times daily.
- Massage 4-6 drops Joy over heart daily.
- Receive a Raindrop Technique on spine 2 times monthly.

SEXUAL DYSFUNCTION

There is an extensive, historical basis that fragrance may amplify desire and create a mood that can overcome frigidity or impotence. In fact, aromas such as rose and jasmine have been used since antiquity to attract the opposite sex and create a romantic atmosphere.

Modern research has shown that the aroma of some essential oils can stimulate the emotional center of the brain. This may explain why essential oils have the potential to help people overcome impotence or frigidity based on emotional factors or inhibitions.

....

Dysfunction (Men)
(See also Prostate Problems, Trauma)

Causes of male sexual dysfunction are divided into two types: physical or psychological problems.

....

Impotence (Men)

Impotence, the inability to perform sexually, may be caused by physical limitations due to an accident or injury or by psychological factors such as inhibitions, trauma, stress, etc.

Male impotence is often linked to problems with the prostate or prostate surgery.

If impotence is related to psychological trauma or unresolved emotional issues, it may be necessary to deal with these issues before any meaningful progress can be made.

Recommendations

Singles: Idaho Blue Spruce, Goldenrod, Sacred Frankincense, Frankincense, Myrrh, Ginger, Nutmeg, Jasmine, Ylang Ylang, Amazonian Ylang Ylang

Blends: Valor, Valor Roll-On, Mister, SclarEssence

Nutritionals: EndoGize, Prostate Health, Ultra Young Plus

Application and Usage
Inhalation

- Diffuse your choice of oils for 15 minutes 2 times daily or as desired.
- Put 2-3 drops of your chosen oil in your hands and rub them together, cup your hands over your nose, and inhale throughout the day as needed.
- Put 8-10 drops of oil on a cotton ball or tissue and put it in an air vent in your house, vehicle, hotel room, etc.
- If diffusing while sleeping, set your timer for the desired length of time for automatic shut off.

Topical

You may apply single oils or blends neat or diluted, depending on the oil or oils being used. Please see the instructions at the beginning of this chapter for more information on applying oils to the skin.

- Apply 2-3 drops neat to Vita Flex points on feet or lower abdomen. Do not apply on sensitive skin in crotch area.

....

Infertility (Men)

Male infertility is the inability of a male to achieve pregnancy in a fertile female. It is commonly due to deficiencies in the semen.

Recommendations

Singles: Idaho Blue Spruce, Sage, Sacred Frankincense, Frankincense, Clary Sage, Goldenrod

Blends: Mister, SclarEssence

Supplements and Implant Oils: Protec, Endo-Gize, Prostate Health

Application and Usage
Topical
You may apply single oils or blends neat or diluted, depending on the oil or oils being used. Please see the instructions at the beginning of this chapter for more information on applying oils to the skin.

- Apply 2-4 drops neat or diluted on the reproductive Vita Flex points of hands and feet inside of wrists, around the front of the ankles in line with the anklebone, on the lower sides of the anklebone, and along the Achilles tendon 1-3 times daily.
- Rub 4-6 drops of Protec on the lower abdomen near the pubic bone and in the area between the scrotum and the rectum.
- Alternatively, use 1 tablespoon of Protec in overnight rectal retention.

....

Lack of Libido (Men)
Lack of libido in men is a much more common complaint than our culture would seem to indicate. The leading reasons men don't want to have sex are medications, usually antidepressants and antihypertensive drugs, drug or alcohol abuse, or low testosterone.

Recommendations
Singles: Idaho Blue Spruce, Pine, Ocotea, Myrrh, Black Pepper, Ylang Ylang, Amazonian Ylang Ylang, Ginger, Nutmeg

Blends: SclarEssence, Valor, Valor Roll-On, Mister, Live with Passion, Transformation, The Gift, En-R-Gee

Nutritionals: EndoGize, MultiGreens, Prostate Health, Sulfurzyme, Essentialzyme, Super B, Mineral Essence, Thyromin, Ultra Young Plus

Body Care Creams: Prenolone Plus Body Cream

Application and Usage
Inhalation
- Diffuse your choice of oils for ½ hour every 4-6 hours or as desired.
- Put 2-3 drops of your chosen oil in your hands and rub them together, cup your hands over your nose, and inhale throughout the day as needed.
- Put 8-10 drops of oil on a cotton ball or tissue and put it in an air vent in your house, vehicle, hotel room, etc.
- If diffusing while sleeping, set your timer for the desired length of time for automatic shut off.

Topical
You may apply single oils or blends neat or diluted, depending on the oil or oils being used. Please see the instructions at the beginning of this chapter for more information on applying oils to the skin.

- Massage 4-6 drops diluted 50:50 on neck, shoulders, and lower abdomen 1-3 times daily.

....

Dysfunction (Women)
Sexual dysfunction can be a result of a physical or psychological problem.

....

Frigidity (Women)
Frigidity is a condition in which women have a lack of libido and tend to become unresponsive to sexual intercourse or are unable to achieve an orgasm. It may leave a woman unhappy, unsatisfied, and depressed.

Recommendations
Singles: Jasmine, Rose, Ylang Ylang, Amazonian Ylang Ylang, Clary Sage, Nutmeg

Blends: En-R-Gee, The Gift, Joy, Valor, Valor Roll-On

Nutritionals: EndoGize, Thyromin, Mineral Essence, Super B, PD 80/20, MegaCal, ImmuPro

Body Care Creams and Serums: Progessence Plus, Prenolone Plus Body Cream

Ylang Ylang (and Amazonian Ylang Ylang) helps balance sexual emotion and sex drive problems. Its aromatic influence elevates sexual energy and enhances relationships.

Clary Sage can help with lack of sexual desire, particularly in women, by regulating and balancing hormones.

Nutmeg supports the nervous system to help overcome frigidity.

Application and Usage
Inhalation

- Diffuse your choice of oils for ½ hour every 4-6 hours or as desired.
- Put 2-3 drops of your chosen oil in your hands and rub them together, cup your hands over your nose, and inhale throughout the day as needed.
- Put 8-10 drops of oil on a cotton ball or tissue and put it in an air vent in your house, vehicle, hotel room, etc.
- If diffusing while sleeping, set your timer for the desired length of time for automatic shut off.

Topical

You may apply single oils or blends neat or diluted, depending on the oil or oils being used. Please see the instructions at the beginning of this chapter for more information on applying oils to the skin.

- Massage 4-6 drops diluted 50:50 on neck, shoulders, and lower abdomen up to 1-3 times daily.

....

Infertility (Women)

Natural progesterone creams when used from the middle to the end of the cycle starting on the day after ovulation, usually day 15 or later, may improve fertility. Some essential oils have hormone-like qualities that can support or improve fertility processes.

Recommendations

Singles: Clary Sage, Ylang Ylang, Amazonian Ylang Ylang, Sage, Anise Seed, Fennel, Yarrow, Geranium

Blends: Dragon Time, Acceptance, Mister, SclarEssence, Lady Sclareol, EndoFlex

Nutritionals: PD 80/20, MultiGreens, Mineral Essence, SuperCal, Thyromin, EndoGize, FemiGen, Estro

MultiGreens: Take 3-8 capsules 2-3 times daily.

Body Care Serums and Creams: Progessence Plus, Prenolone Plus Body Cream

Application and Usage
Topical

You may apply single oils or blends neat or diluted, depending on the oil or oils being used. Please see the instructions at the beginning of this chapter for more information on applying oils to the skin.

- Apply 2-4 drops neat or diluted 50:50 on the lower back and lower abdomen areas 2-3 times daily.
- Apply 2-4 drops on the reproductive Vita Flex points of hands and feet inside of wrists, around the front of the ankles in line with the anklebone, on the lower sides of the anklebone, and along the Achilles tendon 1-3 times daily.
- Rub daily 10 drops Progessence Plus or ½ teaspoon Prenolone Plus Body Cream on lower back area and the lower bowel area near the pubic bone.

Ingestion and Oral

The amount of oil ingested varies with different oils. Whether putting the oils in a capsule or drinking them in a liquid, please refer to the instructions at the beginning of this chapter.

- Take 1 capsule with desired oil 2 times daily.
- Put 2-3 drops of oil in a spoonful of Blue Agave, Yacon Syrup, maple syrup, coconut

oil, milk, etc.
- Put the desired amount of oils in a glass of rice milk, almond milk, goat milk, carrot juice, NingXia Red, or even water and then drink it.

Lack of Libido/Desire (Women)

A woman's sexual desires naturally fluctuate over the years and are affected by a range of physical and emotional factors. Most physical causes of low libido are a result of hormonal imbalance.

Recommendations

Singles: Clary Sage, Nutmeg, Geranium, Ylang Ylang, Amazonian Ylang Ylang, Rose, Idaho Balsam Fir, Lemongrass, Jasmine, Sacred Frankincense, Frankincense, Sage

Blends: SclarEssence, Sensation, Lady Sclareol, Joy, Valor, Valor Roll-On, Live with Passion

Nutritionals: EndoGize, MultiGreens, Estro, Sulfurzyme, PD 80/20, Thyromin, FemiGen

Body Care Creams and Serums: Progessence Plus, Prenolone Plus Body Cream

Ylang Ylang (and Amazonian Ylang Ylang) helps balance sexual emotion and sex drive problems. Its aromatic influence elevates sexual energy and enhances relationships.

Clary Sage can help with lack of sexual desire, particularly with women, by regulating and balancing hormones.

Nutmeg supports the nervous system to help overcome frigidity.

Application and Usage
Inhalation

- Diffuse your choice of oils for ½ hour every 4-6 hours or as desired.
- Put 2-3 drops of your chosen oil in your hands and rub them together, cup your hands over your nose, and inhale throughout the day as needed.
- Put 8-10 drops of oil on a cotton ball or tissue and put it in an air vent in your house, vehicle, hotel room, etc.
- If diffusing while sleeping, set your timer for the desired length of time for automatic shut off.

Topical

You may apply single oils or blends neat or diluted, depending on the oil or oils being used. Please see the instructions at the beginning of this chapter for more information on applying oils to the skin.

- Massage 4-6 drops diluted 50:50 on neck, shoulders, and lower abdomen up to 1-3 times daily or apply 2-3 drops neat to Vita Flex points.

Excessive Sexual Desire (Both Sexes)

Excessive sexual desire is a psychological disorder in which the person is unable to manage his or her sex life and may feel compelled to continually seek sexual activity. Some professionals speculate that it is a form of obsessive-compulsive disorder or a manifestation of the manic phase of bipolar disorder. Excessive sexual desire is best diagnosed and treated by a health-care professional.

Recommendations

Singles: Rose, Myrrh, Marjoram, Valerian, Lavender

Blends: Peace & Calming, Acceptance, Surrender, Joy, Harmony, Gathering

Application and Usage
Inhalation

- Diffuse your choice of oils for ½ hour every 4-6 hours or as desired.
- Put 2-3 drops of your chosen oil in your hands and rub them together, cup your hands over your nose, and inhale throughout the day as needed.
- Put 8-10 drops of oil on a cotton ball or tissue and put it in an air vent in your house,

vehicle, hotel room, etc.

- If diffusing while sleeping, set your timer for the desired length of time for automatic shut off.

Topical

You may apply single oils or blends neat or diluted, depending on the oil or oils being used. Please see the instructions at the beginning of this chapter for more information on applying oils to the skin.

- Massage 4-6 drops diluted 50:50 on neck, shoulders, and lower abdomen up to 1-3 times daily.

SEXUALLY TRANSMITTED DISEASES (See also INFECTIONS)

Sexually transmitted diseases are infections that you can get from having sex with someone who has the infection and are caused by bacteria, parasites, and viruses.

....

Herpes Simplex Type 2

Herpes genitalis is transmitted by sexual contact and results in sores or lesions. Four to seven days after contact with an infected partner, tingling, burning, or persistent itching usually heralds an outbreak. One or two days later, small pimple-like bumps appear over reddened skin. The itching and tingling continue, and the pimples turn into painful blisters, which burst, bleeding with yellowish pus. Five to seven days after the first tingling, scabs form, and healing begins.

Antiviral essential oils have generally been very effective in treating herpes lesions and reducing their onset. Oils such as Melaleuca Alternifolia, Melissa, and Rosemary have been successfully used for this purpose by Daniel Pénoël, MD, in his clinical practice. A study at the University of Buenos Aires found that Sandalwood essential oil inhibited the replication of herpes simplex viruses 1 and 2.41.[35]

Those with herpes should avoid diets high in the amino acid l-arginine, substituting instead l-lysine. Lysine retards the growth of the virus. Foods such as amaranth and plain yogurt are good sources of lysine.

Recommendations

Singles: Melissa, Ravintsara, Dorado Azul Melaleuca Alternifolia, Sandalwood, Blue Cypress, Rosemary

Blends: Melrose, Thieves, Exodus II, Purification

Nutritionals: ImmuPro, Sulfurzyme, Super C, Super C Chewable, ICP, Essentialzyme, Mineral Essence, ComforTone

Ointments and Sprays: Thieves Spray, Rose Ointment

Herpes Blend No. 1 (Topical)

- 4 drops Dorado Azul
- 2 drops Melaleuca Alternifolia
- 1 drop Ravintsara

  Herpes Blend No. 2 (Vaginal)
- 4 drops Dorado Azul
- 3 drops Ravintsara
- 2 drops Sage
- 1 drop Lavender

Application and Usage

Inhalation

- Diffuse your choice of oils for ½ hour every 4-6 hours or as desired.
- Put 2-3 drops of your chosen oil in your hands and rub them together, cup your hands over your nose, and inhale throughout the day as needed.
- Put 8-10 drops of oil on a cotton ball or tissue and put it in an air vent in your house, vehicle, hotel room, etc.
- If diffusing while sleeping, set your timer for the desired length of time for automatic shut off.

Topical

You may apply single oils or blends neat or

diluted, depending on the oil or oils being used. Please see the instructions at the beginning of this chapter for more information on applying oils to the skin.

- Apply single oils or blends neat or diluted, depending on the oils that are used.
- Use Herpes Blend No. 2 diluted 20:80 and put a few drops on a tampon or sanitary pad for nightly applications. If it continues to sting after 5 minutes, remove and change the dilution to 10:90.
- Apply Herpes Blend No.1 on lesions as soon as they appear. Apply 1-2 drops neat 2-3 times daily, alternating between Herpes Blend No. 1 and Melrose each day.
- Receive a Raindrop Technique 1-2 times monthly, as needed.

....

Genital Human Papillomavirus (HPV)

Infection by genital HPV is very common. At least half of the people who are sexually active will contract the virus, yet many will not know it because they will not have any symptoms. There are more than 100 types of HPV, and some types are associated with genital warts, although the warts are not always visible. The longer the virus is in the body, the higher the risk of developing health problems such as cervical cancer or anal cancer.

Recommendations

Singles: Melissa, Dorado Azul, Ravintsara, Palo Santo, Melaleuca Alternifolia, Idaho Tansy, Lavender, Sandalwood
Blends: Melrose, Thieves, ImmuPower, Hope
Nutritionals: ImmuPro, Inner Defense, Life 5
Body Care: Thieves Spray

Application and Usage
Inhalation

- Diffuse your choice of oils for ½ hour every 4-6 hours or as desired.

- Put 2-3 drops of your chosen oil in your hands and rub them together, cup your hands over your nose, and inhale throughout the day as needed.
- Put 8-10 drops of oil on a cotton ball or tissue and put it in an air vent in your house, vehicle, hotel room, etc.
- If diffusing while sleeping, set your timer for the desired length of time for automatic shut off.

Topical

You may apply single oils or blends neat or diluted, depending on the oil or oils being used. Please see the instructions at the beginning of this chapter for more information on applying oils to the skin.

- Apply 1-3 drops neat or dilute 50:50 and apply on location 3-6 times daily.
- Massage 2-4 drops of oil neat on the soles of the feet or on the Vita Flex points of the feet just before bedtime.
- Use Thieves Spray.

Ingestion and Oral

The amount of oil ingested varies with different oils. Whether putting the oils in a capsule or drinking them in a liquid, please refer to the instructions at the beginning of this chapter.

- Take 1 capsule with desired oil diluted 50:50 2 times daily.
- Put 2-3 drops of oil in a spoonful of Blue Agave, Yacon Syrup, maple syrup, coconut oil, milk, etc.
- Put the desired amount of oils in a glass of rice milk, almond milk, goat milk, carrot juice, NingXia Red, or even water and then drink it.

Retention

- Put 2-3 drops of the oil of your choice on a tampon and insert nightly.

Genital Warts/Blisters
(Herpes Simplex Type 2)

Genital warts are a form of viral infection caused by the human papillomavirus (HPV), of which there are more than 100 different types.

One type of HPV virus is among the most common sexually transmitted diseases. Up to 24 million Americans may currently be infected with HPV, which is usually spread through sexual contact. HPV lives only in genital tissue and can later lead to cervical cancer in women.

Recommendations

Singles: Melissa, Dorado Azul, Ravintsara, Palo Santo, Melaleuca Alternifolia, Idaho Tansy, Lavender, Sandalwood
Blends: Melrose, Thieves, ImmuPower, Hope
Nutritionals: ImmuPro, Inner Defense, Life 5
Body Care: Thieves Spray

Application and Usage
Inhalation

- Diffuse your choice of oils for ½ hour every 4-6 hours or as desired.
- Put 2-3 drops of your chosen oil in your hands and rub them together, cup your hands over your nose, and inhale throughout the day as needed.
- Put 8-10 drops of oil on a cotton ball or tissue and put it in an air vent in your house, vehicle, hotel room, etc.
- If diffusing while sleeping, set your timer for the desired length of time for automatic shut off.

Topical

You may apply single oils or blends neat or diluted, depending on the oil or oils being used. Please see the instructions at the beginning of this chapter for more information on applying oils to the skin.

- Apply 1-3 drops neat or dilute 50:50 and apply on location 3-6 times daily.

- Massage 2-4 drops of oil neat on the soles of the feet or on the Vita Flex points of the feet just before bedtime.
- Use Thieves Spray.

Ingestion and Oral

The amount of oil ingested varies with different oils. Whether putting the oils in a capsule or drinking them in a liquid, please refer to the instructions at the beginning of this chapter.

- Take 1 capsule with desired oil diluted 50:50 2 times daily.
- Put 2-3 drops of oil in a spoonful of Blue Agave, Yacon Syrup, maple syrup, coconut oil, milk, etc.
- Put the desired amount of oils in a glass of rice milk, almond milk, goat milk, carrot juice, NingXia Red, or even water and then drink it.

Retention

- Put 2-3 drops of the oil of your choice on a tampon and insert nightly.

Gonorrhea and Syphilis

Gonorrhea is a very common sexually transmitted disease caused by a bacterium *(Neisseria gonorrhoeae)* that can grow and multiply easily in the warm, moist areas of the reproductive tract. It can also grow in the eyes, mouth, throat, and anus.

Syphilis, also a common sexually transmitted disease, is caused by a bacterium *(Treponema pallidum),* and has often been called "the great imitator" because so many of the signs and symptoms are the same as those of other diseases. Sores occur mainly on the external genitals, vagina, anus, or in the rectum. Sores can also occur on the lips and in the mouth.

Note: Seek immediate professional medical attention if you suspect you may have either of these diseases.

Recommendations

Singles: Melissa, Thyme, Mountain Savory, Cinnamon, Oregano

Blends: Melrose, Exodus II, Thieves

Nutritionals: Inner Defense, ImmuPro, Life 5

   Sprays: Thieves Spray

Application and Usage

Topical

You may apply single oils or blends neat or diluted, depending on the oil or oils being used. Please see the instructions at the beginning of this chapter for more information on applying oils to the skin.

Ingestion and Oral

The amount of oil ingested varies with different oils. Whether putting the oils in a capsule or drinking them in a liquid, please refer to the instructions at the beginning of this chapter.

- Take 1 capsule with desired oil 2 times daily for 15 days.
- Put 2-3 drops of oil in a spoonful of Blue Agave, Yacon Syrup, maple syrup, coconut oil, milk, etc.
- Put the desired amount of oils in a glass of rice milk, almond milk, goat milk, carrot juice, NingXia Red, or even water and then drink it.

SHINGLES (HERPES ZOSTER)

Shingles is a short-lived viral infection of the nervous system that starts with fatigue, fever, chills, and intestinal upset. The affected skin areas become sensitive and prone to blistering. One attack usually provides immunity for life. However, for many people, particularly the elderly, pain can persist for months, even years.

Note: Occurrences of shingles around the eyes or on the forehead can cause blindness. Consult an ophthalmologist (eye doctor) immediately if such outbreaks occur.

Recommendations

Singles: Blue Cypress, Elemi, Idaho Tansy, Melaleuca Alternifolia, Oregano, Plectranthus Oregano, Mountain Savory, Sandalwood, Thyme, Peppermint, Ravintsara

Blends: Thieves, Australian Blue, Exodus II

Nutritionals: SuperCal, Sulfurzyme, PD 80/20, MegaCal, Mineral Essence, Essentialzyme

Shingles Blend No. 1

- 10 drops German Chamomile
- 5 drops Lavender
- 4 drops Sandalwood
- 2 drops Geranium

Shingles Blend No. 2

- 10 drops Sandalwood
- 5 drops Blue Cypress
- 4 drops Peppermint
- 2 drops Ravintsara

Application and Usage

Inhalation

- Diffuse your choice of oils for ½ hour every 4-6 hours or as desired.
- Put 2-3 drops of your chosen oil in your hands and rub them together, cup your hands over your nose, and inhale throughout the day as needed.
- Put 8-10 drops of oil on a cotton ball or tissue and put it in an air vent in your house, vehicle, hotel room, etc.
- If diffusing while sleeping, set your timer for the desired length of time for automatic shut off.

Topical

You may apply single oils or blends neat or diluted, depending on the oil or oils being used. Please see the instructions at the beginning of this chapter for more information on applying oils to the skin.

- Apply 6-10 drops neat or diluted 50:50 on affected area, back of the neck, and down the spine 1-3 times daily.

- Apply a compress alternating warm and cold on the spine 1-3 times daily.
- Layering in Raindrop Technique style, apply 3-4 drops each of Oregano (or Plectranthus Oregano), Mountain Savory, and Thyme along the spine.
- Apply 15-20 drops V-6 Vegetable Oil Complex to the spine, massage briefly over the other oils, cover the skin with a dry towel, and apply a warm pack for 15-20 minutes.
- **Note:** Be cautious about warming. If the back becomes too hot, remove the warm pack immediately and add V-6 Vegetable Oil Complex to cool.
- Remove the warm pack and towel, and then layer 4-8 drops each of Melaleuca Alternifolia, Elemi, and Peppermint along the spine.
- Put the dry towel back over the skin and apply an ice pack for 30 minutes.

SHOCK
(See also FAINTING, BURNS)

Shock can be described as a state of profound depression of the vital processes associated with reduced blood volume and pressure. The blood rushes to the vital organs after trauma.

It may be caused by the sudden stimulation of the nerves and convulsive contraction of the muscles caused by the discharge of electricity. Other causes include sudden trauma, terror, surprise, horror, or disgust.

Symptoms or signs

- Irregular breathing
- Low blood pressure
- Dilated pupils
- Cold and sweaty skin
- Weak and rapid pulse
- Dry mouth
- Muscle weakness
- Dizziness or fainting

Any injury that results in the sudden loss of substantial amounts of fluids can trigger shock.

Shock can also be caused by allergic reactions (anaphylactic shock), infections in the blood (septic shock), or emotional trauma (neurogenic shock).

To help someone in shock while waiting for first responders, first cover the victim with a blanket and elevate the feet, unless there is a head or upper torso injury. Inhaling any one of many different essential oils can also help—especially in cases of emotional shock.

Recommendations

Singles: Peppermint, Idaho Balsam Fir, Basil, Sacred Frankincense, Frankincense, Eucalyptus Blue, Dorado Azul, Cardamom, Rosemary, Melissa, Ocotea

Blends: Trauma Life, Clarity, 3 Wise Men, Valor, Valor Roll-On, R.C., Harmony, Present Time

Application and Usage
Inhalation

- Diffuse your choice of oils for ½ hour every 4-6 hours or as desired.
- Put 2-3 drops of your chosen oil in your hands and rub them together, cup your hands over your nose, and inhale throughout the day as needed.
- Put 8-10 drops of oil on a cotton ball or tissue and put it in an air vent in your house, vehicle, hotel room, etc.
- If diffusing while sleeping, set your timer for the desired length of time for automatic shut off.

Topical

You may apply single oils or blends neat or diluted, depending on the oil or oils being used. Please see the instructions at the beginning of this chapter for more information on applying oils to the skin.

- When applying essential oil to the temples, be careful to not get the oil too close to the eyes.
- Apply 1-2 drops diluted 50:50 on temples, back of the neck, and under the nose neat as desired.

- You may also apply 2-3 drops on the Vita Flex points of the feet.
- Applying a single drop under the nose is helpful and refreshing.

SINUS INFECTIONS

A sinus infection is an inflammation of the sinuses and nasal passages. Sinus problems are among the most common chronic ailments.

....

Nasopharyngitis

Nasopharyngitis is an inflammatory condition of the mucous membranes of the back of the nasal cavity where it connects to the throat and the Eustachian tubes.

Recommendations

Singles: Peppermint, Ravintsara, Eucalyptus Blue, Thyme, Rosemary, Blue Cypress, Dorado Azul, Eucalyptus Radiata

Blends: Raven, R.C., Exodus II, Thieves, Breathe Again Roll-On

Nutritionals: Super C, Super C Chewable, ImmuPro, Digest & Cleanse, Inner Defense

Oral Care: Thieves Fresh Essence Plus Mouthwash

Application and Usage
Inhalation

- Diffuse your choice of oils for ½ hour every 4-6 hours or as desired.
- Put 2-3 drops of your chosen oil in your hands and rub them together, cup your hands over your nose, and inhale throughout the day as needed.
- Put 8-10 drops of oil on a cotton ball or tissue and put it in an air vent in your house, vehicle, hotel room, etc.
- If diffusing while sleeping, set your timer for the desired length of time for automatic shut off.

Topical

You may apply single oils or blends neat or diluted, depending on the oil or oils being used. Please see the instructions at the beginning of this chapter for more information on applying oils to the skin.

- Apply 1-2 drops diluted 50:50 just under jawbone on right and left sides 4-8 times daily.
- You may also apply 2-3 drops on the Vita Flex points of the feet

Oral

- Gargle 2-5 times daily with Thieves Fresh Essence Plus Mouthwash or with water that contains 1-2 drops of another oil.
- Put 1 drop of Thieves or Melaleuca Alternifolia at the very back of the tongue and hold it in the mouth, mixing it with saliva for several minutes, and then swallow. This can be very effective if started at the very first indication of infection and repeated 3-4 times for the first hour, then once an hour until symptoms subside.
- Spray inside mouth with Thieves Spray as often as desired.
- Put 1 drop of Exodus II on tongue and swish it around in your mouth before swallowing.

Special Note: In most sinus infections, including nasopharyngitis, rhinitis, sinus congestion, and sinusitis, the nasal irrigation regimen can be extremely effective.

....

Sinus Congestion

Sinus congestion is extremely annoying, and symptoms can last for several days. The most common symptom is difficulty breathing because of blocked nasal passages due to excessive mucus. As a result, the sinuses become inflamed and produce other symptoms such as headaches, fatigue, coughing, sinus pressure or pain, and loss of smell.

Recommendations

Singles: Peppermint, Dorado Azul, Eucalyptus Globulus, Eucalyptus Blue, Palo Santo, Eucalyptus Radiata, Ravintsara, Myrrh, Idaho

Balsam Fir, Thyme, Fennel, Rosemary

Blends: DiGize, Raven, Thieves, Exodus II, Breathe Again Roll-On, Melrose, R.C., Christmas Spirit

Nutritionals: Super C, Super C Chewable, ImmuPro, Thieves Spray

Oral Care: Thieves AromaBright Toothpaste, KidScents Slique Toothpaste, Thieves Lozenges (Hard/Soft), Thieves Fresh Essence Plus Mouthwash, Thieves Spray

Application and Usage
Inhalation

- Diffuse Eucalyptus Blue, Raven, or your choice of oils for ½ hour every 4-6 hours or as desired.
- Put 2-3 drops of your chosen oil in your hands and rub them together, cup your hands over your nose, and inhale throughout the day as needed.
- Put 8-10 drops of oil on a cotton ball or tissue and put it in an air vent in your house, vehicle, hotel room, etc.
- If diffusing while sleeping, set your timer for the desired length of time for automatic shut off.

Topical

You may apply single oils or blends neat or diluted, depending on the oil or oils being used. Please see the instructions at the beginning of this chapter for more information on applying oils to the skin.

- Apply 1-2 drops neat on the temples and back of the neck, as desired.
- Applying a single drop of chosen oil or a swipe of Breathe Again Roll-On under the nose is helpful and refreshing.
- Dilute 50:50 and apply on location 3-6 times daily.
- Massage 2-4 drops of oil neat on the soles of the feet just before bedtime. Children love it.

Nasal Irrigation Regimen *(see box)*

- Place a warm compress with 1-2 drops of chosen oil on the back.

Ingestion and Oral

The amount of oil ingested varies with different oils. Whether putting the oils in a capsule or drinking them in a liquid, please refer to the instructions at the beginning of this chapter.

- Take 1 capsule with desired oil 2 times daily.
- Put 2-3 drops of oil in a spoonful of Blue Agave, Yacon Syrup, maple syrup, coconut oil, milk, etc.
- Put the desired amount of oils in a glass of rice milk, almond milk, goat milk, carrot juice, NingXia Red, or even water and then drink it.
- Gargle with Thieves Fresh Essence Plus Mouthwash 4-6 times daily, as desired.

....

Sinusitis / Rhinitis

Sinusitis is an inflammation of the sinuses and nasal passages. It can cause pressure in the eyes, cheek area, nose, or on one side of the head. A person with a sinus infection may also have a headache, cough, fever, bad breath, and nasal congestion.

Essential oils such as Eucalyptus Radiata and Ravintsara strengthen the respiratory system, open the pulmonary tract, and fight respiratory infection.

Recommendations

Singles: Eucalyptus Blue, Peppermint, Eucalyptus Radiata, Ravintsara, Melaleuca Alternifolia, Idaho Balsam Fir, Thyme, Fennel, Rosemary

Blends: R.C., Melrose, Raven, Thieves, Exodus II, Breathe Again Roll-On

Nutritionals: Super C, Super C Chewable, ImmuPro, Inner Defense

Oral Care: Thieves AromaBright Toothpaste, Thieves Dentarome Plus Toothpaste, Thieves Dentarome Ultra Toothpaste, Thieves Lozenges (Hard/Soft), Thieves Fresh Essence Plus Mouthwash, Thieves Spray

Application and Usage
Inhalation
- Diffuse your choice of oils for ½ hour every 4-6 hours or as desired.
- Put 2-3 drops of your chosen oil in your hands and rub them together, cup your hands over your nose, and inhale 3-8 times throughout the day as needed.
- Put 8-10 drops of oil on a cotton ball or tissue and put it in an air vent in your house, vehicle, hotel room, etc.
- If diffusing while sleeping, set your timer for the desired length of time for automatic shut off.

Topical
You may apply single oils or blends neat or diluted, depending on the oil or oils being used. Please see the instructions at the beginning of this chapter for more information on applying oils to the skin.

- Massage 1-3 drops neat on forehead, nose, cheeks, lower throat, chest, and upper back 3-5 times daily. Be careful not to get oils in or near eyes or eyelids.
- Apply 1-2 drops neat on temples and back of neck as desired.
- Apply 1-3 drops on the Vita Flex points of feet 2-4 times daily.
- Use the Raindrop Technique 1-2 times weekly.
- Bath salts: Mix 4-5 drops of oil with 1 cup of salt in hot water to dissolve salts. Pour into bathtub and then soak for 15-20 minutes or until water cools.
- Place a warm compress with 1-2 drops of chosen oil on the back.

Nasal Irrigation Regimen *(see box above)*
Ingestion and Oral
The amount of oil ingested varies with different oils. Whether putting the oils in a capsule or drinking them in a liquid, please refer to the instructions at the beginning of this chapter.
- Take 1 capsule with desired oil 2 times daily.

Nasal Irrigation Regimen:

Rosemary and Melaleuca Alternifolia oils can be used in a saline solution for very effective nasal irrigation that clears and decongests sinuses. As recommended by Daniel Pénoël, MD, the saline solution is prepared as follows:

- 10 drops Rosemary
- 6 drops Melaleuca Alternifolia
- 8 tablespoons ultra-fine salt

The essential oils are mixed thoroughly in the fine salt and stored in a sealed container. For each nasal irrigation session, 1 teaspoon of this salt mixture is dissolved into 1½ cups distilled water.

This solution is then placed in the tank of an oral irrigator or neti pot to irrigate the nasal cavities, which is done while bending over a sink. This application has brought surprisingly positive results in treating latent sinusitis and other nasal congestion problems.[26]

- Put 2-3 drops of oil in a spoonful of Blue Agave, Yacon Syrup, maple syrup, coconut oil, milk, etc.
- Put the desired amount of oils in a glass of rice milk, almond milk, goat milk, carrot juice, NingXia Red, or even water and then drink it.
- Gargle 2-6 times daily with Thieves Fresh Essence Plus Mouthwash.

SKIN DISORDERS AND PROBLEMS
Essential oils can have powerful antioxidant and antibacterial benefits for the skin. Essential oils used on the skin are often combined with a vegetable carrier oil to:

- Slow evaporation, allowing more time for the oils to penetrate the skin.
- Maintain the lipid barrier of the skin because most essential oils will tend to dry the skin.
- Enhance the effect of the essential oils because many oils work well synergistically in a vegetable oil. Many skin conditions are related to dysfunctions of the liver. It may be necessary to cleanse, stimulate, and condition the liver and colon for 30-90 days before the skin begins to improve.

Abscesses and Boils

Skin abscesses are small pockets of pus that collect under the skin, usually caused by a bacterial or fungal infection.

Any number of essential oils may help reduce inflammation and combat infection, helping to bring an abscess or boil to a head so that the pus will come out and the healing can begin.

Recommendations

Singles: Oregano, Plectranthus Oregano, Clove, Myrrh, Galbanum, Melaleuca Alternifolia, Sacred Frankincense, Frankincense, Lavender, Rosemary, Thyme, Patchouli

Blends: Melrose, Purification, Thieves

Nutritionals: JuvaTone, ComforTone, Essentialzyme, Digest & Cleanse, Inner Defense

Application and Usage

Topical

You may apply single oils or blends neat or diluted, depending on the oil or oils being used. Please see the instructions at the beginning of this chapter for more information on applying oils to the skin.

- Apply 2-3 drops neat (undiluted), depending on which oil you choose.
- Dilute the oil you choose 50:50 with V-6 Vegetable Oil Complex and apply on location 3-6 times daily or as needed.

Acne

Acne results from an excess accumulation of dirt and sebum (oil) produced in the follicles and pores of the skin. As the pores and hair follicles become congested, bacteria begin to feed on the sebum. This leads to inflammation, infection, and the formation of a pimple or a blackhead around the hair follicle.

One of the most common forms of acne, *Acne vulgaris,* occurs primarily in adolescents due to hormone imbalances that stimulate the production of sebum.

Acne may be caused by a hormone imbalance, poor diet, and the use of chemicals found in cleaning products, soaps, cosmetics, lotions, and creams.

Stress may also play a role. According to research conducted by Dr. Toyoda in Japan, acne and other skin problems are a direct result of physical and emotional stress.[36] Essential oils are outstanding for treating acne because of their ability to dissolve sebum, kill bacteria, and preserve the acid mantle of the skin. Natural hormone creams such as Prenolone Plus Body Cream or the gentle Progessence Plus may help with hormone imbalance problems directly affecting the skin.

Recommendations

Singles: Melaleuca Alternifolia, Geranium, Vetiver, Sandalwood, Patchouli, Lavender, German or Roman Chamomile, Cedarwood, Eucalyptus Radiata, Melaleuca Quinquenervia (Niaouli)

Blends: Melrose, Purification, Harmony

Nutritionals: Mineral Essence, Detoxzyme, MultiGreens, ICP, ComforTone, Essentialzyme, Ningxia Wolfberries (Dried), Omega-Gize³, Digest & Cleanse, Balance Complete

Massage Oils, Creams, and Soaps: Boswellia Wrinkle Cream, A·R·T Foaming Cleanser, A·R·T Purifying Toner, Satin Facial Scrub

(Mint), Melaleuca-Geranium Bar Soap, Prenolone Plus Body Cream, Essential Beauty Serum

Application and Usage
Topical

You may apply single oils or blends neat or diluted, depending on the oil or oils being used. Please see the instructions at the beginning of this chapter for more information on applying oils to the skin.

- Gently massage 3-5 drops neat or diluted with V-6 Vegetable Oil Complex into the oily areas 1-3 times daily. Alternate the oils daily for maximum effect.

....

Blisters

Blisters are caused when fluid is trapped under the skin caused by physical injury, chemical burns, sunburns, and microbial infestation caused by fungal and viral diseases such as herpes simplex, athletes foot, etc.

Recommendations

Singles: Melaleuca Alternifolia, Myrrh, Lavender, Roman or German Chamomile, Spikenard, Helichrysum
Blends: Melrose, Purification, Valor
Body Care (Creams, Ointments, and Sprays): LavaDerm Cooling Mist, Rose Ointment, Genesis Hand & Body Lotion

Application and Usage
Topical

You may apply single oils or blends neat or diluted, depending on the oil or oils being used. Please see the instructions at the beginning of this chapter for more information on applying oils to the skin.

- Dilute 50:50 and apply to blistered area 3-6 times daily.
- Spray LavaDerm as often as every 30 minutes as desired.
- Gently apply a little Rose Ointment or lotion to keep skin soft and moist.

....

Boils

Boils and carbuncles (a group of boils) are caused by bacterial infection that creates a pus-filled hair follicle. They can be easily treated with antiseptic essential oils, including Melaleuca Alternifolia and Clove.

Recommendations

Singles: Melaleuca Alternifolia, Myrrh, Clove, Thyme, Oregano
Blends: Melrose, Purification, Thieves

Application and Usage
Topical

You may apply single oils or blends neat or diluted, depending on the oil or oils being used. Please see the instructions at the beginning of this chapter for more information on applying oils to the skin.

- Dilute 2-3 drops of any oil above 50:50 and apply on location 3-6 times daily.

Burns
(See also Shock)

There are three types of burns:

First-degree burns only damage the outer layer of the skin. Sunburn is typically a first-degree burn.

Second-degree burns damage both the outer layer and the underlying layer known as the dermis, manifested by blisters.

Third-degree burns not only destroy or damage skin but can even damage underlying tissues.

Burns can be caused by sunlight, chemicals, electricity, radiation, and heat. Thermal burns are the most common type.

Aloe vera gel (contained in LavaDerm) is used extensively in the treatment of burns and has been studied for its anti-inflammatory and tissue-regenerating properties.

Helichrysum, Lavender, Idaho Balsam Fir, and Frankincense oils support tissue regeneration and reduce scarring and skin discoloration.

Severe burns can result in dehydration and mineral loss. Inflammation often accompanies burns, so dietary protocols should be used to lessen inflammation.

If the burn is large or severe, the individual may go into shock. Inhaling oils may help reduce the shock.

After a burn has started to heal and is drying and cracking, use Rose Ointment or a body lotion with a few drops of Lavender oil to keep skin soft and to promote faster healing.

Seek medical attention for serious burns as necessary.

FIRST-DEGREE BURNS (Sunburn)

The best prevention for sunburn is to avoid prolonged exposure to the sun. When you do go outdoors, always wear sun block or lotion with a SPF greater than 15—especially during the summer and when you expect to be outdoors for a prolonged period of time.

Certain natural vegetable oils and essential oils have been found to provide some protection against the sun. Sesame oil can block or reduce about 30 percent of the burning rays, coconut and olive oils can reduce about 20 percent, and *aloe vera* inhibits about 20 percent. Helichrysum essential oil has been researched for its ability to effectively screen out some of the sun's rays.

Chérie Ross's Sunscreen Blend No. 1
- 10 drops Helichrysum
- 5 drops Lavender
- 3 drops Roman Chamomile
- 1 oz. Sesame Oil
- ½ oz. Coconut Oil
- ½ oz. Olive Oil

Mix and apply before going out in the sun.

Chérie Ross's Sunscreen Blend No. 2
- 30 drops Lavender
- 4 oz. Avocado Oil

Mix and apply before going out in the sun. In the event of a sunburn, LavaDerm Cooling Mist and Lavender, Spikenard, and Idaho Balsam Fir essential oils can offer excellent pain-relieving and healing benefits.

Recommendations

Singles: Spikenard, Lavender, Idaho Balsam Fir, Helichrysum, Rose, Melaleuca Quinquenervia (Niaouli), German Chamomile, Vetiver

Blends: LavaDerm Cooling Mist, Gentle Baby, Australian Blue, Melrose, Valor, Valor Roll-On

Nutritionals: Longevity Softgels, Sulfurzyme, MegaCal, OmegaGize[3], Rose Ointment

Application and Usage
Inhalation
- Diffuse your choice of oils for ½ hour every 4-6 hours or as desired.
- Put 2-3 drops of your chosen oil in your

hands and rub them together, cup your hands over your nose, and inhale throughout the day as needed.

- Put 8-10 drops of oil on a cotton ball or tissue and put it in an air vent in your house, vehicle, hotel room, etc.
- If diffusing while sleeping, set your timer for the desired length of time for automatic shut off.

Topical

You may apply single oils or blends neat or diluted, depending on the oil or oils being used. Please see the instructions at the beginning of this chapter for more information on applying oils to the skin.

- For fast relief of first-degree burns, spray burn immediately with LavaDerm Cooling Mist and continue misting as necessary to cool the area. Spray as often as needed for the first several hours and follow with 2-3 drops of lavender, spikenard, or Idaho balsam fir oil.
- Apply 1-3 drops neat or diluted 50:50 on burn location to cool tissue and reduce inflammation.
- Apply 3-6 times daily or as needed.

SECOND-DEGREE BURNS (Blisters)

Spray burn immediately with LavaDerm Cooling Mist and continue misting when necessary to cool the area. Spray as often as needed for the first several hours and follow with 2-3 drops of Lavender, Spikenard, or Idaho Balsam Fir oil.

- Thereafter, apply LavaDerm every 15-30 minutes during the first day. Apply 2-4 drops of Lavender, Spikenard, or Niaouli oils as needed immediately after each LavaDerm misting.
- On days 2 through 5, mist every hour and follow with 2-4 drops Lavender oil or Niaouli oil.
- Continue using LavaDerm 3 to 6 times daily

The Deadly Dehydration of Burns

Burns tend to swell and blister because of fluid loss from the damaged blood vessels. This is why it is important to keep the burn well hydrated and to drink plenty of water.

In cases of serious burns, fluid loss can become so severe that it sends the victim into shock and requires intravenous transfusions of saline solution to bring up blood pressure.

---

until healed. Apply Rose Ointment to keep tissue soft.

- Mineral Essence: Put 2 droppers full in 3 liters of water and drink throughout the day.

THIRD-DEGREE BURNS

Spray LavaDerm Cooling Mist immediately to hydrate the skin.

Seek medical attention immediately.

....

Chapped, Cracked, or Dry Skin

Dry skin results from loss of the protective lipid layer on the skin surface. It results from exposure to low humidity environments and is often more prevalent during the winter. Dry skin may also crack, creating an opportunity for infection.

Recommendations

Singles: Neroli, Rose, Cedarwood, Roman Chamomile, Palmarosa, Geranium, Lavender, Spikenard, Myrrh, Sandalwood

Body Care Creams, Ointments, and Serums: A·R·T Night Reconstructor, Essential Beauty Serum for Dry Skin, Tender Tush, Sandalwood Moisture Cream, Rose Ointment, KidScents Lotion

Lip Treatment: Lavender Lip Balm, Cinnamint Lip Balm, Grapefruit Lip Balm

Application and Usage
Topical

You may apply single oils or blends neat or diluted, depending on the oil or oils being used. Please see the instructions at the beginning of this chapter for more information on applying oils to the skin.

- Apply 2-3 drops of oil diluted 20:80 in a natural, unperfumed lotion base (V-6 Vegetable Oil Complex or avocado oil) or other high-grade, emollient oil; apply on location as often as needed.
- Combine 3-5 drops of essential oils with 1 teaspoon of Sensation, KidScents Lotion, or Genesis Hand & Body Lotion to create a very effective lotion for rehydrating the skin of chapped hands and maintaining the natural pH balance of the skin.
- Bath and shower gels, such as Dragon Time, Evening Peace, Morning Start, and Sensation are formulated to help balance the acid mantle of the skin. The bar soaps are rich in moisturizers.

....

Clogged Pores

Most skin blemishes begin as clogged pores. To have clean pores, you should maintain a regular skin-care routine. If you keep your pores unclogged and clean, you will have fewer breakouts and more beautiful skin.

Recommendations

Singles: Lemon, Orange, Geranium, Cypress, Lavender
Blends: Melrose, Purification, Inner Child
Skin Care: A·R·T Gentle Foaming Cleanser, Essential Beauty Serum (Acne-Prone Skin), Satin Facial Scrub, Mint

Application and Usage
Topical

You may apply single oils or blends neat or diluted, depending on the oil or oils being used.

Please see the instructions at the beginning of this chapter for more information on applying oils to the skin.

- Apply 2-4 drops neat to affected area and gently remove with cotton ball.
- Use A·R·T Purifying Toner and moisturizing bar soaps.
- Satin Facial Scrub, Mint is a gentle exfoliator designed to clarify skin and reduce acne. If its texture is too abrasive for your skin, mix it with Orange Blossom Facial Wash. This is excellent for those with severe or mild acne.
- Spread scrub over face and let dry for perhaps five minutes to draw out impurities, purifying and toning the skin at the same time. Put a hot towel over face for greater penetration.
- Wash off with warm water by gently patting skin with warm face cloth. If you do not have time to let the mask dry, gently massage in a circular motion for 30 seconds, then rinse. Afterward, apply Sandalwood Moisture Cream. This also works well underneath foundation makeup.

....

Cuts, Scrapes, and Wounds

When selecting essential oils for surface injuries, determine the needs of the entire body, not just of the cut. Think through the cause and type of injury and select oils for each aspect of the trauma. For instance, a wound could encompass muscle damage, nerve damage, ligament damage, inflammation, infection, bone injury, fever, and possibly an emotion. Therefore, select an oil or blend that is specific to each need.

Recommendations

Single Oils: Lavender, Melaleuca Alternifolia, Helichrysum, Rosemary, Eucalyptus Globulus, Dorado Azul, Cypress, Wintergreen, Thyme, Oregano, Plectranthus Oregano, German Chamomile, Mountain Savory, Sacred Frankincense, Frankincense, Myrrh, Spikenard, Eucalyptus Blue

Blends: Melrose, The Gift, 3 Wise Men, Aroma Siez, Aroma Life, Purification, Trauma Life, Peace & Calming, R.C., RutaVaLa, RutaVa-La Roll-On, Stress Away Roll-On, Tranquil Roll-On,

Sprays: Thieves Spray, LavaDerm Cooling Mist

Bruise and Scrape Blend (May be used on infants and children)

- 4 drops Lavender
- 1 drop Cistus
- 1 drop Myrrh

Infected Cut Blend

- 7 drops Geranium
- 5 drops Myrrh
- 3 drops Melaleuca Alternifolia

Application and Usage
Topical

You may apply single oils or blends neat or diluted, depending on the oil or oils being used. Please see the instructions at the beginning of this chapter for more information on applying oils to the skin.

- Dilute recommended oils 50:50 and apply 2-6 drops on location 1-4 times daily.
- Apply LavaDerm Cooling Mist to the affected area.

Note: Peppermint can be helpful in treating wounds but may sting when applied to an open wound. To reduce discomfort, dilute with Lavender or mix in a sealing ointment before applying. When applied to a wound or cut that has a scab, a diluted Peppermint blend will soothe, cool, and reduce inflammation in damaged tissue.

TO DISINFECT

Recommendations

Singles: Melaleuca Alternifolia, Oregano, Plectranthus Oregano, Lemongrass, Melissa, Thyme, Mountain Savory

Blends: Thieves, Melrose, Purification, Citrus Fresh

First Aid Spray

First Aid Recipe:

- 5 drops Lavender
- 3 drops Melaleuca Alternifolia
- 2 drops Dorado Azul

Mix the recipe above thoroughly in ½ teaspoon of salt. Add this to 8 oz. of distilled water, shake vigorously, and pour into a spray bottle. Spray minor cuts and wounds before applying bandage. Repeat 2-3 times daily for 3 days. Continue the healing process by applying 1-2 drops of Melaleuca Alternifolia oil to the wound daily for the next few days. Apply Rose Ointment or Tender Tush to keep the scab soft and to help prevent scarring.

Animal Scents works extremely well for any animal, and it is also very effective for any person who wishes to cover a large area such as the bottom of the feet. When working in rough conditions such as the cold outdoors, construction and building, or anything that is abrasive to the hands, add a few drops of the recipe to a tablespoon of Animal Scents or Rose Ointment and use it throughout the day to relieve the pain and ache of small cuts and scrapes on the skin.

Application and Usage
Topical

You may apply single oils or blends neat or diluted, depending on the oil or oils being used. Please see the instructions at the beginning of this chapter for more information on applying oils to the skin.

- Apply Thieves Spray.
- Dilute recommended oils 50:50 and apply 2-4 drops on the wound 2-5 times daily.

Essential Oils Skin Rejuvenation

Rejuvenate and heal:
- Rose, Sandalwood, Myrrh, Frankincense, Vetiver

Prevent and retard wrinkles:
- Lavender, Spikenard, Myrrh, Frankincense, Sandalwood

Regenerate:
- Geranium, Helichrysum, Spikenard, Melrose Sandalwood

Restore skin elasticity
- Sandalwood with Lavender
- Ylang Ylang with Lavender
- Patchouli with Ylang Ylang

Combat premature aging of the skin
Mix the following recipe into 1 tablespoon V-6 Vegetable Oil Complex, any high-grade vegetable oil, or unscented skin lotion and apply on location 2 times daily.

Skin Rejuvenating Recipe:
- 6 drops Sandalwood
- 4 drops Geranium
- 3 drops Lavender
- 2 drops Sacred Frankincense

TO PROMOTE HEALING

Recommendations

Singles: Sacred Frankincense, Frankincense, Sandalwood, Melissa, Lavender, Idaho Balsam Fir, Palo Santo, Patchouli, Melaleuca Quinquenervia (Niaouli), Myrrh, Helichrysum, Idaho Tansy

Blends: Melrose, Purification, Gentle Baby, Valor

Application and Usage
Topical

You may apply single oils or blends neat or diluted, depending on the oil or oils being used. Please see the instructions at the beginning of

this chapter for more information on applying oils to the skin.

- Dilute recommended oils 50:50 and apply 2-4 drops on the wound 2-5 times daily.

TO REDUCE BLEEDING

Recommendations

Singles: Helichrysum, Cistus, Cypress, Lemon, Geranium, Vetiver, Valerian, Sacred Frankincense, Frankincense, Myrrh

Blends: PanAway, Relieve It, Aroma Siez

Application and Usage
Topical

You may apply single oils or blends neat or diluted, depending on the oil or oils being used. Please see the instructions at the beginning of this chapter for more information on applying oils to the skin.

- Apply a cold compress to the affected area 1-2 times until bleeding stops.

Wound Compress Blend
- 5 drops Geranium
- 5 drops Lemon
- 5 drops German Chamomile
- 2 drops Helichrysum

TO REDUCE SCARRING

Recommendations

Singles: Sacred Frankincense, Frankincense, Lavender, Sandalwood, Cistus, Geranium, Helichrysum, Myrrh

Blends: Gentle Baby, Valor, Melrose

Scar Prevention Blend No. 1
- 3 drops Sandalwood
- 3 drops Sacred Frankincense or Frankincense
- 2 drops Spikenard
- 1 drop Vetiver

Scar Prevention Blend No. 2
- 10 drops Geranium
- 8 drops Helichrysum
- 6 drops Lavender
- 4 drops Patchouli

Application and Usage
Topical

You may apply single oils or blends neat or diluted, depending on the oil or oils being used. Please see the instructions at the beginning of this chapter for more information on applying oils to the skin.

- Dilute recommended oils 50:50 and apply 2-4 drops on the wound 2-5 times daily.

....

Diaper Rash

Dilute all oils when being used for babies. Just 1-2 drops mixed in Tender Tush or Rose Ointment are sufficient for using on diaper rash.

Recommendations

Singles: Lavender, Helichrysum, German Chamomile, Cypress
Blends: Gentle Baby, Purification, Valor
Skin Care: Tender Tush, Rose Ointment, ClaraDerm, LavaDerm Cooling Mist

Application and Usage
Topical

You may apply single oils or blends neat or diluted, depending on the oil or oils being used. Please see the instructions at the beginning of this chapter for more information on applying oils to the skin.

- Apply 1-2 drops diluted 50:50 and/or ointments on location 2-4 times daily during diaper changes.

....

Eczema/Dermatitis

Eczema and dermatitis are both inflammations of the skin and are most often due to allergies, but they also can be a sign of liver disease.

Dermatitis usually results from external factors such as sunburn or contact with poison ivy, metals from wristwatch, earrings, jewelry, etc.; internal factors such as irritant chemicals, soaps, and shampoos; or allergies from gluten and lactose intolerance.

Melaleuca (*M. alternifolia*—tea tree)

During World War II, melaleuca, or tea tree oil (*Melaleuca alternifolia*), was found to have very strong antibacterial properties and worked well in preventing infection in open wounds.

Melrose is a blend containing two types of Melaleuca oil (*M. alternifolia*) and Niaouli (*M. quinquenervia*), plus Rosemary and Clove, making it an exceptional antiseptic and tissue regenerator.

In both dermatitis and eczema, the skin can become red, flaky, and itchy. Small blisters may form, and if they are broken by scratching, they can become infected.

Recommendations

Singles: Lavender, German Chamomile, Myrrh, Blue Cypress, Roman Chamomile, Geranium
Blends: JuvaCleanse, Purification, Melrose, Australian Blue
Nutritionals: Detoxzyme, ICP, ComforTone, Essentialzyme, JuvaTone, JuvaPower, Essentialzymes-4
Body Care: Rose Ointment, KidScents Tender Tush, Regenolone Moisturizing Cream

Application and Usage
Topical

You may apply single oils or blends neat or diluted, depending on the oil or oils being used. Please see the instructions at the beginning of this chapter for more information on applying oils to the skin.

- Apply 1-2 drops diluted 50:50 on location as needed.

Fungal Skin Infections

Fungi and yeast feed on decomposing or dead tissues that exist everywhere such as in our stomachs, on our skin, on food, outside in the lawn, in the garden, on pets, etc. When kept under control, the yeast and fungi populating our bodies are harmless and digest what our bodies cannot or do not use.

When we feed the naturally occurring fungi in our bodies with simple sugars, the fungi are more likely to grow out of control. This condition is known as systemic candidiasis, which invades the blood, gastrointestinal tract, and tissues.

Recommendations

Singles: Melaleuca Alternifolia, Lemongrass, Oregano, Plectranthus Oregano, Lavender, Patchouli

Blends: Melrose, Purification

Skin Care: ClaraDerm

Antifungal Skin Blend
- 10 drops Patchouli
- 5 drops Lemongrass
- 4 drops Melaleuca Quinquenervia (Niaouli)
- 2 drops Melaleuca Alternifolia

Nutritionals: Life 5, Digest & Cleanse, ICP, ComforTone, Essentialzyme, Mineral Essence

Application and Usage
Topical

You may apply single oils or blends neat or diluted, depending on the oil or oils being used. Please see the instructions at the beginning of this chapter for more information on applying oils to the skin.
- Apply 2-4 drops of oil diluted 50:50 on location 3-5 times daily.

Itching

Itching can be due to dry skin, impaired liver function, insects, allergies, or overexposure to chemicals or sunlight.

Recommendations

Singles: Peppermint, Patchouli, Lavender, Oregano, Plectranthus Oregano, Vetiver, Nutmeg, German Chamomile

Blends: Aroma Siez, Purification, Melrose, Thieves, DiGize

Nutritionals: Digest & Cleanse, Life 5, JuvaFlex, JuvaTone, ComforTone, Essentialzyme, Detoxzyme, ICP, JuvaPower

Body Care Ointments and Creams: KidScents Tender Tush, Rose Ointment, Regenolone Moisturizing Cream, LavaDerm Cooling Mist, ClaraDerm

Application and Usage
Topical

You may apply single oils or blends neat or diluted, depending on the oil or oils being used. Please see the instructions at the beginning of this chapter for more information on applying oils to the skin.
- Apply 1-2 drops neat on location several times daily as needed.
- Dilute 50/50 and apply on location 3-6 times daily.
- Spray LavaDerm Cooling Mist or ClaraDerm if condition is evident on the skin.

Moles

Moles appear as small, dark brown spots; come in many colors; and can develop virtually anywhere on your body. Most moles are harmless, but monitoring them is important in detecting skin cancer.

Recommendations

Singles: Oregano, Plectranthus Oregano, Thyme, Melaleuca Alternifolia

Blends: Melrose, Purification

Application and Usage
Topical

You may apply single oils or blends neat or diluted, depending on the oil or oils being used. Please see the instructions at the beginning of this chapter for more information on applying oils to the skin.

- To dry up moles, apply 1-2 drops of Oregano neat (undiluted) on the mole 2-3 times daily.
- Other oils may be used that may also show benefit.

....

Poison Oak/Poison Ivy/Poison Sumac

Poison ivy, poison oak, and poison sumac are plants that contain an irritating, oily sap called urushiol, which triggers an allergic reaction when it comes into contact with skin. An itchy rash can appear within hours of exposure or several days later and usually develops into oozing blisters.

Recommendations

Singles: Peppermint, Myrrh, Patchouli, Vetiver, Eucalyptus Blue, German Chamomile, Roman Chamomile, Rose, Lemon, Idaho Tansy, Melaleuca Alternifolia, Rosemary, Basil, Spikenard

Blends: Melrose, Purification, R.C., Juva-Cleanse

Nutritionals: Detoxzyme, ComforTone, Mineral Essence, Digest & Cleanse, ICP, JuvaPower, OmegaGize³

Body Creams, Ointments, Spray: Rose Ointment, KidScents Tender Tush, Sandalwood Moisture Cream, Thieves Spray, LavaDerm Cooling Mist, ClaraDerm

Application and Usage
Topical

You may apply single oils or blends neat or diluted, depending on the oil or oils being used. Please see the instructions at the beginning of this chapter for more information on applying oils to the skin.

> ### Essential Oils and Skin Vitality
>
> Melaleuca Alternifolia, Dorado Azul, and Lemongrass can help clear acne and balance oily skin conditions. Lemongrass is the predominant ingredient in Morning Start Bath and Shower Gel, which can be used to balance the pH of the skin, decongest the lymphatics, and stimulate circulation.

- Apply 4-6 drops of oil diluted 50:50 to affected areas 2 times daily.
- Apply a cold compress on affected area 2 times daily.

....

Psoriasis

Psoriasis is a noninfectious skin disorder that is marked by skin patches or flaking skin that can occur in limited areas such as the scalp or that can cover up to 80-90 percent of the body.

The overly rapid growth of skin cells is the primary cause of psoriasis. In some cases, skin cells grow four times faster than normal, resulting in the formation of silvery layers that flake off.

Symptoms

- It occurs on elbows, chest, knees, and scalp.
- Slightly elevated reddish lesions are covered with silver-white scales.
- The disease can be limited to one small patch or can cover the entire body.
- Rashes subside after exposure to sunlight.
- Rashes recur over a period of years.

Stop eating sugar!

Recommendations

Singles: Roman Chamomile, Melaleuca Alternifolia, Patchouli, Helichrysum, Rose, Melissa, German Chamomile, Lavender

Blends: Melrose, Gentle Baby, JuvaFlex, Juva-Cleanse

Nutritionals: ICP, ComforTone, Essentialzyme, Life 5, Balance Complete, AlkaLime, JuvaTone, JuvaPower, Sulfurzyme

Body Care Ointments: KidScents Tender Tush, Rose Ointment

Psoriasis Blend
- 4 drops Rosewood
- 2 drops Patchouli
- 2 drops Roman Chamomile
- 2 drops Vetiver
- 2 drops Sandalwood

Application and Usage

Inhalation
- Diffuse your choice of oils for ½ hour every 4-6 hours or as desired.
- Put 2-3 drops of your chosen oil in your hands and rub them together, cup your hands over your nose, and inhale throughout the day as needed.
- Put 8-10 drops of oil on a cotton ball or tissue and put it in an air vent in your house, vehicle, hotel room, etc.
- If diffusing while sleeping, set your timer for the desired length of time for automatic shut off.

Topical
You may apply single oils or blends neat or diluted, depending on the oil or oils being used. Please see the instructions at the beginning of this chapter for more information on applying oils to the skin.
- Apply 2-4 drops neat to affected area 2 times daily.
- Add 6-10 drops to 1 teaspoon of regular skin lotion and apply daily or as needed.
- Place a warm compress with 1-2 drops of chosen oil on the back 3 times weekly.

Ingestion and Oral
The amount of oil ingested varies with different oils. Whether putting the oils in a capsule or drinking them in a liquid, please refer to the instructions at the beginning of this chapter.
- Take 1 capsule with desired oil 1 time daily.
- Put 2-3 drops of oil in a spoonful of Blue Agave, Yacon Syrup, maple syrup, coconut oil, milk, etc.
- Put the desired amount of oils in a glass of rice milk, almond milk, goat milk, carrot juice, NingXia Red, or even water and then drink it.

....

Sagging Skin
Sagging skin is a common problem for many people, especially as they get older. It occurs as the skin loses its elasticity over time.

Recommendations
Singles: Lavender, Helichrysum, Patchouli, Cypress, Tangerine, Sandalwood

Blends: Humility, Inspiration, Joy

Nutritionals: Super C, Super C Chewable, ICP, ComforTone, Essentialzyme, Mineral Essence, JuvaPower

Creams, Toner, and Massage Oil: A·R·T Purifying Toner, Boswellia Wrinkle Cream, Cel-Lite Magic Massage Oil

Skin Firming Blend (Morning)
- 3 drops Tangerine
- 3 drops Cypress

Skin Firming Blend (Evening)
- 8 drops Patchouli
- 5 drops Cypress
- 5 drops Geranium
- 1 drop Sandalwood

Application and Usage
Topical

You may apply single oils or blends neat or diluted, depending on the oil or oils being used. Please see the instructions at the beginning of this chapter for more information on applying oils to the skin.

- Apply 4-6 drops neat or diluted 50:50 on affected area 2 times daily. Use the morning blend before dressing in the morning and the evening blend before bed at night.
- Strength training with weights can also help tighten sagging skin.

....

Scabies

Scabies are caused by eight-legged insects known as itch mites—tiny parasites that burrow into the skin, usually in the fingers and genital areas. The most common variety, *Sarcoptes scabiei,* can quickly infest other people. Although it lives for only one to two months, the female continually lays eggs once it digs into the skin.

The most common remedy for scabies and lice is lindane (gamma benzene hexachloride), a highly toxic polychlorinated chemical that is structurally very similar to hazardous banned pesticides such as DDT and chlordane. It is so dangerous that Dr. Guy Sansfacon, head of the Quebec Poison Control Centre in Canada, has requested that lindane be banned.

Natural, plant-derived essential oils have the same activity as commercial pesticides but are far safer. Essential oils have been studied for their ability to not only repel insects but also to kill them and their eggs as well. Because most oils are nontoxic to humans, they make excellent treatments to combat scabies infestations.

Recommendations
Singles: Palo Santo, Peppermint, Citronella, Rosemary, Palmarosa, Lavandin, Eucalyptus Globulus, Black Pepper, Ginger, Idaho Tansy, Oregano, Plectranthus Oregano, Thyme, Mountain Savory

Blends: Purification, Melrose, Thieves, Exodus II, Abundance

Application and Usage
Topical

You may apply single oils or blends neat or diluted, depending on the oil or oils being used. Please see the instructions at the beginning of this chapter for more information on applying oils to the skin.

- Apply 2-4 drops of recommended oils neat or diluted 50:50 if needed on location 3 times daily.
- To treat hair or scalp, add 3-5 drops of essential oil to 1 teaspoon of shampoo and massage into wet hair. Leave for 5 minutes, then rinse.

....

Skin Ulcers

Skin ulcers are open sores that are often accompanied by the sloughing-off of inflamed tissue. They can be caused by problems with blood circulation, irritation from exposure to corrosive material, exposure to heat, cold, or trauma.

Recommendations
Singles: Helichrysum, Roman Chamomile, Patchouli, Lavender, Clove, Myrrh

Blends: Thieves, Purification, Relieve It, Melrose

Nutritionals: Super C, ICP, ComforTone, Essentialzyme, Power Meal, NingXia Red, Inner Defense, Digest & Cleanse

Body Care Ointments: KidScents Tender Tush, Rose Ointment

Application and Usage
Topical

You may apply single oils or blends neat or diluted, depending on the oil or oils being used. Please see the instructions at the beginning of this chapter for more information on applying oils to the skin.

- Apply 4-6 drops neat or diluted 50:50 on affected area 2 times daily.

....

Stretch Marks

Stretch marks are most commonly associated with pregnancy but can also occur during growth spurts and periods of weight gain.

Recommendations

Singles: Sacred Frankincense, Frankincense, Elemi, Spikenard, Geranium, Lavender, Myrrh

Blends: Gentle Baby, Sensation, Valor, White Angelica

Nutritionals: Sulfurzyme, MegaCal, BLM, Super B, Super C, Super C Chewable, Essentialzyme, Ultra Young Plus, Master Formula HIS or HER

Creams, Lotions, and Ointments: KidScents Tender Tush, Rose Ointment, A·R·T Day Activator, A·R·T Night Reconstructor

Application and Usage
Topical

You may apply single oils or blends neat or diluted, depending on the oil or oils being used. Please see the instructions at the beginning of this chapter for more information on applying oils to the skin.

- Apply 3-6 drops of oil neat or diluted 50:50 2 times daily.

Vitiligo

Vitiligo is a condition in which your skin loses melanin, the pigment that determines the color of your skin, hair, and eyes and occurs when the cells that produce melanin die or no longer form melanin, causing slowly enlarging white patches of irregular shapes to appear on your skin.

The cause has not yet been determined, but there are theories that it may be due to an immune system disorder, heredity possibilities, nutritional deficiencies, overuse of chemicals, and perhaps environmental pollution that affects the proper function of the body that produces melanin.

Some people have reported a single event such as sunburn or emotional distress that triggered the condition. However, none of these theories has been proved to be a definite cause of vitiligo.

Recommendations

Singles: Sandalwood, Myrrh, Vetiver, Patchouli

Blends: Brain Power, Dream Catcher, Humility, Deep Relief Roll-On

Nutritionals: Essentialzyme, Detoxzyme, ICP, JuvaPower, Mineral Essence, Digest & Cleanse, Inner Defense, SleepEssence

Application and Usage
Topical

You may apply single oils or blends neat or diluted, depending on the oil or oils being used. Please see the instructions at the beginning of this chapter for more information on applying oils to the skin.

- Apply 2-4 drops of desired oil neat 2 times daily.
- A cleansing diet might be helpful. Cleansing the liver and digestive system facilitates greater nutritional absorption and waste elimination for proper body function and vibrant health.

Wrinkles

Although wrinkles are a natural part of aging, sun exposure is the major cause. Exposure to heat, wind, and dust, as well as smoking, may also contribute to wrinkling.

Recommendations

Singles: Sacred Frankincense, Frankincense, Myrrh, Vetiver, Helichrysum, Cypress, Rose, Lavender, Patchouli, Geranium, Sandalwood, Neroli, Palmarosa, Spikenard

Blends: Gentle Baby, Sensation, 3 Wise Men, White Angelica, Highest Potential

Nutritionals: MegaCal, Longevity Softgels, NingXia Red, OmegaGize[3], Master Formula HIS or HERS, Sulfurzyme, Super B, Ningxia Wolfberries (Dried)

Skin Care Creams and Ointments: A·R·T Day Activator, A·R·T Night Reconstructor, Boswellia Wrinkle Cream, Wolfberry Eye Cream, A·R·T Gentle Foaming Cleanser, A·R·T Purifying Toner, Rose Ointment, Sandalwood Moisture Cream

Wrinkle-Reducing Blend
- 6 drops Sacred Frankincense or Frankincense
- 5 drops Sandalwood
- 4 drops Geranium
- 3 drops Lavender

Application and Usage
Topical

You may apply single oils or blends neat or diluted, depending on the oil or oils being used. Please see the instructions at the beginning of this chapter for more information on applying oils to the skin.

- Mix 3-4 drops of oil 50:50 in V-6 Vegetable Oil Complex or add to the A·R·T skin-care lotions or moisturizing creams and apply as needed.
- Rose Ointment was developed to keep the skin soft and moist and to supply healing nutrients. It is a natural emollient and contains no chemicals or synthetic ingredients that can cause skin irritation.

  Note: Be careful not to get lotion or oils near the eyes.

SLEEP DISORDERS

Melatonin is the most powerful natural remedy for restoring both quality and quantity of sleep. It improves the length of the time the body sustains deep, stage 4 sleep, the time when the immune system and growth hormone production reaches its maximum.

ImmuPro not only contains melatonin, but it also contains mineral and polysaccharide complexes to restore natural sleep rhythm and eliminate insomnia.

Valerian has been shown to be effective in calming the mind, enabling one to fall asleep easier.

Recommendations

Singles: Lavender, Goldenrod, Valerian, Roman Chamomile, Orange, Mandarin

Blends: RutaVaLa, RutaVaLa Roll-On, Tranquil Roll-On, Peace & Calming, Surrender, Trauma Life, Hope, Humility, Stress Away Roll-On

Nutritionals: SleepEssence, ImmuPro, Essentialzyme, MegaCal, Mineral Essence, OmegaGize[3], Life 5, Thyromin (taken just before getting into bed)

Application and Usage
Inhalation

- Diffuse your choice of oils for ½ hour every 4-6 hours or as desired.
- Put 2-3 drops of your chosen oil in your hands and rub them together, cup your hands over your nose, and inhale throughout the day as needed.
- Put 8-10 drops of oil on a cotton ball or tissue and put it in an air vent in your house, vehicle, hotel room, etc.

- If diffusing while sleeping, set your timer for the desired length of time for automatic shut off.

Topical

You may apply single oils or blends neat or diluted, depending on the oil or oils being used. Please see the instructions at the beginning of this chapter for more information on applying oils to the skin.

- Apply 1-2 drops neat on temples and back of neck, as desired.
- Applying a single drop under the nose is helpful and refreshing.
- Dilute 50:50 and apply on location 3-6 times daily.
- Massage 2-4 drops of oil neat on the soles of the feet just before bedtime. Children love it.

SMOKING CESSATION (See also ADDICTIONS)

Smoking is a difficult habit to break because it involves many aspects of a person's emotions and social life as well as a physical addiction to nicotine. Smoking cessation (quitting smoking) is a vital part of cancer prevention.

Recommendations

Singles: Cinnamon, Clove, Nutmeg, Peppermint, Roman Chamomile, Clary Sage

Blends: Thieves, Harmony, JuvaCleanse, Peace & Calming, GLF

Nutritionals: ICP, ComforTone, Essentialzyme, Life 5, JuvaTone, JuvaPower, JuvaSpice (for salads and cooking)

Application and Usage
Inhalation

- Inhale the oils that work best for you whenever the urge for a cigarette arises.
- Diffuse your choice of oils for ½ hour every 4-6 hours or as desired.
- Put 2-3 drops of your chosen oil in your hands and rub them together, cup your hands over your nose, and inhale throughout the day as needed.
- Put 8-10 drops of oil on a cotton ball or tissue and put it in an air vent in your house, vehicle, hotel room, etc.
- If diffusing while sleeping, set your timer for the desired length of time for automatic shut off.

Topical

You may apply single oils or blends neat or diluted, depending on the oil or oils being used. Please see the instructions at the beginning of this chapter for more information on applying oils to the skin.

Ingestion and Oral

The amount of oil ingested varies with different oils. Whether putting the oils in a capsule or drinking them in a liquid, please refer to the instructions at the beginning of this chapter.

- Take 1 capsule with desired oil 2 times daily.
- Put 2-3 drops of oil in a spoonful of Blue Agave, Yacon Syrup, maple syrup, coconut oil, milk, etc.
- Put the desired amount of oils in a glass of rice milk, almond milk, goat milk, carrot juice, NingXia Red, or even water and then drink it.
- Cleanse colon and liver with ICP, Comfor-Tone, Essentialzyme, and JuvaTone.
- Put 1 drop of Thieves on the tongue every time you have the urge to smoke.
- JuvaTone, JuvaPower, and JuvaSpice (for salads and cooking) detoxify the liver, which in turn help to reduce cravings for nicotine and caffeine. Take 3 tablets of JuvaTone 3 times daily and 2 tablespoon of JuvaPower or JuvaSpice daily.

SNAKE BITES

CAUTION: Get medical attention immediately if you are bitten by a poisonous snake.

Recommendations

Singles: Clove, Eucalyptus Blue, Idaho Balsam Fir, Copaiba, Lemon, Patchouli, Sacred Frankincense, Frankincense, Thyme, Melaleuca Alternifolia

Blends: Purification, Melrose, Thieves

Sprays: Thieves Spray

Application and Usage
Topical

You may apply single oils or blends neat or diluted, depending on the oil or oils being used. Please see the instructions at the beginning of this chapter for more information on applying oils to the skin.

- Apply 2-3 drops diluted 50:50 on location every 15 minutes until professional medical help is available.

SNORING
(See also APNEA)

Just about everyone snores occasionally, but it can affect the quantity and quality of your sleep, which can lead to fatigue, irritability, and increased health problems, in addition to relationship problems with your partner.

Recommendations

Singles: Idaho Balsam Fir, Galbanum, Sandalwood, Rose, Lavender, Valerian, Western Red Cedar, Ylang Ylang, Amazonian Ylang Ylang

Blends: RutaVaLa, RutaVaLa Roll-On, Stress Away Roll-On, The Gift, Harmony, Sacred Mountain, Valor, Transformation

Nutritionals: SleepEssence, MegaCal, Mineral Essence, Detoxzyme, Essentialzyme

Application and Usage
Topical

You may apply single oils or blends neat or diluted, depending on the oil or oils being used. Please see the instructions at the beginning of this chapter for more information on applying oils to the skin.

- Rub 4-6 drops diluted 50:50 on the soles of both feet at bedtime.

Ingestion and Oral

The amount of oil ingested varies with different oils. Whether putting the oils in a capsule or drinking them in a liquid, please refer to the instructions at the beginning of this chapter.

- Take 1 capsule with desired oil 2 times daily.
- Put 2-3 drops of oil in a spoonful of Blue Agave, Yacon Syrup, maple syrup, coconut oil, milk, etc.
- Put the desired amount of oils in a glass of rice milk, almond milk, goat milk, carrot juice, NingXia Red, or even water and then drink it.

SPINA BIFIDA

Spina bifida (SB) is a defect in which the spinal cord of the fetus fails to close during the first month of pregnancy. This results in varying degrees of permanent nerve damage, paralysis in lower limbs, and incomplete brain development. The exact cause is unknown, but scientists suspect that nutritional, genetic, and environmental factors such as exposure to harmful substances may play a role in its cause.

Spina bifida has three different variations:

The most severe form is myelomeningocele, when the spinal cord and its protective sheath (known as the meninges) protrude from an opening in the spine.

Meningocele is when only the meninges protrude from the opening in the spine. The mildest form is occulta, characterized by malformed vertebrae.

Symptoms of this disease range from bowel and bladder dysfunctions to excess build up in the brain of cerebrospinal fluid.

The easiest way to possibly prevent spina bifida is with folic acid supplementation (at least 400 mcg daily, found in Super B) by all women of child-bearing ages.

Recommendations

Singles: Mountain Savory, Helichrysum, Thyme, Melaleuca Alternifolia, Idaho Balsam Fir, Sacred Frankincense, Frankincense

Blends: Melrose, Exodus II, The Gift, Peace & Calming, Deep Relief Roll-On, Tranquil Roll-On, Aroma Siez

Nutritionals: Super B, Balance Complete, Sulfurzyme, MegaCal, JuvaPower, Master Formula HIS or HERS, OmegaGize[3], Essentialzyme, Power Meal

Application and Usage

Topical

You may apply single oils or blends neat or diluted, depending on the oil or oils being used. Please see the instructions at the beginning of this chapter for more information on applying oils to the skin.

- Receive a Raindrop Technique weekly.
- Place a warm compress with 1-2 drops of chosen oil over the affected area.

Ingestion and Oral

The amount of oil ingested varies with different oils. Whether putting the oils in a capsule or drinking them in a liquid, please refer to the instructions at the beginning of this chapter.

- Take 1 capsule with desired oil 2 times daily.
- Put 2-3 drops of oil in a spoonful of Blue Agave, Yacon Syrup, maple syrup, coconut oil, milk, etc.
- Put the desired amount of oils in a glass of rice milk, almond milk, goat milk, carrot juice, NingXia Red, or even water and then drink it.

SPINE INJURIES AND PAIN

According to numerous chiropractors, the Raindrop Technique using therapeutic-grade essential oils is revolutionizing the treatment of many types of back pain, spine inflammation, and vertebral misalignments.

The following essential oils, blends, and supplements are for supporting the structural integrity of the spine and reducing discomfort:

Recommendations

Singles: Idaho Blue Spruce, Dorado Azul, Wintergreen, Marjoram, Idaho Balsam Fir, Helichrysum, Palo Santo, Peppermint, Basil, Copaiba

Blends: PanAway, Aroma Siez, Relieve It, Valor, Valor Roll-On, Deep Relief Roll-On

Nutritionals: MegaCal, SuperCal, Longevity Softgels, BLM, Essentialzyme, Mineral Essence, Power Meal, Sulfurzyme

Application and Usage

Topical

You may apply single oils or blends neat or diluted, depending on the oil or oils being used. Please see the instructions at the beginning of this chapter for more information on applying oils to the skin.

- Apply 6-10 drops diluted 50:50 on location 2 times daily or as needed.
- Place a warm compress with 1-2 drops of desired oil daily (if area is not inflamed).
- Receive a Raindrop Technique 3 times a month.

Ingestion and Oral

The amount of oil ingested varies with different oils. Whether putting the oils in a capsule or drinking them in a liquid, please refer to the instructions at the beginning of this chapter.

- Take 1 capsule with desired oil 2 times daily.
- Put 2-3 drops of oil in a spoonful of Blue Agave, Yacon Syrup, maple syrup, coconut oil, milk, etc.

- Put the desired amount of oils in a glass of rice milk, almond milk, goat milk, carrot juice, NingXia Red, or even water and then drink it.

....

Back Injuries and Pain (Backache) (See also Muscles)

According to numerous chiropractors, the Raindrop Technique using therapeutic-grade essential oils has added tremendous benefit to the treatment of many types of back pain, inflammation, and vertebral misalignments.

Recommendations

Singles: Lavender, Idaho Balsam Fir, Wintergreen, German Chamomile, Basil, Copaiba, Marjoram, Peppermint

Blends: Aroma Siez, PanAway, Relieve It, Deep Relief Roll-On

Nutritionals: BLM, MegaCal, Master HIS or HERS, Power Meal, MultiGreens, NingXia Red

Body Care Massage Oils: Ortho Sport Massage Oil, Ortho Ease Massage Oil

Backache Blend
- 5 drops Wintergreen
- 3 drops Lavender
- 3 drops Idaho Balsam Fir
- 2 drops Marjoram

Application and Usage
Topical

You may apply single oils or blends neat or diluted, depending on the oil or oils being used. Please see the instructions at the beginning of this chapter for more information on applying oils to the skin.

- Apply 2-4 drops neat on specific area 1-3 times daily or as needed.
- Apply 2-4 drops on Vita Flex area of foot.
- Use warm compress with 1-2 drops of chosen oil on the back daily.
- Apply Raindrop Technique 2 times weekly

for 3 weeks.
- Massage with Ortho Ease or Ortho Sport Massage Oil.

....

Herniated Disc/Disc Deterioration

A herniated disc is an abnormal rupture of the central portion of a disc of the spine. For this situation, it is best to consult a specialist.

However, many essential oils can give temporary pain relief.

Recommendations

Singles: Basil, Tarragon, Idaho Blue Spruce, Sacred Frankincense, Frankincense, Idaho Balsam Fir, Helichrysum, Wintergreen, Vetiver, Valerian

Blends: PanAway, Relieve It, Aroma Siez, Deep Relief Roll-On

Nutritionals: Sulfurzyme, BLM, MegaCal, Power Meal, Master HIS or HERS, Essentialzyme, Mineral Essence, OmegaGize[3]

Creams and Massage Oils: Regenolone Moisturizing Cream, Ortho Sport Massage Oil, Ortho Ease Massage Oil

Application and Usage
Topical

You may apply single oils or blends neat or diluted, depending on the oil or oils being used. Please see the instructions at the beginning of this chapter for more information on applying oils to the skin.

- Dilute 50:50 and apply on location for pain relief.
- Place a cold compress on location as needed.
- Receive a Raindrop Technique 2 times weekly.
- Stimulate vertebrae with "pointer technique" *(see box on next page with explanation)*.

....

Lumbago (Lower back pain)

Chronic lower back pain can have many causes, including a damaged or pinched nerve (neuralgia) or a congested colon.

Recommendations

Singles: Basil, Helichrysum, German Chamomile, Elemi, Peppermint, Copaiba, Marjoram, Wintergreen

Blends: Relieve It, PanAway, Deep Relief Roll-On, Stress Away Roll-On

Nutritionals: MegaCal, BLM, ICP, Comfor-Tone, Essentialzyme, Life 5, OmegaGize[3]

Creams and Massage Oils: Regenolone Moisturizing Cream, Ortho Sport Massage Oil, Ortho Ease Massage Oil

Application and Usage

Topical

You may apply single oils or blends neat or diluted, depending on the oil or oils being used. Please see the instructions at the beginning of this chapter for more information on applying oils to the skin.

- Apply 6-10 drops of oil diluted 50:50 on location 2 times daily. Also apply around navel.
- Apply 2-3 drops of desired oil on stomach and intestine and on Vita Flex points of the feet.
- Place a warm compress on lower back 1-2 times daily. If inflamed, use a cool compress.
- Receive a complete Raindrop Technique 3 times each month.

....

Neck Pain and Stiffness

Neck pain and stiffness can be caused by a variety of factors, including stress, injury, tension, everyday activities, or other health problems, some of which may have serious consequences.

Recommendations

Singles: Basil, Marjoram, Idaho Blue Spruce, Helichrysum, Idaho Balsam Fir, Peppermint, Wintergreen, Nutmeg, Copaiba, Elemi, Dorado Azul

Blends: Relieve It, PanAway, Deep Relief Roll-On

Nutritionals: Mineral Essence, MegaCal, Master Formula HIS or HERS, Balance Complete, BLM, OmegaGize[3]

Neck Stiffness Blend
- 5 drops PanAway
- 5 drops Marjoram
- 3 drops Peppermint

Neck Pain Blend
- 7 drops Basil
- 5 drops Wintergreen
- 4 drops Cypress
- 2 drops Peppermint

Application and Usage

Topical

You may apply single oils or blends neat or diluted, depending on the oil or oils being used. Please see the instructions at the beginning of

434

this chapter for more information on applying oils to the skin.

- Apply 4-6 drops diluted 50:50 to neck area and massage 1-3 times daily as needed.
- Place a warm compress on neck area daily or as needed. With inflammation use a cool compress.

....

Sciatica

Sciatica is characterized by pain in the buttocks and down the back of the thigh. The pain worsens during coughing, sneezing, or with flexing and stretching the back. The pain is caused by pressure on the sciatic nerve as it leaves the spine in the lower pelvic region due to spinal misalignment and/or nerve inflammation.

The sciatic nerve is the largest in the body, with branches throughout the legs and feet; sciatica pain can be intense and immobilizing. Acute sciatica has a sudden onset and is usually triggered by a misaligned vertebra pressing against the sciatic nerve due to accident, injury, pregnancy, or inflammation.

Symptoms

- Lower back pain
- Swelling or stiffness in a leg
- Loss of sensation in a leg
- Muscle wasting in a leg

Sulfurzyme, Super B, and OmegaGize³ work well together to help rebuild nerve damage and the myelin sheath.

Recommendations

Singles: Helichrysum, Tarragon, Vetiver, Peppermint, Nutmeg, Thyme, Idaho Blue Spruce, Basil, Rosemary, Copaiba

Blends: Aroma Siez, Relieve It, PanAway

Nutritionals: Sulfurzyme, Super B, Essentialzyme, Master Formula HIS or HERS, OmegaGize³, MegaCal, Mineral Essence

Creams and Massage Oils: Regenolone Moisturizing Cream, Ortho Sport Massage Oil, Ortho Ease Massage Oil

Chiropractors have found that by applying Valor on the bottom of the feet, spinal manipulations are easier to do and last 75 percent longer.

Application and Usage

Topical

You may apply single oils or blends neat or diluted, depending on the oil or oils being used. Please see the instructions at the beginning of this chapter for more information on applying oils to the skin.

- Apply 6-10 drops diluted 50:50 on location 2 times daily or as needed.
- Place a warm compress on affected area 1-2 times daily; cold compress if inflamed.
- Massage 2-3 drops into Vita Flex points of the feet 2-4 times daily.
- Receive a complete Raindrop Technique 3 times monthly.
- Walk backwards for 20 minutes daily with no shoes.

Ingestion and Oral

The amount of oil ingested varies with different oils. Whether putting the oils in a capsule or drinking them in a liquid, please refer to the instructions at the beginning of this chapter.

- Take 1 capsule with desired oil 2 times daily.
- Put 2-3 drops of oil in a spoonful of Blue Agave, Yacon Syrup, maple syrup, coconut oil, milk, etc.
- Put the desired amount of oils in a glass of rice milk, almond milk, goat milk, carrot juice, NingXia Red, or even water and then drink it.

....

Scoliosis

Scoliosis is an abnormal lateral or side-to-side curvature or twist in the spine. It is different from hyperkyphosis (hunchback) or hyperlordosis (swayback), which involve exces-

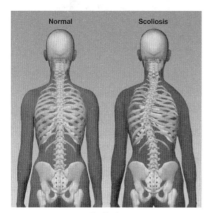

Normal | Scoliosis

Scoliosis

sive front-to-back accentuation of existing spine curvatures.

While some cases of scoliosis can be attributed to congenital deformities such as MS, cerebral palsy, Down syndrome, or Marfan syndrome, the vast majority of scoliosis types are of unknown origin.

Some medical professionals believe that scoliosis may be caused by persistent muscle spasms that pull the vertebrae of the spine out of alignment. Others feel—and there is a growing body of research documenting this hypothesis—that it begins with hard-to-detect inflammation along the spine caused by latent viruses (See citations in this chapter).

Symptoms

- When bending forward, the left side of the back is higher or lower than the right side (the patient must be viewed from the rear).
- One hip may appear to be higher or more prominent than the other.
- Uneven shoulders or scapulas (shoulder blades).
- When the arms are hanging loosely, the distance between the left arm and left side is

different than the distance between the right arm and right side.

The Raindrop Technique is proving to be an effective therapy for helping scoliosis, easing pain, and reducing misalignment.

Recommendations

Singles: Oregano, Plectranthus Oregano, Thyme, Basil, Wintergreen, Cypress, Marjoram, Peppermint

Blends: Aroma Siez, PanAway, Valor, Valor Roll-On

Nutritionals: Mineral Essence, MegaCal, Power Meal, Sulfurzyme, BLM, Master Formula HIS or HERS, NingXia Red

Body Care Massage Oils: Ortho Ease Massage Oil, Ortho Sport Massage Oil

Application and Usage

Topical

You may apply single oils or blends neat or diluted, depending on the oil or oils being used. Please see the instructions at the beginning of this chapter for more information on applying oils to the skin.

- Apply 3-6 drops diluted 50:50 along the spine daily or as needed.
- Receive a Raindrop Technique 2-3 times a week.

Ingestion and Oral

The amount of oil ingested varies with different oils. Whether putting the oils in a capsule or drinking them in a liquid, please refer to the instructions at the beginning of this chapter.

- Take 1 capsule with desired oil 2 times daily.
- Put 2-3 drops of oil in a spoonful of Blue Agave, Yacon Syrup, maple syrup, coconut oil, milk, etc.
- Put the desired amount of oils in a glass of rice milk, almond milk, goat milk, carrot juice, NingXia Red, or even water and then drink it.

SPRAIN

A sprain is an injury to a ligament caused by excessive stretching. The ligament can have a partial tear or be completely torn apart. Sprained ligaments swell rapidly and are painful. Usually, the greater the pain, the more severe the injury is.

Recommendations

Singles: Basil, Dorado Azul, Idaho Blue Spruce, Peppermint, Copaiba, Idaho Balsam Fir, Wintergreen

Blends: PanAway, Relieve It, Aroma Siez, Deep Relief Roll-On

Nutritionals: Sulfurzyme, Mineral Essence, MegaCal, Essentialzyme, Super C, Power Meal, Super B

Creams and Massage Oils: Prenolone Plus Body Cream, Ortho Sport Massage Oil

Application and Usage
Topical

You may apply single oils or blends neat or diluted, depending on the oil or oils being used. Please see the instructions at the beginning of this chapter for more information on applying oils to the skin.

- Apply 4-6 drops diluted 50:50 on location 3-5 times daily.
- Place a cold compress on location 2 times daily.

Ingestion and Oral

The amount of oil ingested varies with different oils. Whether putting the oils in a capsule or drinking them in a liquid, please refer to the instructions at the beginning of this chapter.

- Take 1 capsule with desired oil 2 times daily.
- Put 2-3 drops of oil in a spoonful of Blue Agave, Yacon Syrup, maple syrup, coconut oil, milk, etc.
- Put the desired amount of oils in a glass of rice milk, almond milk, goat milk, carrot juice, NingXia Red, or even water and then drink it.

See the Whole Picture to Produce the Best Results

When selecting oils, particularly for injuries, think through the cause and type of injury and then select oils for each segment.

For instance, a broken bone could encompass muscle damage, nerve damage, ligament strain or tear, inflammation, infection, and bone injury. The emotion of shock, anger, guilt, or suffering from long-time pain is another dimension of the injury that needs to be dealt with through understanding and help on an emotional level. All factors of the injury need to be considered in order to choose the oils that would offer the most benefits.

Select the single oils for each perceived problem, or select a blend that may address all of the needs, and then apply gently in a rotating motion. It would be best to apply the oils first to the feet using the Vita Flex Technique, if that is possible.

STRESS

Stress can be either good or bad. However, long-term stressful situations can produce a lasting, low-level stress that's hard on people. The nervous system pumps out extra stress hormones over an extended period, which can wear out the body's reserves, leaving a person feeling depleted or overwhelmed, weakening the body's immune system, and causing other problems.

Recommendations

Singles: Lavender, Roman Chamomile, Blue Tansy, Cedarwood, Marjoram, Rose, Sandalwood, Sacred Frankincense, Frankincense, Frereana Frankincense, Valerian

Blends: Valor, Valor Roll-On, Peace & Calming, Tranquil Roll-On Trauma Life, Humility, Harmony, RutaVaLa, RutaVaLa Roll-On, The Gift, Common Sense

Nutritionals: Super B, Super C, MultiGreens, Master HIS or HERS, MegaCal, Omega-Gize3, CortiStop Women's

Application and Usage
Inhalation
- Diffuse your choice of oils for ½ hour every 4-6 hours or as desired.
- Put 2-3 drops of your chosen oil in your hands and rub them together, cup your hands over your nose, and inhale throughout the day as needed.
- Put 8-10 drops of oil on a cotton ball or tissue and put it in an air vent in your house, vehicle, hotel room, etc.
- If diffusing while sleeping, set your timer for the desired length of time for automatic shut off.

Topical
You may apply single oils or blends neat or diluted, depending on the oil or oils being used. Please see the instructions at the beginning of this chapter for more information on applying oils to the skin.
- Dilute 50:50 and apply on temples, neck, and shoulders 2 times daily or as needed.
- Use bath salts daily.

Ingestion and Oral
The amount of oil ingested varies with different oils. Whether putting the oils in a capsule or drinking them in a liquid, please refer to the instructions at the beginning of this chapter.
- Take 1 capsule with desired oil 2 times daily.
- Put 2-3 drops of oil in a spoonful of Blue Agave, Yacon Syrup, maple syrup, coconut oil, milk, etc.
- Put the desired amount of oils in a glass of rice milk, almond milk, goat milk, carrot juice, NingXia Red, or even water and then drink it.

THROAT INFECTIONS AND PROBLEMS
(See also COLDS, COUGHS, INFECTIONS, LUNG INFECTIONS)
Throat infection is one of the most common conditions in the world. It is broadly divided into two types, viral and bacterial throat infections.

....

Coughs, Congestive and Dry
Coughs are classified into two categories, acute and chronic. An acute cough is one that has been present for less than three weeks and is divided into infectious and noninfectious causes.

Chronic coughs are those that have been present for more than three weeks and are categorized as conditions within the lungs, conditions within the chest cavity but outside of the lungs, conditions along the passages that transmit air from the lungs to the environment, and digestive causes.

Recommendations
Singles: Eucalyptus Globulus, Peppermint, Melaleuca Alternifolia, Eucalyptus Radiata, Eucalyptus Blue, Myrrh, Goldenrod, Ledum, Mastrante, Spruce, Ravintsara, Cedarwood, Marjoram, Hyssop, Copaiba, Idaho Balsam Fir, Cypress, Melissa

Blends: R.C., Breathe Again Roll-On, Raven, Thieves, Melrose, Peace & Calming, Exodus II

Nutritionals: Inner Defense, Life 5, ImmuPro, Super C, Super C Chewable,

Oral Care: Thieves Fresh Essence Plus Mouthwash, Thieves Lozenges (Hard/Soft), Thieves Spray

Cough Blend
- 10 drops Eucalyptus Globulus
- 1 drop Wintergreen
- 1 drop Peppermint
  The Cough Blend may be ingested, applied topically, and/or diffused as you wish.

Dry Cough Tea Blend

- 3 drops Eucalyptus Radiata
- 2 drops Lemon
- 1 teaspoon Blue Agave or maple syrup
- 4 oz. heated distilled water
  Sip slowly. Repeat as often as needed for relief.

Application and Usage
Inhalation

- Diffuse Eucalyptus Blue, Raven, or your choice of oil for ½ hour every 4-6 hours or as desired.
- Put 2-3 drops of your chosen oil in your hands and rub them together, cup your hands over your nose, and inhale throughout the day as needed.
- Put 8-10 drops of oil on a cotton ball or tissue and put it in an air vent in your house, vehicle, hotel room, etc.
- If diffusing while sleeping, set your timer for the desired length of time for automatic shut off.

Topical

You may apply single oils or blends neat or diluted, depending on the oil or oils being used. Please see the instructions at the beginning of this chapter for more information on applying oils to the skin.

- Place a warm compress with 1-2 drops of chosen oil on the chest, throat, and upper back 2 times daily.
- Apply 1-3 drops to lung Vita Flex points 1-3 times daily.
- Receive a Raindrop Technique 1-2 times weekly.

Ingestion and Oral

The amount of oil ingested varies with different oils. Whether putting the oils in a capsule or drinking them in a liquid, please refer to the instructions at the beginning of this chapter.

- Take 1 capsule with desired oil 2 times daily.

- Put 2-3 drops of oil in a spoonful of Blue Agave, Yacon Syrup, maple syrup, coconut oil, milk, etc.
- Put the desired amount of oils in a glass of rice milk, almond milk, goat milk, carrot juice, NingXia Red, or even water and then drink it.
- Gargle with Thieves Fresh Essence Plus Mouthwash throughout the day as desired.
- Use Thieves Spray as desired.

....

Laryngitis

Laryngitis is inflammation and swelling of the larynx, also known as the voice box. Laryngitis is usually caused by a virus, sometimes by a bacterial infection, or occurs in people who overuse their voice.

Singles: Eucalyptus Radiata, Lemon, Eucalyptus Blue, Palo Santo, Oregano, Plectranthus Oregano, Sacred Frankincense, Frankincense, Frereana Frankincense, Ravintsara, Thyme, Myrrh, Cedarwood, Eucalyptus Globulus, Idaho Ponderosa Pine, Peppermint

Blends: R.C., Thieves, Melrose, Raven, Purification, Exodus II, Breathe Again Roll-On

Nutritionals: Super C, Super C Chewable, Longevity Softgels, MultiGreens, ImmuPro, OmegaGize[3]

Oral Care: Thieves Spray, Thieves Fresh Essence Plus Mouthwash, Thieves Lozenges (Hard/Soft)

Application and Usage
Inhalation

- Diffuse your choice of oils for ½ hour every 4-6 hours or as desired.
- Put 2-3 drops of your chosen oil in your hands and rub them together, cup your hands over your nose, and inhale throughout the day as needed.
- Put 8-10 drops of oil on a cotton ball or tissue and put it in an air vent in your house, vehicle, hotel room, etc.

- If diffusing while sleeping, set your timer for the desired length of time for automatic shut off.
- Add a few drops of oil to a bowl of boiling water. Position the face above the bowl and drape a towel over the head, creating a vaporizing effect. Repeat 2-3 times daily.

Topical

You may apply single oils or blends neat or diluted, depending on the oil or oils being used. Please see the instructions at the beginning of this chapter for more information on applying oils to the skin.

- Apply 1-3 drops diluted 50:50 to throat, chest, and back of neck 2-4 times daily.
- Apply 1-3 drops of selected oil to lung Vita Flex points of the feet 1-3 times daily.
- Receive a Raindrop Technique 2-3 times weekly.

Ingestion and Oral

The amount of oil ingested varies with different oils. Whether putting the oils in a capsule or drinking them in a liquid, please refer to the instructions at the beginning of this chapter.

- Take 1 capsule with desired oil 2 times daily.
- Put 2-3 drops of oil in a spoonful of Blue Agave, Yacon Syrup, maple syrup, coconut oil, milk, etc.
- Put the desired amount of oils in a glass of rice milk, almond milk, goat milk, carrot juice, NingXia Red, or even water and then drink it.
- Put 2 drops of Melrose and 1 drop of Lemon in ½ teaspoon of Blue Agave, Yacon Syrup, or maple syrup, etc., and hold in the back of the mouth for 1-2 minutes and then swallow. Repeat as needed.
- Place a few drops on or under your tongue 2-6 times daily or as often as needed.
- Gargle with a mixture of essential oils and water 4-8 times daily.

- Spray throat with Thieves Spray as often as desired.
- Gargle with Thieves Fresh Essence Plus Mouthwash as needed.

....

Sore Throat

Sore throats are caused by many things such as viruses, bacteria, smoking, breathing polluted air, and allergies to pet dander, pollens, and molds.

Recommendations

Singles: Melaleuca Alternifolia, Ravintsara, Cypress, Eucalyptus Radiata, Lemon, Sacred Frankincense, Frankincense, Thyme, Oregano, Plectranthus Oregano, Peppermint, Myrrh, Wintergreen

Blends: Thieves, Melrose, Raven

Nutritionals: Inner Defense, Super C, Super C Chewable, ImmuPro, Longevity Softgels, OmegaGize[3]

Oral Care: Thieves Lozenges (Hard/Soft), Thieves Fresh Essence Plus Mouthwash, Thieves Spray

Sore Throat Blend No. 1
- 2 drops Thyme
- 2 drops Cypress
- 1 drop Eucalyptus Radiata
- 1 drop Peppermint
- 1 drop Myrrh
- 1 teaspoon honey

Sore Throat Blend No. 2
- 5 drops Lemon
- 2 drops Eucalyptus Globulus
- 2 drops Wintergreen
- 1 drop Peppermint

Application and Usage

Inhalation
- Diffuse your choice of oils for ½ hour every 4-6 hours or as desired.
- Put 2-3 drops of your chosen oil in your hands and rub them together, cup your hands

over your nose, and inhale throughout the day as needed.

- Add a few drops of oil to a bowl of boiling water. Position the face above the bowl and drape a towel over the head, creating a vaporizing effect. Repeat 2-3 times daily.
- If diffusing while sleeping, set your timer for the desired length of time for automatic shut off.

Topical

You may apply single oils or blends neat or diluted, depending on the oil or oils being used. Please see the instructions at the beginning of this chapter for more information on applying oils to the skin.

- Apply 1-3 drops diluted 50:50 to the throat, chest, and back of the neck 2-4 times daily.
- Apply 1-3 drops on the lung Vita Flex points of the foot 1-3 times daily.
- Receive a Raindrop Technique weekly.
- Place a warm compress with 1-2 drops of chosen oil on the throat and chest area 2-3 times daily.

Ingestion and Oral

The amount of oil ingested varies with different oils. Whether putting the oils in a capsule or drinking them in a liquid, please refer to the instructions at the beginning of this chapter.

- Take 1 capsule with desired oil 2 times daily.
- Put 2-3 drops of oil in a spoonful of Blue Agave, Yacon Syrup, maple syrup, coconut oil, milk, etc.
- Put the desired amount of oils in a glass of rice milk, almond milk, goat milk, carrot juice, NingXia Red, or even water and then drink it.
- Place a drop on or under the tongue 2-6 times daily or as often as needed.
- Gargle 4-8 times daily with a mixture of essential oils and water.

Strep Throat

Strep throat is a bacterial throat infection caused by Group A streptococcus and is generally more severe than a viral throat infection. If left untreated, strep throat can lead to kidney inflammation and rheumatic fever.

Recommendations

Singles: Oregano, Plectranthus Oregano, Thyme, Eucalyptus Globulus, Sacred Frankincense, Frankincense, Myrrh, Dorado Azul, Eucalyptus Blue, Mountain Savory, Ocotea, Clove, Cinnamon

Blends: Thieves, Exodus II, Melrose, Raven, R.C., ImmuPower

Nutritionals: Inner Defense, ImmuPro, Super C, Longevity Softgels, Super C Chewable, MultiGreens, ICP, ComforTone, Essentialzyme, OmegaGize[3]

Oral: Thieves Spray, Thieves Lozenges (Hard/Soft), Thieves Fresh Essence Plus Mouthwash

Strep Throat Blend

- 6 drops Lavender
- 2 drops Oregano
- 1 drop Cinnamon
- 1 drop Thyme

Application and Usage

Inhalation

- Diffuse your choice of oils for ½ hour every 4-6 hours or as desired.
- Put 2-3 drops of your chosen oil in your hands and rub them together, cup your hands over your nose, and inhale throughout the day as needed.
- Add a few drops of oil to a bowl of boiling water. Position the face above the bowl and drape a towel over the head, creating a vaporizing effect. Repeat 2-3 times daily.
- If diffusing while sleeping, set your timer for the desired length of time for automatic shut off.

Topical

You may apply single oils or blends neat or diluted, depending on the oil or oils being used. Please see the instructions at the beginning of this chapter for more information on applying oils to the skin.

- Apply 1-3 drops diluted 50:50 to the throat, chest, and back of the neck 2-4 times daily.
- You may also apply 1-3 drops on the lung Vita Flex points of the foot 1-3 times daily.
- Place a warm compress with 1-2 drops of chosen oil on the throat and chest area 2-3 times daily.
- Receive a Raindrop Technique weekly.

Ingestion and Oral

The amount of oil ingested varies with different oils. Whether putting the oils in a capsule or drinking them in a liquid, please refer to the instructions at the beginning of this chapter.

- Take 1 capsule with desired oil 2 times daily.
- Put 2-3 drops of oil in a spoonful of Blue Agave, Yacon Syrup, maple syrup, coconut oil, milk, etc.
- Put the desired amount of oils in a glass of rice milk, almond milk, goat milk, carrot juice, NingXia Red, or even water and then drink it.
- Place a drop on or under the tongue 2-6 times daily or as often as needed.
- Gargle with a mixture of essential oils and water 4-8 times daily.
- Spray throat with Thieves Spray as often as desired.

Regimen for Strep Throat

- ImmuPro: Take 2-4 tablets at bedtime.
- Longevity Softgels: Take 2-4 softgels daily.
- Super C: Take 2-3 tablets 2 times daily or chew Super C Chewable as desired.
- Receive a Raindrop Technique with Immu-Power and/or Exodus II along sides of spine weekly.
- Spray throat with Thieves Spray every 2 hours.

442

....
Tonsillitis

The tonsils are infection-fighting lymphatic tissues at the back of the throat. When they become infected with streptococcal bacteria, they become inflamed, causing a condition known as tonsillitis.

It became popular in the 1960's and 1970's to have the tonsils removed when they became infected. However, tonsillectomies have become much less frequent, as researchers have discovered the important role tonsils play in protecting and fighting infectious diseases and optimizing immune response.

The pharyngeal tonsils located at the back of the throat (known as the adenoids) can also become infected—a condition known as adenitis.

Recommendations

Singles: Clove, Melaleuca Alternifolia, Myrrh, Dorado Azul, Cassia, Ocotea, Goldenrod, Oregano, Plectranthus Oregano, Mountain Savory, Ravintsara, Thyme

Blends: Thieves, Melrose, Exodus II, Immu-Power

Nutritionals: Inner Defense, Super C Chewable, Super C, Detoxzyme, Mineral Essence

Oral Care: Thieves Spray, Thieves Fresh Essence Plus Mouthwash, Thieves Lozenges (Hard/Soft)

Application and Usage
Inhalation

- Diffuse your choice of oils for ½ hour every 4-6 hours or as desired.
- Put 2-3 drops of your chosen oil in your hands and rub them together, cup your hands over your nose, and inhale throughout the day as needed.
- Add a few drops of oil to a bowl of boiling water. Position the face above the bowl and drape a towel over the head, creating a vaporizing effect. Repeat 2-3 times daily.

- If diffusing while sleeping, set your timer for the desired length of time for automatic shut off.

Topical

You may apply single oils or blends neat or diluted, depending on the oil or oils being used. Please see the instructions at the beginning of this chapter for more information on applying oils to the skin.

- Apply 1-3 drops diluted 50:50 to the throat, chest, and back of the neck 2-4 times daily.
- You may also apply 1-3 drops on the lung Vita Flex points of the feet 1-3 times daily.
- Place a warm compress with 1-2 drops of chosen oil on the throat and chest area 2-3 times daily.
- Use the Raindrop Technique weekly.

Ingestion and Oral

The amount of oil ingested varies with different oils. Whether putting the oils in a capsule or drinking them in a liquid, please refer to the instructions at the beginning of this chapter.

- Take 1 capsule with desired oil 2 times daily.
- Put 2-3 drops of oil in a spoonful of Blue Agave, Yacon Syrup, maple syrup, coconut oil, milk, etc.
- Put the desired amount of oils in a glass of rice milk, almond milk, goat milk, carrot juice, NingXia Red, or even water and then drink it. Warm the milk and sip slowly for more soothing relief.
- Place a drop on or under the tongue 2-6 times daily or as often as needed.
- Gargle a mixture of essential oils and water 4-8 times daily.

THYROID PROBLEMS
(See also DEPRESSION, NARCOLEPSY, MALE HORMONE IMBALANCE, MENSTRUAL AND FEMALE HORMONE CONDITIONS)

The thyroid is the energy gland of the human body and produces T3 and T4 thyroid hormones that control the body's metabolism. The thyroid also controls other vital functions such as digestion, circulation, immune function, hormone balance, and emotions.

The thyroid gland is controlled by the pituitary gland, which signals the thyroid when to produce the thyroid hormone.

The hypothalamus gland sends chemical signals to the pituitary gland to monitor hormone levels in the blood stream.

A lack of the thyroid hormone does not necessarily mean that the thyroid is not functioning properly. In some instances, the pituitary gland may be malfunctioning because of its failure to release sufficient TSH (thyroid stimulating hormone) to stimulate the thyroid to make thyroid hormones.

Other cases of thyroid hormone deficiency may be due to the hypothalamus failing to release sufficient TRH (thyrotropin-releasing hormone).

In cases where thyroid hormone deficiency is caused by a malfunctioning pituitary or hypothalamus, supplements or essential oils such as Cedarwood may help stimulate the pituitary or hypothalamus.

People with type-A blood have more of a tendency to have weak thyroid function.

....

Hyperthyroid (Graves' Disease)

When the thyroid becomes overactive and produces excess thyroid hormone, the following symptoms may occur:

- Anxiety
- Restlessness
- Insomnia

- Premature gray hair
- Diabetes mellitus
- Arthritis
- Vitiligo (loss of skin pigment)

Graves' disease, unlike Hashimoto's disease, is an autoimmune disease that results in an excess of thyroid hormone production. MSM has been studied for its ability to reverse many kinds of autoimmune diseases.

MSM is a key component of Sulfurzyme.

Recommendations

Singles: Myrrh, Idaho Blue Spruce, Blue Tansy, Lemongrass, Wintergreen, German Chamomile

Blends: EndoFlex, Brain Power, Clarity, Common Sense

Nutritionals: MultiGreens, Mineral Essence, MegaCal, Essentialzyme, Detoxzyme, Essentialzymes-4, OmegaGize[3], Sulfurzyme, Thyromin (only in the morning), Ultra Young Plus

Application and Usage
Inhalation

- Diffuse your choice of oils for ½ hour every 4-6 hours or as desired.
- Put 2-3 drops of your chosen oil in your hands and rub them together, cup your hands over your nose, and inhale throughout the day as needed.
- Put 8-10 drops of oil on a cotton ball or tissue and put it in an air vent in your house, vehicle, hotel room, etc.
- If diffusing while sleeping, set your timer for the desired length of time for automatic shut off.

Topical

You may apply single oils or blends neat or diluted, depending on the oil or oils being used. Please see the instructions at the beginning of this chapter for more information on applying oils to the skin.

Ingestion

The amount of oil ingested varies with different oils. Whether putting the oils in a capsule or drinking them in a liquid, please refer to the instructions at the beginning of this chapter.

- Take 1 capsule with desired oil 2 times daily.
- Put 2-3 drops of oil in a spoonful of Blue Agave, Yacon Syrup, maple syrup, coconut oil, milk, etc.
- Put the desired amount of oils in a glass of rice milk, almond milk, goat milk, carrot juice, NingXia Red, or even water and then drink it.

....

Hypoglycemia

Hypoglycemia may be caused by low thyroid function.

Excessive consumption of sugar or honey will also cause reactive hypoglycemia, in which a rapid rise in blood sugar is followed by a steep drop to abnormally low levels.

In some cases, hypoglycemia may be a precursor to candida, allergies, chronic fatigue syndrome, depression, and chemical sensitivities.

Signs of hypoglycemia (low blood sugar) include:

- Fatigue, drowsiness, and sleepiness after meals
- Headache or dizziness if times between meals are too long
- Craving for sweets
- Allergic reaction to foods
- Palpitations, tremors, sweats, rapid heartbeat
- Inattentiveness, mood swings, irritability, anxiety, nervousness, inability to cope with stress, and feelings of emotional depression
- Lack of motivation, discipline, and creativity
- Hunger that cannot be satisfied

Often people with some of these symptoms are misdiagnosed as suffering either chronic fatigue or neurosis. Instead, they may be hypoglycemic.

To treat chronic hypoglycemia, it is important to treat the underlying cause such as candida or yeast overgrowth (See Fungal Infections).

Essential oils may reduce hypoglycemic symptoms by helping to normalize sugar cravings, supporting and stabilizing sugar metabolism in the body.

Recommendations

Singles: Lavender, Coriander, Dill, Fennel, Cinnamon Bark

Nutritionals: MultiGreens, NingXia Red, Life 5, Digest & Cleanse, ICP, JuvaPower, Ningxia Wolfberries (Dried)

Application and Usage
Inhalation
- Diffuse your choice of oils for ½ hour every 2 hours or as desired.
- Put 2-3 drops of your chosen oil in your hands and rub them together, cup your hands over your nose, and inhale throughout the day as needed.
- Put 8-10 drops of oil on a cotton ball or tissue and put it in an air vent in your house, vehicle, hotel room, etc.
- If diffusing while sleeping, set your timer for the desired length of time for automatic shut off.

Topical
You may apply single oils or blends neat or diluted, depending on the oil or oils being used. Please see the instructions at the beginning of this chapter for more information on applying oils to the skin.
- Rub 1-2 drops of oil on the temples and back of neck several times daily.
- Place a warm compress with 1-2 drops of chosen oil on the back.

Ingestion and Oral
The amount of oil ingested varies with different oils. Whether putting the oils in a capsule or drinking them in a liquid, please refer to the instructions at the beginning of this chapter.
- Take 1 capsule with desired oil 1 time daily (Coriander, Dill, and Fennel work best through ingestion).
- Put 2-3 drops of oil in a spoonful of Blue Agave, Yacon Syrup, maple syrup, coconut oil, milk, etc.
- Put the desired amount of oils in a glass of rice milk, almond milk, goat milk, carrot juice, NingXia Red, or even water and then drink it.

....

Hypothyroid (Hashimoto's Disease)

This condition occurs when the thyroid is underactive and produces insufficient thyroid hormone. Approximately 40 percent of the U.S. population suffers from milder forms of this disorder to some degree, and these people tend to suffer from hypoglycemia (low blood sugar). In its severe form, it is referred to as Hashimoto's disease.

Hashimoto's disease, like Graves' disease, is an autoimmune condition that affects the thyroid differently, however, by limiting its ability to produce thyroid hormone.

The following symptoms may occur:
- Fatigue
- Yeast infections (candida)
- Lack of energy
- Reduced immune function
- Poor resistance to disease
- Recurring infections
- Low sex hormones

Recommendations

Singles: Lemongrass, Spearmint, Ledum, Myrtle, Peppermint, Myrrh, Clove

Blends: EndoFlex, Brain Power, Clarity

Nutritionals: Thyromin, MultiGreens, Sulfurzyme, Ultra Young Plus, Essentialzyme, Detoxzyme, MegaCal

Application and Usage
Inhalation

- Diffuse your choice of oils for ½ hour every 4-6 hours or as desired.
- Put 2-3 drops of your chosen oil in your hands and rub them together, cup your hands over your nose, and inhale throughout the day as needed.
- Put 8-10 drops of oil on a cotton ball or tissue and put it in an air vent in your house, vehicle, hotel room, etc.
- If diffusing while sleeping, set your timer for the desired length of time for automatic shut off.

Topical

You may apply single oils or blends neat or diluted, depending on the oil or oils being used. Please see the instructions at the beginning of this chapter for more information on applying oils to the skin.

- Apply 3-5 drops neat or diluted 50:50 over the thyroid, the front of the neck, and on both sides of the trachea 1-3 times daily.
- Apply 1-3 drops on the thyroid Vita Flex points of the feet located on the inside edge of the ball of the foot just below the base of the big toe.

Ingestion and Oral

The amount of oil ingested varies with different oils. Whether putting the oils in a capsule or drinking them in a liquid, please refer to the instructions at the beginning of this chapter.

- Take 1 capsule with desired oil 2 times daily.
- Put 2-3 drops of oil in a spoonful of Blue Agave, Yacon Syrup, maple syrup, coconut oil, milk, etc.
- Put the desired amount of oils in a glass of rice milk, almond milk, goat milk, carrot juice, NingXia Red, or even water and then drink it.

TOXEMIA

Toxins or bacteria that accumulate in the bloodstream create a condition called toxemia.

Recommendations

Singles: Clove, Tangerine, Lemon, Cypress, Orange, Patchouli

Blends: Purification, Thieves, Melrose, Citrus Fresh

Nutritionals: Rehemogen, ICP, ComforTone, Essentialzyme, Super C, JuvaTone, JuvaPower, Detoxzyme, Super C Chewable

Application and Usage
Inhalation

- Diffuse your choice of oils for ½ hour every 4-6 hours or as desired.
- Put 2-3 drops of your chosen oil in your hands and rub them together, cup your hands over your nose, and inhale throughout the day as needed.
- Put 8-10 drops of oil on a cotton ball or tissue and put it in an air vent in your house, vehicle, hotel room, etc.
- If diffusing while sleeping, set your timer for the desired length of time for automatic shut off.

Topical

You may apply single oils or blends neat or diluted, depending on the oil or oils being used. Please see the instructions at the beginning of this chapter for more information on applying oils to the skin.

- Dilute 50:50 and apply on location 2-3 times daily or as needed.
- Massage 2-4 drops of oil neat on the soles of the feet just before bedtime.

Ingestion and Oral

The amount of oil ingested varies with different oils. Whether putting the oils in a capsule or drinking them in a liquid, please refer to the instructions at the beginning of this chapter.

- Take 1 capsule with desired oil 3 times daily.

- Put 2-3 drops of oil in a spoonful of Blue Agave, Yacon Syrup, maple syrup, coconut oil, milk, etc.
- Put the desired amount of oils in a glass of rice milk, almond milk, goat milk, carrot juice, NingXia Red, or even water and then drink it.
- Best results may be achieved by eliminating certain foods such as all sugar, white flour, breads, pasta, fried foods, and chlorinated water.

TRAUMA, EMOTIONAL

Emotional trauma can be generated from events that involve loss, abuse, bereavement, accidents, or misfortunes. The scents of essential oils have the ability to cross the blood brain barrier, simulating the amygdala that controls the emotional and memory center of the brain. Certain essential oils help facilitate the processing and release of emotional trauma in a simple way that minimizes psychological turmoil.

Recommendations

Singles: Sacred Frankincense, Frankincense, Idaho Blue Spruce, Idaho Balsam Fir, Western Red Cedar, Spruce, Sandalwood, Rose, Palo Santo, Galbanum, Ocotea, Cedarwood

Blends: The Gift, Trauma Life, Peace & Calming, Hope, RutaVaLa, RutaVaLa Roll-On, Harmony, Gathering, Forgiveness, Release, Envision, Valor, Valor Roll-On, Joy, Oola Balance, Oola Grow, Highest Potential, 3 Wise Men, Sacred Mountain

Nutritionals: Super C, Super C Chewable, Mineral Essence, MegaCal, Essentialzyme, OmegaGize^3, Balance Complete, NingXia Red

Application and Usage
Inhalation

- Diffuse your choice of oils for ½ hour every 4-6 hours or as desired.

- Put 2-3 drops of your chosen oil in your hands and rub them together, cup your hands over your nose, and inhale throughout the day as needed.
- Put 8-10 drops of oil on a cotton ball or tissue and put it in an air vent in your house, vehicle, hotel room, etc.
- If diffusing while sleeping, set your timer for the desired length of time for automatic shut off.

Topical

You may apply single oils or blends neat or diluted, depending on the oil or oils being used. Please see the instructions at the beginning of this chapter for more information on applying oils to the skin.

- Apply 2-4 drops of oil diluted 50:50 or neat to the temples, forehead, crown, and shoulders 1-3 times daily.

TRIGGER FINGER (STENOSING TENOSYNOVITIS)

Tendonitis, often called "tennis elbow" and "golfer's elbow," is a torn or inflamed tendon. Tenosynovitis, sometimes called "trigger finger," is an inflamed tendon being restricted by its sheath (particularly in thumbs and fingers). Repetitive use or infection may be the cause.

When selecting oils for injuries, think through the cause and type of injury and select appropriate oils. For instance, tendonitis could encompass muscle damage, nerve damage, ligament strain/tear, inflammation, infection, and possibly an emotion. The emotional distress may be anger or guilt.

Therefore, select a single oil or blend for each potential cause or a blend to address multiple causes.

Singles: Lemongrass (promotes the repair of connective tissue), Rosewood, Sandalwood

Blends: PanAway, Relieve It, Deep Relief Roll-On

Nutritionals: MegaCal, BLM, Sulfurzyme

MegaCal builds and strengthens bones. Mix 1 teaspoon in water and drink. Taken at night, MegaCal promotes peaceful sleep.

BLM provides critical nutrients for connective tissue and muscle repair and strengthens the bones. Mix 1 teaspoon in water and drink 2 times daily.

Sulfurzyme equalizes water pressure inside the cells and reduces pain. Mix 1-2 teaspoons in water and drink 2 times daily.

Massage Oils: Ortho Sport Massage Oil, Ortho Ease Massage Oil

The oils in Ortho Sport and Ortho Ease massage oils reduce pain and promote healing.

Application and Usage
Inhalation

- Diffuse your choice of oils for ½ hour every 4-6 hours or as desired.
- Put 2-3 drops of your chosen oil in your hands and rub them together, cup your hands over your nose, and inhale throughout the day as needed.
- Put 8-10 drops of oil on a cotton ball or tissue and put it in an air vent in your house, vehicle, hotel room, etc.
- If diffusing while sleeping, set your timer for the desired length of time for automatic shut off.

Topical

You may apply single oils or blends neat or diluted, depending on the oil or oils being used. Please see the instructions at the beginning of this chapter for more information on applying oils to the skin.

- Massage finger with Lavender and Lemongrass.
- Massage Marjoram with Lemongrass for inflamed tendons.
- Single oils or blends may be used singularly or together.

TYPHOID FEVER

Typhoid fever is an infectious disease caused by a bacterium known as *Salmonella typhi*. Usually contracted through infected food or water, typhoid is common in lesser-developed countries.

Some people infected with typhoid fever display no visible symptoms of disease, while others become seriously ill. Both people who recover from typhoid fever and those who remain symptomless are carriers for the disease and can infect others through the bacteria they shed in their feces.

To avoid contracting typhoid fever—especially when traveling overseas—it is essential to drink purified or distilled water and to thoroughly cook foods. Fresh vegetables can be carriers of the bacteria, especially if they have been irrigated with water that has come into contact with human waste.

Symptoms

- Sustained, high fever (101° to 104° F)
- Stomach pains
- Headache
- Rash of reddish spots
- Impaired appetite
- Weakness

Recommendations

Singles: Clove, Thyme, Ravintsara, Cinnamon, Cassia, Peppermint, Black Pepper, Mountain Savory, Oregano, Plectranthus Oregano, Melaleuca Alternifolia

Blends: Thieves, Melrose, Exodus II

Nutritionals: Inner Defense, ImmuPro, Super C, Super C Chewable, NingXia Red

Application and Usage
Inhalation

- Diffuse your choice of oils for ½ hour every 4-6 hours or as desired.
- Put 2-3 drops of your chosen oil in your hands and rub them together, cup your hands

over your nose, and inhale throughout the day as needed.

- Put 8-10 drops of oil on a cotton ball or tissue and put it in an air vent in your house, vehicle, hotel room, etc.
- If diffusing while sleeping, set your timer for the desired length of time for automatic shut off.

Topical

You may apply single oils or blends neat or diluted, depending on the oil or oils being used. Please see the instructions at the beginning of this chapter for more information on applying oils to the skin.

- Apply 4-6 drops of oil diluted 50:50 on lower abdomen 2-4 times daily.

Ingestion and Oral

The amount of oil ingested varies with different oils. Whether putting the oils in a capsule or drinking them in a liquid, please refer to the instructions at the beginning of this chapter.

- Take 1 capsule with desired oil 2 times daily for 10 days.
- Put 2-3 drops of oil in a spoonful of Blue Agave, Yacon Syrup, maple syrup, coconut oil, milk, etc.
- Put the desired amount of oils in a glass of rice milk, almond milk, goat milk, carrot juice, NingXia Red, or even water and then drink it.

ENDNOTES

1. Valnet J, MD. "The Practice of Aromatherapy: A Classic Compendium of Plant Medicines & Their Healing Properties," *Healing Arts Press*. 1990:197.

2. Ammon HP. "Boswellic acids in chronic inflammatory diseases," *Planta Med*. 2006 Oct;72(12):1100-16.

3. Yu MS, et al. "Neuroprotective effects of anti-aging oriental medicine *Lycium barbarum* against beta-amyloid peptide neurotoxicity," *Exp Gerontol*. 2005 Aug-Sep;40(8-9):716-27.

4. Galli RL, et al. "Fruit polyphenolics and brain aging: nutritional interventions targeting age-related neuronal and behavioral deficits," *Ann N Y Acad Sci*. 2002 Apr; 959:128-32.

5. Bickford PC, et al. "Antioxidant-rich diets improve cerebellar physiology and motor learning in aged rats," *Brain Res*. 2000 Jun 2; 866(1-2):211-7.

6. Haze S, Sakai K, Gozu Y. "Effects of fragrance on sympathetic activity in normal adults," *Jpn J Pharmacol*. 2002 Nov;903):247-53.

7. Koo HN, et al. "Inhibition of heat shock-induced apoptosis by peppermint oil in astrocytes," *J Mol Neurosci*. 2001 Dec;17(3):391-6.

8. Ellis Y, et al. "The effect of multi-tasking on the grade performance of business students," *Research in Higher Education*. June 2010. Vol. 8:1-10.

9. Dember WN, et al. "Olfactory Stimulation and Sustained Attention," *Compendium of Olfactory Research,* Ed. Avery N. Gilbert, Kendall Hunt Publishing, 1995:39-46.

10. Vigushin DM, et al. "Phase I and pharmaco-kinetic study of D-limonene in patients with advanced cancer," Cancer Research Campaign Phase I/II Clinical Trials Committee. *Cancer Chemother Pharmacol*. 1998;42(2):111-7.

11. Ionescu JG, et al. "Increased levels of transition metals in breast cancer tissue," *Neuro Endocrinol Lett*. 2006 Dec;27 Suppl 1:36-9.

12. Ghoneum M, Gollapudi S. "Modified arabi-noxylan rice bran (MGN-3/Biobran) enhances yeast-induced apoptosis in human breast cancer cells in vitro," *Anticancer Res*. 2005 Mar-Apr;25 (2A):859-70.

13. Cao GW, Yang WG, Du P. "Observation of the effects of LAK/IL-2 therapy combining with *Lycium barbarum* polysaccharides in the treatment of 75 cancer patients," *Zhonghua Zhong Liu Za Zhi*. 1994 *Psychosomatics*. 2002 Nov-Dec;43(6):508-9.

14. Pace A, et al. "Vitamin E neuroprotection for cisplatin neuropathy: a randomized, placebo-controlled trial," *Neurology*. 2010 Mar 2;74(9):762-6.

15. Banerjee S., Panda CKL, Das S. "Clove (*Syzygium aromaticum* L.), a potential chemopreventive agent for lung cancer," *Carcinogenisis*. 2006 Aug;27(8):1645-54. Epub 2006 Feb 25.

16. Legault J, et al. "Antitumor activity of balsam fir oil: production of reactive oxygen species induced by alpha-humulene as possible mechanism of action," *Planta Med*. 2003 May;69(5):402-7.

17. de Castillo MC, et al. "Bactericidal activity of lemon juice and lemon derivatives against *Vibrio cholerae*," *Biol Pharm Bull*. 2000 Oct;23(10):1235-8.

18. Nasel C, et al. "Functional imaging of effects of fragrances on the human brain after prolonged inhalation," *Chem Senses*. 1994 Aug;19(4):359-64.

19. Komori T, et al. "Effects of citrus fragrance on immune function and depressive states," *Neuro-immunomodulation*. 1995 May-Jun;2(3):174-80.

20. Barrowman JA, et al. "Diarrhoeae in thyroid medullary carcinoma: role of prostaglandins and therapeutic effect of nutmeg," *Br Med J*. 1975 Jul 5;3(5974):11-12.

21. Fawell WN, Thompson G. "Nutmeg for diarrhea of medeatinullary carcinoma of thyroid," *N Eng J Med*. 1973 Jul 12;289(2):108-9.

22. Igimi H, et al. "Medical dissolution of gall-stones. Clinical experience of d-limonene as a simple, safe, and effective solvent," *Dig Dis Sci*. 1991 Feb;36(2):200-8.

23. Igimi H, et al. "A useful cholesterol solvent for medical dissolution of gallstones," *Gastroenterol Jpn*. 1992 Aug;27(4):536-45.

24. Hay IC, Jamieson M, Ormerod AD. "Random-ized trial of aromatherapy. Successful treat-ment for alopecia areata," *Arch Dermatol*. 1998 Nov;134(11):1349-52.

25. Nenoff P, Haustein UF, Brandt W. "Antifungal activity of the essential oil of *Melaleuca alter-nifolia* (tea tree oil) against pathogenic fungi in vitro," *Skin Pharmacol*. 1996;9(6):388-94.

26. Göbel H, et al. "*Effectiveness of Oleum menthae piperitae and paracetamol in therapy of headache of the tension type,*" *Nervenarzt*. 1996 Aug; 67(8):672-81.

27. Göbel H, Schmidt G, Soyka D. "*Effect of peppermint and eucalyptus oil preparations on neurophysiological and experimental algesimetric headache parameters,*" *Cephalalgia*. 1994 Jun; 14(3):228-34; discussion 182.

28. Weydert JA, et al. "Systematic review of treat-ments for recurrent abdominal pain," *Pediatrics*. 2003 Jan;111(1):e1-11.

29. Logan AC, Beaulne TM. "The treatment of small intestinal bacterial overgrowth with enteric-coated peppermint oil: a case report," *Altern Med Rev*. 2002 Oct;7(5):410-7.

30. Sagduyu K. "Peppermint oil for irritable bowel syndrome," *Psychosomatics*. 2002 Nov-Dec;43(6):508-9.

31. Veal L. "The potential effectiveness of essential oils as a treatment for headlice, *Pediculus huma-nus capitis*," *Complement Ther Nurs Midwifery*. 1996 Aug;2(4):97-101.

32. Nasel C, et al. "Functional imaging of effects of fragrances on the human brain after prolonged inhalation," *Chem Senses*. 1994 Aug;19(4):359-64.

33. Hirsch AR, Gomez R. "Inhalation of odorants for weight reduction," *Int. J. Obes*. Vol. 18, Supplement 2, August 1994:79.

34. Göbel H, Schmidt G, Soyka D. "Effect of pep-permint and eucalyptus oil preparations on neurophysiological and experimental algesimet-ric headache parameters," *Cephalalgia*. 1994 Jun;14(3):228-34; discussion 182.

35. Benencia F, Courrèges MC. "Antiviral activity of sandalwood against herpes simplex viruses-1 and -2," *Phytomedicine*. 1999 May;6(2):119-23.

36. Toyoda M, Morohashi M. "Pathenogenesis of acne," *Med Electron Microsc*. 2001 Mar;34(1):29-40.

Appendix A

Product Usage for Body Systems

Product Type Key:

S Essential Oil Single
B Essential Oil Blend
D Dietary Supplement
P Personal Care/Hair and Skin
L Lotions/Creams/Massage Oils
G Bath and Shower Gels/Soaps
A Antiseptic/Sanitizing
O Oral Care

Product	Product Type	Nervous System	Cardiovascular System	Respiratory System	Digestive / Elimination	Immune / Anti-infectious	Glandular / Hormonal	Emotional Balance	Muscle and Bone	Antiaging	Oral Hygiene	Skin and Hair
Abundance	B					●		●				
Acceptance	B	●						●				
AlkaLime	D		●		●				●			
Allerzyme	D				●							
Amazonian Ylang Ylang	S		●				●	●				
Angelica	S	●						●				
Animal Scents Shampoo	G											●
Animal Scents Ointment	L											●
Anise	S				●				●			
AromaGuard Meadow Mist Deodorant	P											●
AromaGuard Mountain Mint Deodorant	P											●
Aroma Life	B		●									
Aroma Siez	B			●					●			
A·R·T Beauty Masque	P											●
A·R·T Creme Masque	P											●
A·R·T Day Activator	P											●
A·R·T Gentle Foaming Cleanser	P											●
A·R·T Night Reconstructor	P											●
A·R·T Purifying Toner	P											●
A·R·T Renewal Serum	P											●
Australian Blue	B							●				
Awaken	B							●				
Balance Complete	D	●	●			●	●				●	
Basil	S		●						●			

Product Type Key:
- **S** Essential Oil Single
- **B** Essential Oil Blend
- **D** Dietary Supplement
- **P** Personal Care/Hair and Skin
- **L** Lotions/Creams/Massage Oils
- **G** Bath and Shower Gels/Soaps
- **A** Antiseptic/Sanitizing
- **O** Oral Care

Product	Product Type	Nervous System	Cardiovascular System	Respiratory System	Digestive / Elimination	Immune / Anti-infectious	Glandular / Hormonal	Emotional Balance	Muscle and Bone	Antiaging	Oral Hygiene	Skin and Hair
Bath & Shower Gel Base	G											●
Believe	B							●				
Bergamot	S				●			●				●
Biblical Sweet Myrrh	S	●				●	●					●
Black Pepper	S	●			●							
BLM (Capsules and Powder)	D								●			
Blue Agave	D						●		●			
Blue Tansy	S	●										
Boswellia Wrinkle Cream	L									●		●
Brain Power	B	●						●				
Breathe Again Roll-On	B			●								
Cajuput	S		●	●								
Cardamom	S				●							
Cassia	S		●		●					●	●	
Cedarwood	S	●		●								
Cel-Lite Magic Massage Oil	L											●
Chocolessence	D				●			●				
Christmas Spirit	B	●	●					●				
Cinnamint Lip Balm	P											●
Cinnamon Bark	S					●						
Cistus	S					●				●		
Citronella	S								●			
Citrus Fresh	B				●			●				
ClaraDerm	P											●
Clarity	B	●						●				
Clary Sage	S						●					
Clove	S		●	●	●	●				●	●	
ComforTone	D				●	●						
Common Sense	B							●				
Canadian Fleabane (Conyza)	S		●				●					
Copaiba	S				●					●	●	
Copaiba Vanilla Moisturizing Conditioner	P											●
Copaiba Vanilla Moisturizing Shampoo	P											●

Product Type Key:
- **S** Essential Oil Single
- **B** Essential Oil Blend
- **D** Dietary Supplement
- **P** Personal Care/Hair and Skin
- **L** Lotions/Creams/Massage Oils
- **G** Bath and Shower Gels/Soaps
- **A** Antiseptic/Sanitizing
- **O** Oral Care

Product	Product Type	Nervous System	Cardiovascular System	Respiratory System	Digestive / Elimination	Immune / Anti-infectious	Glandular / Hormonal	Emotional Balance	Muscle and Bone	Antiaging	Oral Hygiene	Skin and Hair
Coriander	S				●		●					
CortiStop Women's	D						●					
Cumin	S				●	●						
Cypress	S		●						●			
Deep Relief Roll-On	S								●			
Detoxzyme	D				●	●						
Digest & Cleanse	D	●			●	●					●	
DiGize	B				●							
Dill	S				●							
Douglas Fir	S			●					●			
Dragon Time	B						●	●				
Dragon Time Bath & Shower Gel	G						●	●				
Dragon Time Massage Oil	L							●				●
Dream Catcher	B							●				
Egyptian Gold	B	●				●		●				
Einkorn Nuggets	D				●			●				
Elemi	S											●
En-R-Gee	D	●						●				
EndoFlex	B						●					
EndoGize	D						●					
Envision	B							●				
Essential Beauty Serum (Acne-Prone Skin)	P											●
Essential Beauty Serum (Dry Skin)	P											●
Essentialzyme	D				●				●			
Essentialzymes-4	D				●				●			
Estro	D						●	●				
Eucalyptus Blue	S			●					●			
Eucalyptus Citriodora	S			●								
Eucalyptus Dives	S			●								
Eucalyptus Globulus	S			●						●	●	
Eucalyptus Polybractea	S			●								
Eucalyptus Radiata	S			●								●
Evening Peace Bath & Shower Gel	G											●

453

Product	Product Type	Nervous System	Cardiovascular System	Respiratory System	Digestive / Elimination	Immune / Anti-infectious	Glandular / Hormonal	Emotional Balance	Muscle and Bone	Antiaging	Oral Hygiene	Skin and Hair
Exodus II	B					●						
FemiGen	D						●	●				
Fennel	S				●		●					
Forgiveness	B							●				
Frankincense	S	●				●		●			●	●
Frereana Frankincense	S					●		●				
Galbanum	S					●						
Gathering	B							●				
Genesis Hand & Body Lotion	L											●
Gentle Baby	B							●				●
Geranium	S							●				●
German Chamomile	S	●						●				●
Ginger	S	●			●							
GLF	B				●	●						
Goldenrod	S		●				●					
Grapefruit	S		●							●		
Grapefruit Lip Balm	P										●	
Gratitude	B							●				
Grounding	B							●				
Harmony	B							●				
Helichrysum	S		●						●			
Highest Potential	B							●				
Hinoki	S	●		●	●		●					●
Hong Kuai	S			●				●				
Hope	B							●				
Humility	B							●				
Hyssop	S	●	●	●								
ICP	D		●		●							
Idaho Balsam Fir	S	●			●		●					
Idaho Blue Spruce	S			●		●		●	●			
Idaho Ponderosa Pine	S			●	●	●	●					
Idaho Tansy	S					●						
ImmuPower	B					●						

Product Type Key:

S Essential Oil Single
B Essential Oil Blend
D Dietary Supplement
P Personal Care/Hair and Skin
L Lotions/Creams/Massage Oils
G Bath and Shower Gels/Soaps
A Antiseptic/Sanitizing
O Oral Care

Product	Product Type	Nervous System	Cardiovascular System	Respiratory System	Digestive / Elimination	Immune / Anti-infectious	Glandular / Hormonal	Emotional Balance	Muscle and Bone	Antiaging	Oral Hygiene	Skin and Hair
ImmuPro	D					●						
Inner Child	B							●				
Inner Defense	D			●	●	●						
Inspiration	B							●				
Into the Future	B							●				
Jasmine	S						●	●				
Joy	B							●				
Juniper	S				●			●				
JuvaCleanse	B				●					●		
JuvaFlex	B				●			●				
JuvaPower	D				●					●		
JuvaSpice	D				●					●		
JuvaTone	D				●	●						
K&B	D				●							
KidScents Bath Gel	G											●
KidScents Lotion	L											●
KidScents MightyVites	D	●	●	●	●	●	●	●		●		
KidScents Mightyzyme	D			●	●					●		
KidScents Shampoo	P											●
KidScents Slique Toothpaste	O										●	
KidScents Tender Tush	L											●
Lady Sclareol	B						●	●				
Laurus Nobilis (Bay Laurel)	S			●	●	●						
LavaDerm Cooling Mist	P							●				●
Lavender	S	●	●					●				●
Lavender Bath & Shower Gel	G											●
Lavender Conditioner	P											●
Lavender Foaming Hand Soap	G											●
Lavender Hand & Body Lotion	L											●
Lavender Lip Balm	P										●	
Lavender Mint Daily Conditioner	P											●
Lavender Mint Daily Shampoo	P											●
Lavender-Rosewood Moisturizing Bar Soap	G											●

Product Type Key:
- **S** Essential Oil Single
- **B** Essential Oil Blend
- **D** Dietary Supplement
- **P** Personal Care/Hair and Skin
- **L** Lotions/Creams/Massage Oils
- **G** Bath and Shower Gels/Soaps
- **A** Antiseptic/Sanitizing
- **O** Oral Care

Product	Product Type	Nervous System	Cardiovascular System	Respiratory System	Digestive / Elimination	Immune / Anti-infectious	Glandular / Hormonal	Emotional Balance	Muscle and Bone	Antiaging	Oral Hygiene	Skin and Hair
Lavender Shampoo	P											●
Ledum	S				●	●				●		●
Lemon	S			●	●	●				●		
Lemon-Sandalwood Cleansing Bar Soap	G											●
Lemongrass	S					●			●			
Life 5	D				●	●	●			●		
Lime	S			●	●	●				●		
Live with Passion	B							●				
Longevity	B									●		
Longevity Softgels	D		●							●		
M-Grain	B	●										
Magnify Your Purpose	B	●						●				
Mandarin	S				●					●		●
Manuka	S			●	●	●			●			
Marjoram	S		●						●			
Master Formula HERS	D	●	●	●	●	●	●		●	●		
Master Formula HIS	D	●	●	●	●	●	●		●	●		
Mastrante	S	●	●	●		●		●				
MegaCal	D		●						●			
Melaleuca Alternifolia (Tea Tree)	S			●		●			●		●	●
Melaleuca Cajuput	S			●	●	●			●		●	●
Melaleuca Ericifolia	S			●								●
Melaleuca Quinquenervia (Niaouli)	S			●					●			
Melissa	S					●			●			
Melrose	B			●								●
Micromeria	S		●	●	●	●			●			
Mineral Essence	D	●	●			●	●	●	●			
Mister	B							●				
Morning Start Bath & Shower Gel	G											●
Morning Start Moisturizing Bar Soap	G								●			●
Motivation	B	●						●				
Mountain Savory	S					●						
MultiGreens	D	●	●		●	●			●			

456

Product Type Key:
- **S** Essential Oil Single
- **B** Essential Oil Blend
- **D** Dietary Supplement
- **P** Personal Care/Hair and Skin
- **L** Lotions/Creams/Massage Oils
- **G** Bath and Shower Gels/Soaps
- **A** Antiseptic/Sanitizing
- **O** Oral Care

Product	Product Type	Nervous System	Cardiovascular System	Respiratory System	Digestive / Elimination	Immune / Anti-infectious	Glandular / Hormonal	Emotional Balance	Muscle and Bone	Antiaging	Oral Hygiene	Skin and Hair
Myrrh	S	●				●	●					●
Myrtle	S			●	●		●		●			
Neroli	S				●							●
Niaouli	S			●					●			
NingXia Nitro	D	●	●			●	●			●		
NingXia Red	D	●	●			●	●			●		
Ningxia Wolfberries	D	●	●			●	●			●		
Nutmeg	S	●				●						
Ocotea	S					●						
OmegaGize³	D	●	●			●	●		●	●		●
Oola Balance	B							●				
Oola Grow	B							●				
Orange	S				●	●				●		●
Orange Blossom Facial Wash	P											●
Oregano	S			●	●	●			●	●		
Ortho Ease Massage Oil	L								●			●
Ortho Sport Massage Oil	L								●			
Palmarosa	S		●				●					●
Palo Santo	S	●				●						
PanAway	B	●							●			
ParaFree	D				●	●						
Patchouli	S											●
PD 80/20	D						●	●	●			
Peace & Calming	B	●						●				
Peppermint	S	●		●	●				●		●	●
Peppermint-Cedarwood Moisturizing Bar Soap	G								●			●
Petitgrain	S							●				
Pine	S			●				●				
Plectranthus Oregano	S			●	●	●			●	●		
Power Meal	D		●		●	●			●			
Prenolone Plus Body Cream	L	●					●	●	●	●		
Present Time	B							●				
Prostate Health	D						●					

Product Type Key:
- **S** Essential Oil Single
- **B** Essential Oil Blend
- **D** Dietary Supplement
- **P** Personal Care/Hair and Skin
- **L** Lotions/Creams/Massage Oils
- **G** Bath and Shower Gels/Soaps
- **A** Antiseptic/Sanitizing
- **O** Oral Care

Product	Product Type	Nervous System	Cardiovascular System	Respiratory System	Digestive / Elimination	Immune / Anti-infectious	Glandular / Hormonal	Emotional Balance	Muscle and Bone	Antiaging	Oral Hygiene	Skin and Hair
Progessence Plus	P						●					
Protec	B						●					
Pure Protein Complete	D								●	●		
Purification	B				●			●				●
R.C.	B			●								
Raven	B					●						
Ravintsara	S			●		●						
Regenolone Moisturizing Cream	L	●					●		●			●
Rehemogen	D		●		●							
Relaxation Massage Oil	L							●				●
Release	B							●				
Relieve It	B								●			
Roman Chamomile	S	●						●				●
Rose	S							●				●
Rose Ointment	P											●
Rosemary (CT cineol)	S		●		●				●			
Rosewood	S											●
RutaVaLa	B	●						●				
RutaVaLa Roll-On	B	●						●				
Sacred Frankincense	S					●		●				●
Sacred Mountain	B							●				
Sacred Mountain Moisturizing Bar Soap	G							●				●
Sage	S				●	●						
Sandalwood	S	●						●		●		●
Sandalwood Moisture Cream	P											●
SARA	B							●				
Satin Facial Scrub, Mint	P											●
SclarEssence	B/D				●		●					
Sensation	B						●	●				
Sensation Bath & Shower Gel	G											●
Sensation Hand & Body Lotion	L											●
Sensation Massage Oil	L											●
SleepEssence	D							●				

Product Type Key:
- S Essential Oil Single
- B Essential Oil Blend
- D Dietary Supplement
- P Personal Care/Hair and Skin
- L Lotions/Creams/Massage Oils
- G Bath and Shower Gels/Soaps
- A Antiseptic/Sanitizing
- O Oral Care

Product	Product Type	Nervous System	Cardiovascular System	Respiratory System	Digestive / Elimination	Immune / Anti-infectious	Glandular / Hormonal	Emotional Balance	Muscle and Bone	Antiaging	Oral Hygiene	Skin and Hair
Slique Bars	D				●							
Slique Essence	B				●							
Slique Gum	O				●						●	
Slique Slim Caps	D				●							
Slique Tea	D				●							
Spanish Sage	S	●	●	●	●	●	●	●	●	●		●
Spearmint	S				●			●				
Spikenard	S							●				●
Spruce	S	●		●				●				
Stevia Extract	D		●		●	●						
Stress Away	B							●				
Stress Away Roll-On	B							●				
Sulfurzyme (Capsules and Powder)	D	●				●			●	●		●
Super B	D	●	●					●				
Super C (and Chewable)	D				●	●				●		
Super Cal	D	●	●					●	●			
Surrender	B	●						●				
Tangerine	S				●			●		●		●
Tarragon	S	●		●								
The Gift	B	●				●	●	●				
Thieves	A					●				●	●	
Thieves AromaBright Toothpaste	O										●	
Thieves Cleansing Bar Soap	A					●						●
Thieves Dental Floss	O										●	
Thieves Dentarome Plus Toothpaste	O										●	
Thieves Dentarome Ultra Toothpaste	O		●								●	
Thieves Foaming Hand Soap	A					●						●
Thieves Fresh Essence Plus Mouthwash	O					●					●	●
Thieves Household Cleaner	A					●						
Thieves Lozenges (Hard/Soft)	O			●							●	
Thieves Spray	A					●					●	●
Thieves Waterless Hand Purifier	A					●						●
Thieves Wipes	A					●						

Product Type Key:
- **S** Essential Oil Single
- **B** Essential Oil Blend
- **D** Dietary Supplement
- **P** Personal Care/Hair and Skin
- **L** Lotions/Creams/Massage Oils
- **G** Bath and Shower Gels/Soaps
- **A** Antiseptic/Sanitizing
- **O** Oral Care

Product	Product Type	Nervous System	Cardiovascular System	Respiratory System	Digestive / Elimination	Immune / Anti-infectious	Glandular / Hormonal	Emotional Balance	Muscle and Bone	Antiaging	Oral Hygiene	Skin and Hair
Three (3) Wise Men	B							•				
Thyme	S				•				•	•		
Thyromin	D						•					
Trauma Life	B							•				
Tranquil Roll-On	B	•						•				
Transformation	B	•						•	•			
True Source	D	•	•	•	•	•	•	•	•	•		•
Tsuga	S		•	•								
Ultra Young Plus	D						•			•		
V-6 Vegetable Oil Complex	L								•			•
Valerian	S	•										
Valor	B	•						•	•			•
Valor Moisturizing Bar Soap	P	•										•
Valor Roll-On	B	•						•	•			•
Vetiver	S	•					•	•				•
Western Red Cedar	S											•
White Angelica	B							•				
White Fir	S			•				•	•	•		
White Lotus	S		•		•	•	•	•	•		•	
Wintergreen	S								•			
Wolfberry Crisp	D				•	•			•	•		
Wolfberry Eye Cream	L									•		•
Xiang Mao	S					•		•				•
Yacon Syrup	D				•							
Yarrow	S						•	•				
Ylang Ylang	S		•				•	•				
Yuzu	S	•				•		•				

Appendix B

Single Oil Data

Single Oil Name	Botanical Name	Products Containing Single Oil
Amazonian Ylang Ylang	*Cananga odorata Equitoriana*	Oola Balance
Angelica	*Angelica archangelica* (Umbelliferae)	Awaken, Forgiveness, Grounding, Harmony, Live with Passion, Oola Balance, Surrender
Anise	*Pimpinella anisum* (Umbelliferae)	Awaken, ComforTone, Detoxzyme, Digest & Cleanse, DiGize, Dream Catcher, Essentialzyme, Essentialzymes-4, ICP, JuvaPower, JuvaSpice, ParaFree, Power Meal
Basil	*Ocimum basilicum* (Labiatae)	Aroma Siez, Clarity, M-Grain
Bergamot	*Citrus bergamia* (Rutaceae)	A·R·T Renewal Serum, Acceptance, Animal Scents Ointment, AromaGuard Meadow Mist Deodorant, Awaken, Believe, Clarity, Dragon Time Bath & Shower Gel, Dream Catcher, Evening Peace Bath & Shower Gel, Forgiveness, Genesis Hand & Body Lotion, Gentle Baby, Gratitude, Harmony, Humility, Inspiration, Joy, KidScents Lotion, Lady Sclareol, Lavender Conditioner, Lavender-Rosewood Moisturizing Soap, Magnify Your Purpose, Oola Balance, Oola Grow, Prenolone Plus Body Cream, Progessence Phyto Plus, Progessence Plus, Relaxation Massage Oil, Rose Ointment, Sandalwood Moisture Cream, Sensation, Sensation Bath & Shower Gel, Sensation Hand & Body Lotion, Sensation Massage Oil, White Angelica, Wolfberry Eye Cream
Biblical Sweet Myrrh	*Commiphora erythraea*	
Black Pepper	*Piper nigrum* (Piperaceae)	Awaken, Cel-Lite Magic Massage Oil, Dream Catcher, En-R-Gee, NingXia Nitro, Relieve It

Single Oil Name	Botanical Name	Products Containing Single Oil
Blue Cypress	*Callitris intratropica* (Cypressaceae)	Australian Blue, Brain Power, Breathe Again Roll-On, Essential Beauty Serum (Dry Skin), Highest Potential, Oola Grow
Blue Tansy	*Tanacetum annuum* (Compositae)	Acceptance, Australian Blue, Awaken, Dragon Time Bath & Shower Gel, Dream Catcher, Evening Peace Bath & Shower Gel, Highest Potential, JuvaFlex, JuvaTone, KidScents Shampoo, KidScents Tender Tush, Oola Grow, Peace & Calming, Release, SARA, Valor, Valor Moisturizing Soap, Valor Roll-On
Calamus	*Acorus calamus* (Acoraceae)	Exodus II
Canadian Fleabane	*Conyza canadensis* (Compositae)	CortiStop Women's, EndoGize, Ultra Young Plus
Cardamom	*Elettaria cardamomum* (Zingiberaceae)	Clarity, Transformation
Carrot Seed	*Daucus carota* (Apiaceae or Umbelliferae)	Animal Scents Ointment, Rose Ointment
Cassia	*Cinnamomum cassia* (Lauraceae)	Exodus II, EndoGize
Cedarwood	*Cedrus atlantica* (Pinaceae)	A·R·T Beauty Masque, Australian Blue, Brain Power, Cel-Lite Magic Massage Oil, Egyptian Gold, Essential Beauty Serum (Acne-Prone Skin), Essential Beauty Serum (Dry Skin), Grounding, Highest Potential, Inspiration, Into the Future, KidScents Bath Gel, KidScents Lotion, Live with Passion, Oola Grow, Peppermint-Cedarwood Moisturizing Soap, Progessence Plus, Progessence Phyto Plus, Sacred Mountain, Sacred Mountain Moisturizing Soap, SARA, Stress Away Roll-On, Tranquil Roll-On
Celery Seed	*Apium graveolens* (Umbelliferae)	GLF, JuvaCleanse

Single Oil Name	Botanical Name	Products Containing Single Oil
Cinnamon Bark	*Cinnamomum zeylanicum (Syn. C. verum)* (Lauraceae)	Abundance, Christmas Spirit, Cinnamint Lip Balm, Egyptian Gold, Exodus II, Gathering, Highest Potential, Inner Defense, KidScents Slique Toothpaste, Magnify Your Purpose, Mineral Essence, Oola Grow, Slique Bars, Thieves, Thieves AromaBright Toothpaste, Thieves Cleansing Soap, Thieves Dental Floss, Thieves Dentarome Plus Toothpaste, Thieves Dentarome Ultra Toothpaste, Thieves Foaming Hand Soap, Thieves Fresh Essence Plus Mouthwash, Thieves Household Cleaner, Thieves Lozenges (Hard/Soft), Thieves Spray, Thieves Waterless Hand Purifier, Thieves Wipes
Cistus	*Cistus ladanifer* (Cistaceae)	ImmuPower, KidScents Tender Tush, Oola Balance, The Gift
Citronella	*Cymbopogon nardus* (Gramineae)	Animal Scents Shampoo, Purification
Cistrus Hystrix	*Citrus hystrix* (Rutaceae)	Trauma Life
Clary Sage	*Salvia sclarea* (Labiatae)	Cel-Lite Magic Massage Oil, CortiStop Women's, Dragon Time, Dragon Time Bath & Shower Gel, Dragon Time Massage Oil, EndoGize, Estro, Evening Peace Bath & Shower Gel, FemiGen, Into the Future, Lady Sclareol, Lavender Conditioner, Lavender Shampoo, Live with Passion, Oola Grow, Prenolone Plus Body Cream, SclarEssence, Transformation
Clove	*Syzygium aromaticum* (Oleaceae)	Abundance, AromaGuard Meadow Mist Deodorant, AromaGuard Mountain Mint Deodorant, BLM, Deep Relief Roll-On, En-R-Gee, Essential Beauty Serum (Dry Skin), Essentialzyme, Essentialzymes-4, ImmuPower, Inner Defense, K&B, KidScents Slique Toothpaste, Longevity, Longevity Softgels, Melrose, OmegaGize[3], PanAway, ParaFree, Progessence Phyto Plus, Progessence Plus, Thieves, Thieves AromaBright Toothpaste, Thieves Cleansing Soap, Thieves Dental Floss, Thieves Dentarome Plus Toothpaste, Thieves Dentarome Ultra Toothpaste, Thieves Foaming Hand Soap, Thieves Fresh Essence Plus Mouthwash, Thieves Household Cleaner, Thieves Lozenges (Hard/Soft), Thieves Spray, Thieves Waterless Hand Purifier, Thieves Wipes

Single Oil Name	Botanical Name	Products Containing Single Oil
Copaiba	*Copaifera reticulata/ langsdorfii* and/or *Multijuga* (Caesalpiniacea)	A·R·T Beauty Masque, Breathe Again Roll-On, Copaiba Vanilla Moisturizing Conditioner, Copaiba Vanilla Moisturizing Shampoo, Deep Relief Roll-On, Progessence Phyto Plus, Progessence Plus, Stress Away Roll-On
Coriander	*Coriandrum sativum* (Umbelliferae)	A·R·T Renewal Serum, Acceptance, Animal Scents Ointment, AromaGuard Meadow Mist Deodorant, Awaken, Believe, Clarity, Dragon Time Bath & Shower Gel, Evening Peace Bath & Shower Gel, Forgiveness, Genesis Hand & Body Lotion, Gentle Baby, Gratitude, Harmony, Humility, Inspiration, Joy, KidScents Lotion, Lady Sclareol, Lavender-Rosewood Moisturizing Soap, Magnify Your Purpose, Oola Balance, Oola Grow, Relaxation Massage Oil, Rose Ointment, Sandalwood Moisture Cream, Sensation, Sensation Bath & Shower Gel, Sensation Hand & Body Lotion, Sensation Massage Oil, Wolfberry Eye Cream
Cumin	*Cuminum cyminum* (Umbelliferae)	Detoxzyme, ImmuPower, ParaFree, Protec
Cypress	*Cupressus sempervirens* (Cupressaceae)	Aroma Life, Aroma Siez, Cel-Lite Magic Massage Oil, R.C.
Davana	*Artemisia pallens* (Compositae)	A·R·T Creme Masque, Lavender Bath & Shower Gel, Trauma Life
Dill	*Anethum graveolens* (Umbelliferae)	
Dorado Azul	*Hyptis suaveolens* (Lamiaceae)	Common Sense
Douglas Fir	*Pseudotsuga menziesii* (Abietaceae)	Regenolone Moisturizing Cream
Elemi	*Canarium luzonicum* (Burseraceae)	Ortho Sport Massage Oil

Single Oil Name	Botanical Name	Products Containing Single Oil
Eucalyptus Blue	*Eucalyptus bicostata* (Myrtaceae)	Breathe Again Roll-On
Eucalyptus Citriodora	*Eucalyptus citriodora* (Myrtaceae)	R.C.
Eucalyptus Dives	*Eucalyptus dives* (Myrtaceae)	
Eucalyptus Globulus	*Eucalyptus globulus* (Myrtaceae)	Breathe Again Roll-On, Ortho Ease Massage Oil, Ortho Sport Massage Oil, R.C., Thieves Dentarome Ultra Toothpaste
Eucalyptus Polybractea	*Eucalyptus polybractea* (Myrtaceae)	
Eucalyptus Radiata	*Eucalyptus radiata* (Myrtaceae)	AromaGuard Mountain Mint Deodorant, Breathe Again Roll-On, Inner Defense, KidScents Slique Toothpaste, Ortho Ease Massage Oil, Raven, R.C., Thieves, Thieves AromaBright Toothpaste, Thieves Cleansing Soap, Thieves Dental Floss, Thieves Dentarome Plus Toothpaste, Thieves Dentarome Ultra Toothpaste, Thieves Foaming Hand Soap, Thieves Fresh Essence Plus Mouthwash, Thieves Household Cleaner, Thieves Lozenges (Hard/Soft), Thieves Spray, Thieves Waterless Hand Purifier, Thieves Wipes
Eucalyptus Staigeriana	*E. staigeriana* (Myrtaceae)	Breathe Again Roll-On, Essential Beauty Serum (Acne-Prone Skin)
Fennel	*Foeniculum vulgare* (Umbelliferae)	Allerzyme, CortiStop Women's, Detoxzyme, Digest & Cleanse, DiGize, Dragon Time, Dragon Time Bath & Shower Gel, Dragon Time Massage Oil, Essentialzyme, Essentialzymes-4, Estro, FemiGen, ICP, JuvaFlex, JuvaPower, JuvaSpice, K&B, Mister, ParaFree, Power Meal, Prenolone Plus Body Cream, Prostate Health, SclarEssence

Single Oil Name	Botanical Name	Products Containing Single Oil
Frankincense	*Boswellia carterii* (Burseraceae)	Abundance, Acceptance, A·R·T Day Activator, A·R·T Gentle Foaming Cleanser, A·R·T Night Reconstructor, A·R·T Purifying Toner, Awaken, Believe, Boswellia Wrinkle Cream, Brain Power, ClaraDerm, Common Sense, CortiStop Women's, Egyptian Gold, Exodus II, Forgiveness, Gathering, Gratitude, Harmony, Highest Potential, Humility, ImmuPower, Inspiration, Into the Future, KidScents Tender Tush, Longevity, Longevity Softgels, Oola Balance, Oola Grow, Progessence Plus, Protec, 3 Wise Men, Transformation, Trauma Life, Valor, Valor Moisturizing Soap, Valor Roll-On, Wolfberry Eye Cream
Frereana Frankincense	*Boswellia frereana*	Slique Gum
Geranium	*Pelargonium graveolens* (Geraniaceae)	A·R·T Creme Masque, A·R·T Renewal Serum, Acceptance, Animal Scents Ointment, Animal Scents Shampoo, AromaGuard Meadow Mist Deodorant, Awaken, Believe, Boswellia Wrinkle Cream, Clarity, Copaiba Vanilla Moisturizing Conditioner, Copaiba Vanilla Moisturizing Shampoo, Dragon Time Bath & Shower Gel, EndoFlex, Envision, Evening Peace Bath & Shower Gel, Forgiveness, Gathering, Genesis Hand & Body Lotion, Gentle Baby, Gratitude, Harmony, Highest Potential, Humility, Inspiration, Joy, JuvaFlex, JuvaTone, K&B, KidScents Bath Gel, KidScents Lotion, Lady Sclareol, Lavender-Rosewood Moisturizing Soap, Magnify Your Purpose, Melaleuca-Geranium Moisturizing Soap, Oola Balance, Oola Grow, Prenolone Plus Body Cream, Prostate Health, Relaxation Massage Oil, Release, SARA, Sandalwood Moisture Cream, Sensation, Sensation Bath & Shower Gel, Sensation Hand & Body Lotion, Trauma Life, White Angelica, Wolfberry Eye Cream
German Chamomile	*Matricaria recutita* (Compositae)	A·R·T Day Activator, A·R·T Night Reconstructor, ComforTone, EndoFlex, JuvaTone, OmegaGize³, Surrender
Ginger	*Zingiber officinale* (Zingiberaceae)	Abundance, Allerzyme, ComforTone, DiGize, Digest & Cleanse, EndoGize, Essentialzymes-4, ICP, Live with Passion, Magnify Your Purpose, Ultra Young Plus

Single Oil Name	Botanical Name	Products Containing Single Oil
Goldenrod	*Solidago canadensis* (Asteraceae)	Common Sense
Grapefruit	*Citrus paradisi* (Rutaceae)	Cel-Lite Magic Massage Oil, Citrus Fresh, GLF, Grapefruit Lip Balm, KidScents Slique Toothpaste, Power Meal, Slique Essence, Super C
Helichrysum	*Helichrysum italicum* (Compositae)	Aroma Life, Awaken, Brain Power, ClaraDerm, Deep Relief Roll-On, Forgiveness, GLF, JuvaCleanse, JuvaFlex, Live with Passion, M-Grain, PanAway, Trauma Life
Hinoki	*Chamaecyparis obtusa* (Hinoki)	
Hong Kuai	*Chamaecyparis formosensis*	
Hyssop	*Hyssopus officinalis* (Labiatae)	Awaken, Egyptian Gold, Exodus II, GLF, Harmony, ImmuPower, Oola Balance, Relieve It, White Angelica
Idaho Balsam Fir	*Abies balsamea* (Pinaceae)	Animal Scents Ointment, Believe, BLM, Deep Relief Roll-On, En-R-Gee, Egyptian Gold, Gratitude, Oola Balance, Sacred Mountain, Sacred Mountain Moisturizing Soap, Slique Slim Caps, The Gift, Transformation
Idaho Blue Spruce	*Picea pungens*	Believe, Evergreen Essence, Transformation
Idaho Ponderosa Pine	*Pinus ponderosa* (Pinus)	
Idaho Tansy	*Tanacetum vulgare* (Compositae)	ImmuPower, Into the Future, Lady Sclareol, Oola Grow, ParaFree
Ishpingo	*Ocotea quixos,* (Lauraceae)	Chocolessence

Single Oil Name	Botanical Name	Products Containing Single Oil
Jasmine	*Jasminum officinale* (Oleaceae)	A·R·T Creme Masque, A·R·T Renewal Serum, Awaken, Clarity, Dragon Time, Dragon Time Bath & Shower Gel, Dragon Time Massage Oil, Evening Peace Bath & Shower Gel, Forgiveness, Genesis Hand & Body Lotion, Gentle Baby, Harmony, Highest Potential, Inner Child, Into the Future, Joy, Lady Sclareol, Lavender Conditioner, Lavender Shampoo, Live with Passion, Oola Balance, Oola Grow, Sensation, Sensation Hand & Body Lotion, Sensation Massage Oil, Sensation Bath & Shower Gel, The Gift
Juniper	*Juniperus osteosperma* and *J. scopulorum* (Cupressaceae)	Allerzyme, Awaken, Cel-Lite Magic Massage Oil, DiGize, Dream Catcher, En-R-Gee, Grounding, Hope, Into the Future, K&B, Morning Start Bath & Shower Gel, Morning Start Moisturizing Soap, Oola Grow, Ortho Ease Massage Oil, 3 Wise Men
Laurus Nobilis (Bay Laurel)	*Laurus nobilis* (Lauraceae)	Breathe Again Roll-On, ParaFree
Lavandin	*Lavandula x hybrida* (Labiatae)	Animal Scents Shampoo, Purification, Release
Lavender	*Lavandula angustifolia* (Labiatae)	A·R·T Beauty Masque, A·R·T Gentle Foaming Cleanser, A·R·T Purifying Toner, AromaGuard Meadow Mist Deodorant, Aroma Siez, Awaken, Brain Power, ClaraDerm, Copaiba Vanilla Moisturizing Conditioner, Copaiba Vanilla Moisturizing Shampoo, Dragon Time, Dragon Time Bath & Shower Gel, Dragon Time Massage Oil, Egyptian Gold, Envision, Essential Beauty Serum (Dry Skin), Estro, Forgiveness, Gathering, Gentle Baby, Harmony, Highest Potential, KidScents Tender Tush, LavaDerm Cooling Mist, Lavender Bath & Shower Gel, Lavender Conditioner, Lavender Foaming Hand Soap, Lavender Hand & Body Lotion, Lavender Lip Balm, Lavender Mint Daily Conditioner, Lavender Mint Daily Shampoo, Lavender-Rosewood Moisturizing Soap, Lavender Shampoo, M-Grain, Mister, Motivation, Oola Balance, Oola Grow, Orange Blossom Facial Wash, Prostate Health, R.C., Relaxation Massage Oil, RutaVaLa, RutaVaLa Roll-On, Sandalwood Moisture Cream, SARA, SleepEssence, Stress Away Roll-On, Surrender, Tranquil Roll-On, Trauma Life, Wolfberry Eye Cream

Single Oil Name	Botanical Name	Products Containing Single Oil
Ledum	*Ledum groenlandicum* (Ericaceae)	GLF, JuvaCleanse
Lemon	*Citrus limon* (Rutaceae)	A·R·T Gentle Foaming Cleanser, A·R·T Purifying Toner, AlkaLime, Animal Scents Shampoo, AromaGuard Meadow Mist Deodorant, AromaGuard Mountain Mint Deodorant, Awaken, Citrus Fresh, Clarity, Digest & Cleanse, Deep Relief Roll-On, Dragon Time Bath & Shower Gel, Evening Peace Bath & Shower Gel, Forgiveness, Genesis Hand & Body Lotion, Gentle Baby, Harmony, Inner Defense, Joy, JuvaTone, KidScents Bath Gel, KidScents Shampoo, KidScents Slique Toothpaste, Lavender Bath & Shower Gel, Lavender Conditioner, Lavender Foaming Hand Soap, Lavender Hand & Body Lotion, Lavender Shampoo, Lemon-Sandalwood Cleansing Soap, Master Formula HERS, Master Formula HIS, MegaCal, Mineral Essence, MultiGreens, NingXia Red, Oola Balance, Orange Blossom Facial Wash, Power Meal, Raven, Sensation Hand & Body Lotion, Slique Essence, Super C, Surrender, Thieves, Thieves AromaBright Toothpaste, Thieves Cleansing Soap, Thieves Dental Floss, Thieves Dentarome Plus Toothpaste, Thieves Dentarome Ultra Toothpaste, Thieves Foaming Hand Soap, Thieves Fresh Essence Plus Mouthwash, Thieves Household Cleaner, Thieves Lozenges (Hard/Soft), Thieves Spray, Thieves Waterless Hand Purifier, Thieves Wipes, Transformation
Lemongrass	*Cymbopogon flexuosus* (Gramineae)	DiGize, En-R-Gee, Essentialzymes-4, ICP, Inner Child, Inner Defense, Morning Start Bath & Shower Gel, Morning Start Moisturizing Soap, MultiGreens, Ortho Ease Massage Oil, Ortho Sport Massage Oil, Purification, Slique Slim Caps, Super C, Super Cal
Lemon Myrtle	*Backhousia citriodora* (Myrtaceae)	Slique Slim Caps
Lime	*Citrus aurantifolia* (Rutaceae)	A·R·T Beauty Masque, AlkaLime, Common Sense, Copaiba Vanilla Moisturizing Conditioner, Copaiba Vanilla Moisturizing Shampoo, Stress Away Roll-On
Mandarin	*Citrus reticulata* (Rutaceae)	Awaken, Citrus Fresh, Dragon Time Bath & Shower Gel, Joy

Single Oil Name	Botanical Name	Products Containing Single Oil
Manuka	*Leptospermum scoparium* (Myrtaceae)	Essential Beauty Serum (Acne-Prone Skin)
Marjoram	*Origanum majorana* (Labiatae)	Aroma Life, Aroma Siez, Dragon Time, Dragon Time Bath & Shower Gel, M-Grain, Ortho Ease Massage Oil, R.C., SuperCal
Mastrante	*Lippia alba*	
Melaleuca Alternifolia (Tea Tree)	*Melaleuca alternifolia* (Myrtaceae)	Animal Scents Ointment, AromaGuard Meadow Mist Deodorant, ClaraDerm, Essential Beauty Serum (Acne-Prone Skin), Melaleuca-Geranium Moisturizing Soap, Melrose, ParaFree, Purification, Rehemogen, Rose Ointment
Melaleuca Cajuput	*Melaleuca leucadendron* (Myrtaceae)	
Melaleuca Ericifolia	*Melaleuca ericifolia* (Myrtaceae)	Melaleuca-Geranium Moisturizing Soap
Melaleuca Quinquenervia (Niaouli)	*Melaleuca quinquenervia* (Myrtaceae)	AromaGuard Meadow Mist Deodorant, Melrose
Melissa	*Melissa officinalis* (Labiatae)	A·R·T Gentle Foaming Cleanser, A·R·T Purifying Toner, Awaken, Brain Power, Forgiveness, Hope, Humility, Live with Passion, MultiGreens, White Angelica
Micromeria	*Micromeria fruticosa*	
Mountain Savory	*Satureja montana* (Labiatae)	ImmuPower, Surrender
Mugwort	*Artemisia vulgaris* (Asteraceae)	ComforTone, Inspiration

Single Oil Name	Botanical Name	Products Containing Single Oil
Myrrh	*Commiphora myrrha* (Burseraceae)	Abundance, Animal Scents Ointment, Boswellia Wrinkle Cream, ClaraDerm, Egyptian Gold, EndoGize, Essential Beauty Serum (Dry Skin), Exodus II, Gratitude, Hope, Humility, Lavender Bath & Shower Gel, Lavender Foaming Hand Soap, Lavender Hand & Body Lotion, Oola Balance, Protec, Rose Ointment, Sandalwood Moisture Cream, The Gift, 3 Wise Men, Thyromin, White Angelica
Myrtle	*Myrtus communis* (Myrtaceae)	Breathe Again Roll-On, EndoFlex, Inspiration, JuvaTone, Mister, Prostate Health, Purification, R.C., Super Cal, Thyromin
Neroli	*Citrus sinensis* (Rutaceae)	Acceptance, Awaken, Humility, Inner Child, Live with Passion, Oola Grow, Present Time
Nutmeg	*Myristica fragrans* (Myristicaceae)	EndoFlex, En-R-Gee, Magnify Your Purpose, NingXia Nitro, ParaFree, Power Meal
Ocotea	*Ocotea quixos* (Lauraceae)	A·R·T Beauty Masque, A·R·T Creme Masque, Common Sense, KidScents Slique Toothpaste, Oola Balance, Slique Essence, Slique Tea, Stress Away Roll-On, Thieves AromaBright Toothpaste, Transformation
Orange	*Citrus sinensis* (Rutaceae)	Abundance, Awaken, Balance Complete, Christmas Spirit, Cinnamint Lip Balm, Citrus Fresh, Envision, Harmony, ImmuPro, Inner Child, Into the Future, Lady Sclareol, Longevity, Longevity Softgels, NingXia Red, Oola Balance, Oola Grow, Peace & Calming, Power Meal, Pure Protein Complete, SARA, Slique Bars, Super C, Super C Chewable, Thieves Foaming Hand Soap, Thieves Lozenges (Soft)
Oregano	*Origanum compactum* (Labiatae)	ImmuPower, Inner Defense, Ortho Sport Massage Oil, Regenolone Moisturizing Cream
Palmarosa	*Cymbopogon martini* (Gramineae)	Animal Scents Ointment, Awaken, Clarity, Dragon Time Bath & Shower Gel, Evening Peace Bath & Shower Gel, Forgiveness, Genesis Hand & Body Lotion, Gentle Baby, Harmony, Joy, Oola Balance, Rose Ointment, Sensation Hand & Body Lotion
Palo Santo	*Bursera graveolens* (Burseraceae)	Deep Relief Roll-On, Transformation

Single Oil Name	Botanical Name	Products Containing Single Oil
Patchouli	*Pogostemon cablin* (Labiatae)	Abundance, Allerzyme, Animal Scents Ointment, DiGize, Live with Passion, Magnify Your Purpose, Orange Blossom Facial Wash, Peace & Calming, Rose Ointment
Peppermint	*Mentha piperita* (Labiatae)	Allerzyme, Aroma Siez, AromaGuard Mountain Mint Deodorant, BLM, Breathe Again Roll-On, Chocolessence, Cinnamint Lip Balm, Clarity, ComforTone, CortiStop Women's, Deep Relief Roll-On, DiGize, Digest & Cleanse, Einkorn Nuggets, Essentialzyme, Essentialzymes-4, Mightyzyme, Lavender Mint Daily Conditioner, Lavender Mint Daily Shampoo, M-Grain, Mineral Essence, Mister, Morning Start Bath & Shower Gel, Morning Start Moisturizing Soap, NingXia Nitro, Ortho Ease Massage Oil, Ortho Sport Massage Oil, PanAway, Peppermint-Cedarwood Moisturizing Soap, Progessence Phyto Plus, Progessence Plus, Prostate Health, R.C., Raven, Regenolone Moisturizing Cream, Relaxation Massage Oil, Relieve It, Satin Facial Scrub Mint, SclarEssence, Slique Gum, Thieves AromaBright Toothpaste, Thieves Dental Floss, Thieves Dentarome Plus Toothpaste, Thieves Dentarome Ultra Toothpaste, Thieves Fresh Essence Plus Mouthwash, Thieves Lozenges (Hard/Soft), Thieves Waterless Hand Purifier, Thyromin, Transformation
Petitgrain	*Citrus sinensis* (Rutaceae)	
Pine	*Pinus sylvestris* (Pinaceae)	Evergreen Essence, Grounding, R.C.
Plectranthus Oregano	*Plectranthus amboinicus*	
Ravintsara	*Cinnamomum camphora* (Lauraceae)	ImmuPower, Raven
Roman Chamomile	*Chamaemelum nobile* (Compositae)	A·R·T Creme Masque, Awaken, ClaraDerm, Clarity, Dragon Time Bath & Shower Gel, Evening Peace Bath & Shower Gel, Forgiveness, Genesis Hand & Body Lotion, Gentle Baby, Harmony, Joy, JuvaFlex, K&B, KidScents Tender Tush, M-Grain, Motivation, Oola Balance, Oola Grow, Rehemogen, Satin Facial Scrub, Sensation Hand & Body Lotion, Surrender, Tranquil Roll-On, Wolfberry Eye Cream

Single Oil Name	Botanical Name	Products Containing Single Oil
Rose	*Rosa damascena* (Rosaceae)	Awaken, Egyptian Gold, Envision, Forgiveness, Gathering, Gentle Baby, Harmony, Highest Potential, Humility, Joy, Oola Balance, Oola Grow, Rose Ointment, SARA, Trauma Life, White Angelica
Rosemary	*Rosmarinus officinalis* CT cineole (Labiatae)	AromaGuard Meadow Mist Deodorant, AromaGuard Mountain Mint Deodorant, Clarity, ComforTone, En-R-Gee, Essentialzymes-4, ICP, Inner Defense, JuvaFlex, JuvaTone, KidScents Slique Toothpaste, Melrose, Morning Start Bath & Shower Gel, Morning Start Moisturizing Soap, MultiGreens, Orange Blossom Facial Wash, Purification, Rehemogen, Sandalwood Moisture Cream, Satin Facial Scrub, Thieves, Thieves AromaBright Toothpaste, Thieves Cleansing Soap, Thieves Dental Floss, Thieves Dentarome Plus Toothpaste, Thieves Dentarome Ultra Toothpaste, Thieves Foaming Hand Soap, Thieves Fresh Essence Plus Mouthwash, Thieves Household Cleaner, Thieves Lozenges (Hard/Soft), Thieves Spray, Thieves Waterless Hand Purifier, Thieves Wipes, Transformation
Rosewood	*Aniba rosaeodora* (Lauraceae)	Gentle Baby, KidScents Tender Tush, Lavender-Rosewood Moisturizing Soap, Oola Grow, Progessence Phyto Plus, Progessence Plus, Valor, Valor Moisturizing Soap, Valor Roll-On, White Angelica
Ruta	*Ruta graveolens* (Rutaceae)	Common Sense, RutaVaLa, RutaVaLa Roll-On, SleepEssence
Sacred Frankincense	*Boswellia sacra* (Burceraceae)	Oola Balance, The Gift, Transformation
Sage	*Salvia officinalis* (Labiatae)	Dragon Time Bath & Shower Gel, Dragon Time Massage Oil, EndoFlex, Envision, FemiGen, K&B, Magnify Your Purpose, Mister, Prenolone Plus Body Cream, Protec

Single Oil Name	Botanical Name	Products Containing Single Oil
Sandalwood	*Santalum album* (Santalaceae)	Acceptance, A·R·T Day Activator, A·R·T Gentle Foaming Cleanser, A·R·T Night Reconstructor, A·R·T Purifying Toner, Awaken, Boswellia Wrinkle Cream, Brain Power, Dream Catcher, Essential Beauty Serum (Dry Skin), Evening Peace Bath & Shower Gel, Forgiveness, Gathering, Harmony, Highest Potential, Inner Child, Inspiration, KidScents Tender Tush, Lady Sclareol, Lemon-Sandalwood Cleansing Soap, Live with Passion, Magnify Your Purpose, Oola Balance, Oola Grow, Release, Sandalwood Moisture Cream, 3 Wise Men, Transformation, Trauma Life, Ultra Young Plus, White Angelica
Spanish Sage (Sage Lavender)	*Salvia lavandulifolia* (Lamiaceae)	Awaken, Harmony, Lady Sclareol, Oola Balance, SclarEssence
Spearmint	*Mentha spicata* (Labiatae)	Cinnamint Lip Balm, Citrus Fresh, Einkorn Nuggets, EndoFlex, GLF, KidScents Slique Toothpaste, Lavender Mint Daily Conditioner, Lavender Mint Daily Shampoo, NingXia Nitro, OmegaGize^3, Relaxation Massage Oil, Slique Essence, Slique Gum, Thieves AromaBright Toothpaste, Thieves Fresh Essence Plus Mouthwash, Thyromin
Spikenard	*Nardostachys jatamansi* (Valerianaceae)	Animal Scents Shampoo, Egyptian Gold, Exodus II, Humility, Inspiration, LavaDerm Cooling Mist, Oola Balance, The Gift
Spruce	*Picea mariana* (Pinaceae)	Abundance, Awaken, Christmas Spirit, Envision, Gathering, Grounding, Harmony, Highest Potential, Hope, Inner Child, Inspiration, Motivation, Oola Balance, Oola Grow, Present Time, R.C., Relieve It, Sacred Mountain, Sacred Mountain Moisturizing Soap, Surrender, 3 Wise Men, Trauma Life, Valor, Valor Moisturizing Soap, Valor Roll-On, White Angelica
Tangerine	*Citrus reticulata* (Rutaceae)	Awaken, Citrus Fresh, ComforTone, Dream Catcher, Inner Child, Joy, KidScents Shampoo, KidScents Slique Toothpaste, NingXia Red, Peace & Calming, Relaxation Massage Oil, SleepEssence, Slique Essence, Super C
Tarragon	*Artemisia dracunculus* (Compositae)	Allerzyme, ComforTone, DiGize, Essentialzyme, Essentialzymes-4, ICP

Single Oil Name	Botanical Name	Products Containing Single Oil
Thyme	*Thymus vulgaris* (Labiatae)	Essential Beauty Serum (Acne-Prone Skin), Inner Defense, Longevity, Longevity Softgels, Ortho Ease Massage Oil, Ortho Sport Massage Oil, ParaFree, Rehemogen, Thieves Dentarome Ultra Toothpaste
Tsuga	*Tsuga canadensis* (Pinaceae)	
Valerian	*Valeriana officinalis* (Valerianaceae)	RutaVaLa, RutaVaLa Roll-On, SleepEssence, Trauma Life
Vanilla	*(Vanilla planifolia)*	A·R·T Beauty Masque, A·R·T Creme Masque, Chocolessence, Copaiba Vanilla Moisturizing Conditioner, Copaiba Vanilla Moisturizing Shampoo, NingXia Nitro, Slique Bars, Slique Tea, Slique Tea (International), Stress Away Roll-On
Vetiver	*Vetiveria zizanoides* (Gramineae)	A·R·T Creme Masque, Deep Relief Roll-On, Inspiration, Lady Sclareol, Melaleuca-Geranium Moisturizing Soap, Ortho Ease Massage Oil, Ortho Sport Massage Oil, ParaFree, SleepEssence, Thieves Fresh Essence Plus Mouthwash
Vitex	*(Vitex agnus-castus)* (Lamiaceae)	Progessence Phyto Plus
Western Red Cedar	*Thuja plicata* (Cupressaceae)	Evergreen Essence, KidScents Lotion
White Fir	*Abies concolor* (Pinaceae)	AromaGuard Mountain Mint Deodorant, Australian Blue, Grounding, Highest Potential, Into the Future, Oola Grow
White Lotus	*Nymphaea lotus*	Into the Future, Oola Grow, SARA
Wintergreen	*Gaultheria procumbens* (Ericaceae)	BLM, Deep Relief Roll-On, Ortho Ease Massage Oil, Ortho Sport Massage Oil, PanAway, Raven, Regenolone Moisturizing Cream, Super Cal, Thieves Dentarome Ultra Toothpaste
Xiang Mao	*Cymbopogon citratus*	

Single Oil Name	Botanical Name	Products Containing Single Oil
Yarrow	*Achillea millefolium* (Compositae)	Dragon Time, Dragon Time Massage Oil, Mister, Prenolone Plus Body Cream
Ylang Ylang	*Cananga odorata* (Annonaceae)	A·R·T Creme Masque, A·R·T Renewal Serum, Acceptance, Animal Scents Ointment, Aroma Life, AromaGuard Meadow Mist Deodorant, Australian Blue, Awaken, Believe, Boswellia Wrinkle Cream, Clarity, Common Sense, Dragon Time Bath & Shower Gel, Dragon Time Massage Oil, Dream Catcher, Evening Peace Bath & Shower Gel, FemiGen, Forgiveness, Gathering, Genesis Hand & Body Lotion, Gentle Baby, Gratitude, Grounding, Harmony, Highest Potential, Humility, Inner Child, Inspiration, Into the Future, Joy, KidScents Lotion, Lady Sclareol, Lavender-Rosewood Moisturizing Soap, Magnify Your Purpose, Motivation, Oola Grow, Peace & Calming, Prenolone Plus Body Cream, Present Time, Relaxation Massage Oil, Release, Rose Ointment, Sacred Mountain, Sacred Mountain Moisturizing Soap, Sandalwood Moisture Cream, SARA, Sensation, Sensation Bath & Shower Gel, Sensation Hand & Body Lotion, Sensation Massage Oil, White Angelica, Wolfberry Eye Cream
Yuzu	*Citrus junos* (Rutaceae)	NingXia Red

Appendix C

Essential Oil Blends Data

Blend Name	Single Oil Contents	Uses/Application Areas
Abundance	Orange, Frankincense, Patchouli, Clove, Ginger, Myrrh, Cinnamon Bark, Spruce	Diffuse; inhale; dilute for topical use and apply on location.
Acceptance	Coriander, Geranium, Bergamot, Frankincense, Sandalwood, Blue Tansy, Neroli, Ylang Ylang (Carrier: Almond Oil)	Diffuse; apply over heart and thymus; on wrists, neck, or temples; or behind ears.
Aroma Life	Cypress, Marjoram, Ylang Ylang, Helichrysum (Carrier: Sesame Seed Oil)	Diffuse; inhale; apply over heart, abdomen, or spine.
Aroma Siez	Basil, Marjoram, Lavender, Peppermint, Cypress	Apply to sore muscles, ligaments, or areas of poor circulation.
Australian Blue	Blue Cypress, Ylang Ylang, Cedarwood, Blue Tansy, White Fir	Diffuse; inhale; apply to wrists, neck, temples, or Vita Flex points.
Awaken	Joy, Forgiveness, Present Time, Dream Catcher, Harmony (Carrier: Fractionated Coconut Oil)	Diffuse; inhale; apply over heart, on wrists, neck, temples, forehead, or Vita Flex points.
Believe	Idaho Balsam Fir, Coriander Seed, Bergamot, Frankincense, Idaho Blue Spruce, Ylang Ylang, Geranium	Diffuse; inhale; apply over heart, on wrists, neck, temples, forehead, or Vita Flex points.
Brain Power	Sandalwood, Cedarwood, Frankincense, Melissa, Blue Cypress, Lavender, Helichrysum	Diffuse; inhale; apply on neck, throat, temples, or under nose.
Breathe Again Roll-On	Eucalyptus Staigeriana, Eucalyptus Globulus, Eucalyptus Radiata, Laurus Nobilis, Peppermint, Copaiba, Myrtle, Blue Cypress, Eucalyptus Blue (Azul) (*Eucalyptus spp.*) (Carrier: Fractionated Coconut Oil, Rose Hip Seed Oil)	Apply on throat, neck, or chest.

Blend Name	Single Oil Contents	Uses/Application Areas
Christmas Spirit	Orange, Cinnamon Bark, Spruce	Diffuse; inhale; apply over heart, on wrists, neck, temples, or Vita Flex points.
Citrus Fresh	Orange, Tangerine, Grapefruit, Lemon, Mandarin, Spearmint	Diffuse; inhale; apply on edge of ears, wrists, neck, temples, or Vita Flex points.
Clarity	Basil, Cardamom, Rosemary, Peppermint, Coriander, Geranium, Bergamot, Lemon, Ylang Ylang, Jasmine, Roman Chamomile, Palmarosa	Diffuse; inhale; apply on edge of ears, wrists, neck, forehead, temples, or Vita Flex points.
Common Sense	Frankincense, Ylang Ylang, Ocotea, Goldenrod, Ruta, Dorado Azul, Lime	Diffuse; wear as a fragrance.
Deep Relief Roll-On	Peppermint, Lemon, Idaho Balsam Fir, Clove, Copaiba, Wintergreen, Helichrysum, Vetiver, Palo Santo (Carrier: Fractionated Coconut Oil)	Apply directly on desired location.
DiGize	Tarragon, Ginger, Peppermint, Juniper, Fennel, Anise, Patchouli, Lemongrass	Massage or use as a compress on the stomach; apply on Vita Flex points on feet and ankles; take as a dietary supplement in a capsule.
Dragon Time	Fennel, Clary Sage, Marjoram, Lavender, Yarrow, Jasmine	Diffuse; inhale; apply on wrists, neck, temples, or Vita Flex points.
Dream Catcher	Sandalwood, Tangerine, Ylang Ylang, Black Pepper, Bergamot, Juniper, Anise, Blue Tansy	Diffuse; inhale; apply on location as needed.
Egyptian Gold	Frankincense, Lavender, Idaho Balsam Fir, Myrrh, Spikenard, Hyssop, Cedarwood, Rose, Cinnamon Bark	Diffuse; inhale; apply over heart, on wrists, neck, temples, or Vita Flex points; take as a dietary supplement in a capsule.
EndoFlex	Spearmint, Sage, Geranium, Myrtle, German Chamomile, Nutmeg (Carrier: Sesame Seed Oil)	Diffuse; inhale; apply over lower back, thyroid, kidneys, liver, feet, glandular areas, and Vita Flex points for these organs; take as a dietary supplement in a capsule.

Blend Name	Single Oil Contents	Uses/Application Areas
En-R-Gee	Rosemary, Juniper, Lemongrass, Nutmeg, Idaho Balsam Fir, Clove, Black Pepper	Diffuse; inhale; apply on desired location.
Envision	Spruce, Geranium, Orange, Lavender, Sage, Rose	Diffuse; inhale; apply on forehead, edge of ears, wrists, neck, temples, or Vita Flex points.
Evergreen Essence	Idaho Blue Spruce, Idaho Ponderosa Pine, Scotch Pine, Red Fir, Western Red Cedar, White Fir, Black Pine, Pinyon Pine, Lodgepole Pine	Diffuse; inhale directly.
Exodus II	Myrrh, Cassia, Cinnamon Bark, Calamus, Hyssop, Galbanum, Spikenard, Frankincense (Carrier: Olive Oil)	Diffuse; inhale; apply on ears, wrists, Vita Flex points, or spine.
Forgiveness	Melissa, Geranium, Frankincense, Sandalwood, Coriander, Angelica, Lavender, Bergamot, Lemon, Ylang Ylang, Jasmine, Helichrysum, Roman Chamomile, Palmarosa, Rose (Carrier: Sesame Seed Oil)	Diffuse; inhale; apply behind ears, on wrists, neck, temples, navel, solar plexus, or over heart.
Gathering	Lavender, Geranium, Galbanum, Frankincense, Sandalwood, Ylang Ylang, Spruce, Cinnamon Bark, Rose	Diffuse; inhale; apply on edge of ears, wrists, neck, temples, or spine.
Gentle Baby	Geranium, Rosewood, Coriander, Palmarosa, Lavender, Ylang Ylang, Roman Chamomile, Lemon, Jasmine, Rose	Diffuse; apply on desired location.
GLF	Ledum, Helichrysum, Celery Seed, Grapefruit, Hyssop, Spearmint	Take as a dietary supplement in a capsule.
Gratitude	Idaho Balsam Fir, Frankincense, Coriander, Myrrh, Ylang Ylang, Galbanum, Bergamot, Geranium	Diffuse; inhale; apply behind ears, over heart, on wrists, base of neck, temples, or base of spine.
Grounding	White Fir, Spruce, Ylang Ylang, Pine, Cedarwood, Angelica, Juniper	Diffuse; inhale; apply behind ears, on wrists, base of neck, temples, or base of spine.

Blend Name	Single Oil Contents	Uses/Application Areas
Harmony	Sandalwood, Lavender, Ylang Ylang, Frankincense, Orange, Angelica, Geranium, Hyssop, Spanish Sage, Spruce, Coriander, Bergamot, Lemon, Jasmine, Roman Chamomile, Palmarosa, Rose	Diffuse; inhale; apply on edge of ears, wrists, neck, temples, over heart, or chakra/Vita Flex points.
Highest Potential	Australian Blue, Gathering, Jasmine, Ylang Ylang	Diffuse; inhale; apply on edge of ears, wrists, neck, or temples.
Hope	Melissa, Juniper, Myrrh, Spruce (Carrier: Almond Oil)	Diffuse; inhale; apply on edge of ears, wrists, neck. temples, over heart, or chakra/Vita Flex points.
Humility	Coriander, Ylang Ylang, Bergamot, Geranium, Melissa, Frankincense, Myrrh, Spikenard, Neroli, Rose (Carrier: Fractionated Coconut Oil)	Diffuse; inhale; apply over heart, on neck, forehead, or temples.
ImmuPower	Hyssop, Mountain Savory, Cistus, Ravintsara, Frankincense, Oregano, Clove, Cumin, Idaho Tansy	Diffuse; inhale; apply on navel, chest, temples, wrists, under nose, or Vita Flex points.
Inner Child	Orange, Tangerine, Ylang Ylang, Jasmine, Sandalwood, Lemongrass, Spruce, Neroli	Diffuse; inhale; apply on edge of ears, wrists, neck, or temples.
Inspiration	Cedarwood, Spruce, Myrtle, Coriander, Sandalwood, Frankincense, Bergamot, Spikenard, Vetiver, Ylang Ylang, Geranium	Diffuse; inhale; apply on edge of ears, wrists, neck, temples, forehead, crown of head, bottom of feet, or spine.
Into the Future	Clary Sage, Ylang Ylang, White Fir, Idaho Tansy, Frankincense, Jasmine, Juniper, Orange, Cedarwood, White Lotus (Carrier: Almond Oil)	Diffuse; inhale; apply on edge of ears, over heart, on wrists, neck, or temples.
Joy	Bergamot, Ylang Ylang, Geranium, Lemon, Coriander, Tangerine, Jasmine, Roman Chamomile, Palmarosa, Rose	Diffuse; inhale; apply over the heart, thymus, temples, and wrists; massage on the lower back, abdomen, and on the heart and brain Vita Flex points.
JuvaCleanse	Helichrysum, Celery Seed, Ledum	Apply over the liver and on the liver and kidney Vita Flex points; take as a dietary supplement in a capsule.

Blend Name	Single Oil Contents	Uses/Application Areas
JuvaFlex	Fennel, Geranium, Rosemary, Roman Chamomile, Blue Tansy, Helichrysum (Carrier: Sesame Seed Oil)	Apply over liver area and massage on the Vita Flex points or along the spine.
Lady Sclareol	Coriander, Geranium, Vetiver, Orange, Clary Sage, Bergamot, Ylang Ylang, Sandalwood, Spanish Sage, Jasmine, Idaho Tansy	Apply on ankle Vita Flex points or at the clavicle notch; wear as a fragrance.
Live with Passion	Sandalwood, Clary Sage, Ginger, Jasmine, Patchouli, Cedarwood, Helichrysum, Angelica, Melissa, Neroli	Diffuse; apply on wrists, temples, chest, or forehead.
Longevity	Thyme, Orange, Clove, Frankincense	Take as a dietary supplement.
M-Grain	Basil, Marjoram, Lavender, Roman Chamomile, Peppermint, Helichrysum	Diffuse; inhale; apply over brain stem, on forehead, crown of head, shoulders, back of neck, temples, and Vita Flex points.
Magnify Your Purpose	Sandalwood, Sage, Coriander, Patchouli, Nutmeg, Bergamot, Cinnamon Bark, Ginger, Ylang Ylang, Geranium	Diffuse; inhale; apply over heart, solar plexus, or thymus, on temples, ears, or wrists.
Melrose	Rosemary, Melaleuca Alternifolia, Clove, Niaouli	Diffuse; inhale; apply on broken skin, cuts, scrapes, burns, rashes, or infection.
Mister	Sage, Fennel, Lavender, Myrtle, Yarrow, Peppermint (Carrier: Sesame Seed Oil)	Diffuse; inhale; apply on ankle Vita Flex points, lower pelvis, or areas of concern.
Motivation	Roman Chamomile, Spruce, Ylang Ylang, Lavender	Diffuse; inhale; apply on feet, chest, nape of neck, behind ears, wrists, or around navel.
Oola Balance	Lavender, Frankincense, Ylang Ylang, Sacred Frankincense, Idaho Balsam Fir, Jasmine, Sandalwood, Galbanum, Orange, Angelica, Geranium, Myrrh, Hyssop, Ocotea, Spanish Sage, Spruce, Cistus, Spikenard, Coriander, Bergamot, Lemon, Roman Chamomile, Palmarosa, Rose	Diffuse; inhale; topical: dilute 1 drop with 1 drop of V-6 or olive oil and apply on temples, back of neck, forehead, or other areas as needed.

Blend Name	Single Oil Contents	Uses/Application Areas
Oola Grow	Sweet Almond, Roman Chamomile, Spruce, Blue Cypress, Coriander, Clary Sage, Ylang Ylang, Geranium, Bergamot, Jasmine, Rosewood, Cedarwood, White Fir, Lavender, Frankincense, Galbanum, Juniper, Orange, Sandalwood, Blue Tansy, Idaho Tansy, Neroli, Cinnamon Bark, Rose, White Lotus (Carrier: Coconut Oil)	Diffuse; inhale; topical: dilute 1 drop with 1 drop of V-6 or olive oil and apply to desired area as needed.
PanAway	Wintergreen, Helichrysum, Clove, Peppermint	Diffuse; inhale; apply on temples, back of neck, forehead, or other areas.
Peace & Calming	Tangerine, Orange, Ylang Ylang, Patchouli, Blue Tansy	Diffuse; inhale; apply on wrists, edge of ears, or Vita Flex points.
Present Time	Neroli, Spruce, Ylang Ylang (Carrier: Almond Oil)	Diffuse; inhale; apply on sternum and thymus area, neck, and forehead.
Purification	Citronella, Lemongrass, Rosemary, Melaleuca Alternifolia, Lavandin, Myrtle	Diffuse; inhale; apply on cuts, sores, bruises, or wounds.
Raven	Ravintsara, Lemon, Wintergreen, Peppermint, Eucalyptus Radiata	Diffuse; inhale; apply on throat and lung area and Vita Flex points.
R.C.	Myrtle, Eucalyptus Globulus, Marjoram, Pine, Eucalyptus Citriodora, Lavender, Cypress, Eucalyptus Radiata, Spruce, Peppermint	Diffuse; inhale; apply on chest, neck, throat, or over sinus area.
Release	Ylang Ylang, Lavandin, Geranium, Sandalwood, Blue Tansy (Carrier: Olive Oil)	Diffuse; inhale; apply over liver or anywhere trauma has occurred; massage on bottoms of feet and behind ears.
Relieve It	Spruce, Black Pepper, Hyssop, Peppermint	Apply on desired location.
RutaVaLa	Lavender, Valerian, Ruta	Diffuse; inhale.
RutaVaLa Roll-On	Lavender, Valerian, Ruta (Carrier: Fractionated Coconut Oil)	Apply on wrists, temples, neck, bottom of feet, or other area as needed.

Blend Name	Single Oil Contents	Uses/Application Areas
Sacred Mountain	Spruce, Ylang Ylang, Idaho Balsam Fir, Cedarwood	Diffuse; inhale, apply on crown of head, back of neck, behind ears, on thymus and wrists.
SARA	Ylang Ylang, Geranium, Lavender, Orange, Blue Tansy, Cedarwood, White Lotus, Rose (Carrier: Almond Oil)	Apply over energy centers and areas of abuse, on navel, lower abdomen, temples, nose, and Vita Flex points.
SclarEssence	Clary Sage, Spanish Sage, Peppermint, Fennel	Take 1 capsule daily, as needed.
Sensation	Coriander, Ylang Ylang, Bergamot, Jasmine, Geranium	Diffuse; apply on location, neck, or wrists.
Slique Essence	Grapefruit, Tangerine, Spearmint, Lemon, Ocotea (Sweetener: Stevia)	
Stress Away Roll-On	Copaiba, Lime, Cedarwood, Vanilla, Ocotea, Lavender	Inhale; apply on location or on arms, back, shoulders, chest or abdomen, or elsewhere as needed.
Surrender	Lavender, Lemon, Roman Chamomile, Spruce, Angelica, German Chamomile, Mountain Savory	Diffuse; inhale; apply on forehead, solar plexus, along ear rim, chest, and nape of neck.
The Gift	Sacred Frankincense, Idaho Balsam Fir, Jasmine, Galbanum, Myrrh, Cistus, Spikenard	Diffuse; massage on bottoms of feet; wear as a fragrance.
Thieves	Clove, Lemon, Cinnamon Bark, Eucalyptus Radiata, Rosemary	Diffuse; apply on bottoms of feet.
3 Wise Men	Sandalwood, Juniper, Frankincense, Spruce, Myrrh (Carrier: Almond Oil)	Diffuse; inhale; apply on crown of head, behind ears, over eyebrows, on chest, over thymus, and at back of neck.
Tranquil Roll-On	Lavender, Cedarwood, Roman Chamomile (Carrier: Fractionated Coconut Oil)	Apply on temples, neck, or wrists.

Blend Name	Single Oil Contents	Uses/Application Areas
Transformation	Lemon, Peppermint, Clary Sage, Sandalwood, Idaho Blue Spruce, Sacred Frankincense, Cardamom, Palo Santo, Ocotea	Diffuse; apply on Vita Flex points or other desired locations.
Trauma Life	Sandalwood, Frankincense, Valerian, Spruce, Davana, Lavender, Geranium, Helichrysum, Citrus Hystrix, Rose	Diffuse; inhale; apply on bottom of feet, chest, forehead, nape of neck, behind ears, and along spine using the Raindrop Technique.
Valor	Spruce, Rosewood, Blue Tansy, Frankincense (Carrier: Fractionated Coconut Oil)	Diffuse; inhale; apply on wrists, chest, and base of neck, bottom of feet, or along spine using the Raindrop Technique.
Valor Roll-On	Spruce, Rosewood, Frankincense, Blue Tansy (Carrier: Fractionated Coconut Oil)	Apply on feet, wrists, or back of the neck; wear as a fragrance.
White Angelica	Myrrh, Bergamot, Sandalwood, Geranium, Ylang Ylang, Spruce, Rosewood, Coriander, Hyssop, Melissa, Rose, Angelica (Carrier: Fractionated Coconut Oil)	Diffuse; inhale; apply on shoulders, spine, crown of head, wrists, behind ears, base of neck, or Vita Flex points.

NOTES

NOTES

NOTES

NOTES

NOTES

NOTES

NOTES

NOTES

NOTES

NOTES

NOTES

NOTES